Bradford Teaching Hospitals **NHS**

NHS Foundation Trust

Health Library & Information Service
Bradford Royal Infirmary, BD9 6RJ

Tel: 01274 364130   Email: medical.library2@bthft.nhs.uk

Search, Reserve & Renew books by logging into our
Online Catalogue: **http://bradford.nhslibraries.com**
(call us for your Reader and Pin Number)

Fines are chargeable on this book if you keep it beyond the
agreed date.
10p per day / 50p per week

Uropathology

HIGH-YIELD PATHOLOGY

Uropathology

Ming Zhou, MD, PhD
Associate Professor and Director
Surgical Pathology and Urologic Pathology
NYU Medical Center Tisch Hospital
New York City, New York

George J. Netto, MD
Associate Professor of Pathology, Urology and Oncology
Director of Surgical Pathology Molecular Diagnostics
The Johns Hopkins Medical Institutions
Baltimore, Maryland

Jonathan I. Epstein, MD
Professor of Pathology, Urology, Oncology
Reinhard Professor of Urologic Pathology
Director of Surgical Pathology
Department of Pathology
The Johns Hopkins Medical Institutions
Baltimore, Maryland

ELSEVIER
SAUNDERS

1600 John F. Kennedy Blvd.
Ste 1800
Philadelphia, PA 19103-2899

UROPATHOLOGY: HIGH-YIELD PATHOLOGY　　　　　　　　ISBN: 978-1-4377-2523-0

Notices

Knowledge and best practice in this field are constantly changing. As new research and experience broaden our understanding, changes in research methods, professional practices, or medical treatment may become necessary.

Practitioners and researchers must always rely on their own experience and knowledge in evaluating and using any information, methods, compounds, or experiments described herein. In using such information or methods, they should be mindful of their own safety and the safety of others, including parties for whom they have a professional responsibility.

With respect to any drug or pharmaceutical products identified, readers are advised to check the most current information provided (i) on procedures featured or (ii) by the manufacturer of each product to be administered to verify the recommended dose or formula, the method and duration of administration, and contraindications. It is the responsibility of practitioners, relying on their own experience and knowledge of their patients, to make diagnoses, to determine dosages and the best treatment for each individual patient, and to take all appropriate safety precautions.

To the fullest extent of the law, neither the Publisher nor the authors, contributors, or editors assume any liability for any injury and/or damage to persons or property as a matter of products liability, negligence, or otherwise, or from any use or operation of any methods, products, instructions, or ideas contained in the material herein.

Library of Congress Cataloging-in-Publication Data

Uropathology : high-yield pathology / [edited by] Ming Zhou, George Netto, Jonathan Epstein.
  p. ; cm.
ISBN 978-1-4377-2523-0
I. Zhou, Ming, MD, PhD. II. Netto, George J. III. Epstein, Jonathan I.
[DNLM: 1. Male Urogenital Diseases—pathology. WJ 141]
617.4'6—dc23

　　　　　　　　　　　　　　　　　　　　　　　　　　　2011053082

Executive Content Strategist: William Schmitt
Senior Content Specialist: Katie DeFrancesco
Publishing Services Manager: Anne Altepeter
Senior Project Manager: Doug Turner
Designer: Steve Stave

Printed in the People's Republic of China

Last digit is the print number: 9 8 7 6 5 4 3 2

To my wife, Lan, and daughters, Grace and Rebecca, for their love and support.
Ming Zhou

To my truest friend and anchor—my wife, Ruby!
George Netto

Dilek Baydar, MD
Professor of Pathology
Department of Pathology
Hacettepe University School of Medicine
Ankara, Turkey

Fadi Brimo, MD
Pathologist and Assistant Professor
Departments of Pathology and Urology
Montreal General Hospital
McGill University Health Center
Montreal, Quebec, Canada

Alcides Chaux, MD
Post-Doctoral Research Fellow
Department of Pathology
The Johns Hopkins Medical Institutions
Baltimore, Maryland;
Professor of Pathology
Universidad del Norte
Asunción, Paraguay

Ying-Bei Chen, MD, PhD
Assistant Attending Pathologist
Department of Pathology
Memorial Sloan-Kettering Cancer Center
New York City, New York

Charles Guo, MD
Assistant Professor
Department of Pathology
The University of Texas MD Anderson
   Cancer Center
Houston, Texas

Donna Hansel, MD, PhD
Associate Professor
Department of Anatomic Pathology
Cleveland Clinic
Cleveland, Ohio

Mathieu Latour, MD, FRCPC
Assistant Professor
Director, Residency Training Program in Anatomic
   Pathology
Département de Pathologie et Biologie cellulaire
Centre Hospitalier de l'Université de Montréal
Montréal, Québec, Canada

Tamara Lotan, MD
Assistant Professor
Department of Pathology
The Johns Hopkins Medical Institutions
Baltimore, Maryland

Cristina Magi-Galluzzi, MD, PhD
Associate Professor
Department of Anatomic Pathology
Cleveland Clinic
Cleveland, Ohio

Adeboye Osunkoya, MD
Assistant Professor of Pathology and Urology
Director, Genitourinary Pathology
Department of Pathology
Emory University School of Medicine
Atlanta, Georgia

Chin-Chen Pan, MD
Professor and Director of General Pathology
Department of Pathology
Taipei Veterans General Hospital
Taipei, Taiwan

Anil Parwani, MD, PhD
Division Director
Pathology Informatics;
Associate Professor
Pathology and Biomedical Informatics
UPMC Shadyside
Pittsburgh, Pennsylvania

Brian D. Robinson, MD
Assistant Professor of Pathology and Laboratory
   Medicine
Assistant Professor of Pathology in Urology
Weill Medical College of Cornell University
New York City, New York

**Hemamali Samaratunga, MBBS, LRCP,
   MRCS, FRCPA**
Associate Professor
University of Queensland;
Anatomical Pathologist
Aquesta Specialized Uropathology
Brisbane, Queensland, Australia

Puay Hoon Tan, FRCPA
Head and Senior Consultant
Department of Pathology
Singapore General Hospital
Singapore

Fabio Tavora, MD
Director
Argos Laboratory
Fortaleza, Brazil;
Visiting Professor
Escola Paulista de Medicina
São Paulo, Brazil

Toyonori Tsuzuki, MD, PhD
Director
Department of Pathology
Nagoya Daini Red Cross Hospital
Nagoya, Japan

Ximing Yang, MD, PhD
Professor of Pathology and Chief of Urologic
    Pathology
Department of Surgical Pathology
Northwestern Memorial Hospital
Northwestern University Feinberg School
    of Medicine
Chicago, Illinois

Huihui Ye, MD
Staff Pathologist
Department of Pathology
Beth Israel Deaconess Medical Center
Boston, Massachusetts

Ming Zhou, MD, PhD
Associate Professor and Director
Surgical Pathology and Urologic Pathology
NYU Medical Center Tisch Hospital
New York City, New York

Today's pathologists, in practice and in training, all face a similar challenge: too much to learn but too little time. When the decision comes to buying a textbook, pathologists want one that is comprehensive yet easy to read and features many good images.

This book fits the bill. It has a unique format. Rather than combining many topics into one lengthy chapter that readers have to wade through, each chapter covers one specific disease entity or diagnostic issue, such as staging and grading. Each chapter provides excellent images of gross and microscopic pathology, along with highly templated and bulleted text. The clinical, pathologic, immunohistochemical, and molecular features of each disease entity are succinctly discussed and up to date. Emphasis is placed on the pathologic features and diagnostic criteria. Pertinent differential diagnoses are provided, along with diagnostically important clinical, gross, microscopic, and immunohistochemical clues.

A book is only as good as its writers. We are very fortunate to have assembled a team of internationally known surgical pathologists who not only understand the issues practicing pathologists face in their daily work but also have a vision for the future of genitourinary pathology.

Acknowledgments
We are enormously grateful to the contributors of this book. They spent countless hours out of their very busy schedules to make this textbook possible.

We thank Margaret LaPlaca for her secretarial assistance. We also want to thank our publisher, Elsevier, and executive content strategist, William Schmitt, for his support and encouragement during the production of this book. A special thanks is given to Katie DeFrancesco, our content development specialist at Elsevier, for her patience and persistence in keeping this book on track.

Ming Zhou, MD, PhD
George J. Netto, MD
Jonathan I. Epstein, MD

CONTENTS

M. SOFT TISSUE TUMORS AND LYMPHOMAS   513

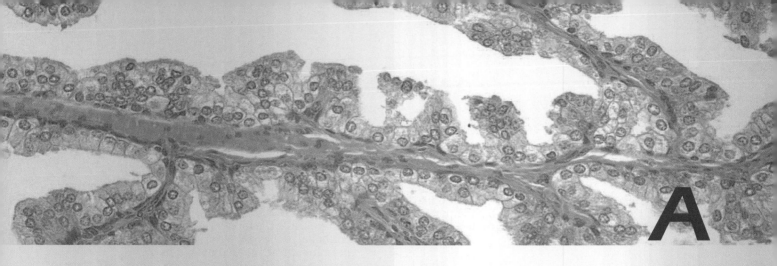

A

NONNEOPLASTIC DISEASE OF THE PROSTATE

ANATOMY AND HISTOLOGY OF THE PROSTATE

Definition
- In an adult man, the prostate gland is shaped like an inverted cone, with the base at the bladder neck and the apex at the urogenital diaphragm. It weighs 30 to 40 g.

Anatomy
- Located within the pelvis, the prostate is anterior to the rectum.
- The prostatic urethra runs through the center of the prostate, with a 35-degree anterior angle at the verumontanum, and serves as an important reference landmark.
- Anatomically, the prostate is composed of three zones (peripheral, central, and transition zone) with different volume, histology, and disease preference.
- The anterior fibromuscular stroma covers the anterior-medial surface.
- The central zone (approximately 25% of the prostate volume) is an inverted cone surrounding ejaculatory ducts and forms part of the prostate base.
- The transition zone (approximately 5% of the volume of the normal prostate) lies anterolateral to the proximal prostatic urethra; it often enlarges together with the anterior fibromuscular stroma to a massive size owing to benign prostatic hyperplasia.
- The peripheral zone (approximately 70% of the prostate volume) extends posterolaterally around the central zone and distal prostatic urethra.

Pathology
Histology
- Prostate glands are medium to large in size and form a lobulated architecture with intervening fibromuscular stroma.
- The contour of the glands is irregular with luminal undulation and papillary infolding.
- Glands are lined mainly with two types of cells: secretory and basal cells.
  - Secretory cells are cuboidal or columnar shaped with clear to pale cytoplasm and reddish granular pseudostratified nuclei (nuclei are perpendicular to basal lamina).
  - Basal cells are situated at the periphery of the glands beneath the secretory cells, with blue-gray, smooth nuclei (spindle shaped and parallel to the basement membrane).
- Epithelial cells with neuroendocrine differentiation are rarely seen; urothelial cells are commonly seen in proximity to the urethra.
- Corpora amylacea, which are round, concentrically laminated structures, are present within the glandular lumen.
- Lipofuscin pigment, considered a product of wear and tear in aging cells, may be seen in secretory cells.
- Peripheral zone acini are simple, round to oval, and set in a loose stroma of smooth muscle and collagen.
- Transition zone glands are similar to those in the peripheral zone, but are embedded in a compact stroma that forms a distinctive boundary with the loose stroma of the peripheral zone.
- Central zone acini are large and complex, with intraluminal ridges, papillary infolding, and occasional epithelial arches and cribriform glands mimicking prostatic intraepithelial neoplasia (PIN).
- The ratio of epithelium to stroma is higher in the central zone than the rest of the prostate, and the stroma is composed of compact interlacing smooth muscle bundles.
- The secretory cells of the central zone have eosinophilic cytoplasm and stratified nuclei; the basal cell layer is prominent.
- Seminal vesicles/ejaculatory ducts
  - Central irregular lumen with surrounding clusters of smaller glands
  - Scattered cells showing prominent degenerative nuclear atypia
  - Golden-brown lipofuscin pigments
- Verumontanum mucosal gland
  - Closely packed small acini beneath urethral mucosa
  - Orange-brown dense luminal secretion
  - Lipofuscin pigment often present
- Cowper glands
  - Extraprostatic structures found within the urogenital diaphragm
  - Dimorphic population of ducts and mucinous acini
  - Intermixed with skeletal muscle fibers
  - Acini with voluminous, pale cytoplasm
  - Noninfiltrative, lobular pattern
- Paraganglia
  - Small cluster or nest of cells with prominent vascular pattern
  - Intimately associated with nerve
  - Most common in periprostatic soft tissue
  - Clear or amphophilic, granular cytoplasm
  - Inconspicuous nucleoli

Immunopathology (including immunohistochemistry)
- Benign prostatic secretory and basal cells are immunoreactive for antibodies to broad-spectrum and low-molecular-weight cytokeratin.
- Secretory cells are considered to be terminally differentiated and are positive for prostate-lineage–specific markers such as prostate-specific antigen (PSA), prostate-specific acid phosphatase (PAP), and prostate-specific membrane antigen (PSMA).
- Basal cells are prostate stem cells and less differentiated; they are negative for prostate-specific markers but positive for high-molecular-weight cytokeratin (34βE12 or cytokeratin 5/6) and p63.
- PSA is not expressed in seminal vesicle/ejaculatory duct epithelium or prostatic urothelial cells.
- Neuroendocrine cells coexpress PSA and androgen receptors, suggesting a common cell of origin for epithelial cells and neuroendocrine cells; most neuroendocrine cells of the prostate contain chromogranin A.

Main differential diagnosis
- Seminal vesicles/ejaculatory ducts
  - High-grade prostatic intraepithelial neoplasia
  - Radiation changes
- Verumontanum mucosal gland
  - Prostate carcinoma
- Cowper glands
  - Foamy gland carcinoma
- Paraganglia
  - High-grade, high-stage prostate carcinoma

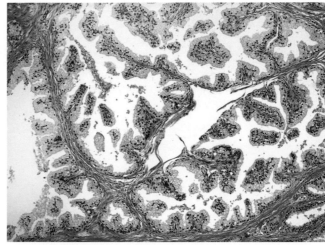

Fig 3. At scanning power, benign prostate glands are medium to large in size and show a lobulated architecture with intervening fibromuscular stroma.

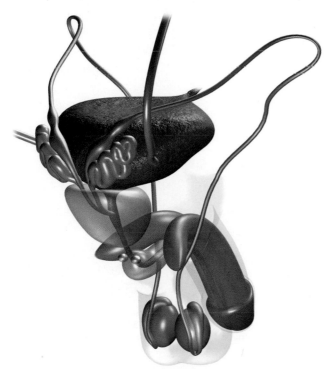

Fig 1. Diagram of male genitourinary system anatomy.

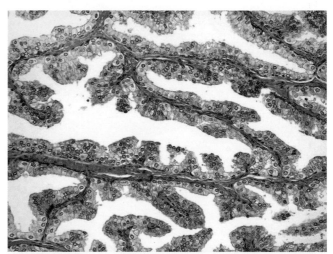

Fig 4. Normal prostate glands have irregular contour with luminal undulation and papillary infolding.

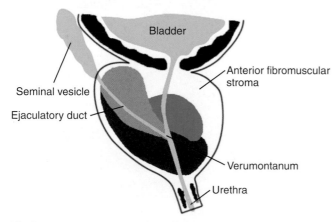

Fig 2. Diagram of the prostate showing the location of the anatomic zones (peripheral zone [purple], transition zone [green], central zone [pink]) in relation to the proximal urethra, ejaculatory duct, and verumontanum.

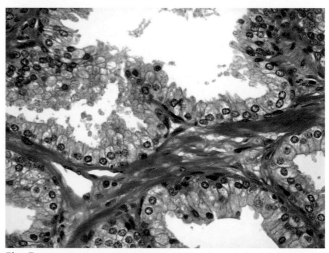

Fig 5. Normal prostate glands comprise mainly two types of cells: secretory cells and basal cells. Secretory cells are cuboidal or columnar-shaped with clear to pale cytoplasm and pseudostratified nuclei. Basal cells are situated at the periphery of the gland beneath the secretory cells.

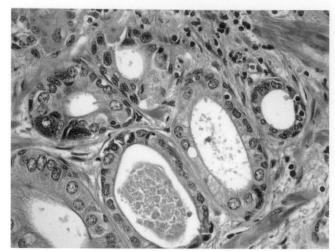

Fig 6. Neuroendocrine cells cannot be appreciated on routine H&E-stained sections in benign prostate tissue. In some cancers, neuroendocrine cells have red cytoplasmic granules, termed paneth cell–like neuroendocrine differentiation.

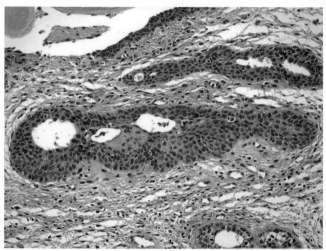

Fig 7. Urothelial cells in proximity to the prostatic urethra.

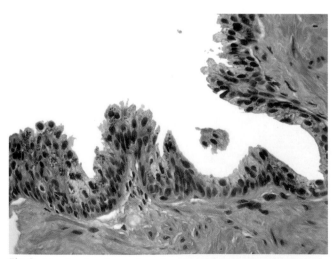

Fig 8. Lipofuscin pigment can be seen in benign prostate glands.

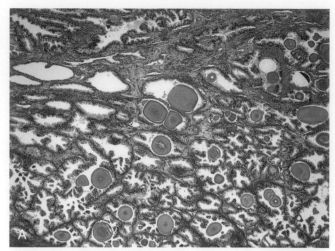

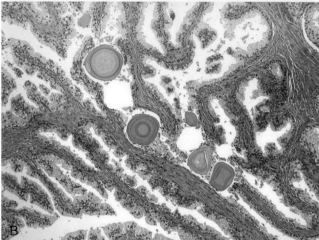

Fig 9. A, Corpora amylacea are noted within the lumen of numerous benign prostatic glands. **B,** Most corpora amylacea are round; the presence of concentric laminations is variable.

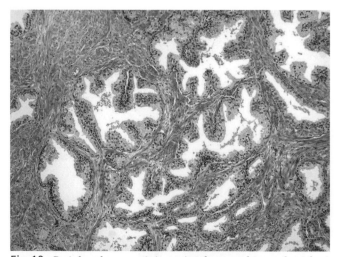

Fig 10. Peripheral zone acini are simple, round to oval, and set in a loose stroma of smooth muscle and collagen.

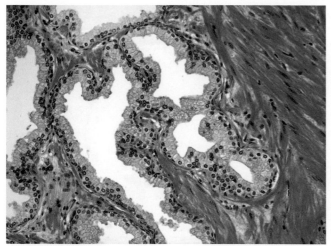

Fig 11. Transition zone glands are embedded in a compact stroma that forms a distinctive boundary with the loose stroma of the peripheral zone.

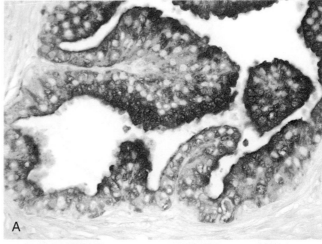

A

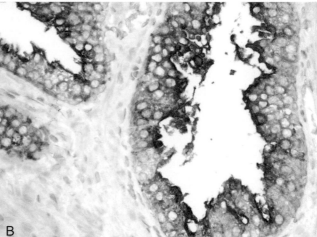

B

Fig 14. Secretory cells are positive for prostate-specific acid phosphatase **(A)** and prostate-specific membrane antigen **(B)**. Basal cells are negative for prostate-specific markers.

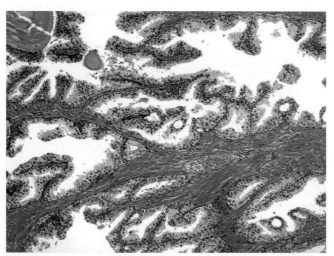

Fig 12. Central zone prostate glands are large and complex, with intraluminal ridges, papillary infolding, and occasional epithelial arches (Roman bridges). The stroma is composed of compact interlacing smooth muscle bundles.

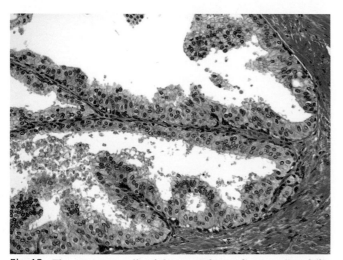

Fig 13. The secretory cells of the central zone have eosinophilic cytoplasm and stratified nuclei. A prominent basal cell layer is a common finding.

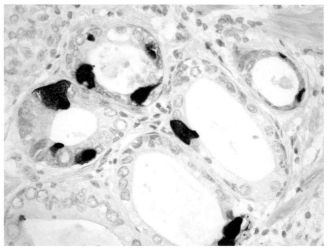

Fig 15. Adenocarcinoma of the prostate (same case as Fig 6) positive for chromogranin A.

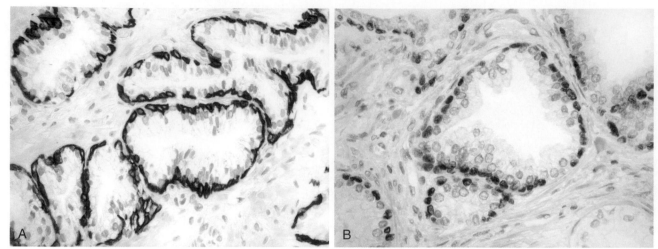

Fig 16. Basal cells are positive for high-molecular-weight cytokeratin (34BE12, cytoplasmic staining) **(A)** and p63 (nuclear staining) **(B)**.

Definition
- Seminal vesicles are a pair of male sex accessory glands posterolateral to the base of urinary bladder.
- The excretory duct of the seminal vesicle and ampulla of the vas deferens join to form ejaculatory ducts bilaterally, which converge and open into prostatic urethra at the verumontanum.
- It develops from the Wolffian (mesonephric) duct.

Clinical features
- Congenital agenesis (unilateral or bilateral)
  - It is often associated with agenesis or ectopia of the vas deferens.
  - A subset of patients has mutations in the cystic fibrosis *CFTR* gene, and agenesis occurs as a result of luminal blockade by thick secretions.
  - Other patients have abnormal development of the mesonephric duct during embryogenesis because of unknown reasons, often associated with ipsilateral renal agenesis if it occurs before 7 weeks gestation.
  - Infertility is seen in patients with bilateral agenesis or unilateral agenesis and contralateral obstruction despite intact testicular spermatogenesis.
- Cysts
  - Congenital cysts are often associated with ipsilateral renal agenesis or dysplasia, reflecting maldevelopment of distal mesonephric duct, faulty ureteral budding, or atresia of the ejaculatory ducts.
  - Acquired cysts are associated with obstruction secondary to chronic prostatitis.
- Amyloidosis
  - Common; incidence increases with age
  - Usually a localized finding without systemic disease; frequently also involves the vas deferens and ejaculatory ducts
  - Amyloid derived from semenogelin I, the major secretory product of the seminal vesicles
- Primary carcinoma of seminal vesicle
  - Exceedingly rare
  - Must rule out invasion from prostate or other sites

Pathology
Histology
- Complex mucosal folds are present in reproductive years, with dilatation and blunted epithelium with advanced age.
- Architecture is characterized by a central, large, dilated lumina with numerous small glands clustered around the periphery, often located at the end of cores on a needle biopsy specimen.
- The epithelium is composed of two cell layers: columnar and basal cells. Columnar cells have short microvilli and characteristically contain a large amount of lipofuscin (golden-brown pigment).
- Scattered cells show prominent nuclear atypia with bizarre shape, marked hyperchromasia, and sometimes intranuclear inclusions ("monster" cells); atypia appears to be degenerative in nature without mitotic activity.
- Lumens contain eosinophilic secretions, often with crystalloids. Occasionally spermatozoa are present.
- Thick muscular wall in seminal vesicle separates it from the prostate. The outer portion of the ejaculatory duct has a thin muscle coat that progressively attenuates when it gets closer to verumontanum, surrounded by prostate tissue.
- The seminal vesicle and ejaculatory duct tissue are often indistinguishable on a needle biopsy specimen.
- The amyloid appears as a subepithelial nodular deposit. There is usually no amyloid deposit around blood vessels or in the prostatic parenchyma.
- Squamous or intestinal metaplasia of epithelium can occur.
- Stromal spindle cell proliferation ranging in extent from focal to mass forming rarely occurs.

Immunohistochemistry
- There is negative or focal weak immunoreactivity to prostate markers PSA, PSAP in seminal vesicle; ejaculatory duct epithelium may show stronger staining.
- MUC6 labels seminal vesicle/ejaculatory duct epithelium, but not prostatic glands.
- There is nuclear expression of PAX2, a marker of mesonephric origin.
- Stromal spindle cell proliferation is positive for estrogen receptor and progesterone receptor

Main differential diagnosis
- Prostatic adenocarcinoma
  - Bizarre nuclear atypia uncommon
  - Architectural pattern often infiltrative, rarely appearing as small glands clustered near a large lumen
  - Can rarely have type 2 lipofuscin pigment (nonrefractile, gray, brown, blue, variable in size), but not the type 1 golden-brown and refractile lipofuscin granules
  - Immunohistochemistry: high-molecular-weight cytokeratin negative, PSA positive, PAX2 negative
- High-grade PIN
  - Homogenous nuclear atypia with enlarged and hyperchromatic nuclei and nucleoli visible at intermediate-high power (20× objective)
  - No golden-brown pigment

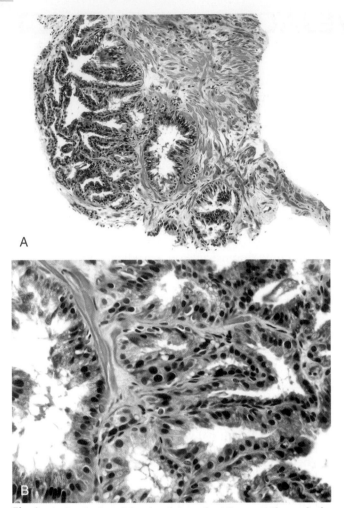

Fig 1. **A,** Seminal vesicle–ejaculatory duct tissue at the end of a biopsy core. **B,** Golden-brown lipofuscin granules and scattered hyperchromatic cells are apparent.

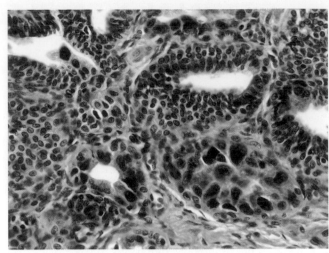

Fig 3. Seminal vesicle–ejaculatory duct glands with marked atypia. Golden-brown pigment can be seen in scattered cells.

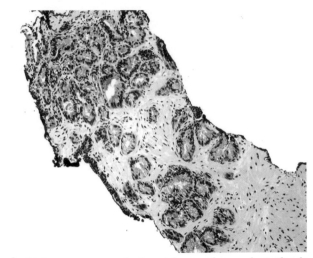

Fig 4. At low power, seminal vesicle–ejaculatory duct glands appear as crowed small glands with enlarged nuclei, mimicking prostatic adenocarcinoma.

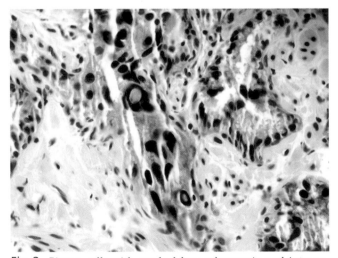

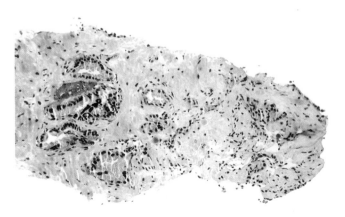

Fig 2. Bizarre cells with marked hyperchromasia and intranuclear inclusion.

Fig 5. Seminal vesicle–ejaculatory duct glands can appear to be relatively infiltrative, but marked atypia is uncommon for prostate cancer.

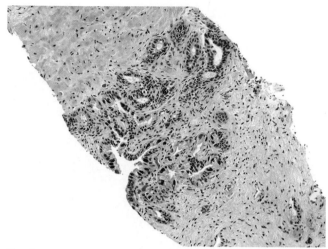

Fig 6. Seminal vesicle–ejaculatory duct glands mimic prostatic intraepithelial neoplasia and associated small glands.

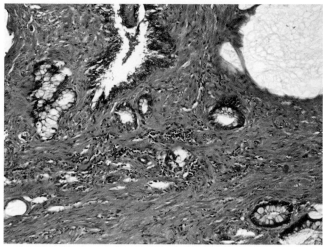

Fig 9. Intestinal metaplasia with goblet cells is a rare variant.

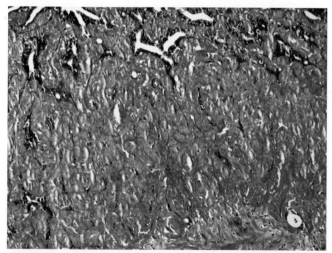

Fig 7. Amyloid present in seminal vesicle as diffuse subepithelial nodular deposits.

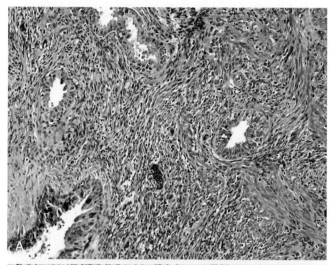

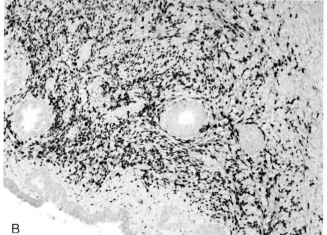

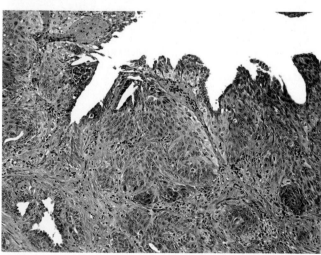

Fig 8. Squamous metaplasia can rarely be seen in seminal vesicle–ejaculatory duct tissue.

Fig 10. **A,** Unusual case of spindle cell proliferation with ovarian-like stroma involving the seminal vesicle–ejaculatory duct. **B,** The spindle cell proliferation is immunoreactive to ER (shown) and PR (not shown).

Definition
- Also called *bulbourethral gland;* paired, pea-shaped small exocrine glands in males, homologous to Bartholin's glands in females
- Deeply located posterolateral to the membranous (or bulbous) urethra in the urogenital diaphragm
- Lobular pattern of dimorphic population of mucinous acini and excretory ducts

Clinical features
Epidemiology
- Normal anatomic structure rarely present on transurethral resection or needle biopsy specimen of prostate that can mimic prostate cancer

Pathology
Histology
- Well-demarcated lobules composed of crowded, uniform mucinous acini with scattered duct structures situated in skeletal muscle
- Acini lined by distended epithelial cells with abundant intracytoplasmic mucin and basally oriented small nuclei with inconspicuous nucleoli
- Totally or subtotally occluded gland lumina and attenuated basal cell layer
- Separate from prostatic tissue

Immunopathology (including immunohistochemistry)
- Mucicarmine, periodic acid Schift (PAS)-D, and Alcian blue positive
- PSAP, S-100 typically negative; PSA may show focal clumped positivity in acinar cells
- High-molecular-weight cytokeratin highlights ductal epithelium and attenuated peripheral basal cells

Main differential diagnosis
- Mucin cell metaplasia of prostatic glands
  - Mucin-filled goblet cells usually involve only a portion of a prostatic gland or a few glands.
  - Mucin cell metaplasia glands are intermixed with prostatic tissue as opposed to skeletal muscle.
- Foamy gland prostatic adenocarcinoma
  - Abundant, foamy cytoplasm, lacking globoid distended goblet cells
  - Well-formed lumina with slightly rigid laminar border, often with numerous dense pink intraluminal amorphous secretions
  - Basally oriented nuclei, although small, with usually hyperchromatic and scattered visible nucleoli
  - PSA and PSAP positive, high-molecular-weight cytokeratin, p63 negative, and mucicarmine negative

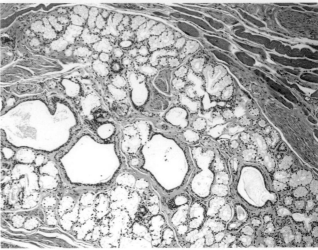

Fig 1. Cowper glands appear as lobules of acini with mucin-containing cells and centrally located excretory ducts, surrounded by skeletal muscle on transurethral resection.

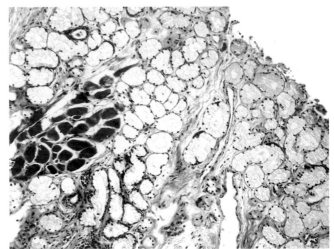

Fig 2. Dimorphic population of mucinous acini and scattered ducts, and adjacent skeletal muscle are diagnostic for Cowper gland on needle biopsy.

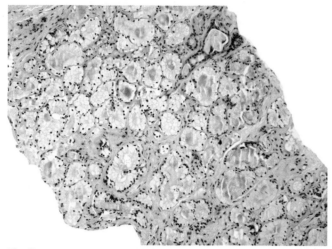

Fig 3. Cowper glands sometimes contain eosinophilic luminal secretions, mimicking foamy gland prostate adenocarcinoma.

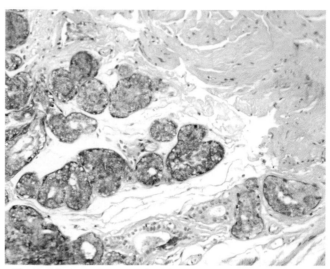

Fig 5. Mucicarmine stain highlights the intracellular mucin.

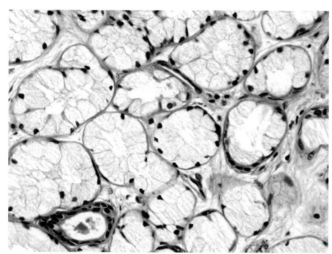

Fig 4. Acini are lined by distended epithelial cells with abundant intracytoplasmic mucin and basally oriented small nuclei with inconspicuous nucleoli. Attenuated basal cells only focally present.

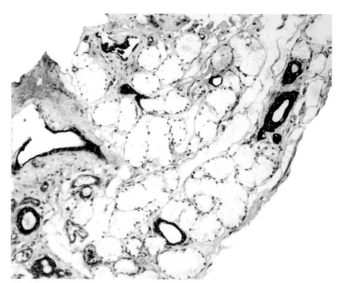

Fig 6. Ductal epithelial cells are strongly positive for high-molecular-weight cytokeratin. Scattered basal cells at the periphery of acini are also positive.

Definition
- Nodular hyperplasia or benign prostatic hyperplasia (BPH) consists of a nonmalignant enlargement of the prostate because of overgrowth of the epithelium and fibromuscular tissue of the transition zone and periurethral area.
- It occurs commonly in men after 50 years of age, sometimes leading to compression of the urethra and obstruction of the flow of urine.

Clinical features
Epidemiology
- The cause of BPH is not well understood, but it has been proposed that it could be caused by:
  - Aging process
  - Decreased testosterone levels
  - Accumulation of dihydrotestosterone

Presentation
- The obstructive symptoms of BPH, referred to as *lower urinary tract symptoms,* are:
  - Difficulty initiating a urine stream
  - Hesitant, interrupted, and weak stream
  - Urgency and leaking or dribbling
- As the urethra becomes narrower, the bladder wall becomes thicker and the bladder itself becomes smaller, causing:
  - Difficulty initiating
  - Frequent urination
  - Bladder irritability
  - Sudden strong urge to urinate, especially at night
  - Urge incontinence

Prognosis and treatment
- Low symptom index score (mild symptoms): usual procedure is watchful waiting
- Mid-range symptom index score (moderate symptoms): usual procedure is pharmaceutical intervention
  - α-Receptor blockers (tamsulosin hydrochloride [Flomax]) relax the prostatic-urethral muscle, thereby improving urinary flow.
  - 5-α-Reductase inhibitors (finasteride and dutasteride [Avodart]) help to shrink the prostate.
- High symptom index score (severe symptoms): usual procedure is the use of invasive techniques
  - Nonsurgical invasive treatments include transurethral microwave thermotherapy and transurethral needle ablation.
  - Surgical treatments include transurethral resection of the prostate, transurethral incision of the prostate, laser prostatectomy, and open prostatectomy.

Pathology
- Development of nodular hyperplasia includes three pathologic changes: nodule formation, diffuse enlargement of the transition zone and periurethral tissue, and enlargement of nodules.
- The proportion of epithelium to stroma increases as symptoms become more severe.

- Nodular hyperplasia usually involves the transition zone, but occasionally nodules arise from the periurethral tissue at the bladder neck.
- Protrusion of bladder neck nodules into the bladder lumen is referred to as *median lobe hyperplasia.*

Histology
- Grossly, nodular hyperplasia consists of variably sized nodules that are rubbery, firm or soft, and yellow-gray, with a bulging cut surface.
- Nodular hyperplasia is composed of varying proportions of epithelium and stroma (fibrous connective tissue and smooth muscle).
- If there is prominent epithelial hyperplasia in addition to stromal hyperplasia, the numerous luminal spaces create soft and grossly spongy nodules that ooze a pale-white watery fluid upon sectioning.
- If nodular hyperplasia is predominantly fibromuscular, there may be diffuse enlargement or numerous trabeculations without prominent nodularity.
- Degenerative changes include calcification and infarction, probably related to vascular insufficiency.
- Benign prostatic hyperplasia frequently occurs concurrently with chronic inflammatory infiltrates, mainly composed of chronically activated T cells and macrophages.
- Focal acinar atrophy can be seen within nodular hyperplasia and significantly increases with patient age.

Immunopathology (including immunohistochemistry)
- Same as normal prostatic glands

Main differential diagnoses
- Most common variants of nodular hyperplasia
  - Atypical adenomatous hyperplasia
  - Cribriform clear cell hyperplasia
  - Basal cell hyperplasia
- Pseudohyperplastic cancer
- Prostatic stromal tumor of uncertain malignant potential

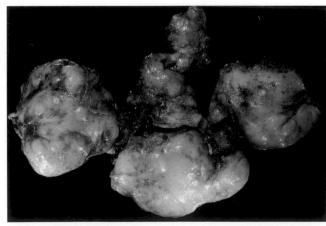

Fig 1. Nodular hyperplasia, gross appearance.

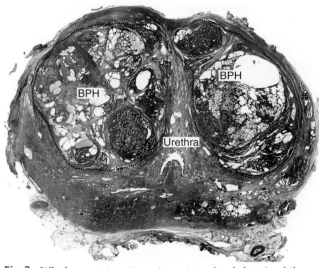

Fig 2. Whole-mount section of prostate gland showing bilateral nodules of benign prostatic hyperplasia (BPH) involving transition zone.

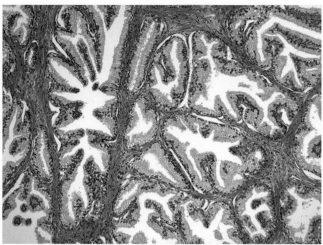

Fig 4. Epithelial hyperplasia in addition to stromal hyperplasia. The hyperplastic glands have irregular contour with luminal undulation and papillary infolding.

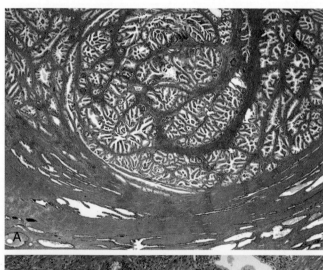

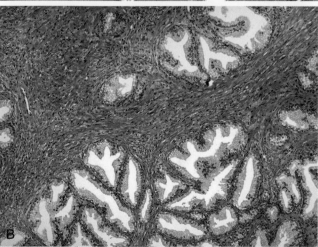

Fig 3. **A,** Mixed epithelial-stromal nodule of nodular hyperplasia. **B,** Note the dense fibromuscular stroma that forms the boundary of the nodule with the transition zone stroma.

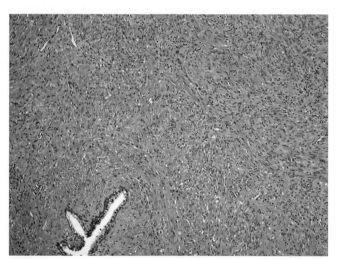

Fig 5. Predominantly fibromuscular nodular hyperplasia. The nodule consists of stromal fibroblasts with scattered lymphocytes.

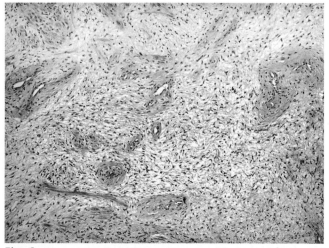

Fig 6. Pure stromal nodule with myxoid degeneration and prominent vessels.

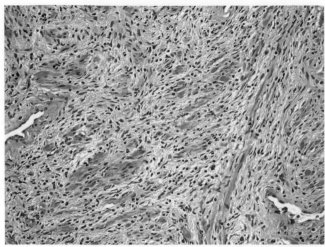

Fig 7. Stromal nodule with smooth muscle fibers, fibroblasts, vessels, and sprinkled lymphocytes.

Definition
- Presence of acute inflammatory cells in the prostate tissue, with or without clinical symptoms

Clinical features
Epidemiology
- Prostatitis syndrome is one of the most common encounters in urologic practice; it is more likely to affect younger men than are nodular hyperplasia and prostate cancer.
- Acute bacterial prostatitis is the most common form of acute inflammation, often caused by gram-negative organisms (*Escherichia coli* in 80% of infections).

Presentation
- Symptomatic patients often have fever, chills, irritative and obstructive voiding symptoms, and lower back and perineal pain. Urine or prostatic secretion culture positive for organisms.
- Patchy acute inflammation is frequently found in needle biopsy specimens of asymptomatic patients for cancer screening.

Prognosis and treatment
- Prostate biopsy is contraindicated in patients with acute symptoms.
- Course is benign; most respond to antimicrobial treatment. Surgical drainage may be required for abscess.

Pathology
Histology
- Sheets of neutrophils within or around glands, intraductal cellular debris, and stromal edema are present. Focal necrosis and microabscess formation may be present.
- Reactive changes seen in glands involved by acute inflammation include atrophy and mild nuclear atypia with focally prominent nucleoli.
- Acute inflammation encountered in prostate biopsy specimens should be diagnosed as prostate tissue with acute inflammation—and not as acute prostatitis—because the presence of focal acute inflammation on a biopsy specimen does not correlate with clinical symptomatology.

Immunopathology (including immunohistochemistry)
- Inflamed glands are generally positive for high-molecular-weight cytokeratin and p63; however, some glands involved by inflammation focally can be negative for basal cell markers.

Main differential diagnosis
- Reactive changes with acute inflammation can mimic prostatic adenocarcinoma.
  - Rarely, prostate cancer glands are associated with acute inflammation. To make this diagnosis, the architectural pattern should be overtly infiltrative with significant nuclear atypia beyond that seen in adjacent obviously benign glands. Typically, the diagnosis should also be verified using basal cell markers.

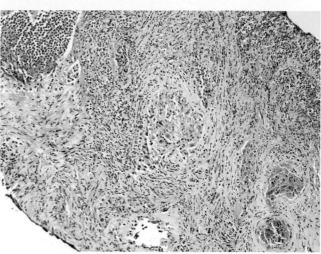

Fig 1. Prominent acute inflammatory infiltrate involves prostatic glands and stroma. Necrosis of glands and microabscess are present in the case of clinical acute prostatitis.

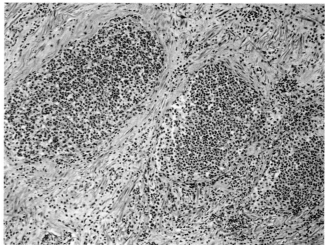

Fig 2. Microabscess replaces the normal prostatic ducts on transurethral resection in the case of clinical acute prostatitis.

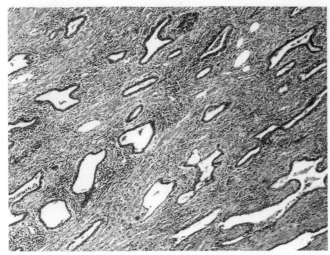

Fig 3. Mixed acute and chronic inflammation is associated with atrophy. This is a common finding and should not be diagnosed as prostatitis.

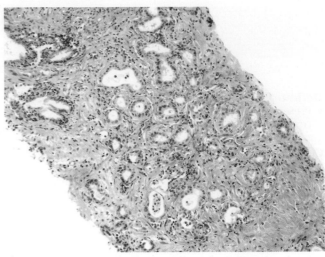

Fig 4. Crowded small glands with scattered nuclei showing prominent nucleoli, seen in the spectrum of reactive changes of acute inflammation, mimic prostatic adenocarcinoma.

CHRONIC INFLAMMATION OF THE PROSTATE

Definition
- Presence of chronic inflammatory cells in the prostate tissue, with or without clinical symptoms

Clinical features
Epidemiology
- Clinically can be divided into chronic bacterial prostatitis, chronic prostatitis/chronic pelvic pain syndrome inflammatory type, and asymptomatic chronic inflammatory prostatitis
- Asymptomatic chronic inflammation commonly present in prostate biopsy specimens

Presentation
- Nonspecific symptoms such as lower back pain; urine or prostatic secretion culture positive for organisms in bacterial prostatitis; serum PSA possibly elevated

Prognosis and treatment
- Antimicrobial therapy and α-blocker therapy

Pathology
Histology
- Periglandular, perilobular or diffuse infiltrate of lymphocytes, plasma cells, and some histiocytes are present.
- Atrophy is commonly seen in association with chronic inflammation.
- Reactive changes, including architectural change mimicking cancer, can be seen.
- Chronic inflammation encountered in prostate biopsies should not be called *chronic prostatitis;* it is common in benign prostatic hyperplasia and benign prostates without hyperplasia and does not correlate with the clinical symptomatology.

Immunopathology (including immunohistochemistry)
- Lymphocytes are mainly T cells.
- Inflamed glands are generally positive for high-molecular-weight cytokeratin and p63; however, some glands involved by inflammation focally can be negative for basal cell markers.

Main differential diagnosis
- Nonspecific granulomatous inflammation (NSGP)
  - NSGP consists of a periglandular expansile infiltrate composed of epithelioid histiocytes, lymphocytes, plasma cells, neutrophils, and variable eosinophils. Often, discrete granulomas are not seen.
- Reactive changes with chronic inflammation can mimic prostatic adenocarcinoma.
  - Rarely, prostate cancer glands are associated with chronic inflammation. To make this diagnosis, the architectural pattern should be overtly infiltrative with significant nuclear atypia beyond that seen in adjacent obviously benign glands. Typically the diagnosis should also be verified using basal cell markers.

- Cords or single cells of Gleason pattern 5 adenocarcinoma can mimic crushed chronic inflammatory cells, but pleomorphism and nuclear atypia can be appreciated at high power. CAM5.2 is the best immunohistochemical marker to label high-grade prostate cancer as opposed to inflammation, because some high-grade cancers may not express prostate-specific markers (i.e., PSA).
- Chronic lymphocytic leukemia/small lymphocytic lymphoma
  - Monotonous population of small lymphocytes, often diffuse without periglandular distribution
- CD5, CD23, and CD20 positive, CD10 and cyclin D1 negative

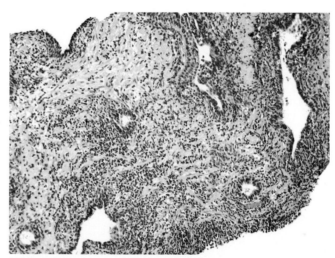

Fig 1. Periglandular and stromal chronic inflammatory infiltrate composed of lymphocytes and plasma cells.

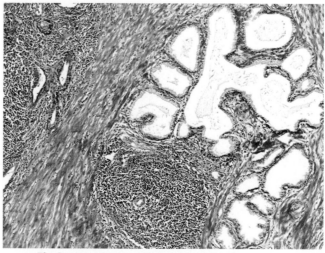

Fig 2. Prominent perilobular lymphoid aggregate.

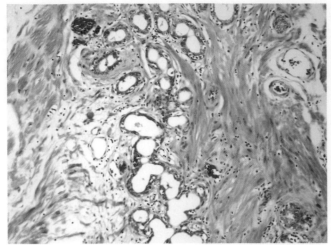

Fig 3. Glandular atrophy and scattered chronic inflammatory cells.

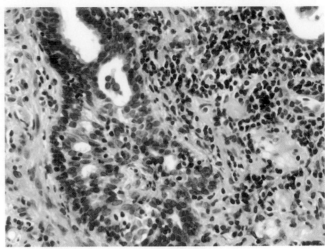

Fig 4. Pseudocribriform glands and adjacent prominent chronic inflammation.

NONSPECIFIC GRANULOMATOUS PROSTATITIS

Definition
- Mixed inflammatory response owing to extravasated prostatic fluid, bacterial toxins, and cell debris

Clinical features
Epidemiology
- Most commonly seen in men 50 to 69 years old, with a range of 18 to 86 years
- Present in 0.5% to 3.4% of prostate specimens and accounts for approximately two thirds of all granulomatous processes of the prostate

Presentation
- There is irritative voiding symptoms, fever, chills, hematuria, and obstructive voiding symptoms.
- The patient may be asymptomatic.
- Most men report urinary tract infection within the month preceding diagnosis.
- Prostate gland may be fixed, firm, and nodular on digital rectal examination (DRE), mimicking prostate cancer.
- Serum PSA level is often elevated.

Prognosis and treatment
- Most symptoms resolve within a few months.
- Abnormal DRE may persist for up to 8 years in many men.
- Treatment consists of warm sitz baths, fluids, and antibiotics if concomitant urinary tract infection is documented.
- Surgical intervention may be necessary to relieve persistent obstructive symptoms.

Pathology
Histology
- Dense, lobular, or nodular inflammation centered on ducts and acini is present.
- Mixed inflammatory infiltrate contains epithelioid histiocytes, lymphocytes, plasma cells, eosinophils, and scattered neutrophils.
- Well-formed, nonnecrotic granulomata are uncommon; multinucleated giant cells are only seen in 50% of cases on needle biopsy specimen.
- Early lesions show dilated or ruptured ducts and acini containing neutrophils, debris, desquamated epithelial cells, and foamy histiocytes.
- Older lesions show a more prominent fibrous component.

Immunopathology (including immunohistochemistry)
- Positive for histiocytic markers (CD68)
- Negative for cytokeratins (CAM5.2) and prostatic markers (PSA, PSMA)

Molecular diagnostics
- Noncontributory

Main differential diagnosis
- An unusual epithelioid variant of NSGP can closely mimic high-grade prostate cancer. In contrast to cancer, there are other admixed, more readily recognizable acute and chronic inflammatory cells. In difficult cases, immunohistochemistry for CAM5.2 and CD68 should be performed. CAM5.2 is better than prostate-specific markers for demonstrating epithelial differentiation, because the latter may be negative in very high-grade prostate cancer.
- Infectious granulomatous prostatitis starts as well-formed, nonnecrotizing granulomas that are adjacent to intact prostate glands, as opposed to NSGP, which forms around ruptured acini. As infectious granulomas expand, they can destroy prostate glands and develop caseous necrosis. In contrast, NSGP lacks caseous necrosis; in a minority of cases, there may be neutrophils within the center of the granulomatous inflammation.
- Allergic granulomatous prostatitis is rare and is characterized by small, uniform eosinophilic areas of necrosis with sheets of eosinophils both surrounding the necrosis and extending into the stroma in areas distant from the necrosis. Although NSGP can have numerous eosinophils, they are seen in the setting of a polymorphous inflammatory infiltrate.
- Malakoplakia tends not to have much of a polymorphous inflammatory infiltrate. Michaelis-Gutmann bodies are unique to malakoplakia.

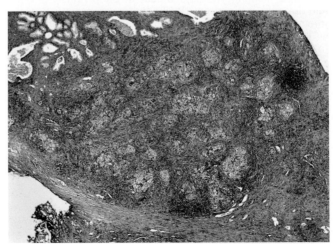

Fig 1. Low-power view showing the lobular architecture and periductal nature of nonspecific granulomatous prostatitis.

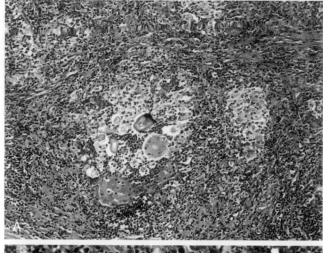

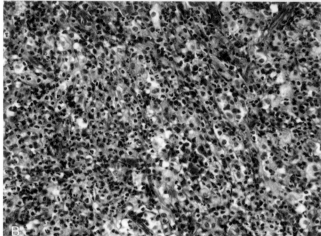

Fig 2. **A,** In the earlier and more active phases of nonspecific granulomatous inflammation, neutrophils, eosinophils, and foamy macrophages fill the duct lumen, and occasional foreign body–type giant cells may be seen in association with corpora amylacea. Lymphocytes predominate at the periphery of ducts and throughout the stroma. **B,** On high-power examination, the inflammatory infiltrate is composed of a mixture of neutrophils, eosinophils, lymphocytes, histiocytes, and plasma cells.

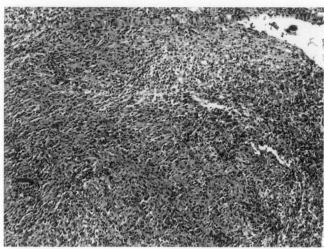

Fig 3. Older lesions of nonspecific granulomatous inflammation may show a more prominent fibrous component.

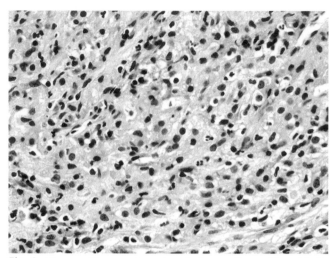

Fig 4. Nonspecific granulomatous inflammation with epithelioid histiocytes mimicking cancer. Note the admixed inflammation, which would be unusual in adenocarcinoma of the prostate.

Definition
- Granulomatous inflammatory response seen after transurethral resection or needle core biopsy of the prostate gland

Clinical features
Epidemiology
- It is common in repeated transurethral resection (TUR) if performed within a few months of the initial inciting TUR.
- It rarely can be seen after prostate needle biopsy.
- Less than 1% of benign specimens contain granulomata, with post-biopsy granulomatous inflammation comprising approximately one quarter of these lesions.

Presentation
- Typically an incidental finding

Prognosis and treatment
- Benign; no treatment necessary

Pathology
Histology
- It resembles rheumatoid nodules in that granulomata are variably sized, often serpiginous, and contain central fibrinoid necrosis (necrobiosis) with peripheral palisading histiocytes.
- The perimeters of the granulomata often have lymphocytic infiltrate.
- If seen following a recent (less than 3 months) TUR, numerous eosinophils may be seen.
- Adjacent areas may show nonnecrotizing granulomata and multinucleated giant cells.

Immunopathology (including immunohistochemistry)
- Noncontributory

Molecular diagnostics
- Noncontributory

Main differential diagnosis
- Allergic granulomatous prostatitis is rare and is characterized by small, uniform eosinophilic areas of necrosis with sheets of eosinophils both surrounding the necrosis and extending into the stroma in areas distant from the necrosis. In postbiopsy granulomas, the eosinophils are only localized around the granulomas. The granulomas in postbiopsy lesions are also more variably shaped than allergic granulomas.
- In infectious granulomatous prostatitis, granulomas often have caseous necrosis as opposed to the coagulative necrosis seen in postbiopsy granulomas. Whereas in caseous necrosis there is only necrotic debris, outlines of prostatic stroma and glands may still be visible in coagulative necrosis of postbiopsy granulomas.

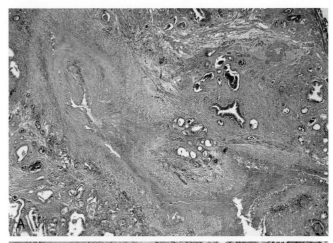
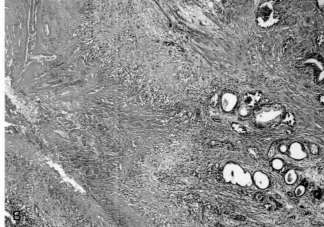
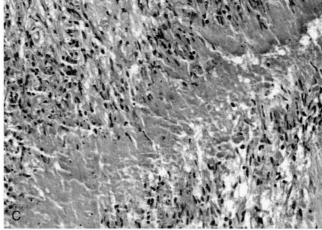

Fig 1. **A,** The borders of a post-TUR granuloma are often irregular and serpiginous, creeping around benign ducts and lobules. **B,** The center of the granuloma is necrotic, and the "ghosts" of glands and vessels can often be seen within the fibrinoid necrosis. **C,** Epithelioid histiocytes line the periphery of a post-TUR granuloma.

Definition
- Aggregate of lipid-laden histiocytes found within the prostatic stroma

Clinical features
Epidemiology
- Incidence is low; fewer than 50 cases have been reported, although many cases are not reported (i.e., not as rare as appears).
- There is no association with increased serum lipid levels.

Presentation
- Typically an incidental diagnosis on prostate needle biopsies performed to rule out carcinoma
- Rarely found on samples from TUR of the prostate (TURP)
- Rarely associated as an incidental finding with adjacent carcinoma

Prognosis and therapy
- No treatment is required for this incidental finding.

Pathology
Histology
- Well-circumscribed nodular collection of foamy histiocytes
- Typically a single focus in biopsy specimen, smaller than 0.5 mm
- Occasionally, histiocytes arranged in cords and individual cells with an infiltrative pattern
- Abundant, vacuolated foamy cytoplasm
- Small, uniform, and benign-appearing nuclei with inconspicuous nucleoli
- Absence of mitotic figures

Immunopathology
- Diffusely positive for histiocytic marker CD68
- Negative for keratins (CAM5.2, pan-cytokeratin)
- Generally negative for prostatic markers PSA, PSAP

Main differential diagnosis
- High-grade foamy gland adenocarcinoma: typically, carcinoma has a more infiltrative appearance. It would be rare for foamy gland carcinoma to have no glandular differentiation; CD68 would be negative in carcinoma.
- Hormone-treated adenocarcinoma: changes in surrounding benign prostate (atrophy, basal cell hyperplasia, squamous metaplasia) are clues to hormonal therapy; residual glandular carcinoma may be present.
- Nonspecific granulomatous prostatitis typically contains a mixed inflammatory background with neutrophils and lymphocytes.

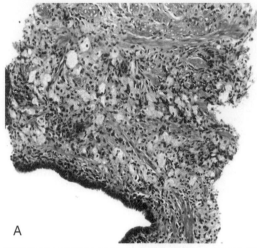
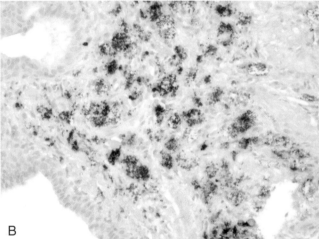
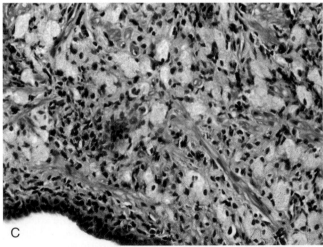

Fig 1. **A,** Collections of pale-staining single cells are interspersed throughout prostatic stroma. **B,** Immunohistochemical stain for CD68 is positive and helpful to rule out high-grade foamy gland carcinoma or carcinoma with hormonal treatment effect. **C,** At higher power, foamy cytoplasm is evident and nuclear atypia is absent. Admixed lymphocytes are also appreciated.

GRANULOMATOUS INFLAMMATION OF INFECTIOUS ETIOLOGY

Definition
- Granulomatous prostatitis induced by infectious agents

Clinical features
Epidemiology
- It is rare compared with noninfectious granulomatous prostatitis.
- It can be caused by bacteria, fungi, parasites, and viruses.
- Mycobacterial prostatitis can occur in patients with systemic tuberculosis or as a complication of Bacillus-Calmette-Guerin (BCG) therapy.
- It is seen frequently in immunocompromised hosts in the abscence of BCG therapy.

Pathology
Histology
- Granulomas with or without necrosis
- Multinucleate giant cells
- Caseating necrosis in tuberculosis
- Acinar destruction
- Microorganisms demonstrated with proper histo-chemical stains

Main differential diagnosis
- NSGP shows ruptured acini with associated granulomatous reaction. Although there may be central neutrophils, the lesion lacks necrosis. In contrast, infectious granulomas start as nonnecrotizing granulomas adjacent to intact acini. As the granulomas expand, they can develop necrosis and destroy acini.

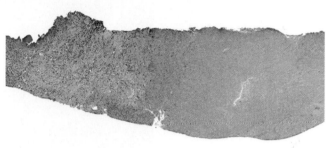

Fig 2. Tuberculosis characterized by caseous necrosis and chronic granulomatous inflammation.

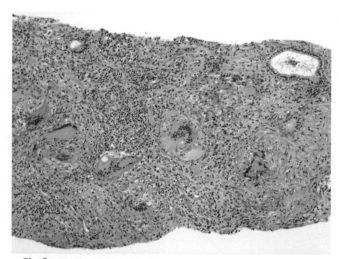

Fig 3. Numerous multinucleated giant cells in tuberculosis.

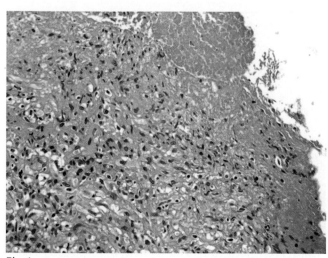

Fig 1. Caseating granuloma composed of epithelioid histiocytes in tuberculosis.

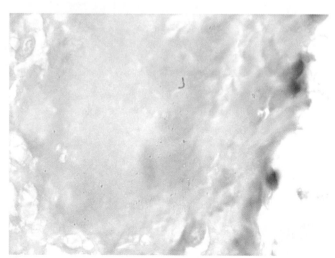

Fig 4. A *Mycobacterium* spp. bacillus demonstrated using acid-fast stain.

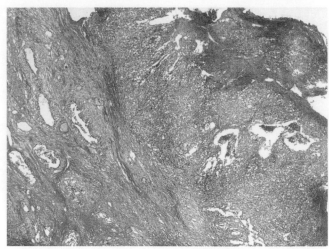

Fig 5. Cryptococcal prostatitis showing extensive acinar destruction and granulomatous inflammation.

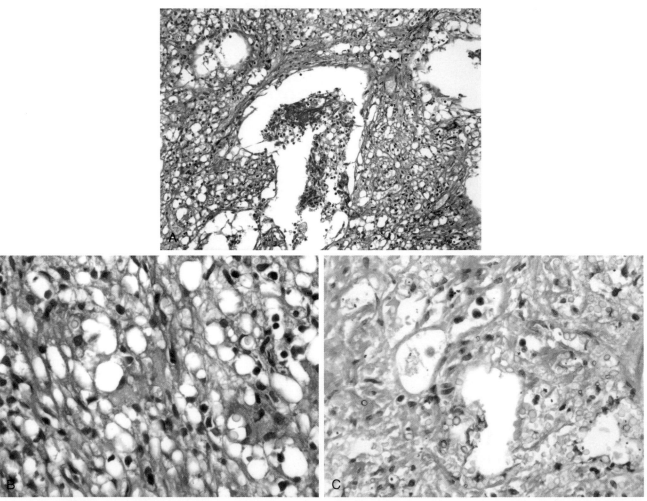

Fig 6. A, Destruction of prostatic acini with exudate in the glandular lumen in cryptococcosis of the prostate. **B,** Cryptococci among histiocytes. **C,** Mucinous capsule of cryptococci demonstrated with mucicarmine stain.

Definition
- Small benign glands are arranged in nests with reduced cytoplasmic volume in luminal epithelial cells; simple atrophy maintains relatively normal glandular spacing and luminal diameter.

Clinical features
Epidemiology
- Typically affects elderly, with prevalence and extent of gland involvement increasing with age
- Has been reported in at least 70% of men aged 19 to 29 years

Presentation
- Typically an incidental histologic finding, but may cause prostatic induration or a hypoechoic lesion on transrectal ultrasound

Prognosis and treatment
- Benign process with no treatment necessary

Pathology
Histology
- At low power, architecturally there are relatively normal caliber glands spaced similarly apart as adjacent nonatrophic glands.
- Luminal cells have reduced cytoplasmic volume resulting in an increased nuclear-to-cytoplasmic ratio; a high ratio imparts a basophilic appearance at low power.
- Nuclei are often hyperchromatic and occasionally enlarged mildly; nucleoli may be present, although they should not be as prominent as in carcinoma.

Immunopathology (including immunohistochemistry)
- Basal cell markers, such as p63 and high-molecular-weight cytokeratin, are invariably positive and typically show complete circumferential staining.

Molecular diagnostics
- Noncontributory

Main differential diagnosis
- Prostatic adenocarcinoma with atrophic features: simple atrophy is not a close mimicker of prostate cancer, because it does not appear infiltrative, and the glands are not that crowded as long as it is recognized that small nucleoli may be visible.

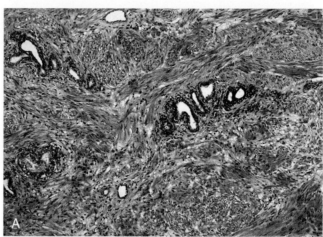

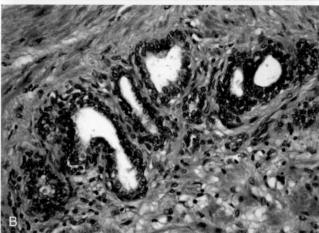

Fig 1. **A,** Simple atrophy consists of relatively normal-sized glands lined by secretory cells with scant cytoplasm, leading to an increased nuclear-to-cytoplasmic ratio, nuclear crowding, and a blue appearance at low power. **B,** High-power examination shows uniformly bland nuclei without prominent nucleoli.

Definition
- A distinct form of glandular atrophy characterized by cystically dilated glands with sharp luminal borders

Pathology
Histology
- Atrophic prostatic glands show cystic dilatation.
- Glands have sharp luminal borders without papillary infolding.
- Cells show clear scant cytoplasm, increased nuclear-to-cytoplasmic ratio, and bland monotonous mildly enlarged nuclei.
- Nucleoli can be conspicuous, but not to the degree seen in prostatic adenocarcinoma.

Immunohistochemistry
- Basal cell markers such as p63 and high-molecular-weight cytokeratin highlight the presence of basal cells around the glands (usually complete circumferential staining, but can be incomplete and patchy).

Main differential diagnosis
- Prostatic adenocarcinoma (Gleason score 3 + 3 = 6) has the following differentiating features:
  - Infiltrative pattern of growth
  - Often amphophilic cytoplasm
  - Cytologic atypia with prominent nucleoli
  - Lack of basal cells

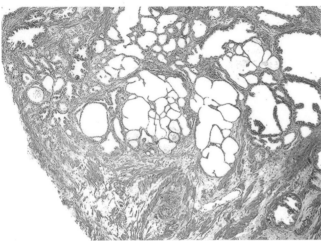

Fig 1. Cystic atrophy is a collection of atrophic and cystically dilated prostatic glands.

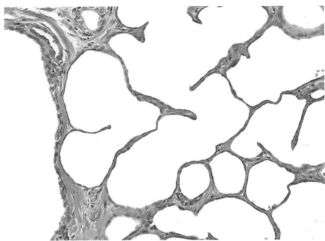

Fig 3. Cells lining the glands are flattened to low cuboidal and show clear scant cytoplasm, increased nuclear-to-cytoplasmic ratio, and bland monotonous nuclei with occasional conspicuous, but not prominent nucleoli.

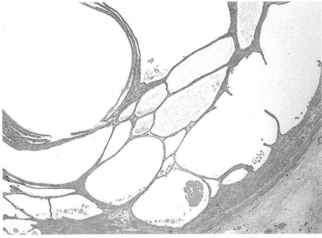

Fig 2. In contrast to the nonatrophic benign prostatic glands, atrophic glands have sharp luminal borders without papillary infolding.

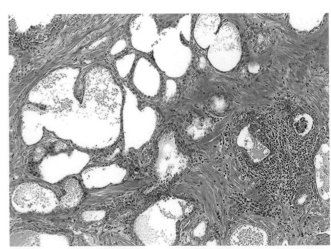

Fig 4. Cystic atrophy is often accompanied by chronic inflammation.

Definition
- Morphologically distinct subtype of focal atrophy

Clinical features
Epidemiology
- Commonly seen in prostatic needle biopsy and radical prostatectomy specimens
- Typically occurs in the elderly; common in young men

Presentation
- Usually asymptomatic
- May cause total or free PSA elevation, prostatic induration, or hypoechoic lesions on transrectal ultrasound

Prognosis and treatment
- Not associated with an increased risk of cancer on subsequent biopsy

Pathology
Histology
- Small, round acini compactly arranged in a lobular pattern often surrounding a dilated duct
- Scanty cytoplasm and crowded small glands imparting a basophilic appearance
- Mild nuclear enlargement and small nucleoli at times present
- May be seen in close proximity to partial atrophy
- Inflammatory changes in some cases (proliferative inflammatory atrophy)
- Elastosis or fibrosis in some cases (sclerotic atrophy)
- Sclerotic lesions can appear infiltrative

Immunohistochemistry and special studies
- Overexpression of COX2, BCL2, and proliferation markers PCNA and Ki-67 (MIB-1)
  - 34β E12 and p63 reveal intact basal cells
  - Racemase expression rare
  - Frequency of p53 mutations similar to that in high-grade PIN (HGPIN) lesions

Molecular diagnostics
- Hypermethylation of cytosine residues in the upstream "CpG island" in the *GSTP1* gene, higher than in normal tissues
- In situ shortening of CAG repeat lengths commonly found
- Chromosome 8 centromeric gain, significantly greater than in benign prostate

Main differential diagnosis
- Prostatic adenocarcinoma: postatrophic hyperplasia (PAH) tends to have a lobular configuration in many cases. A truly infiltrative pattern of isolated acini among and between more typical benign glands is not seen. PAH is basophilic at low power because of a lack of both apical and lateral cytoplasm, whereas most adenocarcinomas of the prostate have more cytoplasm (either eosinophilic or amphophilic) with a paler appearance at low magnification. Sclerosis is not a feature seen with adenocarcinoma. Markedly prominent nucleoli, as seen in some carcinomas, are not present in PAH. Basal cell markers are typically positive in most glands of PAH.

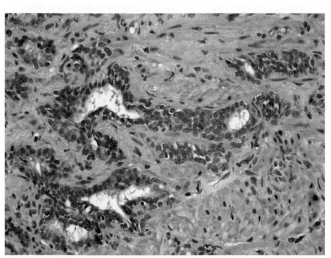

Fig 1. Postatrophic hyperplasia; some glands cut tangentially.

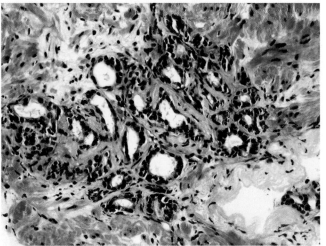

Fig 2. Postatrophic hyperplasia with crowded glands in a lobular configuration.

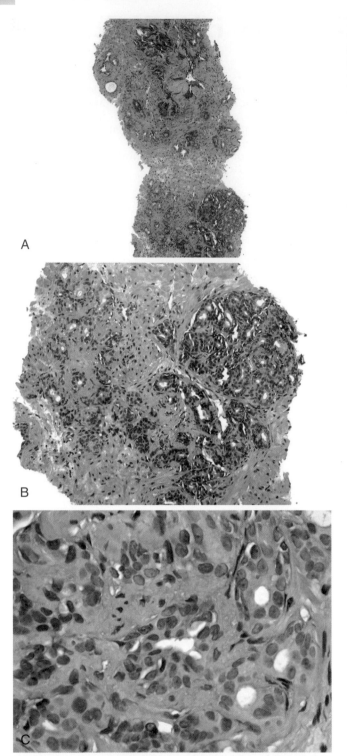

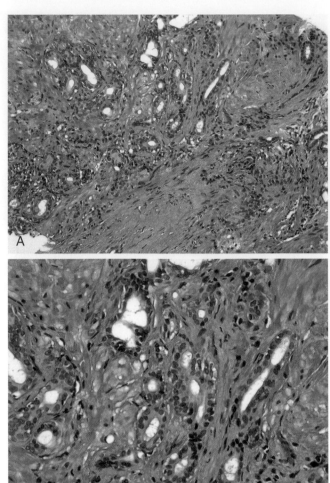

Fig 4. A, Postatrophic hyperplasia with lobular appearance and basophilic collagen. **B,** Glands with atrophic cytoplasm lined by bland nuclei.

Fig 3. A, Postatrophic hyperplasia (PAH) with basophilic glands with well-formed lumina seen at low magnification. **B,** Lobular appearance of some foci of PAH. Note basophilic collagen around some of the glands, which is characteristic and not associated with prostate cancer. **C,** PAH glands have scant cytoplasm laterally and apically, accounting for their basophilic appearance at low magnification. At higher power, some small to medium-sized nucleoli may be visible.

Definition
- Benign glands with pale and diminished cytoplasm, differing from simple atrophy and PAH in that the glands do not appear basophilic at low magnification; can mimic prostate cancer (Gleason scores 4 to 6)

Clinical features
Epidemiology
- Affects adult men of all age groups

Presentation
- Clinically asymptomatic or present with lower urinary tract symptoms of bladder outlet obstruction

Prognosis and treatment
- Benign lesion that does not require specific treatment

Pathology
Histology
- Benign glands have scant and pale cytoplasm, differing from PAH in which the glands do not appear dark at low magnification, owing to more abundant pale cytoplasm lateral to the nuclei.
- Glands are crowded with many having slightly undulating tufted luminal border in contrast to the straight luminal border seen in many prostate cancers.
- Irregular crinkled nuclei of luminal/secretory cells are present.
- Small nucleoli are occasionally discernible.
- Basal cells can be scant to absent.

Immunopathology (including immunohistochemistry)
- Basal cells can be patchily highlighted with p63 and 34βE12.
- Some glands may be entirely negative for basal cell markers.
- α-Methyl–coenzyme A racemase can decorate the cytoplasm of glandular lining cells of partial atrophy, albeit at weak to moderate intensity.

Molecular diagnostics
- No specific information available

Main differential diagnosis
- Atypical adenomatous hyperplasia/adenosis: adenosis has a more lobular appearance with more crowded glands. Individual cells of adenosis have more abundant cytoplasm. Partial atrophy and adenosis have identical immunohistochemical staining patterns.
- Acinar adenocarcinoma (Gleason scores 4 to 6) usually has more abundant apical cytoplasm and straighter luminal borders. Although small nucleoli can be seen in partial atrophy, they are not as large as can be seen in some adenocarcinomas. Partial atrophy is not infiltrative in between benign glands. A patchy basal cell layer rules out adenocarcinoma. However, because a limited focus of partial atrophy may have an absence of a basal cells, the presence of negative basal cells in a small focus of glands with scant luminal cytoplasm is not diagnostic of cancer.

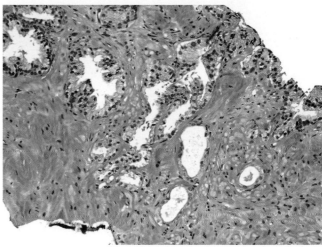

Fig 1. Partial atrophy at low magnification features pale glands that can appear slightly more crowded but maintain a lobular architecture.

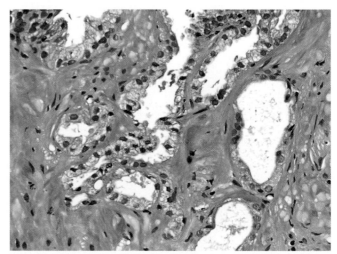

Fig 2. Medium magnification shows lining epithelial cells to contain nuclei that are dark to vesicular with slightly irregular crinkled outlines, reaching the luminal surface of the cytoplasm in some cells. The cytoplasm is pale and delicate with more abundant cytoplasm lateral to the nuclei. Note that several of the glands have slight ruffling to the luminal border.

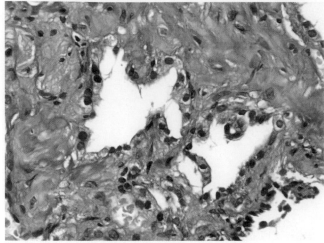

Fig 3. High magnification shows variably shrunken pale cytoplasm and nuclei that sometimes reach the cell surface.

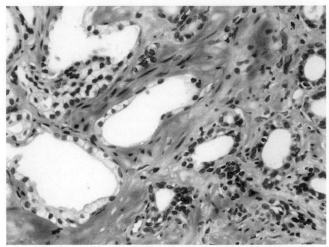

Fig 4. Glands with partial atrophy *(left)* merging with those of postatrophic hyperplasia (PAH; *right*). Note the lack of both apical and lateral cytoplasm in PAH as opposed to partial atrophy, where there is abundant cytoplasm lateral to the nuclei.

Definition
- Adenosis of the prostate is a pseudoneoplastic lesion usually in the transition zone that can mimic prostate adenocarcinoma and consists of a proliferation of crowded glands, arranged in a nodule but without significant cytologic atypia. A synonym is *atypical adenomatous hyperplasia.*

Clinical features
Presentation
- It is usually seen in transurethral resections of prostate or radical prostatectomy specimens, but it can also been seen in a needle biopsy specimen.
- Patients are usually asymptomatic.
- It is an incidental histologic finding.
- Some patients may have raised serum prostate-specific antigen levels as an unrelated finding.

Prognosis and treatment
- No treatment is needed.
- Following a diagnosis of adenosis (benign mimicker of cancer), a repeated biopsy is not indicated, unless clinically indicated.

Pathology
Histology
- Lobular lesions are composed of crowded glands.
- Lesions are partially circumscribed with a pushing rather than infiltrating border, although the small acini may show a limited degree of infiltrative features at the margins.
- Individual glands are closely packed but separate and show no evidence of fusion.
- Glands have variable sizes and shapes, although they are typically smaller than benign hyperplastic glands.
- Cuboidal to low columnar cells are present with moderate to abundant clear or lightly eosinophilic cytoplasm.
- The basal cells are usually recognized, at least focally in some of the glands.
- The luminal borders are often irregular, in contrast to the smooth luminal borders of prostatic adenocarcinoma.
- Lumens are usually empty with variable amount of corpora amylacea or eosinophilic crystalloids, or both.
- Nuclei are round to oval, slightly enlarged, and have uniform fine chromatin and inconspicuous or small nucleoli.

Immunohistochemistry
- Patchy basal cells are present and can be demonstrated by incomplete immunostaining for high-molecular-weight cytokeratin (CK903/34βE12) or p63.
- Racemase (p504s) is focally expressed in 10% of cases and diffusely positive in approximately 7.5% of cases of adenosis.

Molecular diagnostics
- Abnormalities of chromosome 8 in a very small proportion (4% to 7%) of adenosis cases

Main differential diagnosis
- Adenosis can be difficult to distinguish from low-grade prostatic adenocarcinoma (Gleason pattern 1 or 2), because both are located in the transition zone and show small acinar proliferation and intraluminal crystalloids.
- Histologic features of adenosis of the prostate in needle biopsy specimens have significant overlap with prostatic adenocarcinoma.
  - Major differentiating features are: (1) absent huge nucleoli; (2) small glands sharing cytoplasmic and nuclear features with admixed larger benign glands; (3) pale, clear cytoplasm; (4) rare blue-tinged mucinous secretions; (5) common corpora amylacea; (6) occasional glands with basal cells; and (7) lobular growth.
  - Features that overlap with carcinoma are: (1) crowded (back-to-back glands); (2) intraluminal crystalloids; (3) medium-sized nucleoli; (4) scattered poorly formed glands and single cells; and (5) minimal infiltration at periphery of nodule.

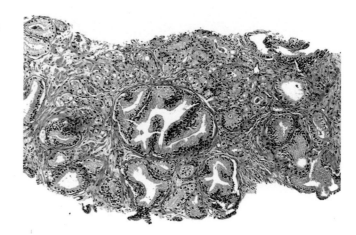

Fig 1. Crowded, variably sized glands with infiltrative appearance of glands at the edges from a case of adenosis diagnosed on needle biopsy. More benign-appearing glands with papillary infoldings and branching are admixed with glands of adenosis. Some glands have dense amphophilic cytoplasm and luminal eosinophilic crystalloids.

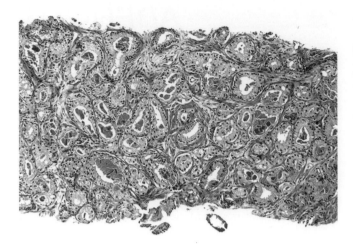

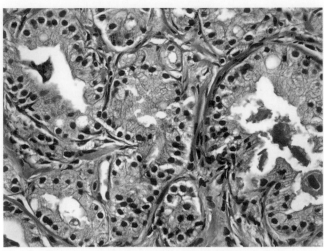

Fig 2. Variably sized glands lined by epithelial secretory cells with clear to eosinophilic cytoplasm and minimal cytologic atypia. Many of the glands have luminal eosinophilic crystalloids and dense secretions.

Fig 4. Higher magnification of Fig 3 showing predominantly large glands lined by epithelial secretory cells with clear eosinophilic cytoplasm, minimal cytologic atypia with inconspicuous nucleoli, few focally prominent basally located cells with dense amphophilic cytoplasm, and luminal eosinophilic crystalloids.

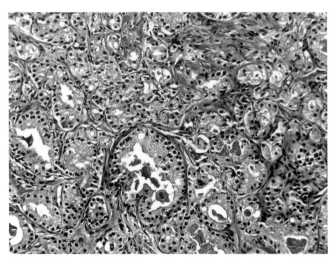

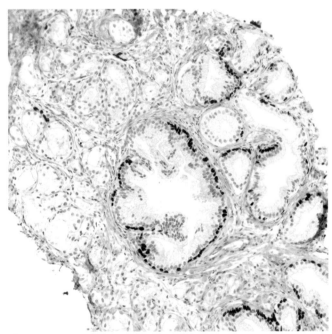

Fig 3. Higher magnification showing glands of adenosis with minimal cytologic atypia. Some glands show recognizable basal cells and have small pinpoint nucleoli within the nuclei.

Fig 5. Immunohistochemical findings of adenosis of the prostate with patchy reactivity for p63 in both small and large glands.

Definition
- Benign lesion of the prostate characterized by a biphasic population of small-sized glands and a cellular spindled cell stroma showing myoepithelial differentiation

Clinical features
Epidemiology
- The incidence has been estimated in approximately 2% of any prostatic specimens, but is much less common in needle biopsy specimens than transurethral resections.
- Usually only one or two microscopic foci are found in any given case, although rare cases may be extensive.

Presentation
- These lesions are incidental findings in prostate specimens (TUR, biopsies, prostatectomies).
- There is no association with increased PSA levels.
- Sclerosing adenosis may occasionally be found adjacent to prostatic adenocarcinoma.

Prognosis and therapy
- No treatment is required for this benign incidental condition.

Pathology
Histology
- Sclerosing adenosis consists of a proliferation of glands and stroma forming ill-defined microscopic nodules.
- The glandular element, which is virtually always present, demonstrates crowding and an infiltrative pattern and can show nuclear enlargement with prominent nucleoli.
- In some areas the glandular pattern resembles usual adenosis.
- In some cases, a hyaline rim of connective tissue surrounds some of the glands, which is distinctive.
- The stromal component is variably cellular, but lacks pleomorphism or mitotic figures.
- There seems to be a continuum between the glandular and stromal component.

Immunopathology
- The glandular component in sclerosing adenosis is positive for prostate-specific markers, such as PSA, PAP, and PSMA.
- The glands are benign and thus also contain basal cells, which are positive for antibodies, such as p63, CK5/6, or high-molecular-weight cytokeratin cocktails.
- The stromal component is positive for muscle-specific actin, weakly with S-100, and can also express high-molecular-weight cytokeratin.
- Overexpression of AMACR in the glandular component has not been reported.

Main differential diagnosis
- Prostatic adenocarcinoma, usual type—sclerosing adenosis is a common mimicker of adenocarcinoma because of the population of small crowded glands with occasional nuclear atypia and somewhat infiltrative borders. Sclerosing adenosis does not, however, widely infiltrate between benign prostatic glands, although it may do so focally, in contrast to usual adenosis. The cellular stromal component is virtually absent in prostatic adenocarcinoma, where only mild stromal response is seen. The hyaline collar around glands in sclerosing adenosis is absent in prostatic adenocarcinoma. In most cases, needle biopsy specimens containing foci of sclerosing adenosis should be analyzed with immunohistochemical studies to exclude malignancy.
- Sarcomatoid prostatic adenocarcinoma—given the biphasic population in sclerosing adenosis, one might consider the diagnosis of sarcomatoid carcinoma. In sclerosing adenosis, the lesions are usually small as opposed to sarcomatoid carcinoma. The stromal component is bland, in contrast to the overt malignant morphology in the spindle cell component of sarcomatoid carcinomas. The glandular component also does not show as much atypia as is usually seen in high-grade carcinomas with sarcomatoid differentiation.

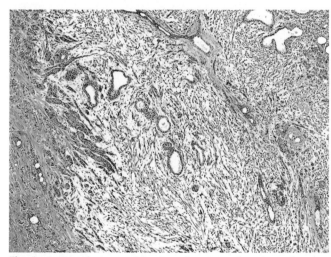

Fig 1. Low-power magnification showing sclerosing adenosis. The lesion lacks the lobular appearance of usual adenosis. A biphasic appearance with glandular and myxoid areas is visible.

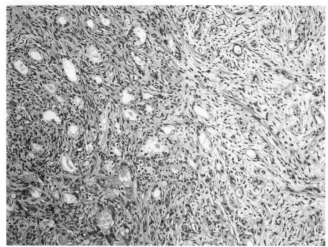

Fig 2. Higher magnification shows well-formed glands *(left)* merging with cellular myxoid areas *(right)*.

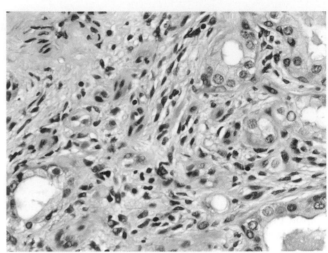

Fig 5. High magnification of cellular stromal areas. Cellularity is much greater than seen in a prostate with adenosis or carcinoma.

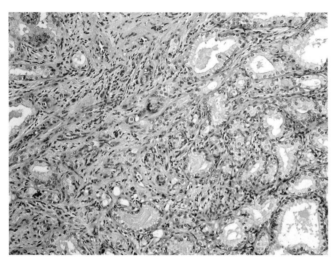

Fig 3. Areas resemble usual adenosis consisting of crowded pale glands *(right)* blending in with more cellular spindle cell areas.

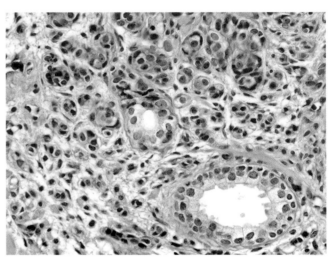

Fig 6. Transition from benign-appearing glands *(lower right)* to poorly formed glands and single epithelioid cells with prominent nucleoli *(top)* to spindle cells *(lower left)*.

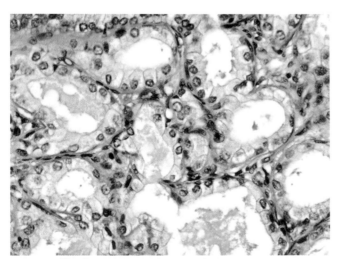

Fig 4. High magnification of adenosis areas.

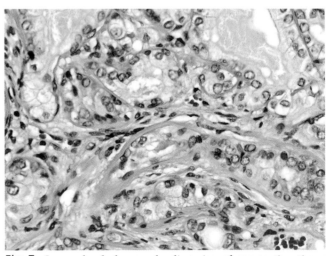

Fig 7. Some glands have a hyaline rim of connective tissue around the glands.

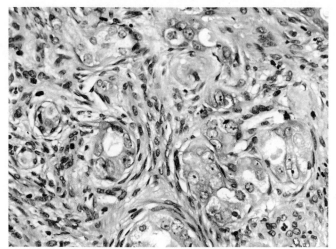

Fig 8. Some glands have prominent nucleoli. Note the cellular stroma.

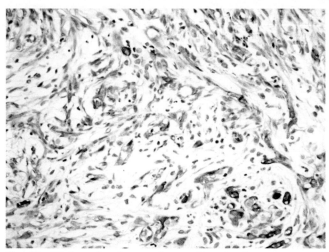

Fig 10. High-molecular-weight cytokeratin shows positivity around individual epithelioid and spindle cells.

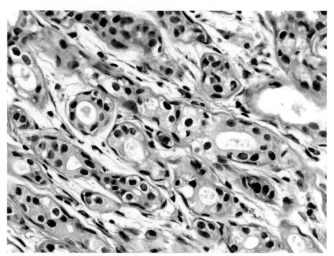

Fig 9. Glands with prominent nucleoli mimic prostate cancer. Many of the glands have a hyaline rim of connective tissue around them, a feature typical of sclerosing adenosis and not seen in prostate cancer.

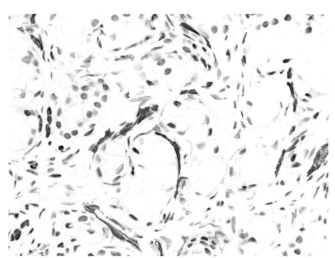

Fig 11. Muscle-specific actin labels some of the basal cells, in contrast to usual adenosis in which basal cells do not show myoepithelial differentiation.

CLEAR CELL CRIBRIFORM HYPERPLASIA

Definition
- A form of benign prostatic hyperplasia characterized by proliferation of benign glands with cribriform architecture in the transition zone of the prostate

Clinical features
Epidemiology
- Mean age, 64 to 72 years

Presentation
- Involves the transition zone
- Mostly seen in TURP specimens removed for urinary obstructive symptoms in patients with benign prostatic hyperplasia

Prognosis and treatment
- Benign entity
- No treatment needed

Pathology
Histology
- Usually nodular pattern of growth, but rarely can look infiltrative
- Crowded cribriform glands with uniform and round lumina
- Cuboidal to low columnar cells with pale-clear cytoplasm, small bland nuclei, and inconspicuous nucleoli
- Prominent basal cell layer around many glands consisting of a row of cuboidal dark cells beneath the clear cells; small knots of basal cells seen less frequently; rarely, basal cells not readily visible on routine sections

Immunohistochemistry
- Basal cell markers, such as p63 and high-molecular-weight cytokeratin, highlight the presence of basal cells around the glands (often incomplete staining).

Main differential diagnosis
- Cribriform HGPIN has the following differentiating features:
  - Cytologic atypia with prominent nucleoli
  - Usually amphophilic cytoplasm
  - Inconspicuous basal cell layer on sections stained with hematoxylin and eosin
  - Immunohistochemistry not useful because both lesions have patchy basal cell layer
- Cribriform adenocarcinoma (Gleason score, 4 + 4 = 8) has the following differentiating features:
  - Cytologic atypia with prominent nucleoli
  - Usually amphophilic cytoplasm
  - Lack of basal cells
  - Usually accompanied by small infiltrative malignant glands

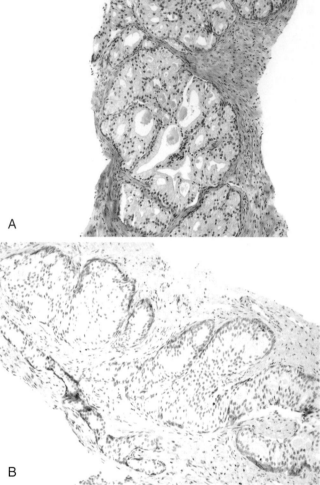

A

B

Fig 1. **A,** An example of clear cell cribriform hyperplasia in a prostate needle core biopsy specimen. The differential diagnosis includes high-grade prostatic intraepithelial neoplasia and prostatic acinar adenocarcinoma with cribriform architecture (Gleason score 4 + 4 = 8). **B,** Basal cell markers (high-molecular-weight cytokeratin in this example) highlight the presence of basal cells around the glands.

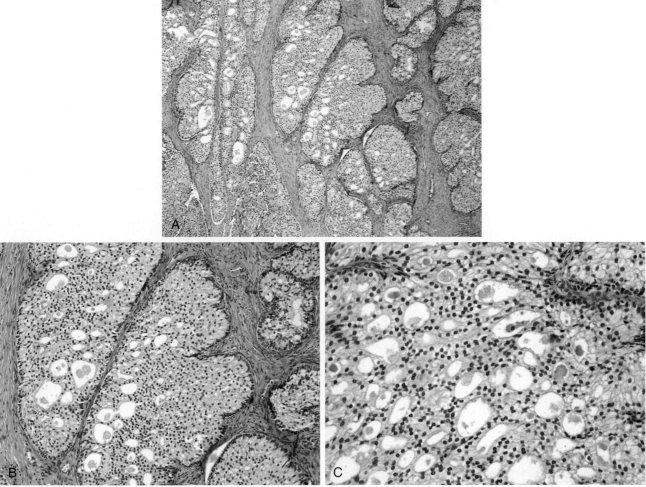

Fig 2. A, Low-power view of clear cell cribriform hyperplasia showing nodular growth of crowded cribriform glands with clear cytoplasm. **B,** A prominent basal cell layer around many glands is commonly seen. **C,** The glands are composed of cribriform structures lined by cuboidal cells with pale to clear cytoplasm, small bland nuclei, and inconspicuous nucleoli.

Definition
- Rare benign lesion characterized by tubular or acinar proliferation of mesonephric remnants

Clinical features
Epidemiology
- Very rare
- Mean age, 67 years

Presentation
- Incidental finding seen either on TURP or radical prostatectomy specimens

Prognosis and treatment
- Benign entity
- No treatment needed

Pathology
Histology
- Located within the prostatic parenchyma, especially around the prostatic base, or in the bladder neck or periprostatic tissue
- Usually lobular pattern of growth, but can look infiltrative
- Crowded small tubules with one of the following histologic patterns:
  - Atrophic tubules containing colloid-like secretions
  - Atrophic tubules with empty lumina and occasional micropapillary projections
- Tubules lined with a single layer of cuboidal bland cells with small monotonous nuclei and inconspicuous nucleoli (rarely prominent)
- Tubules lacking basal cells
- Tubules seen intimately associated with nerves and ganglia

Immunohistochemistry
- Positive staining for p63 and high-molecular-weight cytokeratin
- Negative staining for PSA, PSAP, and AMACR

Main differential diagnosis
- Prostatic adenocarcinoma (Gleason score 3 + 3 = 6) has the following differentiating features:
  - Cytologic atypia with prominent nucleoli
  - Presence of luminal loose granular secretion rather than colloidlike material
  - Positive staining for PSA, PSAP, and AMACR and negative staining for p63 and high-molecular-weight cytokeratin
    - Note that a small subset of prostatic adenocarcinoma shows aberrant staining for p63, but not high-molecular-weight cytokeratin.
- Nephrogenic adenoma has the following differentiating features:
  - Mainly periurethral location
  - Peritubular hyaline rim
  - Hobnail cells with focal degenerative atypia
  - Positive staining for PAX2 and PAX8

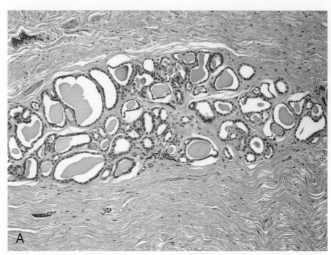

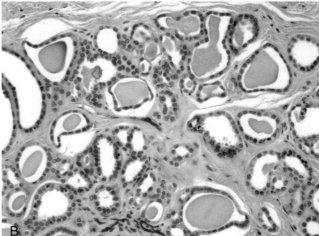

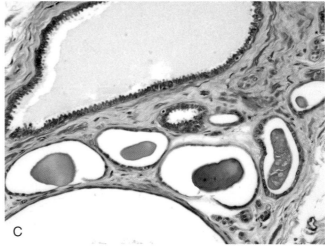

Fig 1. **A,** Mesonephric remnant hyperplasia generally shows a vaguely lobular pattern of growth in some areas. **B,** Mesonephric remnant hyperplasia composed of atrophic tubules containing colloidlike secretions. **C,** Tubules are lined by a single layer of cuboidal bland cells with small, monotonous nuclei and inconspicuous nucleoli. Basal cells are absent.

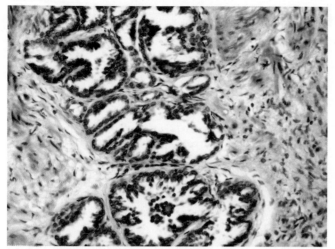

Fig 2. Occasionally the tubules contain micropapillary projections.

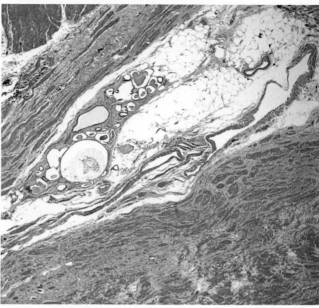

Fig 4. Mesonephric remnant hyperplasia can have an infiltrative appearance. The tubules are atrophic and have no associated stromal reaction.

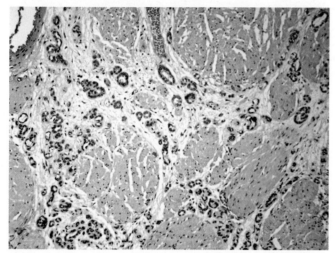

Fig 3. Mesonephric remnant hyperplasia located at the base of the prostate adjacent to the bladder in perivesicle adipose tissue.

Definition
- Proliferation of basal cells ranging from focal incomplete involvement of prostatic glands to florid growth completely lacking luminal cells

Clinical features
Epidemiology
- Uncommon histologic pattern of benign hyperplasia
- Most common in transition zone; can also be found in the peripheral zone
- In association with squamous metaplasia and atrophy, occurring after hormonal treatment

Pathology
Histology
- It usually develops as proliferation of small glands, occasionally as solid nests or forming pseudocribriform or true cribriform (adenoid basal form) structures.
- The incomplete form has residual luminal secretory cells surrounded by multilayered basal cells; the complete form has only basal cells.
- Basal cells are recognized by their basophilic nuclei with scant cytoplasm. Nuclei often stream parallel to basement membrane and show inconspicuous to prominent nucleoli.
- Rare mitotic figures can be seen.
- Well-formed lamellar calcifications are present.
- Unique intracytoplasmic eosinophilic globules are present.
- Desmoplastic stroma reaction is absent; however, it can appear infiltrating when intermixed with benign prostatic glands.
- Squamous metaplasia is not uncommonly seen in basal cell hyperplasia.
- The term *atypical basal cell hyperplasia* used in cases with nucleoli more prominent than typical cases is no longer used as the atypia is not associated with adverse outcome.

Immunopathology (including immunohistochemistry)
- Strong positivity with high-molecular-weight cytokeratin and p63, often more in peripherally located cells; negative for AMACR
- PSA and PSAP showing weak and focal reactivity

Main differential diagnosis
- Prostate adenocarcinoma
  - Prostate cancer cells are usually not as basophilic because they contain more cytoplasm. Prostate cancer also uncommonly consists of multilayered small glands and does not manifest as solid nests.
  - Calcification in cancer is often more granular and is associated with necrosis.
  - Cancer is negative for high-molecular-weight cytokeratin and p63.
- HGPIN
  - HGPIN consists architecturally of large glands without crowding.

- In HGPIN, the atypical nuclei are in columnar cells that reach the luminal border with an underlying inconspicuous basal cell layer. In basal cell hyperplasia, the multilayered cells have rounder nuclei. If basal cell hyperplasia with prominent nucleoli is present, there are often overlying secretory cells with benign-appearing nuclei.
- In HGPIN, the atypical cells are negative for high-molecular-weight cytokeratin and p63, whereas underlying flattened basal cells are positive.

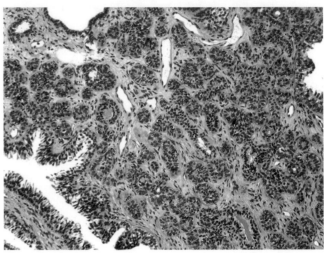

Fig 1. Basal cell hyperplasia appears as a proliferation of uniform, basophilic small glands in normal-appearing stroma between benign prostatic glands.

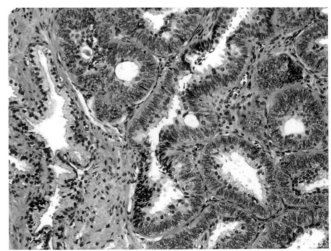

Fig 2. Incomplete form is characterized by residual luminal secretory cells undermined by multiple layers of basal cells with basophilic nuclei and scant cytoplasm.

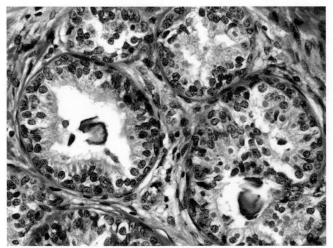

Fig 3. Well-formed lamellar calcifications are seen in up to half of the cases. Note the scattered intracytoplasmic eosinophilic globules, a unique feature of basal cell hyperplasia.

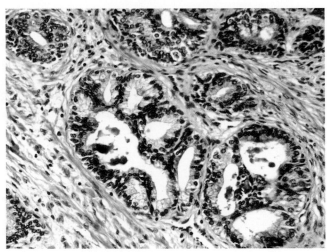

Fig 6. Basal cell hyperplasia with pseudocribriform formation mimicking prostatic intraepithelial neoplasia, but glands are more back-to-back than true cribriform. The presence of lamellar calcification is another clue.

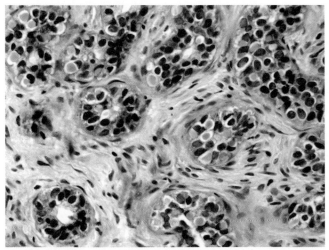

Fig 4. Another example of intracytoplasmic eosinophilic globules involving small nests of basal cells.

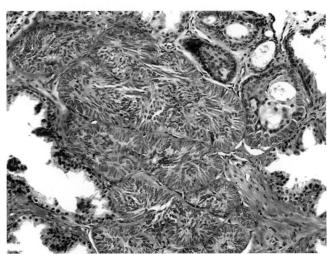

Fig 7. Squamous metaplasia *(right)* occurs in association with basal cell hyperplasia. The longitudinal nuclei of basal cells appear streaming parallel to the basement membrane.

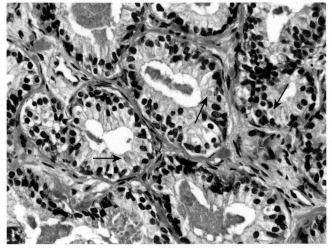

Fig 5. Crowded small glands of basal cell hyperplasia mimic prostate adenocarcinoma. However, the multiple layering of atypical basophilic cells is unusual for cancer. Note the presence of a few scattered intracytoplasmic eosinophilic globules *(arrows)*.

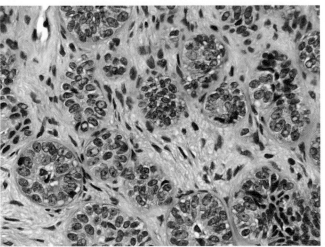

Fig 8. Basal cell hyperplasia with prominent nucleoli is identical to other ordinary types.

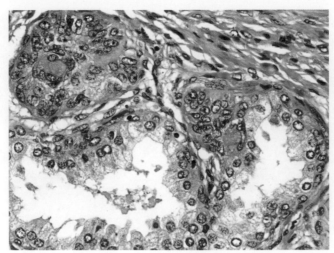

Fig 9. Basal cells display prominent nucleoli and focal blue mucin. Adjacent areas show more typical basal cell hyperplasia.

Definition
- Replacement of benign cuboidal epithelium of peripheral prostatic ducts and acini with benign urothelium

Pathology
Histology
- Epithelium of ducts and acini are replaced or undermined by pseudostratified, spindle-shaped cells with occasional longitudinal nuclear grooves.
- It can be seen throughout the prostate in infants, neonates, and adults.

Main differential diagnosis
- Urothelial carcinoma involving the prostate—occasionally, urothelial metaplasia can be extensive and mimic urothelial carcinoma based on the architecture; however, in contrast to urothelial carcinoma, urothelial metaplasia lacks cytologic atypia and necrosis.

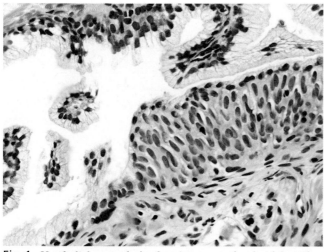

Fig 1. Urothelial metaplasia showing normal cuboidal epithelium undermined by metaplastic urothelial cells.

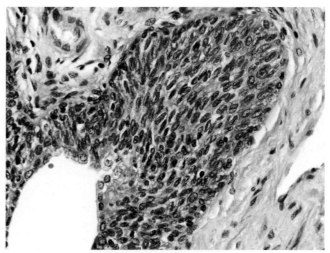

Fig 2. Urothelial metaplasia.

Definition
• Replacement of normal cuboidal epithelium of prostatic ducts and acini with benign squamous epithelium

Pathology
Histology
• Glands lined with squamous epithelium, with or without keratinization
• Typically seen either in an infarct (may be complicated with reactive atypia; see Chapter 25, "Prostratic Infarct," in this section) or following hormonal treatment

Main differential diagnosis
• Primary squamous cell carcinoma of prostate—in contrast to squamous cell carcinoma, squamous metaplasia following hormonal therapy lacks cytologic atypia. Furthermore, the squamous metaplasia following hormonal therapy is diffuse throughout the prostate and often also has features of basal cell hyperplasia. The only situation in which there may be diffuse squamous metaplasia with atypia is in the setting of prior combined radiation and hormonal therapy.

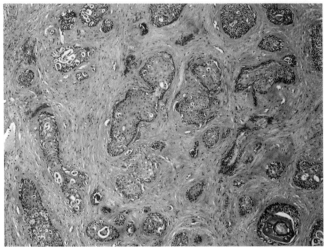

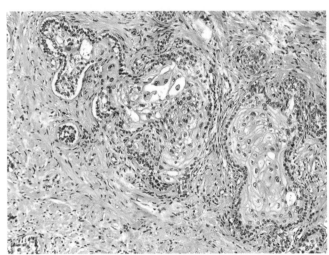

Fig 2. Squamous metaplasia following hormonal treatment, with unremarkable stroma.

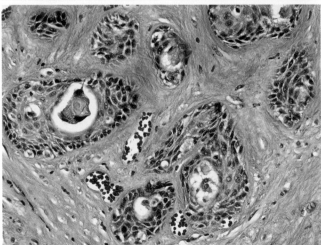

Fig 1. Squamous metaplasia in an infarct showing evenly distributed squamous islands in densely fibrotic stroma with extravasated red blood cells.

Definition
- Replacement of normal cuboidal epithelium of prostatic ducts and acini with goblet cells

Pathology
Histology
- Glands are lined by goblet cells that have mucin-filled cytoplasm and small, dark, basally located nuclei.
- Metaplasia may involve individual cells, an entire acini, or a cluster of acini.
- It may involve normal glands or hyperplastic glands, rarely seen in high-grade PIN, not associated with prostate cancer.

Immunopathology (including immunohistochemistry)
- Positive for PAS, PAS-D, mucicarmine, and Alcian blue
- Negative for PSA and PSAP
- Basal cells positive for high-molecular-weight cytokeratin and p63

Main differential diagnosis
- Cowper glands are extraprostatic and located in skeletal muscle. In addition, Cowper glands have dimorphic glands with ducts and mucinous glands.
- In foamy gland adenocarcinoma of prostate, foamy gland carcinoma cells are columnar, lack distinct cell borders, and have a fine microvesicular (xanthomatous) appearance, whereas the cells in mucin cell metaplasia are globoid goblet cells with distinct cell borders. Foamy gland adenocarcinoma lacks mucin, typically has abundant dense intraluminal eosinophilic secretions, and lacks a basal cell layer.

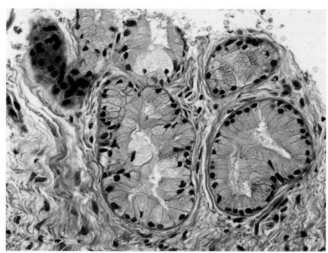

Fig 1. Mucin cell metaplasia is easily recognized when normal cuboidal epithelium is replaced by scattered goblet cells.

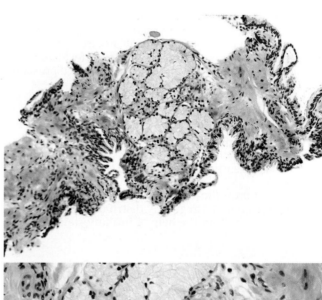

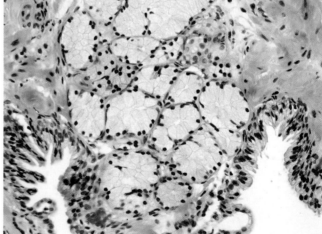

Fig 2. Mucin cell metaplasia, showing a cluster of acini completely replaced by mucin-secreting cells. They are not Cowper glands because the mucinous glands are located in between normal prostatic glands.

NEUROENDOCRINE CELLS INVOLVING THE PROSTATE

Definition
- Neuroendocrine cells of the prostate are intraepithelial regulatory cells that regulate both growth and differentiation, as well as the exocrine secretory activity of the prostate (part of the amine precursor uptake and decarboxylation [APUD] system of endocrine-paracrine cells).
- These cells are rich in serotonin-containing granules and can secrete a variety of peptide hormones.

Clinical features
Prognosis and treatment
- Neuroendocrine differentiation can occur in prostatic carcinoma and may have prognostic significance, mostly in androgen independent cancer.
- However, the prognostic significance of focal neuroendocrine differentiation in primary untreated prostatic carcinoma is controversial.

Pathology
Histology
- Neuroendocrine cells can occasionally be observed under light microscopy when they show fine intracytoplasmic eosinophilic granules (Paneth cell–like change).
- In normal prostatic parenchyma, neuroendocrine cells are scattered, irregularly distributed, and easily overlooked without the help of immunostains.
- Neuroendocrine cells are usually more common near the verumontanum but are seen in all zones.
- Neuroendocrine cells rest on the basal cell layer between secretory cells.
- Neuroendocrine differentiation can occur in HGPIN and in prostatic carcinoma.
- Three forms are described:
  - Focal neuroendocrine differentiation in conventional prostatic adenocarcinoma
  - Carcinoid tumor (well-differentiated neuroendocrine tumor)
  - Small-cell neuroendocrine carcinoma

Immunopathology
- Immunostaining with neuroendocrine markers helps to identify neuroendocrine cells in normal prostatic tissue and neuroendocrine differentiation in tumors.
- Antibodies against synaptophysin, chromogranin A, CD56, neuron-specific enolase, bombesin-gastrin–releasing peptide, and serotonin are the most frequently used.
- Androgen receptor, PSA, and PAP are not found in neuroendocrine cells.
- Five percent to 10% of prostatic carcinomas have focal zones with a large number of single or clustered neuroendocrine cells detected by chromogranin A.

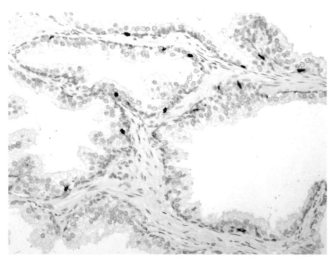

Fig 1. Chromogranin A immunostain in normal prostatic parenchyma of the peripheral zone showing isolated positive cells along the basal layer.

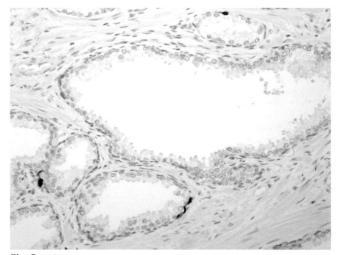

Fig 2. Chromogranin A immunostain showing a different region of the peripheral zone with less common positive cells.

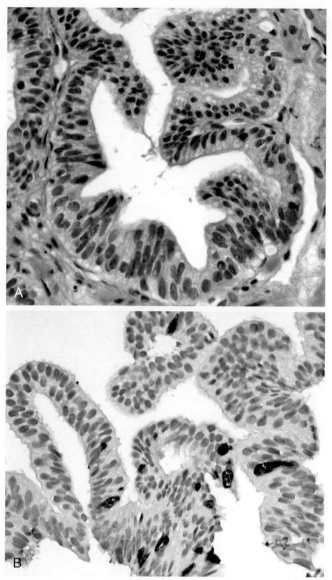

Fig 3. **A,** Neuroendocrine cells with Paneth cell–like change observed in a focus of high-grade prostatic intraepithelial neoplasia. **B,** Chromogranin A immunostain confirming the neuroendocrine nature of these cells.

Definition
- Benign, small, acinar proliferation of prostatic glands that occurs exclusively in the verumontanum and adjacent prostatic urethra; a potential mimic of prostate adenocarcinoma

Clinical features
Epidemiology
- Incidental finding in 14% of radical prostatectomy specimens in men aged 47 to 87 years

Presentation
- Mostly incidental lesion in the verumontanum, utricle, or adjacent prostatic urethra
- Often multifocal

Prognosis and treatment
- Not a risk factor for malignancy
- No treatment necessary

Pathology
Histology
- Lobular proliferation of uniform, tightly packed, round, small acini with preserved basal cell layer
- Benign cytology with small or mildly enlarged uniform nuclei
- Inconspicuous nucleoli
- Basophilic or clear cytoplasm
- Frequent intraluminal corpora amylacea and distinct red-brown-orange concretions
- Lipofuscin pigment in the cytoplasm of luminal cells
- Adjacent and continuous with urothelium

Immunohistochemistry
- PSA expression by luminal secretory cells
- Immunoreactivity for 34βE12 and p63 by basal cells, negative S100

Molecular diagnostics
- Not contributory

Main differential diagnosis
- Low-grade prostatic adenocarcinoma: verumontanum mucosal gland hyperplasia mimics prostate cancer in that the glands are crowded. However, as with adenosis, the glands (1) have a lobular configuration, (2) lack cytologic atypia, (3) have distinctively colored corpora amylacea, and (4) have a readily recognizable basal cell layer in at least some of the glands.

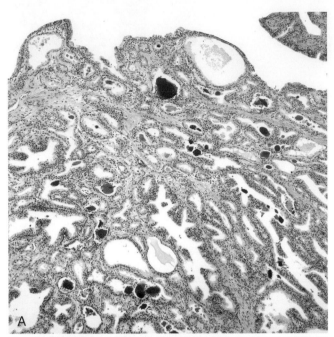
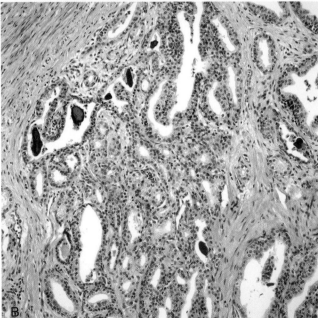

Fig 1. **A,** Verumontanum mucosal gland hyperplasia. Small and tightly packed acini may mimic well-differentiated prostatic adenocarcinoma. Corpora amylacea–like frequent intraluminal concretions are present and are often red-orange-brown. **B,** Acini exhibit lobular proliferation and no cytologic atypia.

Definition
- Area of ischemic stromal and glandular tissue damage typically associated with BPH

Clinical features
Epidemiology
- It is most frequently associated with BPH and typically seen in TURP, suprapubic prostatectomies, and enucleation specimens.
- Incidence ranges from 3% to 12% in totally sampled autopsy prostates and is as high as 25% in BPH specimens.
- It is encountered rarely in biopsy specimens (less than 0.1%).
- Association with cardiovascular risk factors (e.g., recent cardiovascular surgery, smoking) has been reported.

Presentation
- Urinary symptoms are frequent (e.g., acute urinary retention, hematuria).
- Elevated PSA is common (levels up to 287 ng/mL have been reported).

Prognosis and therapy
- Therapy is similar to that for BPH and acute urinary retention.

Pathology
Histology
- Most commonly seen in transition zone
- Typically a single focus in biopsy specimen, up to 1 cm in size; multiple foci may be seen in resection specimens
- Early-age infarcts: discrete foci of coagulative stromal and glandular necrosis with typical histologic zonation and recent hemorrhage
- Intermediate-age infarcts: reactive stroma and epithelium without necrosis
- Remote infarcts: replacement of stroma with dense fibrosis and squamous metaplasia in glands, cyst formation
- Frequently associated with immature squamous–urothelial metaplasia in surrounding glands, which may show overt cytologic atypia with mitoses

Immunopathology
- Metaplastic glands are positive for high-molecular-weight keratins.

Main differential diagnosis
- Urothelial carcinoma involving prostate: although immature squamous–urothelial metaplasia in a prostatic infarct may show overt cytologic atypia, recognition of surrounding areas of stromal necrosis and hemorrhage, combined with the histologic zonation typical of infarction (progressively less severe changes away from the center of the lesion), helps to distinguish this benign entity from urothelial carcinoma involving prostatic glands.
- Prostatic granulomas secondary to infection: infectious granulomas are often accompanied by grumous cellular debris and epithelioid histiocytes.
- Post-TURP granulomas: history is helpful. Post-TURP granulomas often show central fibrinoid necrosis with palisading epithelioid histiocytes.
- Prior cryotherapy: history is helpful. Cryotherapy may show similar stromal necrosis with glandular squamous metaplasia for up to 3 months after therapy, followed by stromal hyalinization and fibrosis. Areas of necrosis are more diffuse than in localized infarcts.

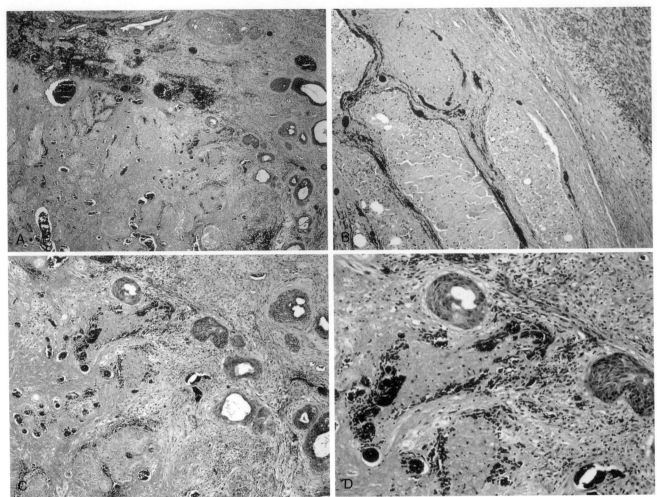

Fig 1. A, Recent infarct with zonation showing central necrosis surrounded by reactive urothelial metaplasia. **B,** Central area of coagulative necrosis. **C,** Interface between areas of necrosis and surrounding urothelial–squamous metaplasia. **D,** Urothelial–squamous metaplasia in surrounding glands may be mildly or severely atypical. Note the extravasated erythrocytes in surrounding stroma as a clue that this is reactive adjacent to an infarct; this is especially useful in needle biopsy when the central area of necrosis is not sampled.

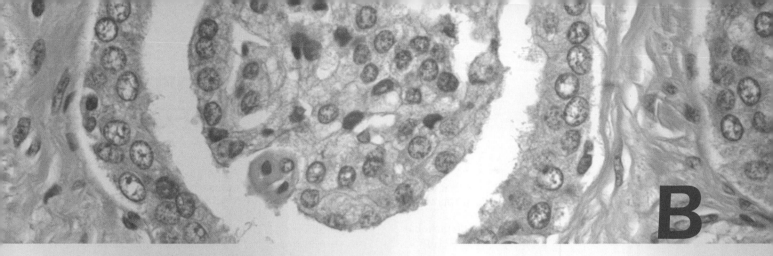

NEOPLASTIC DISEASE
OF THE PROSTATE

B

Definition
- Proliferation of secretory epithelial cells that displays significant architectural and cytologic atypia within the pre-existing acini and ducts
- Categorized into low-grade prostatic intraepithelial neoplasia (LGPIN) and high-grade (HGPIN) types

Clinical features
Epidemiology
- Increased prevalence of HGPIN with age
- Considerable variation in different ethnic background with higher prevalence and more extensive HGPIN in African Americans compared with whites
- HGPIN diagnosed in 4% to 6% in prostate needle biopsy, 2% to 3% in transurethral resection of the prostate (TURP) specimens, and 85% to 100% of radical prostatectomies

Presentation
- Does not result in abnormal findings on digital rectal examination or elevated serum prostate-specific antigen (PSA)
- Diagnosed only by histologic examination of prostate tissue

Prognosis and treatment
- HGPIN is a precursor to some prostate carcinomas.
- HGPIN in needle biopsy carries approximately a 25% risk of finding cancer in subsequent repeated biopsy compared with a 19% risk if initial biopsy specimen is benign. Consider repeated biopsy within 12 months only when the initial biopsy specimen is six-core sextant or if there is multifocal HPGIN.
- If unifocal HPGIN, repeated biopsy is recommended within 2 to 3 years.
- LGPIN should not be diagnosed because of the lack of diagnostic reproducibility and association with cancer detection in subsequent repeat biopsy.

Pathology
Histology
- Darker-appearing glands with benign architecture at low scanning magnification
- Nuclear enlargement, crowding, irregular spacing, and stratification with chromatin hyperchromasia, clumping, and variably prominent nucleoli
- LGPIN: no prominent nucleoli
- HGPIN: prominent nucleoli at 20× magnification
- Four major architectural patterns: tufting, micropapillary, flat, and cribriform
- Minor histologic variants: signet-ring, mucinous, inverted, and small-cell neuroendocrine

Immunohistochemistry
- Secretory cells positive for pan-cytokeratin and low-molecular-weight cytokeratin; positive but often reduced expression of PSA and prostate-specific acid phosphatase (PAP)
- HGPIN often has discontinuous basal cell layer marked with HMWCK (34βE12, CK5/6) and p63; LGPIN has complete basal cell layers

- Sixty percent to 80% HGPIN + α-methylacyl–coenzyme A (CoA) racemase (AMACR)
- Twenty percent of HGPIN are ERG positive.

Main differential diagnosis
- Normal structure (central zone glands, seminal vesicle–ejaculatory duct epithelium)
- Benign lesions (reactive atypia owing to inflammation, infarction or radiation, metaplasia [transitional cell, squamous cell])
- Hyperplasia (clear cell cribriform hyperplasia, basal cell hyperplasia)
- Prostate carcinoma with cribriform pattern
- Intraductal carcinoma of the prostate
- Ductal prostatic carcinoma

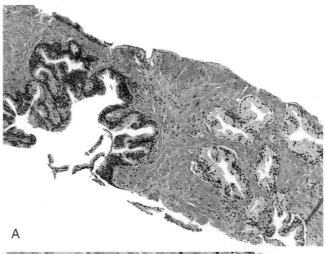

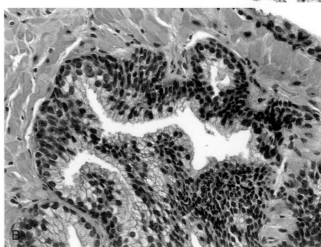

Fig 1. Low-grade prostatic intraepithelial neoplasia (PIN). **A,** At scanning magnification, the low-grade PIN gland is architecturally similar to, but appears darker than, the adjacent benign glands. **B,** At higher magnification (×20), the secretory cells have crowded, stratified, and enlarged nuclei. No prominent nucleoli are appreciated at this magnification.

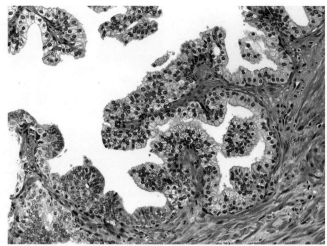

Fig 2. High-grade prostatic intraepithelial neoplasia partially involves a prostate gland.

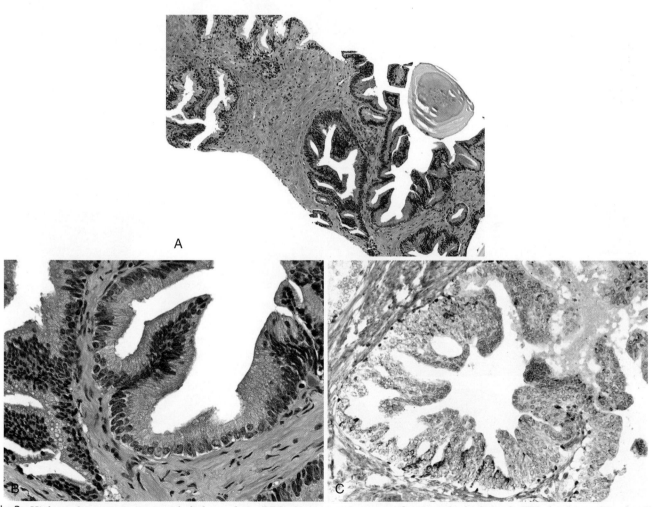

Fig 3. High-grade prostatic intraepithelial neoplasia (PIN). **A,** At scanning magnification, the high-grade PIN gland is architecturally similar to, but appears darker than, the adjacent benign glands. **B,** At higher magnification (×20), the secretory cells have crowded, stratified, and enlarged nuclei with coarse and clumpy chromatin. Large and conspicuous nucleoli are visible in the secretory cells at this magnification. **C,** High-grade PIN glands often have discontinuous basal cell layer, or even absent basal cell layer (p63), and a majority are positive for α-methylacyl–coenzyme A racemase.

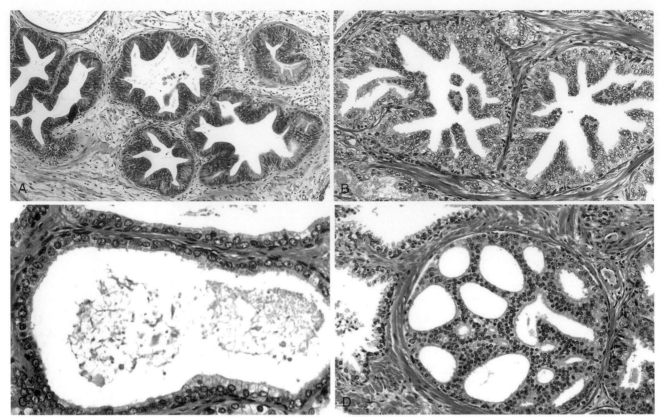

Fig 4. Four major architectural patterns of high-grade prostatic intraepithelial neoplasia, including tufting **(A)**, micropapillary **(B)**, flat **(C)**, and cribriform **(D)**. These patterns often coexist. Different architectural patterns have no significant clinical difference.

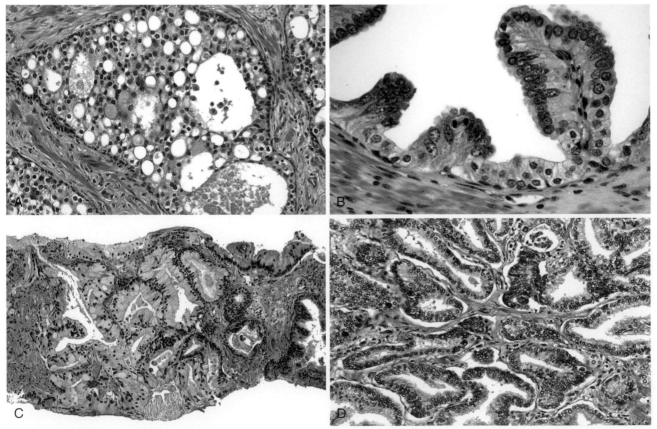

Fig 5. Unusual histologic patterns of high-grade prostatic intraepithelial neoplasia (PIN), including signet-ring PIN with mucin vacuoles inside cells **(A)**, inverted PIN with nuclei polarized towards the luminal surface of the gland **(B)**, foamy gland PIN with abundant foamy cytoplasm **(C)**, and PIN with pineth cell–like neuroendocrine differentiation. **(D).**

INTRADUCTAL CARCINOMA OF THE PROSTATE

Definition
- Typically characterized by the spread of prostatic adenocarcinoma into benign prostatic ducts or acini; intraductal solely in rare cases

Clinical features
Epidemiology
- Common in radical prostatectomy, especially those with a large tumor volume, more than 30% of the cases with a tumor volume of 4 to 10 cm³
- Rare in prostate biopsies; less than 0.1%

Presentation
- Most patients are symptomatic with elevated serum PSA.
- Some may have abnormality on digital rectal examination.

Prognosis and treatment
- Typically, it indicates poor clinical outcome and accelerated disease progression.
- It usually is associated with aggressive prostate cancer in radical prostatectomy: high Gleason score, large tumor volume, extraprostatic tumor expansion, and positive surgical margin.
- For localized disease, treat with radical prostatectomy, radiation therapy, and others.
- For metastatic disease, treat with hormonal and chemotherapy therapy.
- Rarely, cases can have only intraductal growth. This can only be diagnosed at radical prostatectomy with an entirely submitted specimen; the prognosis would be expected to be excellent.

Pathology
Histology
- Malignant epithelial cells fill and expand nonneoplastic prostatic ducts and acini.
- The contour and branching architecture of prostatic ducts are often recognizable.
- Basal cells may be often observed on hematoxylin and eosin (H&E) staining, although usually they are not.
- Four patterns have been described:
  - Solid pattern: sheets of tumor cells fill large acini and prostatic ducts.
  - Dense cribriform pattern: tumor cells form closely packed cribriform structures with small round lumens.
  - Loose cribriform pattern: tumor cells form cribriform structures with large irregular lumens, yet distinguished from prostatic intraepithelial neoplasia (PIN) by either marked pleomorphism or necrosis.
  - Micropapillary pattern: tumor cells form tufts or micropapillary structures, yet distinguished from PIN by either marked pleomorphism or necrosis.
- Often there is marked pleomorphism with large hyperchromatic nuclei and frequent mitotic activity.
- Sometimes comedonecrosis is present.

Immunopathology
- Nonneoplastic ducts or acini are positive for high-molecular-weight cytokeratin and p63.
- Prostatic adenocarcinoma cells inside the ducts are usually positive for racemase and negative for high-molecular-weight cytokeratin and p63.

Main differential diagnosis
- Prostatic ductal adenocarcinoma: cribriform glands with large, slitlike lamina, tall columnar tumor cells, papillary fronds with true fibrovascular cores, usually lacking basal cells
- Cribriform prostatic acinar adenocarcinoma: lack contour or branching of prostatic ducts, irregular infiltrating border, lack basal cells
- High-grade prostatic intraepithelial neoplasia: lacks solid or dense cribriform patterns, rarely have comedonecrosis, and lacks marked pleomorphism
- Intraductal spread of urothelial carcinoma: rarely form glandular or cribriform structures, negative for PSA and PAP, positive for p63 and high-molecular-weight cytokeratin in two thirds of cases

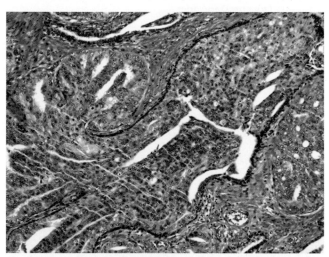

Fig 1. Prostatic adenocarcinoma spreads into and expands a prostatic duct. The intraductal carcinoma shows solid and densely packed cribriform patterns. The contour of duct and basal cells can be recognized.

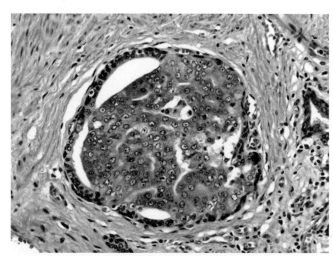

Fig 2. Prostatic adenocarcinoma spreads into and expands a large prostatic gland. The intraductal carcinoma is characterized by densely packed cribriform glands, and basal cells of the benign gland are visible.

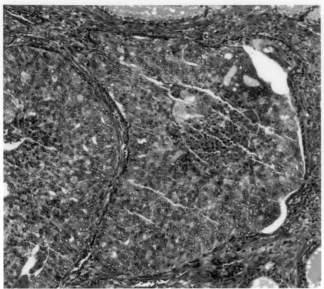

Fig 3. Intraductal carcinoma of the prostate shows comedone-crosis in a large prostatic duct.

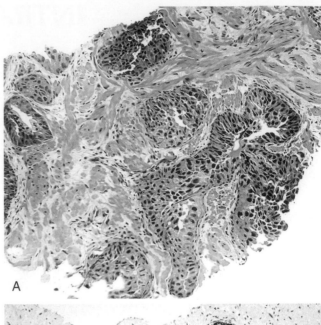

A

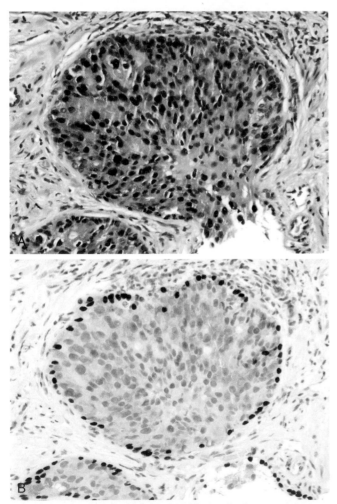

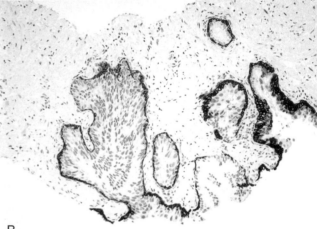

B

Fig 5. **A,** Intraductal carcinoma of the prostate shows marked nuclear atypia. **B,** The nonneoplastic ducts and glands show the presence of basal cells on immunostaining for high-molecular-weight cytokeratin.

Fig 4. **A,** Intraductal carcinoma of the prostate is characterized by a solid pattern. **B,** The nonneoplastic glands show the presence of basal cells on immunostaining for p63.

PROSTATIC CARCINOMA, USUAL VARIANT

Definition
- Acinar adenocarcinoma of the prostate gland is the most frequently diagnosed form of cancer in the United States. The National Cancer Institute estimates that almost 200,000 new cases will develop in 2010.

Clinical features
Epidemiology
- Prostate cancer is the third leading cause of cancer-related death in men in developing countries.
- Multiple genetic and environmental factors are involved in prostate carcinogenesis.
- Age, family history, and race are definitive risk factors.
- The degree of risk is related to the age and the number of the affected relatives, with the greatest risk conferred by a father or brother, with an onset before 40 years of age.
- Racial background, with American blacks having higher incidence, higher grade, and more extensive cancer, may be related to different genetic and environmental factors.
- Dietary fat and sex hormone levels are probable risk factors for prostate carcinoma.
- Many susceptibility loci and several candidate genes have been identified for hereditary prostate cancer.
- Linkage analysis has identified few candidate loci for hereditary prostate cancer. Of them, three genes have been cloned as RNaseL on 1q24-25, HPC2 on 17p, and MSR1 on 8p22-23.

Presentation
- Most prostate carcinoma is asymptomatic.
- Approximately 70% of prostate carcinoma arise in the peripheral zone, and some can result in abnormal findings on digital rectal examination.
- Rarely, prostate carcinoma can lead to urinary obstruction when a large tumor arises in the transition zone or extends into the transition zone from the peripheral zone or invades the bladder neck.
- Locally aggressive prostate carcinoma involves the bladder and rectum and can cause hematuria, rectal bleeding, or obstruction.
- Rarely, patients exhibit symptoms and signs that are related to metastatic prostate carcinoma to different anatomic sites, most commonly bone, regional lymph nodes, lung, and brain.
- Currently, most prostate carcinomas are clinically detected by serum PSA screening and digital rectal examination.

Prognosis and treatment
- Treatment for prostate cancer depends on the stage of the disease and the grade of the tumor; other important factors in planning treatment are the man's age and general health and his feelings about the treatments and their possible side effects.
- Prostate cancer can be managed in a number of ways:
  - Active surveillance (watchful waiting)
  - Surgery (radical prostatectomy)
  - Radiation therapy (external beam radiotherapy or implantation of radioactive seeds [brachytherapy])
  - Hormonal therapy (surgical castration [orchiectomy] or pharmacologic blockade of androgen effect with lutenizing hormone–releasing hormone analogs or antiandrogen compounds)
  - Cryotherapy
- Radical prostatectomy is considered to be the most reliable method of eradication of localized prostate cancer.
- Locally advanced prostate carcinoma is frequently managed by a combination of radiation and hormonal ablation.
- The prognosis for patients with prostate carcinoma is highly variable and depends on a variety of host, tumor, and treatment parameters:
  - For prostate cancer, limited to the prostate (stages I or II) and well or moderately differentiated (Gleason score 3 + 4 = 7 or less), the 5-year outcome is considered to be excellent.
  - Biochemical recurrence occurs in approximately 11% to 13% of patients with clinically localized prostate cancer treated with radical prostatectomy.
  - The overall PSA recurrence-free survival rates are 84% and 83% at 3 and 5 years, respectively.
  - The actuarial probability of remaining progression-free at 5 and 8 years postoperatively is 78% and 71%, respectively.
  - When stratified by pathologic stage, 5-year freedom from progression of disease after RP was 83% and 69% for pT2 and pT3, node-negative prostate cancer, respectively.

Pathology
Histology
- Three histologic features are diagnostic (cancer-specific) of prostate carcinoma, because they have not been described in benign glands:
  - Mucinous fibroplasia (collagenous micronodules) occurs as delicate fibrous tissue with ingrowth of fibroblasts within or adjacent to cancer glands.
  - Glomeruloid formation is created by intraluminal cribriform proliferation of malignant cells and often surrounded by a crescentic space, resembling a renal glomerulus.
  - Perineural invasion with cancer glands encircling the entire circumference of a nerve is pathognomonic of prostate carcinoma. (Benign glands can occasionally be found to abut a nerve; however, circumferential extension of benign glands entirely around a nerve has not been described.)
- Prostate carcinoma has a constellation of architectural, cytoplasmic, nuclear, and intraluminal features:
  - Architecture
    - Gland-forming prostate carcinomas are more crowded than benign glands and typically exhibit haphazard growth pattern and infiltrative growth pattern, with malignant glands situated between or flanking benign glands.

- In contrast to benign glands with irregular and undulating luminal borders, prostate carcinoma glands are smaller and have straight luminal borders.
- When prostate carcinoma becomes less differentiated, it loses glandular differentiation and forms cribriform structures, fused glands, poorly delineated glands, solid sheets or cords, or even single tumor cells.
- Cytoplasm
  - Prostate carcinoma glands may have amphophilic cytoplasm.
  - Low-grade prostate carcinoma often has pale, clear cytoplasm, indistinct from benign glands.
  - Prostate carcinoma typically lacks lipofuscin pigment.
- Nuclei
  - Typically, prostate carcinoma displays enlarged nuclei and prominent nucleoli.
  - Some prostate carcinomas lack prominent nucleoli yet have enlarged and hyperchromatic nuclei.
  - Cancer nuclei, even in poorly differentiated ones, show little variation in size and shape.
  - Mitoses and apoptotic bodies are more common in prostate carcinoma and rarely found in benign glands.
- Lumina
  - Crystalloids are dense, eosinophilic, crystal-like structures commonly found within the glandular lumens of cancer glands.
  - Intraluminal, pink, acellular, dense secretions and blue-tinged mucin are additional findings seen preferentially in prostate carcinoma.
  - Corpora amylacea are common in benign glands and are seen rarely in prostate carcinoma.
- Stroma
  - Ordinary prostate carcinoma does not elicit a prominent stromal inflammatory or desmoplastic response.

Immunopathology (including immunohistochemistry)
- The majority of prostate carcinomas express PSA, although there is considerable intratumoral and intertumoral heterogeneity, and the expression is decreased in a minority of high-grade prostate carcinoma.
- Prostate-specific acid phosphatase (PSAP) has a diagnostic utility similar to PSA, although it is in general more sensitive and less specific than the latter.
- Prostate cancer can occasionally show negative staining for cytokeratin (CK) 7, which can be useful to differentiate prostate carcinoma from urothelial carcinoma, which is typically positive.
- Prostate carcinoma uniformly lacks a basal cell layer and therefore is negative for high-molecular-weight cytokeratin (HMWCK). However, prostate carcinoma can occasionally contain sparse tumor cells positive for HMWCK, yet not in a basal cell distribution, especially after radiation or hormonal therapy.
- p63 is a nuclear protein expressed in basal cells of pseudostratified epithelia, including the prostate. p63 is negative in prostate cancer.
- AMACR is an enzyme involved in the metabolism of branched chain fatty acids and bile acid intermediates; it is overexpressed in approximately 80% of prostate carcinoma in needle biopsy specimens. AMACR is not entirely specific for prostate carcinoma, as it is present in high-grade prostatic intraepithelial neoplasia (>90%), adenosis (17.5%), partially atrophic glands,

and occasionally morphologically benign glands. AMACR can be used as a confirmatory staining, in conjunction with H&E histology and basal cell markers, for prostate carcinoma.

Main differential diagnosis
- Partial atrophy
- Postatrophic hyperplasia
- Adenosis
- Sclerosing adenosis
- Basal cell hyperplasia
- Seminal vesicle–ejaculatory duct tissue
- Verumontanum mucosal gland hyperplasia
- Cowper glands
- Paraganglia
- Mesonephric remnants
- Nonspecific granulomatous prostatitis
- Benign prostatic hyperplasia
- High-grade prostatic intraepithelial hyperplasia
- Radiation effect

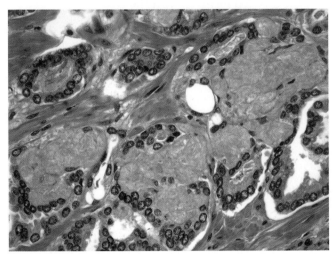

Fig 1. Mucinous fibroplasia (collagenous micronodules) consists of delicate loose fibrous tissue with an ingrowth of fibroblasts within or adjacent to cancer glands.

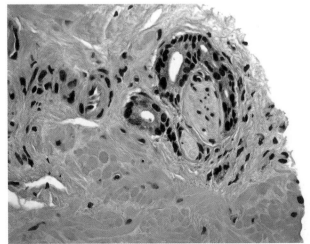

Fig 2. Perineural invasion with cancer glands encircling the entire circumference of a nerve is pathognomonic of prostate carcinoma.

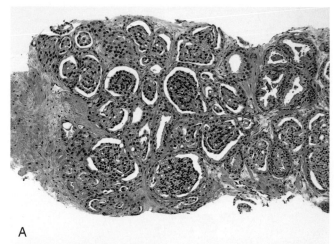

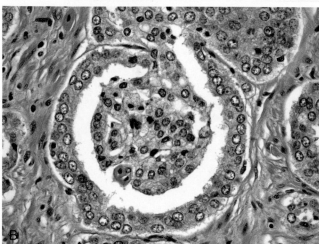

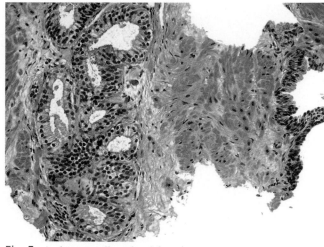

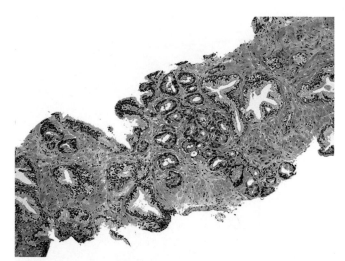

Fig 5. Architecturally, gland-forming prostate carcinomas are more crowded than benign glands.

Fig 3. **A,** Glomeruloid formation is created by intraluminal proliferation of malignant cells. **B,** Glomeruloid structure is often surrounded by a crescentic space resembling a renal glomerulus.

Fig 6. Typically, prostate cancer glands exhibit an infiltrative growth pattern, with malignant glands situated between or flanking benign glands.

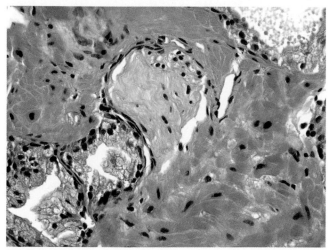

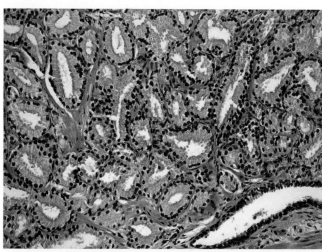

Fig 4. Benign prostatic glands can occasionally be found to abut a nerve; however, circumferential extension of benign glands entirely around a nerve has not been described.

Fig 7. In contrast to benign glands with irregular and undulating luminal borders, prostate carcinoma glands are smaller and have straight luminal borders.

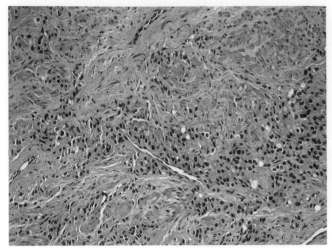

Fig 8. When prostate carcinoma becomes less differentiated, it loses glandular differentiation and forms poorly delineated fused glands, cords, or even single tumor cells.

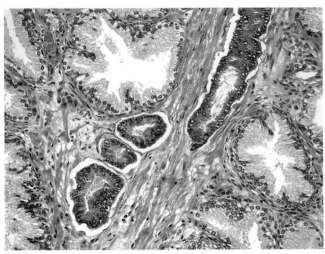

Fig 9. Prostate carcinoma glands may have amphophilic cytoplasm. Notice the intense cytoplasmic staining compared with the surrounding benign glands.

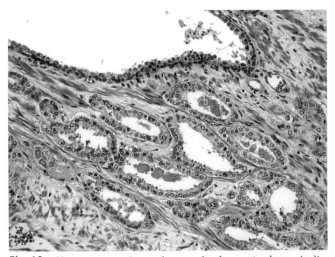

Fig 10. Gleason score 6 may have pale-clear cytoplasm, indistinct from benign glands.

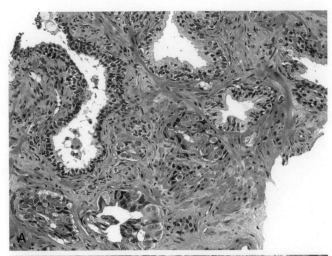

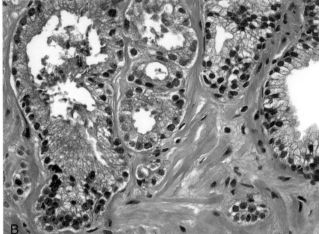

Fig 11. Typically, prostate carcinoma displays nucleomegaly **(A)** and prominent nucleoli **(B).**

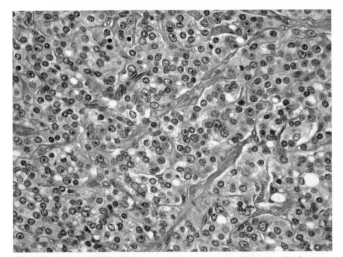

Fig 12. Poorly differentiated prostate cancer showing little variation in nuclear size and shape.

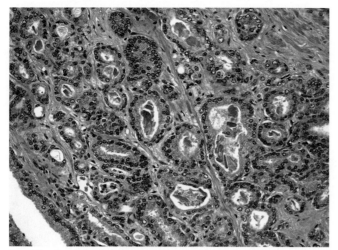

Fig 13. Crystalloids are dense eosinophilic crystal-like structures commonly found within the glandular lumens of cancer glands.

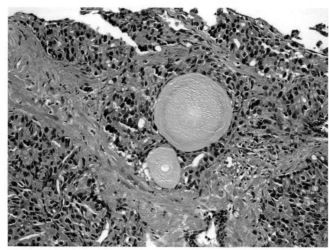

Fig 16. Corpora amylacea are common in benign glands and only rarely seen (as in this case) in prostate carcinoma.

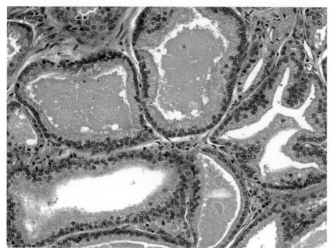

Fig 14. Intraluminal pink acellular dense secretions are findings seen preferentially in prostate carcinoma.

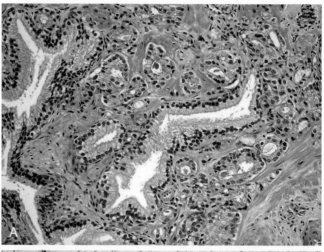

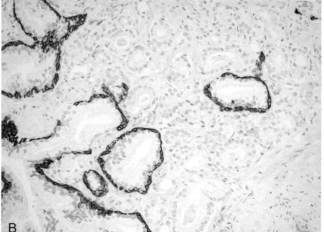

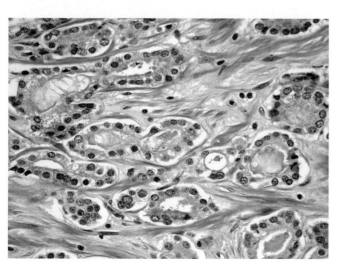

Fig 15. Blue-tinged mucin can be seen within the lumen of prostate carcinoma glands.

Fig 17. A, Small glands of prostate carcinoma infiltrating between larger benign glands. B, Prostate cancer glands uniformly lack a basal cell layer and therefore are negative for HMWCK; in contrast, benign glands show strong cytoplasmic staining in the basal cells.

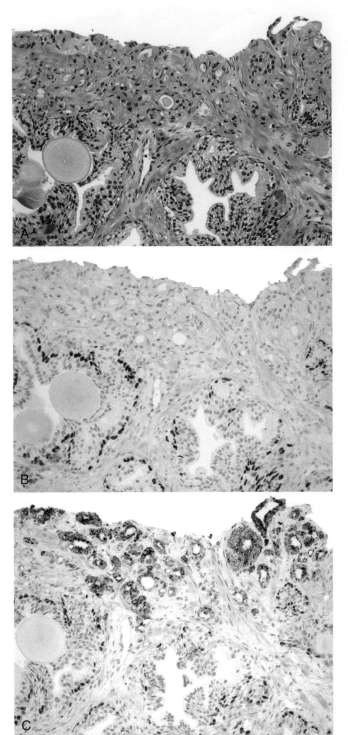

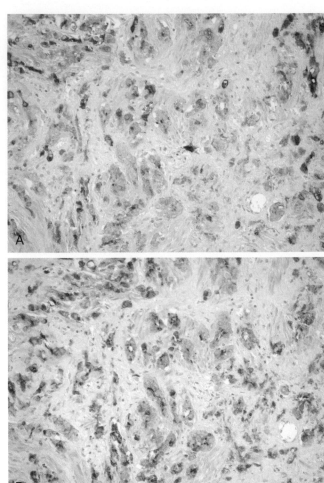

Fig 19. High-grade prostate cancer. PSAP **(A)** has a diagnostic utility similar to PSA **(B),** although it is in general more sensitive and less specific than PSA.

Fig 18. A, Small focus of prostate cancer on needle biopsy *(top).* **B,** p63 nuclear staining is expressed in basal cells of benign prostatic glands, but is negative in prostate cancer. **C,** Prostate carcinoma shows strong cytoplasmic staining with AMACR. p63 nuclear staining is positive in basal cells of adjacent benign glands, but negative in neoplastic glands (p63/AMACR cocktail).

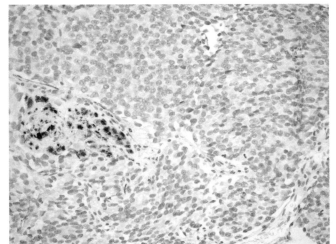

Fig 20. High-grade prostate cancer. Notice that most of the tumor cells show negative staining for CK7. CK7 can sometimes be useful to differentiate prostate carcinoma from urothelial carcinoma, which is typically diffusely positive for CK7.

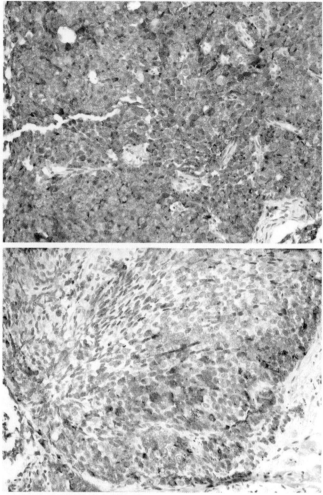

Fig 21. The majority of prostate carcinomas express PSA although there is considerable intratumoral heterogeneity. There is variable intensity of staining in two different areas of the same tumor.

Definition
- The variant of prostatic adenocarcinoma with cancer glands having scant volume of cytoplasm, which can be mistaken for atrophy or postatrophic hyperplasia

Clinical features
Epidemiology
- Makes some component of adenocarcinomas in 3% of radical prostatectomy specimens, 2% of prostate needle biopsy specimens

Presentation
- Not different from ordinary prostate adenocarcinoma

Prognosis and treatment
- Not different from ordinary prostate adenocarcinoma

Pathology
Histology
- Glands with round dilated or distorted lumina
- Flattened neoplastic lining of the glands with scant atrophic cytoplasm
- Significant cytologic atypia with nuclear enlargement and prominent nucleoli
- Can contain luminal eosinophilic proteinaceous secretions, blue mucin, crystalloids, apocrine blebs, collagenous micronodules, and adjacent high-grade prostatic intraepithelial neoplasia
- Infiltrative growth pattern
- Usually Gleason score 6
- Often intermixed with ordinary nonatrophic prostate carcinoma

Immunohistochemistry and special studies
- Like usual prostatic adenocarcinoma
  - Negative basal cell markers
  - Positive PSA, PSAP and AMACR

Main differential diagnosis
- Postatrophic hyperplasia: to diagnose atrophic adenocarcinoma of the prostate, one of three criteria must be satisfied: (1) glands must have an infiltrative growth pattern, requiring atrophic glands to be present to be situated as isolated acini on both sides of benign glands; this differs from the pseudo-infiltrative appearance seen with atrophy where there is a single patch of atrophic glands that appears disorganized and going off in different directions; (2) atrophic glands merge with neoplastic glands that have more cytoplasm (i.e., usual nonatrophic cancer); (3) atrophic glands have large, prominent nucleoli beyond the small yet visible nucleoli that may occasionally be seen with postatrophic hyperplasia.

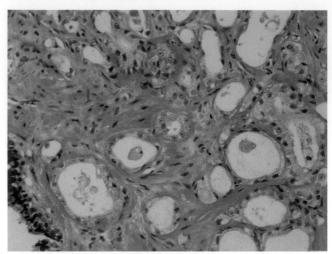

Fig 1. Atrophic adenocarcinoma with very prominent nucleoli diagnostic of carcinoma.

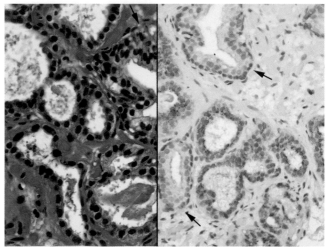

Fig 2. Atrophic adenocarcinoma (*left*) where cancer glands have atrophic cytoplasm with enlarged nuclei. Note benign gland (*arrow*). Immunohistochemical stain (*right*) for high-molecular-weight cytokeratin (brown) and AMACR (red) showing retention of basal cell layer in benign glands (*arrows*). Atrophic adenocarcinoma shows absence of basal cells and is positive for AMACR.

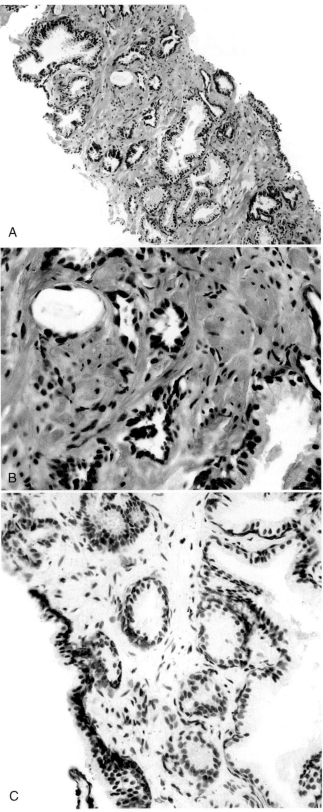

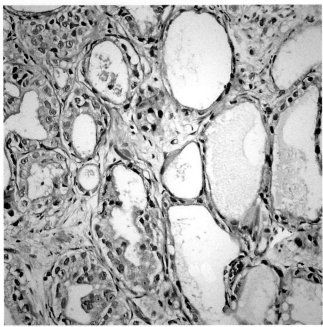

Fig 4. Prostatic adenocarcinoma with mixed atrophic and usual (nonatrophic) patterns.

Fig 3. A, Atrophic prostate adenocarcinoma with atrophic glands infiltrating on both sides of benign glands with abundant pale cytoplasm, an architectural feature not seen with benign atrophy. **B,** At higher magnification, the glands are cytologically indistinguishable from benign atrophic glands. **C,** Immunohistochemistry for high-molecular-weight cytokeratin reveals an absence of basal cells in the atrophic cancer glands.

Definition
- A morphologically distinct variant of prostatic adeno-carcinoma characterized by abundant foamy cyto-plasm

Clinical features
Epidemiology
- Uncommon
- Older age group similar to usual prostatic adenocarci-noma (mean age, 65 years)

Presentation
- PSA can be normal or elevated
- Sometimes an indurated nodule on digital rectal examination
- Can produce hypoechoic lesions on ultrasound

Prognosis and treatment
- Not low grade despite deceivingly benign histologic appearance
- Behavior dependent on Gleason score and stage of presentation
- Treatment modalities similar to those for usual acinar adenocarcinoma (e.g., radical prostatectomy, radio-therapy, hormone ablation therapy)

Pathology
Histology
- Crowded or infiltrating glands with abundant xantho-matous cytoplasm are present.
- Typically, nuclei are small and nucleoli are inconspic-uous.
- Typically glands are well formed, with a Gleason score of 3 + 3 = 6.
- High-grade foamy gland cancer (Gleason patterns 4 and 5) displays architectural patterns of cribriform, fused, and poorly formed glands, cords, single cells, or solid sheets. Nuclei are commonly enlarged in these cases. Nucleoli can be prominent and mitotic figures may be observed.
- Intraluminal, dense, pink secretions are sometimes found.
- Stromal desmoplasia can be prominent.
- Perineural invasion and extraprostatic extension is present in some cases.
- Rarely, relatively bland cytologic features and an exu-berant stromal reaction can be particularly difficult to recognize as malignant in a needle biopsy specimen.
- There can be associated usual or foamy gland high-grade prostatic intraepithelial neoplasia.
- Intraductal carcinoma can be produced.
- Often there is coexistent usual acinar adenocarci-noma.

Immunohistochemistry and special studies
- Positive for PSA, PSAP
- α-Methyl-CoA racemase is commonly positive.
- 34βE12 and p63 are usually negative, although some-times positive in a patchy basal or nonbasal distribu-tion, particularly in higher-grade cancers.
- Neutral mucin and lipid stains negative; colloidal iron and Alcian blue stains positive.
- Ultrastructurally, the foamy cells display numerous intracytoplasmic vesicles and numerous polyribo-somes.

Molecular diagnostics
- *TMPRSS2-ERG* fusion present in 29% of cases

Main differential diagnosis
- Benign glands: foamy gland cancers architecturally are abnormal, typically composed of crowded glands with an infiltrative appearance. They have distinctive cytoplasm with a foamy, xanthomatous, microvesicu-lar appearance. The cytoplasm is voluminous relative to the size of the nuclei, much more so than seen in benign glands. Occasional nuclei in foamy gland cancer have more recognizable malignant features. Numerous dense, pink, amorphous secretions further distinguish foamy gland cancer from benign glands, having rounded corpora amylacea with concentric rings.
- Mucinous metaplasia: crowded glands of mucinous metaplasia differs from foamy gland cancer in that most cases of mucin metaplasia have a lobular appear-ance and only partially involved benign glands. In cases with extensive mucinous metaplasia, the glandular lumina are occluded with the mucinous cytoplasm, as opposed to the open lumina with pink, dense secretions in foamy gland cancers. The cells of mucinous metaplasia are rounded, globoid goblet cells, whereas foamy gland cancer cells lack these features. Mucin stains are strongly positive in muci-nous metaplasia and negative in foamy gland cancer. Immunohistochemically, mucinous metaplasia is surrounded by a basal cell layer.
- Cowper glands: all the features described previously for mucinous metaplasia apply to Cowper glands. In addition, Cowper glands are exterior to the prostate and situated in skeletal muscle distal to the prostate, compared with foamy gland cancer, which is typically intraprostatic. Depending on the plane of section, it is sometimes possible to visualize the ducts of Cowper glands admixed with mucinous glands, giving it a characteristic dimorphic appearance similar to normal mucinous salivary gland tissue.

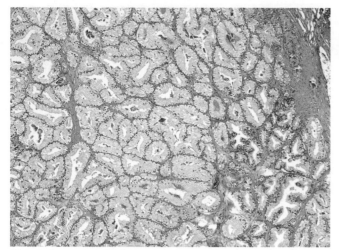

Fig 1. Low magnification of foamy gland carcinoma with crowded glands containing abundant cytoplasm.

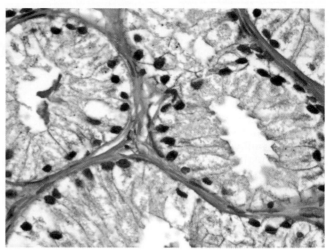

Fig 4. Nuclei in foamy gland carcinoma are typically bland without prominent nucleoli.

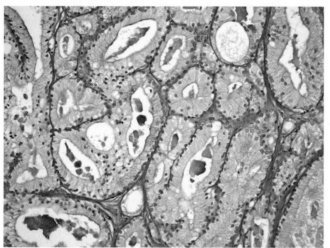

Fig 2. Foamy gland carcinoma with open lumina often containing crystalloids and dense eosinophilic secretions.

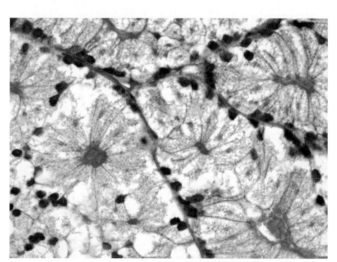

Fig 5. Foamy gland carcinoma with bland nuclei.

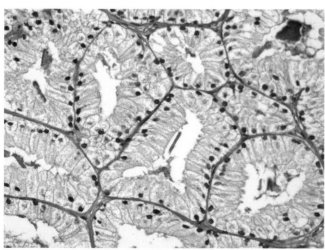

Fig 3. Foamy gland carcinoma.

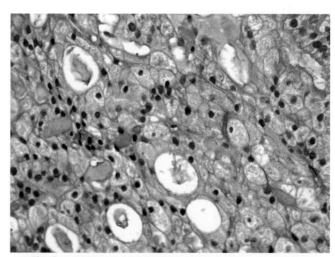

Fig 6. Cribriform higher-grade foamy gland carcinoma.

Definition
- A histologic variant of prostatic adenocarcinoma that resembles benign glandular hyperplasia because of large caliber glands with papillary infoldings and branching and occasional presence of corpora amylacea

Clinical features
Epidemiology
- Affects adult men of all age groups

Presentation
- May be clinically asymptomatic with raised serum prostate-specific antigen on screening, with prostate cancer identified on prostate core biopsies
- May develop with lower urinary tract symptoms of bladder outlet obstruction, with prostate cancer discovered incidentally on transurethral resection specimens

Prognosis and treatment
- As it is often accompanied by conventional forms of adenocarcinoma, the prognosis depends on the overall Gleason score of the accompanying cancer.
- If present as the sole pattern, it should be graded as Gleason score 3 + 3 = 6.
- Treatment options depend on a combination of preoperative prostate-specific antigen levels, extent of tumor, and overall Gleason scores, and can be aided by available nomograms.

Pathology
Histology
- Architecturally benign-appearing glands with large caliber and sometimes complex architecture, papillary infoldings, branching, and occasional corpora amylacea are present.
- Clues to malignant nature are crowded glands at low magnification and nuclear and nucleolar enlargement with pink amorphous secretions and crystalloids at higher magnification.
- Blue-tinged mucin and mitoses may be present.
- Accompanying high-grade prostatic intraepithelial neoplasia and perineural invasion may be seen in the same frequency as conventional prostate cancer.
- Adjacent conventional acinar adenocarcinoma may be present.
- There may be foamy cytoplasm showing the combined features of foamy gland pseudohyperplastic cancer.

Immunopathology (including immunohistochemistry)
- Antibodies to basal cells (p63, 34βE12) are negative, confirming the absence of basal cells in these glands and corroborating malignancy.
- Because occasional HGPIN glands can be negative for basal cell markers, the diagnosis of pseudohyperplastic cancer can only be made when numerous atypical glands are negative.
- α-Methyl-CoA racemase decorates the cytoplasm of the lining epithelial cells supporting their malignant nature, although this stain has to be interpreted in conjunction with basal cell markers because α-methyl-CoA racemase may be observed in high-grade prostatic intraepithelial neoplasia, adenosis (atypical adenomatous hyperplasia), and benign glands.

Molecular diagnostics
- No specific information available on this variant

Main differential diagnosis
- Benign glandular hyperplasia: pseudohyperplastic cancer glands are more crowed at low magnification and have more cytologic atypia at high magnification.
- HGPIN: pseudohyperplastic cancer glands tend to be more crowded than HGPIN and lack basal cells.

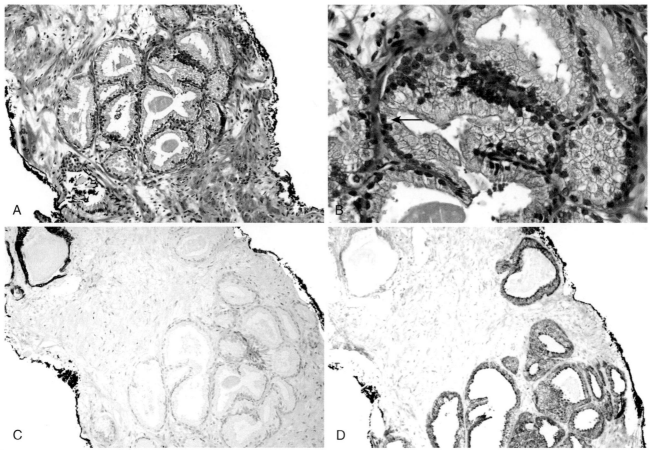

Fig 1. **A,** Prostate core biopsy showing crowded focus of glands that are about the same size as usual benign glands. Some of the glands have papillary infoldings and corpora amylacea. **B,** Higher magnification of the glands shows numerous prominent nucleoli *(arrow).* **C,** Immunohistochemistry for the basal cell marker 34βE12 shows absent basal cells in these glands. Note the benign gland with intact basal cell layer in the upper left. **D,** Immunohistochemistry for the α-methylacyl–coenzyme A racemase is positive in the pseudohyperplastic focus.

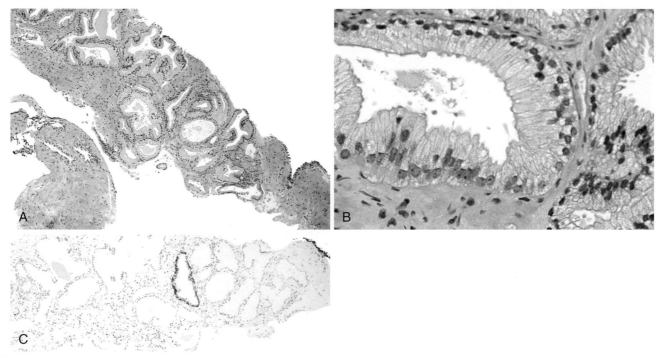

Fig 2. **A,** Large glands with papillary infolding resemble benign glands. In some areas the glands are crowded, raising the possibility of pseudohyperplastic cancer. **B,** High magnification of the abnormal glands shows multiple epithelial cell nuclei with prominent nucleoli. **C,** Immunohistochemistry for basal cells using 34βE12 antibodies shows their absence in these glands, confirming cancer.

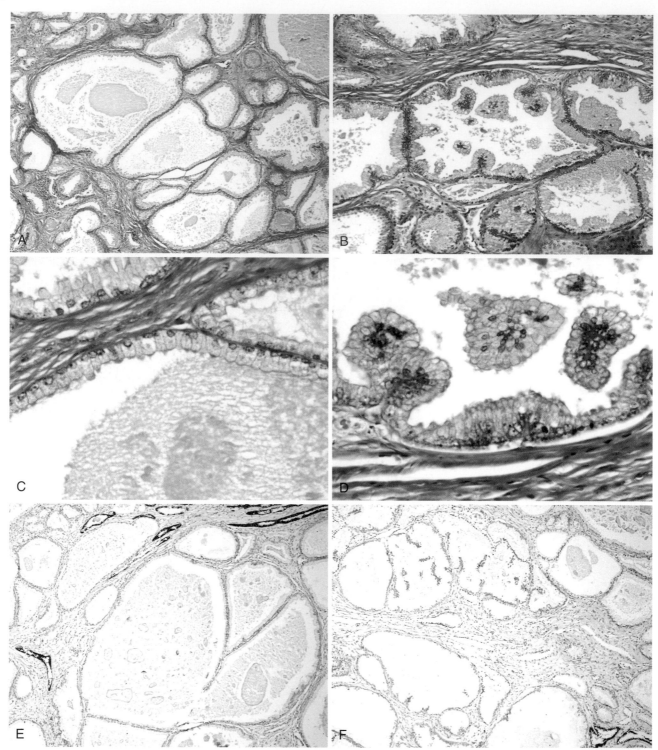

Fig 3. **A,** Cystic pattern of pseudohyperplastic carcinoma in which the neoplastic glands resemble cystically dilated benign glands. Features at low power suggestive of pseudohyperplastic cancer are that many of the glands have a straight luminal border despite having abundant cytoplasm. In addition, the glands are more crowded than benign glands. **B,** Other glands in the focus were large with papillary infolding further mimicking benign glands. **C,** Prominent nucleoli are present in the flat lining of the cystically dilated glands. **D,** Areas with papillary infolding also show prominent nucleoli. **E,** Numerous glands with cystic dilatation and a flat lining are negative for 34βE12, which is consistent with pseudohyperplastic prostate cancer. **F,** Pseudohyperplastic prostate cancer with papillary infolding is also negative for 34βE12. Note the benign glands with an intact basal cell layer in the *lower right*.

PROSTATIC ADENOCARCINOMA, MUCINOUS VARIANT

Definition
- The diagnosis of mucinous adenocarcinoma of the prostate is established only when extracellular mucin is secreted in sufficient quantity to result in pools of mucin involving more than 25% of the tumor volume on radical prostatectomy.

Clinical features
Epidemiology
- It is rare and one of the least common morphologic variants of prostatic adenocarcinoma.
- Incidence is 0.2% of all prostatic adenocarcinomas.
- Mean patient age is 56 years (range, 44 to 69 years).

Presentation
- Elevated PSA
- Positive digital rectal examination

Prognosis and treatment
- Mucinous adenocarcinoma of the prostate treated with radical prostatectomy is not more aggressive than usual nonmucinous prostatic adenocarcinoma and is potentially less aggressive.
- There are no data to determine whether overall mucinous adenocarcinoma of the prostate differs in prognosis relative to usual prostate cancer.
- It is treated the same as nonmucinous prostate cancer.

Pathology
Gross pathology
- Mucinous pools occasionally identified in tumor nodules grossly

Histology
- Epithelium is typical of nonmucinous adenocarcinoma of the prostate and shows relatively uniform cytology.
- Typically cribriform glands (Gleason pattern 4) floating in pools of mucin are present.
- Also seen are clusters of well-formed glands floating in pools of mucin (Gleason pattern 3).
- At least 25% of the tumor must be composed of mucin pools; diagnosis can be made only on radical prostatectomy specimens.
- When less than 25% of the tumor on radical prostatectomy is composed of mucin pools, or when seen on needle core biopsy or transurethral resection specimens, the term *prostatic adenocarcinoma with mucinous features* should be used.
- Tumors are typically admixed with nonmucinous prostatic adenocarcinoma.
- High-grade prostatic intraepithelial neoplasia may also be identified.

Immunopathology (including immunohistochemistry)
- Positive: PSA, PSAP, AMACR, prostein (P501S), MUC2

Main differential diagnosis
- Mucinous colonic adenocarcinoma or mucinous adenocarcinoma of the urachus/bladder involving the prostate: both of these entities would have the same morphology. Typically, strips of glandular epithelium are present, lining mucinous lakes. The epithelium has varying degrees of cytologic atypia, although in areas there is greater nuclear pleomorphism than is seen in mucinous adenocarcinoma of the prostate. Mucin-positive signet cells may be seen, which rules out mucinous prostate cancer with exceedingly rare exception. Immunohistochemical stains for prostatic markers are negative and tumors may express CDX2 or diffuse nuclear beta catenin, which are negative in mucinous adenocarcinoma of the prostate.
- Mucinous adenocarcinoma of the prostate arising from the prostatic urethra: mucinous adenocarcinomas can rarely arise from glandular metaplasia of the prostatic urethra, either from flat glandular metaplasia or from villous adenomatous glandular metaplasia. Through a process of dysplasia, analogous to what is seen in the gastrointestinal tract, the metaplastic epithelium can develop into a mucinous adenocarcinoma identical in morphology and immunohistochemistry to that described for mucinous adenocarcinoma of the urachus and bladder. These tumors may be restricted to the prostate, mimicking mucinous adenocarcinoma of the prostate.

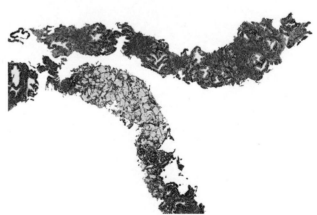

Fig 1. Prostate needle core biopsy specimen with prostatic adenocarcinoma with mucinous features. Note that the diagnosis of mucinous prostatic adenocarcinoma can be made only on radical prostatectomy.

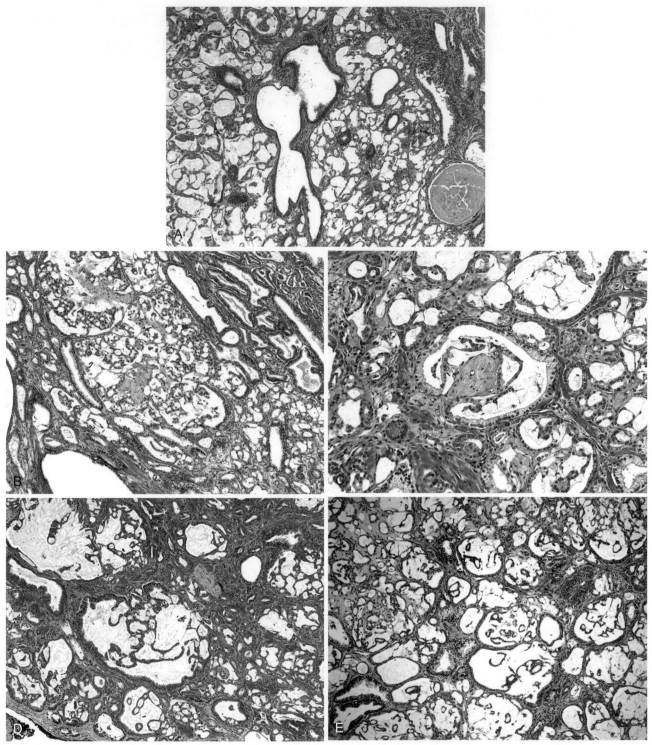

Fig 2. **A,** Mucinous prostatic adenocarcinoma infiltrating inbetween benign glands. **B,** Mucinous prostatic adenocarcinoma with focal mucinous fibroplasia. **C,** Mucinous prostatic adenocarcinoma with mucinous fibroplasia mimicking perineural invasion. **D,** Mucinous prostatic adenocarcinoma with adjacent usual type prostatic adenocarcinoma. **E,** Mucinous prostatic adenocarcinoma in which some of the mucinous areas contain well-formed individual glands. Foci such as these should be considered Gleason pattern 3.

Definition
- A variant of prostatic carcinoma that is morphologically characterized by pseudostratified columnar epithelium, typically arranged in dilated glands with flat or tufted pattern with morphologic features that resemble HGPIN

Clinical features
Epidemiology
- These tumors are uncommon, although it is difficult to estimate incidence because these lesions have only recently been recognized.

Presentation
- Patients with this variant of prostatic carcinoma exhibit increased PSA or a palpable lesion on digital rectal examination, similar to other prostatic carcinomas.
- PSA levels do not seem to differ from conventional forms of prostatic adenocarcinoma.

Prognosis and treatment
- Treatment of this variant of prostatic carcinoma should follow the same guidelines of conventional acinar tumors.
- In the few studies reported to date, the behavior of these tumors is not different from acinar forms, when compared with tumors with similar Gleason grades.
- Whereas most studies consider ductal morphology (see Chapter 13, "Ductal Adenocarcinoma," in this section) as a more aggressive tumor with comparable behavior to Gleason score 8 tumors, PIN-like ductal adenocarcinomas are more akin to Gleason score 6 acinar adenocarcinoma.
- Most reported cases with available follow-up were organ-confined at radical prostatectomy.

Pathology
Histology
- As the term implies, PIN-like ductal adenocarcinomas resemble high-grade PIN with some cytologic features of ductal adenocarcinoma of the prostate.
- Analogous to the architectural patterns seen in HGPIN, PIN-like ductal adenocarcinoma typically displays flat and tufted patterns. A pattern with small tufts of epithelium is a common finding. Because PIN-like ductal adenocarcinoma often is composed of dilated cystic glands, it is not unusual to see strips of the PIN-like epithelium along the edge of the core on a needle biopsy specimen.
- PIN-like carcinoma usually shows less prominent nucleoli than HGPIN.
- The cytology of the epithelium is of ductal type, with pseudostratified columnar cells, basally located nuclei, and amphophilic cytoplasm; therefore the term *PIN-like ductal adenocarcinoma* can also be used for this variant.

Immunopathology
- Similar to acinar adenocarcinoma, PIN-like carcinomas are by definition uniformly negative for basal cell markers (p63 and high-molecular-weight cytokeratin). AMACR is positive in the majority of tumor glands.
- This feature is helpful in distinguishing PIN-like carcinoma from ductal adenocarcinoma and HGPIN, both of which show patchy basal cell staining.

Main differential diagnosis
- HGPIN: PIN-like ductal carcinoma is distinguished from HGPIN by the higher prevalence of flat epithelium, more crowded glands, and often large dilated glands. Cytologic atypia seems to be less intense in cases of carcinoma than in HGPIN. Absence of basal cells by immunohistochemistry is essential to establish the diagnosis of PIN-like ductal carcinoma. However, as HGPIN glands can occasionally be negative for basal cell markers, the diagnosis of PIN-like ductal adenocarcinoma requires multiple glands that are negative for the basal cell markers.
- Usual ductal adenocarcinoma of the prostate: if not otherwise specified, the term *ductal adenocarcinoma* is used for cribriform or papillary variants of ductal adenocarcinoma in contrast to the flat and tufted appearance of PIN-like ductal adenocarcinoma. In most studies, ductal adenocarcinomas have a behavior similar to those of prostatic carcinomas (Gleason score 4 + 4 = 8). PIN-like ductal adenocarcinomas are uniformly negative for basal cell markers, whereas ductal adenocarcinomas may show patchy basal cell staining.

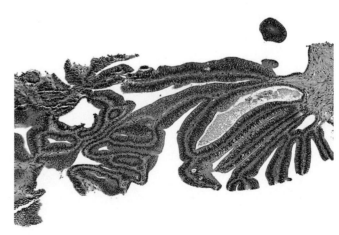

Fig 1. Medium-power view of prostatic intraepithelial neoplasia–like ductal adenocarcinoma with typical cytology of ductal adenocarcinoma. Glands are lined by pseudostratified columnar epithelium with mild to moderate nuclear atypia and amphophilic cytoplasm.

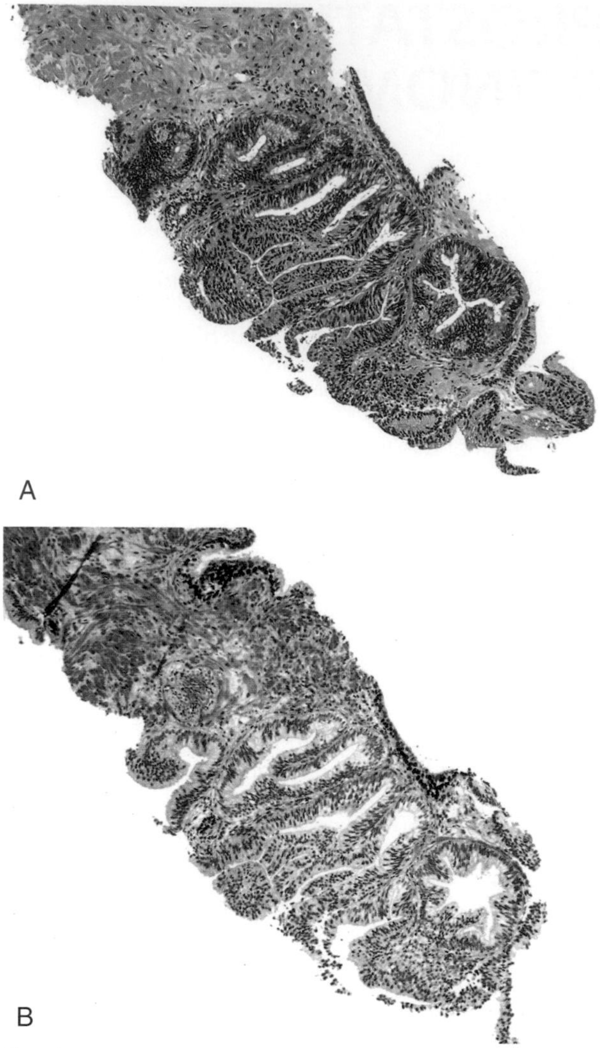

A

B

Fig 2. **A,** Prostatic intraepithelial neoplasia (PIN)-like ductal adenocarcinoma. Glands are lined by a pseudostratified columnar epithelium. Although the glands are similar in size to those seen in high-grade PIN, the glands are more crowded than in high-grade PIN. **B,** This p63 immunohistochemical study shows the absence of basal cells in PIN-like ductal adenocarcinoma glands.

A

B

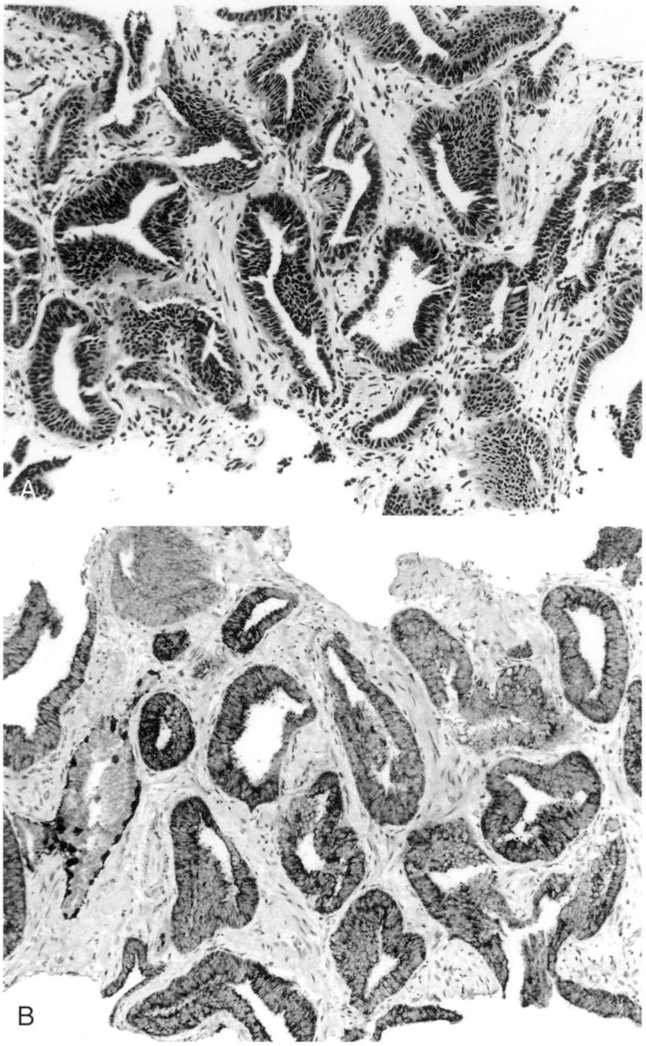

Fig 3. **A,** Prostatic intraepithelial neoplasia (PIN)-like ductal adenocarcinoma, mostly with flat morphology. The glands are crowded. At this power, one cannot appreciate nuclear atypia. Immunohistochemical studies are essential to distinguish from high-grade PIN. **B,** Triple antibody cocktail with intense α-methylacyl–coenzyme A racemase positivity in PIN-like ductal adenocarcinoma and an absence of basal cells (p63 and high-molecular-weight cytokeratin).

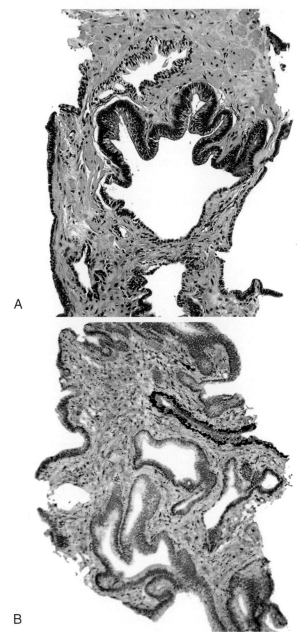

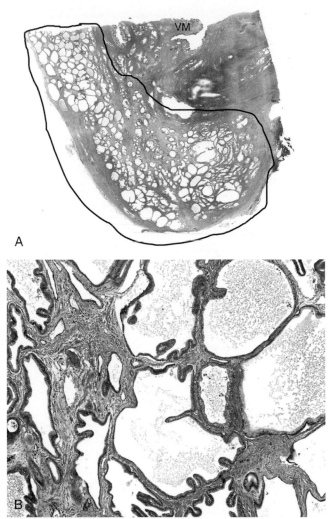

Fig 5. **A,** Low-power view of a posterolateral section of a radical prostatectomy showing a tumor forming cystically dilated glands *(area inside black line)*. **B,** Higher-power view showing typical prostatic intraepithelial neoplasia–like ductal adenocarcinoma morphology of glands with flat and micropapillary epithelium. *VM,* Verumontanum.

Fig 4. **A,** Prostatic intraepithelial neoplasia (PIN)-like ductal adenocarcinoma. Glands with a flat epithelium and small tufts closely resembling high-grade PIN. Note the strip of epithelium on the left side, which is the lining of a larger cyst. **B,** This p63 immunohistochemical study shows the absence of basal cells in PIN-like ductal adenocarcinoma glands.

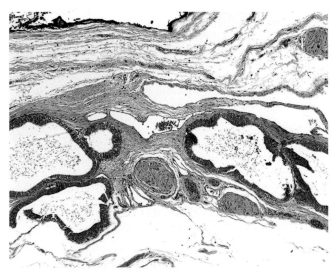

Fig 6. A rare case of prostatic intraepithelial neoplasia–like ductal adenocarcinoma in an area of focal extraprostatic extension.

Definition
- Malignant epithelial neoplasm of the prostate that demonstrates epithelial and sarcomatoid components (formerly called *carcinosarcoma*)

Clinical features
Epidemiology
- Incidence is rare (fewer than 100 cases reported).
- Average age is 70 years, with a range of 47 to 91 years.
- Patients often have a precedent history of acinar adenocarcinoma that can be as remote as 16 years prior.
- A history of radiation or hormone treatment for the original acinar adenocarcinoma is common.

Presentation
- Obstructive voiding symptoms may be present.
- Elevated PSA may be present.
- Metastatic disease may be a first sign.

Prognosis and treatment
- Prognosis is poor.
- Distant metastases to bone, liver, and lung occur in approximately one third of patients.
- Five-year cancer-specific survival is 41%.
- Actuarial risk of death is 20% at 1 year.
- Treatment is based on stage.

Pathology
Histology
- Carcinoma appears grossly as a gray-white mass with necrosis and hemorrhage.
- A prominent sarcomatoid component may consist of undifferentiated spindled cells ranging from 5% to 99% of the mass.
- Sarcomatoid component may be storiform, fascicular, or without pattern.
- Bizarre tumor giant cells may be present within the sarcomatoid component.
- Heterologous elements such as osteosarcoma, chondrosarcoma, and rhabdomyosarcoma may be present.
- Virtually all patients will have a concurrent high-grade acinar adenocarcinoma or unusual variant of prostate cancer present, even in small amounts.
- Unusual concurrent forms of prostate cancer include squamous cell carcinoma and carcinomas with enteric-type glands, basaloid carcinoma, or foamy micropapillary carcinoma.

Immunopathology
- The sarcomatous component is positive for cytokeratin or Cam5.2 in virtually all cases, whereas PSA and PSAP are positive in only approximately 50% of cases.
- The carcinomatous component is generally positive for cytokeratin and PSA or PSAP.
- Heterologous elements variably stain for mesenchymal markers, including desmin, S100, and smooth-muscle actin.

Molecular diagnostics
- Light microscopy and immunohistochemistry are most important in the diagnosis.

Main differential diagnosis
- Primary prostatic sarcoma, such as malignant phyllodes tumor, leiomyosarcoma, and malignant solitary fibrous tumor
  - Lacks epithelial component
  - Lesions characterized by well-defined histology

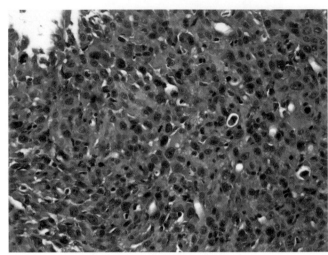

Fig 1. Sarcomatoid carcinoma demonstrates a variable proportion of undifferentiated slightly spindled, cells with frequent mitotic activity.

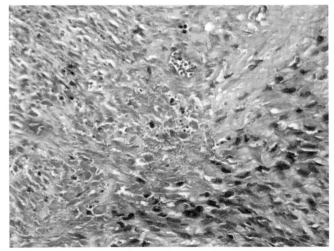

Fig 2. The finding of necrosis is common in these lesions.

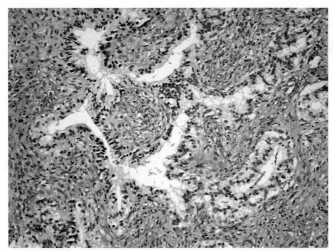

Fig 3. Unusual variants of prostate cancer may occur in sarcomatoid carcinoma, including carcinoma with enteric-type features as shown here.

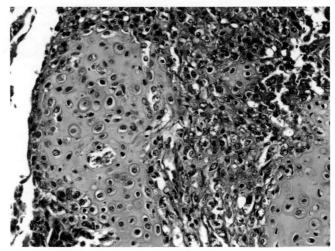

Fig 5. Heterologous elements may be present and include chondrosarcoma (shown here), osteosarcoma, and rhabdomyosarcoma.

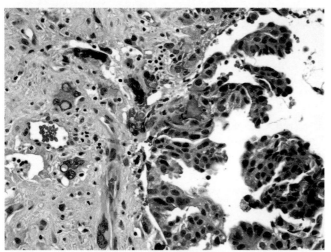

Fig 4. Bizarre tumor giant cells may be present within the sarcomatoid component, seen here adjacent to an unusual form of prostate cancer with micropapillary features.

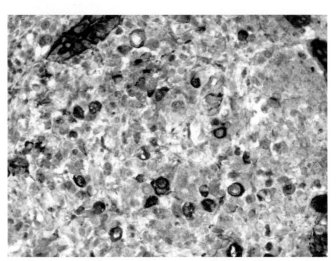

Fig 6. Cytokeratin immunostains are at least focally positive in virtually all cases.

PLEOMORPHIC GIANT CELL CARCINOMA OF THE PROSTATE

Definition
- A rare and aggressive variant of prostate carcinoma with pleomorphic and anaplastic features with bizarre and pleomorphic giant cells

Clinical features
Epidemiology
- Average age is 65.8 years, with a range of 59 to 76 years.

Presentation
- Elevated PSA
- Urinary symptoms

Prognosis and treatment
- Prognosis is poor.
- Treatment is dependent on stage, grade, and coexistent histologic subtypes.

Pathology
Histology
- Presence of giant, bizarre, anaplastic cells with abundant cytoplasm
- Marked pleomorphism
- Aggregates or sheets of mononucleate and multinucleate giant cells
- Discohesive tumor cells with extensive necrosis
- Atypical mitotic figures
- Multiple coexistent histologic components possibly seen, including conventional prostate cancer, small cell carcinoma, squamous carcinoma, or ductal adenocarcinoma

Immunohistochemistry and special studies
- Positive for cytokeratins AE1/AE3 or Cam 5.2, or both
- PSA possibly positive in the pleomorphic giant cells

Main differential diagnosis
- Radiation atypia: atypical changes seen in the radiated benign nuclei have a more degenerative and smudgy appearance, compared with the nuclear atypia seen in the pleomorphic giant cell carcinoma.
- Sarcomatoid carcinoma of the prostate: prominent spindle cell morphology occasionally may contain neoplastic giant cells. The bizarre cells in pleomorphic giant cell carcinoma appear epithelial and are seen typically in glands or cohesive nests, whereas atypical cells in sarcomatoid carcinoma appear as isolated spindle cells in the stroma.
- Urothelial carcinoma with pleomorphic giant cells can be difficult to distinguish. The key is identifying the bizarre cells admixed with more typical adenocarcinoma of the prostate and the use of immunohistochemistry for prostate markers, if necessary.

- Metastatic carcinoma from other sites has bizarre giant cells and pleomorphism. A battery of immunostains including melanoma, lymphoid, and epithelial markers, and antibodies against thrombomodulin and PSA should be performed. Clinical history will be critical to arrive at a correct diagnosis.

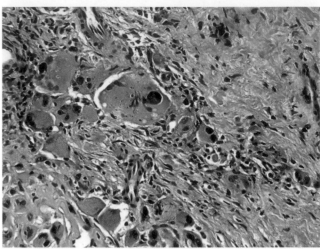

Fig 1. Characteristic giant pleomorphic cells with abundant cytoplasm from a radical prostatectomy specimen.

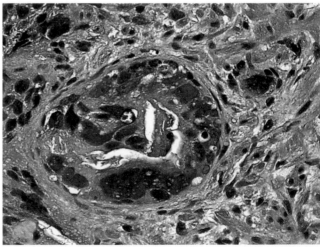

Fig 2. High-power view of bizarre multinucleated giant cells with marked pleomorphism and atypia.

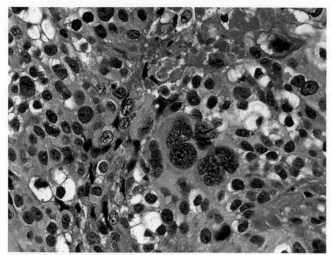

Fig 3. Giant pleomorphic giant cells with marked pleomorphism and bizarre atypia. Note the smaller acinar prostatic carcinoma cells with round nuclei and prominent nucleoli in the background.

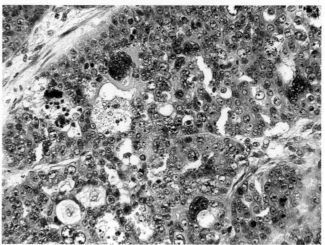

Fig 4. High-magnification view of bizarre multinucleated giant cells.

Definition
- A rare variant of prostate carcinoma with a prominent lymphoid infiltrate

Clinical features
Epidemiology
- There is only one series of five patients, with age ranging from 69 to 82 years (mean, 76 years). An additional case report exists.

Presentation
- Elevated PSA
- Urinary obstructive symptoms
- Hematuria

Prognosis and treatment
- Prognosis was poor for all four patients in the series with follow-up; they were dead within 8 to 26 months.
- Most of the patients had advanced disease (cT3 or cT4).
- The one case report had 50% lymphoepithelioma-like carcinoma of the prostate (LELC) admixed with prostate cancer (Gleason score 4 + 3 = 7) treated with radical prostatectomy. The patient was free of disease within a short follow-up period (15 months).

Pathology
Histology
- Prostatic adenocarcinoma that can be admixed with ductal or squamous differentiation
- LELC with undifferentiated carcinoma cells having indistinct cell borders arranged as individual or clusters of cells
- Admixed heavy lymphocytic infiltrate with occasional plasma cells, neutrophils, or eosinophils

Immunohistochemistry and special studies
- LELC positive for cytokeratin and EMA
- LELC positive for PSA and PSAP and AMACR
- Most cases of LELC are aneuploid
- Negative for Epstein-Barr virus by in situ hybridization
- Lymphocytes mark primarily as T cells

Main differential diagnosis
- Large cell lymphoma: distinction must be made on identifying admixed usual prostate carcinoma component as well as performing immunohistochemistry for lymphoid and epithelial markers.
- LELC of the bladder may have identical histology, although some cases of bladder LELC are associated with noninvasive and invasive urothelial carcinoma. LELC of the prostate can be diagnosed in the presence of intimately admixed usual prostate cancer. LELC of the prostate will label immunohistochemically with PSA and PSAP in contrast to LELC arising in the bladder.

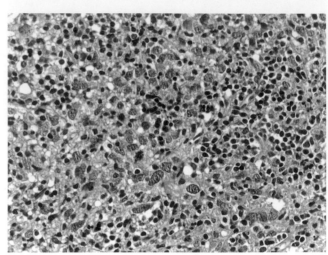

Fig 1. Lymphoepithelioma-like carcinoma of the prostate with scattered malignant cells with enlarged nuclei within dense lymphoid infiltrate. (Courtesy Rodolfo Montironi, Institute of Pathological Anatomy, University of Ancona School of Medicine, Ancona, Italy.)

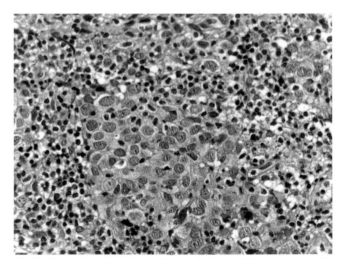

Fig 2. Lymphoepithelioma-like carcinoma of the prostate with a more cohesive nest of undifferentiated prostate cancer among dense lymphoid backgrounds. (Courtesy Rodolfo Montironi, Institute of Pathological Anatomy, University of Ancona School of Medicine, Ancona, Italy.)

PROSTATE CARCINOMA WITH SQUAMOUS DIFFERENTIATION

Definition
- Squamous differentiation in prostate cancer is exceedingly rare and is more often, yet not exclusively, seen in cases of prior hormone or radiation therapy, and is usually associated with a poor prognosis. In general, the adenocarcinoma component is typically high grade, whereas the squamous component has a wider range of differentiation.

Clinical features
Epidemiology
- Mean age at diagnosis is 68 years (range, 49 to 86 years).
- Risk factors include a prior history of prostatic adenocarcinoma.
- Prior hormonal or radiation therapy is often present.
- It may appear with no prior adenocarcinoma or any history of treatment.

Presentation
- Bladder outlet obstruction and dysuria (most common)
- Hematuria
- Bone pain from metastatic disease

Prognosis and treatment
- More aggressive than prostatic acinar adenocarcinoma
- Limited therapeutic success with surgery, radiation, or hormonal therapy
- Metastatic disease in one third of cases

Pathology
Histology
- Squamous carcinomas may be pure.
- The most common pattern among prostate carcinoma with squamous differentiation is adenosquamous carcinoma.
- It can also coexist with sarcomatoid carcinoma.
- The squamous carcinoma component of mixed cases can range from 5% to 95%.
- The squamous component has varying degrees of cytologic atypia.
- In cases with adenocarcinoma, the glandular component is typically high grade.
- In the squamous component, the nuclei are larger and more pleomorphic.

Immunohistochemistry and special studies
- Prostate-specific acid phosphatase and prostate-specific antigen are positive in a large percentage of the adenocarcinomas and only focally positive in the squamous carcinomas.
- High-molecular-weight cytokeratins are diffusely positive in more than 95% of the squamous carcinomas.

Main differential diagnosis
- Squamous metaplasia in the setting of an adjacent infarct: if the center of the infarct is not seen on biopsy, the clues to an adjacent infarct are stromal hemorrhage and hemosiderin deposition. The squamous metaplasia adjacent to an infarct may have considerable atypia and mitotic figures, such that attention to the intervening stroma or adjacent visible necrotic tissue is key to differentiation from squamous carcinoma.
- Squamous change in benign prostate tissue following hormonal therapy: in contrast to squamous carcinoma or adenosquamous carcinoma, squamous metaplasia following hormone therapy is bland and diffuse throughout the gland.
- Direct extension of squamous cell carcinoma from the bladder or anal canal or from urothelial carcinoma of the urinary bladder with squamous cell differentiation: pure squamous carcinoma of the prostate cannot be differentiated from these secondary tumors coming from the bladder or intestine on morphologic grounds and must be done on clinical grounds.

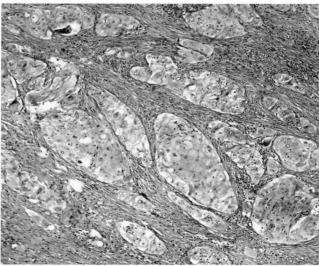

Fig 1. Moderately differentiated pure squamous cell carcinoma from a radical prostatectomy specimen. The patient has a history of prostatic adenocarcinoma (Gleason score, 3 + 3 = 6) that was subsequently treated with radiation.

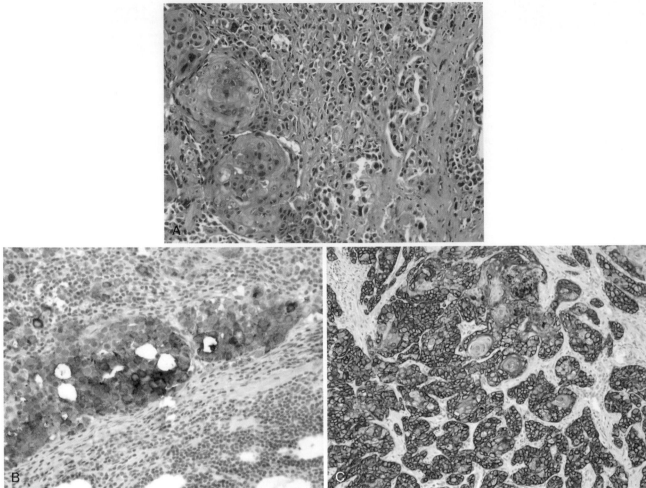

Fig 2. **A,** Adenosquamous carcinoma with squamous carcinoma component *(left)* and adenocarcinoma *(right)*. **B,** The adenocarcinoma component of adenosquamous carcinoma is positive for prostate-specific antigen. **C,** Squamous carcinoma component labels with antibodies to high-molecular-weight cytokeratin.

Definition
- Morphologically distinct variant of prostatic adeno-carcinoma

Clinical features
Epidemiology
- In pure form, ductal adenocarcinoma accounts for fewer than 1% and is associated with acinar adenocarcinoma in approximately 5% of prostate cancers.
- It occurs in an older age group similar to that for acinar adenocarcinoma.
- It can arise in large primary periurethral ducts or in peripheral ducts.

Presentation
- Most peripheral zone tumors are asymptomatic and detected on transrectal ultrasound (TRUS) biopsy specimen.
- Peripheral zone tumors may cause prostatic enlargement or induration on digital rectal examination.
- Periurethral tumors can appear with hematuria and obstructive lower urinary tract symptoms.
- Carcinoma may appear as friable white to gray polypoid lesions protruding from the urethra or ducts near the verumontanum on cystoscopic or urethroscopic examination.
- Serum PSA is variable and may occasionally be normal. PSA is elevated in most cases.

Prognosis and treatment
- Usual ductal adenocarcinoma has a high risk of presenting at an advanced stage and is known to display aggressive clinical behavior.
- The presence of any ductal adenocarcinoma component on a needle biopsy specimen is an adverse prognostic feature.
- Conflicting studies exist whether any proportion of ductal adenocarcinoma in radical prostatectomy specimens is a significant predictor for stage pT3 disease. In one study, any ductal component correlated with aggressive behavior, whereas in another only cancers in which the ductal component occupied more than 10% behaved more aggressively.
- Five-year actuarial risk of progression of cases treated by radical prostatectomy is approximately 50%.
- Usual ductal adenocarcinoma composed of cribriform or papillary formation is analogous to Gleason pattern 4 cancer. PIN-like ductal adenocarcinoma behaves more like Gleason pattern 3 carcinoma.
- Treatment modalities include transurethral resection, radical prostatectomy, androgen ablation therapy, chemotherapy, or radiotherapy or a combination of any of these.
- A small subset of periurethral tumors can be eradicated with transurethral resection.

Pathology
Histology
- Ductal adenocarcinoma of usual type
  - Several architectural patterns including cribriform, papillary, solid, and invasive glandular composed of tall columnar cells displaying nuclear pseudo-stratification
  - An admixture of patterns usually observed, with the most common patterns being papillary and cribriform
  - Abundant amphophilic, eosinophilic, or clear cytoplasm
  - Cytologic atypia varying from minimal, resembling adenomatous epithelium in the gastrointestinal tract, to more prominent with prominent nucleoli
  - Gleason grade of at least 4 as recommended by the ISUP modified Gleason grading system. Solid tumor or cribriform tumor with comedonecrosis graded as pattern 5
  - Metastases exhibiting purely ductal morphology or mixed with acinar adenocarcinoma
- Rare histologic patterns
  - PIN-like ductal adenocarcinoma (see Chapter 8, "Prostatic Ductal Adenocarcinoma, PIN-Like," in this section)
  - Ductal adenocarcinoma with mucinous and goblet cell features
  - Foamy gland ductal adenocarcinoma
  - Ductal adenocarcinoma with Paneth cell–like neuroendocrine features
  - Micropapillary ductal adenocarcinoma
  - Ductal adenocarcinoma with cystic papillary features

Immunohistochemistry and special studies
- Immunostaining for PSA and PSAP in most tumors
- α-Methylacyl-CoA racemase positive in a high percentage of cases
- Basal cell markers positive in a basal cell distribution, usually as patchy staining in approximately 30% of cases
- CEA, CK7, and CK20 focally positive
- High Ki-67 labeling index
- CDX2 rarely positive

Molecular diagnostics
- *TMPRSS2-ERG* fusion found in approximately 50% of cases

Main differential diagnosis
- Colorectal adenocarcinoma: colon cancer can mimic ductal adenocarcinoma composed of individual glands, especially those with necrosis. In contrast to most colonic adenocarcinomas containing mucin, only rare ductal adenocarcinomas do so. The presence of cribriform and papillary components is typical of ductal adenocarcinoma and would be exceedingly uncommon in adenocarcinoma of the colon. Immunohistochemistry for prostatic markers is diagnostic. CDX2 is rarely positive in prostate cancer compared with colonic adenocarcinoma, in which it is usually positive.
- Urothelial carcinoma: solid nests of ductal adenocarcinoma can resemble infiltrating urothelial carcinoma, although these more solid, poorly differentiated components will always be accompanied by a glandular component typical of ductal adenocarcinoma.

Papillary ductal adenocarcinoma can be confused with papillary noninvasive urothelial carcinoma. The pseudostratified columnar lining of ductal adenocarcinoma differs from papillary urothelial carcinoma.

- Prostatic acinar adenocarcinoma, including intraductal acinar adenocarcinoma, is composed of cuboidal to short columnar cells that lack the pseudostratified columnar appearance of ductal adenocarcinoma. Acinar adenocarcinoma lacks papillary formation and cribriform glands with slit-like spaces; acinar cribriform cancer has rounded lumina.
- Villous adenoma, as in the differential diagnosis of colonic adenocarcinoma, contains mucin and is immunohistochemically positive for intestinal markers (e.g., CDX2, nuclear β catenin) and negative for prostatic antigens.
- Prostatic urethral polyps, other than arising in the prostatic urethra, lack any similarity to prostatic ductal adenocarcinomas. Prostatic urethral polyps are composed of crowded entirely benign glands that are polypoid rather than papillary growths. The surface lining is either benign prostatic or urothelial cells.
- Cribriform HGPIN is uncommon and fits within the normal architecture whereas cribriform ductal adenocarcinoma glands tend to be more crowded, infiltrative, and often have central necrosis. Although ductal adenocarcinomas can have a patchy basal cell layer, most cases lack a basal cell layer. In contrast to HGPIN, which may have micropapillary features, the papillary structures in ductal adenocarcinoma have true papillary fronds with well-established fibrovascular cores. In limited specimens it may be impossible to distinguish the two entities with a recommendation for additional tissue sampling.

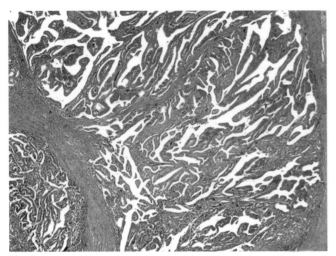

Fig 1. Papillary prostatic ductal adenocarcinoma in the transition zone.

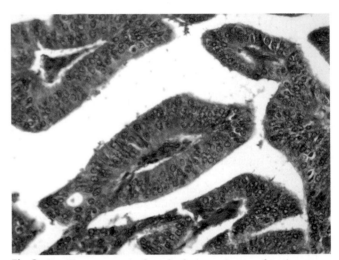

Fig 3. Papillary prostatic ductal adenocarcinoma showing pseudostratified columnar epithelium.

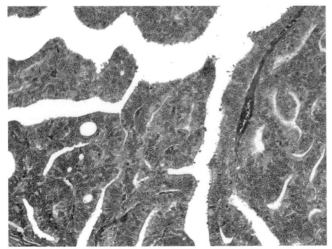

Fig 2. Papillary prostatic ductal adenocarcinoma.

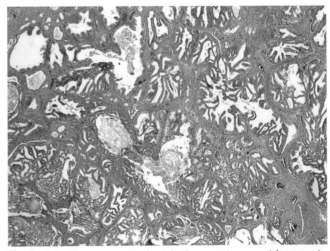

Fig 4. Cribriform prostatic ductal adenocarcinoma with necrosis.

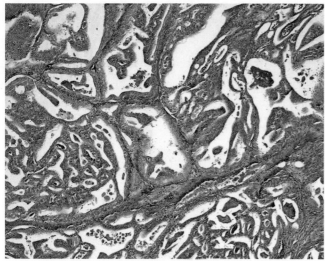

Fig 5. Cribriform prostatic ductal adenocarcinoma.

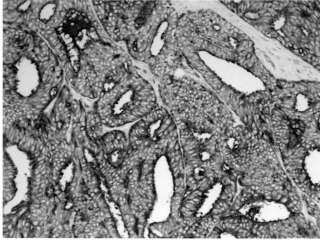

Fig 8. Prostate-specific antigen immunoreactivity in prostatic ductal adenocarcinoma.

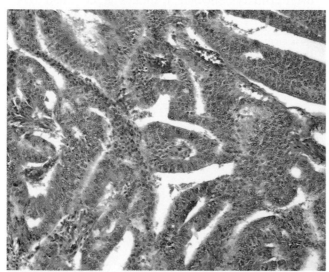

Fig 6. Cribriform and papillary prostatic ductal adenocarcinoma.

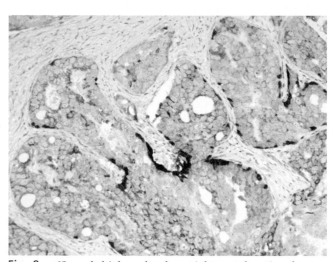

Fig 9. p63 and high-molecular-weight cytokeratin show a patchy basal cell layer in prostatic ductal adenocarcinoma that expresses α-methylacyl–coenzyme A racemase.

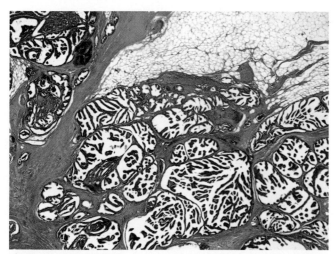

Fig 7. Prostatic ductal adenocarcinoma extending into periprostatic adipose tissue.

Definition
- A rare histologic variant of prostatic carcinoma morphologically akin to those diagnosed in the lung

Clinical features
Epidemiology
- Affects adult men of older age, range 44 to 92 years (mean, 69 years)

Presentation
- By itself does not result in elevated serum PSA levels, although may be associated with usual prostatic adenocarcinoma and elevated serum PSA
- May develop with lower urinary tract symptoms of bladder outlet obstruction, with prostate cancer discovered on transurethral resection specimens
- May develop with distant metastases
- May have prior prostate adenocarcinoma
- Uncommonly associated with Cushing syndrome from ectopic adrenocorticotropic hormone production
- Uncommonly with hypercalcemia
- Infrequently with syndrome of inappropriate ADH secretion
- Rarely with Lambert-Eaton myasthenic syndrome

Prognosis and treatment
- Aggressive disease with poor prognosis even when localized, although prognosis correlates with stage
- Usually advanced stage at presentation
- Poor response to antiandrogen therapy
- Typically treated with same combination chemotherapy regimen as small cell carcinoma of the lung; tumors may initially respond, but then rapidly relapse
- Rare cases cured by chemotherapy
- Elevated serum LDH and lowered albumin levels predict worse survival

Pathology
Histology
- Classic "oat cell" and intermediate cell morphology
- Necrosis
- Occasionally can see large pleomorphic giant cells
- Linear cords of small cells
- Rosette formation
- Vacuolated cytoplasm
- Desmoplasia may be seen

Immunopathology (including immunohistochemistry)
- Neuroendocrine markers (usually at least one) are positive.
- Prostate-specific antigen, prostein (p501S), and prostate-specific membrane antigen are typically negative; when positive, they are focal.
- TTF-1 is positive in 50% of cases.
- CD44 is positive in small cell prostatic carcinoma, but negative in small cell carcinoma of nonprostate origin, and present in only rare scattered cells in conventional adenocarcinoma.

Molecular diagnostics
- Transcriptomic profiling shows upregulation of proliferative, neuroendocrine, and tyrosine kinase receptors and downregulation of cell adhesion molecules.
- A clonal relationship is demonstrated with concurrent adenocarcinoma with sequencing of the *TP53* gene.
- Approximately 50% of cases are positive for *TMPRSS2-ERG* fusion by fluorescence in situ hybridization, whereas small cell carcinomas arising from other sites are negative.

Main differential diagnosis
- Gleason pattern 5 adenocarcinoma: prominent nucleoli and abundant cytoplasm favor usual high-grade prostate cancer. Nuclear molding with numerous mitotic figures and apoptotic bodies favor small cell carcinoma. Immunohistochemically, absent staining for prostatic markers, greater than 50% Ki-67 indices, diffuse CD44 staining, and more than focal neuroendocrine marker expression favor small cell carcinoma.
- Metastatic small cell carcinoma from other primary organs: if tumor develops in the prostate without an overt primary elsewhere, it should be presumed to be of small cell origin. Typically, there is no need to do immunohistologic or molecular workup to verify prostatic origin, because small cell carcinomas are treated the same regardless of site of origin.

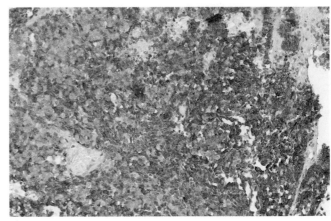

Fig 1. Immunohistochemical analysis for synaptophysin reveals diffuse positive cytoplasmic reactivity.

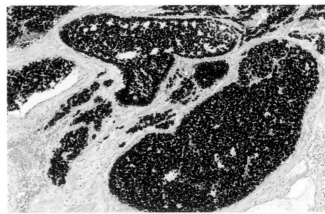

Fig 2. TTF-1 nuclear reactivity in the tumor cells of smallcell prostate carcinoma.

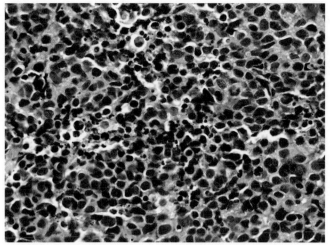

Fig 3. High magnification shows classic small cell features with a high nuclear-to-cytoplasmic ratio, indistinct nucleoli, and numerous apoptotic bodies.

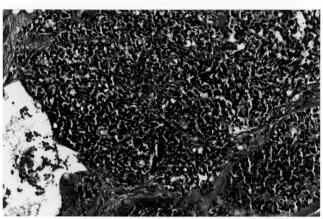

Fig 6. Expansile sheet of tumor cells with rare interspersed rosettes.

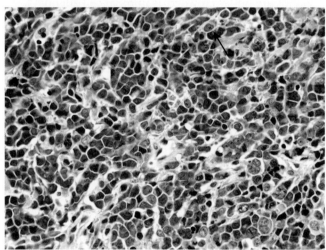

Fig 4. Some small cell carcinomas can have slightly more open vesicuwith discernible but small nucleoli *(arrow)*. Cells still have high nuclear-to-cytoplasmic ratios, nuclear molding, many nuclei without nucleoli, and numerous mitotic figures typical of small cell carcinoma.

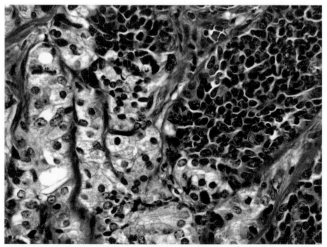

Fig 7. Prostatic chips from transurethral resection, showing several chips containing cellular sheets of tumor seen at low magnification.

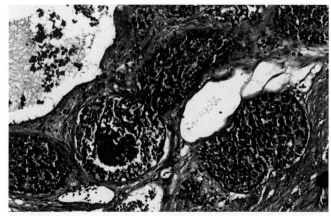

Fig 5. An area of necrosis is noted within a tumor island. Other islands show a focal rosette formation.

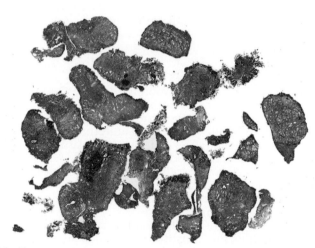

Fig 8. Smallcell carcinoma admixed with usual high-grade acinar adenocarcinoma of the prostate.

Definition

- A well-formed distinct nodule of basaloid nests in the prostate gland, also referred to as *adenoid basal cell hyperplasia, adenoid cystic–like tumor,* and *basal cell tumor*

Clinical features

Epidemiology

- Affects adult men of older age groups

Presentation

- May be clinically asymptomatic
- May appear with lower urinary tract symptoms of bladder outlet obstruction

Prognosis and treatment

- Benign condition without any specific treatment apart from the accompanying symptoms

Pathology

Histology

- Transition zone lesion
- Basal cell hyperplasia involving adenomatous nodules
- Circumscribed nodule with an expansile growth pattern compressing the surrounding gland
- Clusters of small, cytologically uniform bland cells with oval-round nuclei and scant cytoplasm, forming acinar structures and solid nests
- Acinar structures typically with scant atrophic luminal cytoplasm
- Variably sized nucleoli, including prominent ones, and occasional mitoses
- Basaloid nests with peripheral palisading and cribriform architecture constituting the adenoid basal cell pattern
- Cylindroma-like areas present
- May contain well-formed calcifications

Immunopathology (including immunohistochemistry)

- Antibodies to basal cells (p63, 34βE12) are positive in the constituent cells of basal cell adenoma, although often only the peripheral cells are positive.
- Ki-67 and bcl2 can be used to distinguish basal cell adenoma from basal cell carcinoma, with basal cell adenoma showing lower expression of both these biological markers than the basal cell carcinoma.

Molecular diagnostics

- No specific information available on this variant

Main differential diagnosis

- Basal cell hyperplasia can be considered a variant of nodular basal cell hyperplasia; it is a benign lesion regardless of the term used.
- HGPIN is composed of glands that fit within the normal architectural pattern of the prostate, such that the glands are not as crowded as in basal cell adenoma. HGPIN also does not form a nodule. The glands of HGPIN tend to have more columnar nuclei with more apical cytoplasm; nuclei within both HGPIN and basal cell hyperplasia may have very prominent nucleoli.
- Basal cell adenoma consists of a relatively circumscribed nodule, whereas basal cell carcinoma is infiltrative. There are also certain patterns seen in benign basal cell proliferations, as opposed to basal cell carcinoma (see Chapter 16, "Basal Cell Hyperplasia," in this section). Overexpression of Bcl2 or an elevated Ki-67 above 5% also favors basal cell Carcinoma.

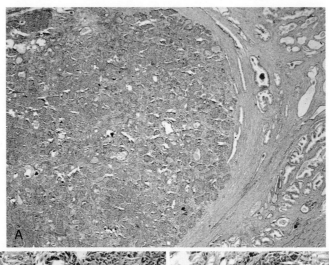

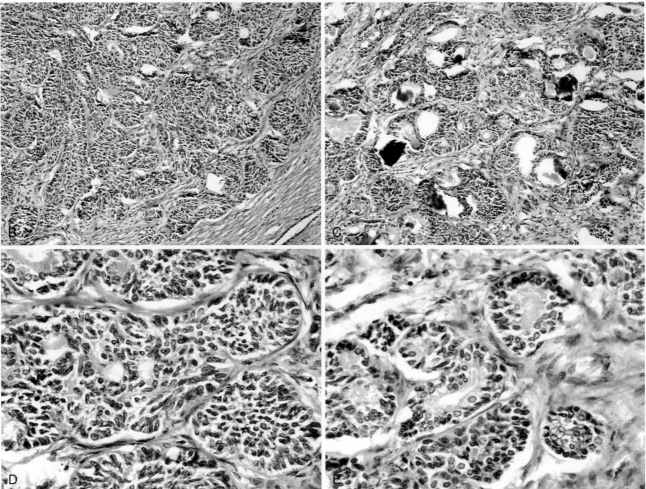

Fig 1. **A,** Well-circumscribed nodule of basal cell adenoma. **B,** Basal cell adenoma consisting of crowded solid basaloid nests. **C,** Many of the nests contain well-formed calcifications. **D,** Higher magnification of basaloid nests with ovoid to slightly spindled nuclei with scant cytoplasm. Occasional small nucleoli are identified. **E,** Area of basal cell adenoma with gland formation. Glands are lined by multilayered basaloid cells with scant cytoplasm. Glands have atrophic cytoplasm at the luminal border in contrast to usual prostatic carcinoma.

Definition
- A variant of cancer that shows basal cell differentiation with multiple patterns: (1) resembling its namesake in the skin, comprising large basaloid nests with peripheral palisading and necrosis; (2) histologic similarity to adenoid cystic carcinoma of salivary gland origin, sometimes termed *adenoid cystic carcinoma;* (3) resembling basal cell hyperplasia; and (4) composed of variably sized and shaped basaloid nests

Clinical features
Epidemiology
- Affects elderly men with rare cases reported in younger patients

Presentation
- May be clinically asymptomatic
- May appear with lower urinary tract symptoms of bladder outlet obstruction

Prognosis and treatment
- Distant metastases are most frequently associated with cases composed of solid basaloid nests with central necrosis.
- Locally infiltrative growth is seen with other patterns of basal cell carcinoma.
- Therapeutic options are radical prostatectomy, radiotherapy, and chemotherapy.

Pathology
Histology
- Histologic findings are variable.
- Solid basaloid nests and islands with peripheral palisading and areas with central necrosis are present.
- An adenoid cystic pattern with cribriform glands closely resembles its namesake in the salivary gland.
- Medium-sized and large basaloid nests are variable in size and shape.
- Histology is identical to basal cell hyperplasia, with the exception of evidence of malignancy such as a highly infiltrative pattern between benign glands, perineural invasion, or extraprostatic extension.
- Stromal desmoplasia is a useful finding in some basal cell carcinomas because it is absent in basal cell hyperplasia, which at most can have a myxoid background.
- Some basal cell carcinomas have a dual cell population, with inner glands having abundant eosinophilic cytoplasm, a feature not seen in basal cell hyperplasia.

Immunopathology (including immunohistochemistry)
- Immunoreactivity for 34βE12 is observed in the malignant cells, confirming their relationship with prostatic basal cells.
- S-100 staining is reported as weak to intensely positive in approximately 50% of tumor cells.
- Anti-smooth muscle actin (HHF35) reactivity is absent.
- Strong Bcl-2 positivity and high Ki-67 indices are found in some basal cell carcinomas compared with basal cell hyperplasia, in which Ki-67 indices are usually less than 5%.

Molecular diagnostics
- No specific information available on this variant

Main differential diagnosis
- Basal cell hyperplasia: see Histology.

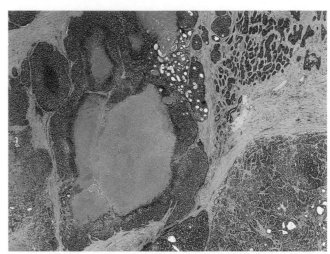

Fig 1. Solid nest of basal cell carcinoma with central necrosis.

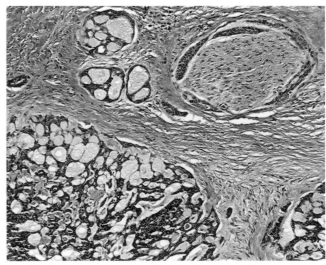

Fig 2. Adenoid cystic pattern with perineural invasion.

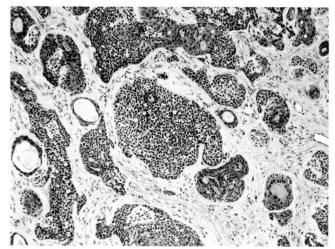

Fig 3. Variably sized and shapes of basaloid nests. Note inner glands with eosinophilic cytoplasm.

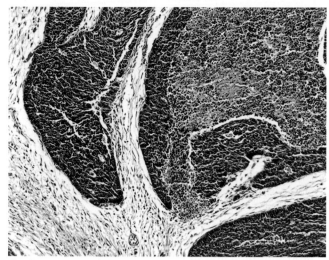

Fig 6. Solid nests of basal cell carcinoma with desmoplastic stromal reaction.

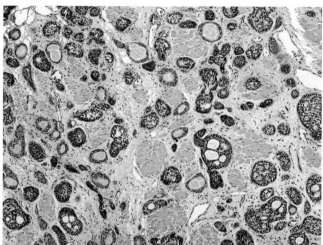

Fig 4. Individual nests and small glands with focal cribriform formation resembling basal cell hyperplasia, except for the invasion of thick muscle bundles consistent with bladder neck invasion.

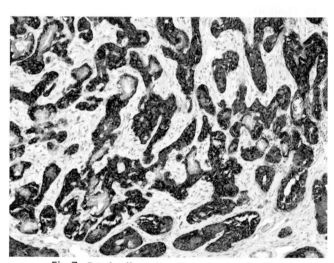

Fig 7. Basal cell carcinoma expressing 34βE12.

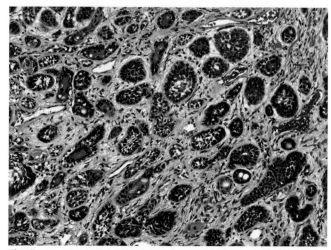

Fig 5. Small nests and tubules resembling basal cell hyperplasia. Note that some have inner cells with abundant eosinophilic cytoplasm, which is diagnostic of basal cell carcinoma.

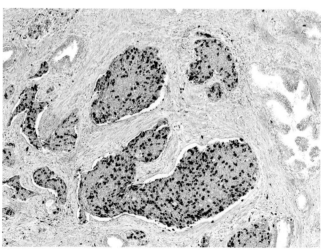

Fig 8. Solid pattern of basal cell carcinoma with elevated Ki-67. Basal cell hyperplasia typically shows less than 5% positivity.

Definition

- Urothelial carcinoma can involve the prostatic tissue by direct extension from an invasive bladder cancer (pT4), or CIS can extend to involve the prostatic urethra with growth down the prostatic ducts and acini, with or without prostatic stromal invasion.

Clinical features

Epidemiology

- Patient age ranges from 45 to 90 years.
- Primary urothelial carcinoma of the prostate is rare, accounting for 0.7% to 2.8% of all prostate cancers.
- Secondary spread from a bladder primary is much more common and can be seen in up to 45% of the cystoprostatectomy specimens from patients with invasive urothelial carcinoma.

Presentation

- Patients often have urinary obstruction and hematuria.
- Digital rectal examination may show irregularity in the prostate.
- PSA may be slightly elevated.

Prognosis and treatment

- Treatment depends on the presence or absence of prostatic stromal invasion.
  - In the absence of tumor prostatic stromal invasion, patients are usually treated with cystoprostatectomy. Intravesical BCG or mitomycin may be tried in some older patients, those with significant comorbidity, or those having radical transurethral resection because of patient preference.
  - In the presence of tumor prostatic stromal invasion, patients are usually treated with radical cystoprostatectomy and regional lymph node dissection.
- Prognosis depends on the presence or absence of prostatic stromal invasion.
  - With stromal invasion, the prognosis is poor with a mean survival of 18 months.
  - Without stromal invasion, the prognosis depends on the stage of the bladder cancer.

Pathology

Histology

- Noninvasive cancer
  - Usually urothelial carcinoma fills and expands periurethral glands, prostatic ducts, and acini, with frequent central comedonecrosis.
  - Usually high-grade urothelial carcinoma shows marked nuclear pleomorphism and frequent mitotic activity.
  - There may be pagetoid spread or burrowing of tumor cells between the basal cell and secretory cell layers in the prostate glands.
  - There is commonly involvement of the prostatic tissue at the 5- and 7-o'clock positions at the verumontanum level.
- Invasive cancer
  - Stromal invasion is characterized by irregular stromal infiltration of neoplastic nests, sheets, or single cells, often associated with a prominent desmoplastic stromal response.

Immunopathology

- Positive for CK7, variably for CK20
- p63, high-molecular-weight cytokeratin, and thrombomodulin are positive in approximately two thirds of cases.
- Uroplakin may be positive but can be lost in poorly differentiated urothelial carcinoma.
- PSA, PAP, prostate-specific membrane antigen (PSMA), and P501S are negative.

Main differential diagnosis

- Poorly differentiated prostatic adenocarcinoma is in the differential with a poorly differentiated tumor involving both the prostate and bladder. Prostate adenocarcinomas tend to have less pleomorphic nuclei or overt, glandular, vague microacinar differentiation. However, rare prostate cancers can be highly pleomorphic and indistinguishable from urothelial cancer, for which immunostains are needed. Adenocarcinomas are positive for PSA, PSMA, and p501S and are negative for p63, high-molecular-weight cytokeratin, and thrombomodulin. As noted previously, one third of urothelial carcinomas can also be negative for prostatic basal cell markers.
- Intraductal carcinoma of the prostate can mimic intraductal spread of urothelial carcinoma. Typically, in addition to solid nests, intraductal carcinoma of the prostate also shows cribriform glandular structures and is accompanied by small glands of prostate cancer. Intraductal carcinoma of the prostate has the same immunohistochemistry as infiltrating high-grade prostate cancer.

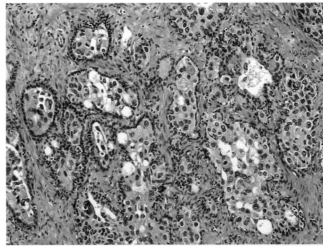

Fig 1. Urothelial carcinoma involves prostatic ducts and acini, but does not invade prostatic stroma.

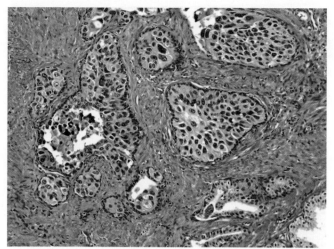

Fig 2. Urothelial carcinoma involves and expands prostatic ducts and acini with focal necrosis.

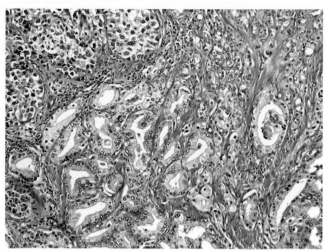

Fig 5. Collision tumor with both urothelial carcinoma *(upper left)* and prostatic adenocarcinoma.

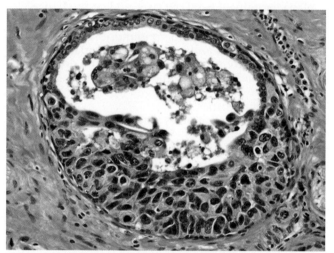

Fig 3. Urothelial carcinoma burrows between the secretory cell and basal cell layers.

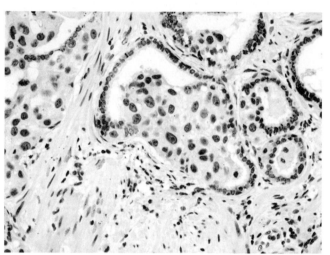

Fig 6. Urothelial carcinoma cells are negative for prostein (p501S), but prostatic glandular cells are positive.

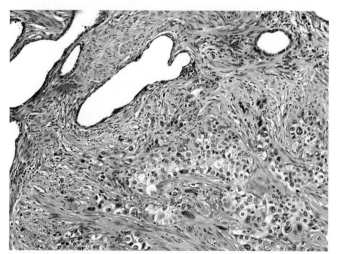

Fig 4. Urothelial carcinoma invades prostatic stroma and induces desmoplastic reaction.

PROSTATIC STROMAL TUMORS OF UNCERTAIN MALIGNANT POTENTIAL

Definition
- Stromal tumors of uncertain malignant potential (STUMPs) are tumors arising from the specialized prostatic stroma. Prior synonyms include *atypical stromal (smooth muscle) hyperplasia, phyllodes type of atypical stromal hyperplasia, phyllodes tumor,* and *cystic epithelial-stromal tumor.*

Clinical features
Epidemiology
- Affects adult men of older age groups

Presentation
- Symptoms of lower urinary tract obstruction followed by abnormal findings on digital rectal examination, hematuria, hematospermia, rectal fullness, or a palpable rectal mass are most common.
- The patient may be clinically asymptomatic.

Prognosis and treatment
- STUMPs can recur frequently and rapidly after incomplete excision.
- They often involve the peripheral zone, where they can be adherent to the rectum.
- Rarely STUMPs can be associated with stromal sarcoma concurrently or with progression to stromal sarcoma over time. Histologic subtypes of STUMP do not correlate with clinical behavior or association to sarcoma.
- Most STUMPs are confined to the prostate and rarely progress to sarcoma, such that in general they are associated with a good prognosis.
- Patient age, treatment preference, presence and size of the lesion on rectal examination or imaging studies, and extent of the lesion on tissue sampling are all factors to consider in deciding whether to proceed with definitive resection for STUMPs diagnosed on biopsy or treat with expectant management.

Pathology
- The most common pattern seen in approximately 50% of STUMPs is hypercellular stroma with scattered stromal cells containing pleomorphic yet degenerative-appearing nuclei admixed with benign prostatic glands. Stromal mitotic figures are typically absent, and atypical mitoses should not be seen.

- The second pattern of STUMP comprises hypercellular stroma composed of bland fusiform stromal cells with eosinophilic cytoplasm admixed with benign glands.
- The phyllodes pattern is another pattern with leaf-like hypocellular fibrous stroma covered by benign-appearing prostatic epithelium.
- The final pattern of STUMP is composed of extensive myxoid stroma containing bland stromal cells, often lacking admixed glands.
- Mixtures of the various patterns can be seen.
- The glands in a STUMP are histologically benign, although they may be more crowded with papillary infolding than acini in the surrounding uninvolved prostate. Other benign epithelial proliferations seen in STUMPs include urothelial metaplasia, squamous metaplasia, basal cell hyperplasia, adenosis, cribriform hyperplasia, prominent basal cell layer, and cystic change.

Immunopathology (including immunohistochemistry)
- Positive for CD34 and vimentin with variable immunoreactivity for smooth muscle actin and desmin
- Progesterone receptor frequently present

Molecular diagnostics
- No specific information available on this variant

Main differential diagnosis
- Stromal sarcoma: see Chapter 19, "Prostatic Stromal Sarcoma," in this section.
- Stromal nodular hyperplasia: a pure stromal nodule of benign prostate hyperplasia (BPH) consists of nodules, whereas the myxoid variant of STUMP is composed of sheets of stroma without nodularity. In addition, stromal nodules of BPH characteristically have thick-walled arterioles when viewed in cross-section.
- Crowded glands of BPH: because of the associated benign glandular proliferations seen with STUMP, it may be confused with glandular predominant BPH. The presence of marked increased cellularity of the intervening stroma is diagnostic of STUMP.

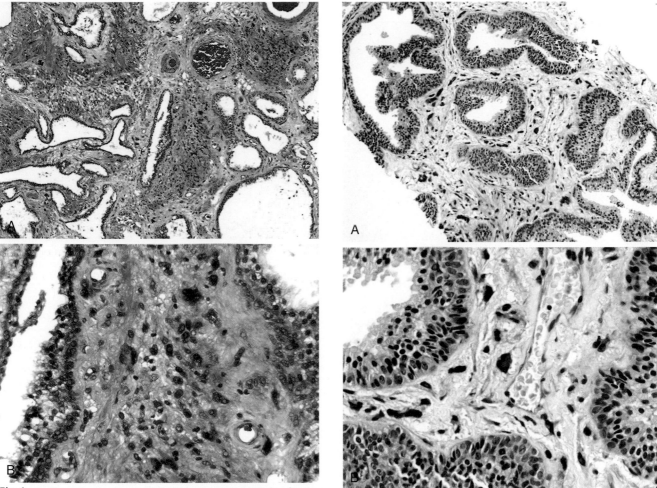

Fig 1. **A,** Transurethral resection of the prostate with focal areas of increased stromal cellularity and scattered atypical nuclei. **B,** Higher magnification shows degenerative atypia.

Fig 2. **A,** Needle biopsy specimen with scattered cells showing hyperchromatic yet degenerative-appearing nuclei. Cellularity is not increased overall. **B,** Higher magnification demonstrates hyperchromatic nuclei with smudged chromatin and lack of mitotic activity.

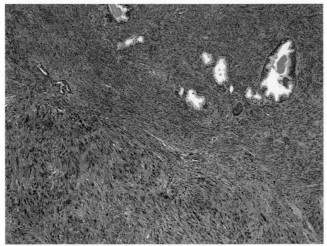

Fig 3. Stromal tumor of uncertain malignant potential with areas showing degenerative atypia *(bottom)* and others with markedly hypercellular stroma without atypia and with eosinophilic cytoplasm between benign prostate glands *(top).*

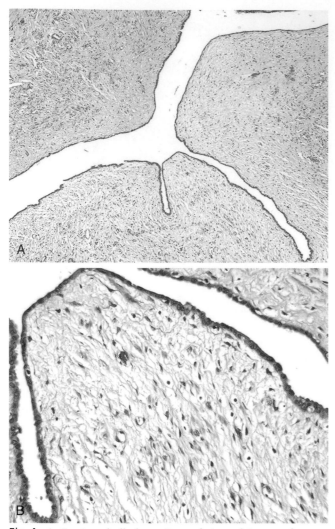

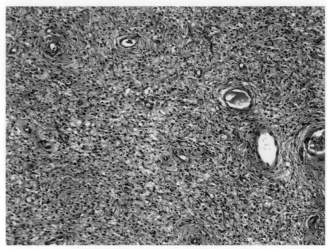

Fig 5. Myxoid pattern of stromal tumor of uncertain malignant potential from a 60-g transurethral resection of the prostate that was diffusely involved without the nodularity seen in stromal nodular benign prostatic hyperplasia.

Fig 4. **A,** Benign phyllodes pattern of stromal tumor of uncertain malignant potential. **B,** Hypocellular fibrous stroma of benign phyllodes tumor beneath benign atrophic prostate epithelium.

Definition
- Stromal sarcomas are malignant tumors arising from the specialized prostatic stroma. It includes malignant phyllodes tumor.

Clinical features
Epidemiology
- Affects adult men of older age groups

Presentation
- Symptoms include lower urinary tract obstruction, abnormal findings on digital rectal examination, hematuria, hematospermia, rectal fullness, or a palpable rectal mass.

Prognosis and treatment
- Stromal sarcomas can extend out of the prostate and metastasize to distant sites, such as bone, lung, abdomen, and retroperitoneum.
- Treatment for stromal sarcoma is typically radical prostatectomy depending on the age of the patient.
- There are few data regarding the use of radiotherapy or chemotherapy.

Pathology
- Stromal sarcomas have variable histology with phyllodes, storiform, epithelioid, or fibrosarcomatous patterns, or they may be patternless.
- Lesions may be circumscribed or infiltrate between benign prostatic glands.
- Stromal sarcomas have one or more of the following features within the spindle cell component: hypercellularity, cytologic atypia, mitotic figures, or necrosis.
- Stromal sarcomas can be subclassified into low and high grades, with high-grade tumors being defined by marked pleomorphism and hypercellularity often with increased mitotic activity and occasional necrosis.
- As with STUMP, a variety of benign glandular proliferations may accompany the stromal sarcoma (see Chapter 18, "Prostatic Stromal Tumors of Uncertain Malignant Potential," in this section).

Immunopathology (including immunohistochemistry)
- Positive for CD34 and vimentin with variable immunoreactivity for smooth muscle actin and desmin
- Progesterone receptor frequently present

Molecular diagnostics
- No specific information available on this variant

Main differential diagnosis
- STUMP: low-grade stromal sarcomas are distinguished from STUMP by the variable presence of moderately marked hypercellularity, moderate nuclear pleomorphism (excluding degenerative atypia), and mitotic activity.
- Other sarcomas: in general, if a sarcoma primary in the prostate does not have the morphology of a specific sarcoma (i.e., lacks the organized fascicular growth pattern of leiomyosarcoma), and especially if it expresses CD34 and progesterone receptor, it can be classified as stromal sarcoma.

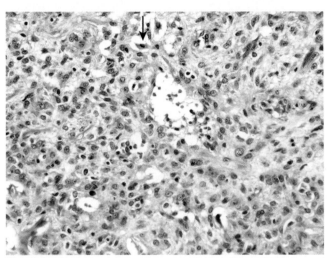

Fig 1. Stromal sarcoma that is patternless. Note the increased cellularity and scattered mitotic figures *(arrow)*.

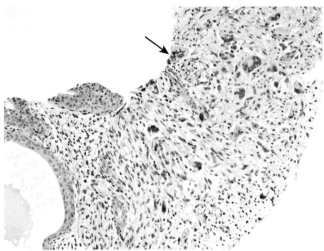

Fig 2. Stromal sarcoma, which differs from stromal tumor of uncertain malignant potential by marked increased stromal cellularity and atypical mitotic figure *(arrow)*.

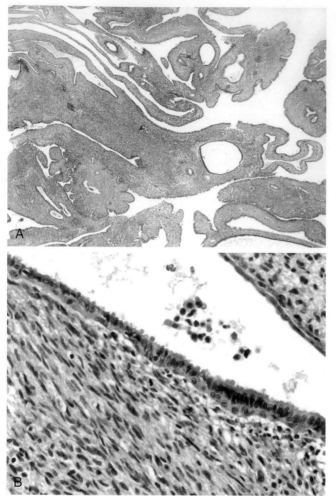

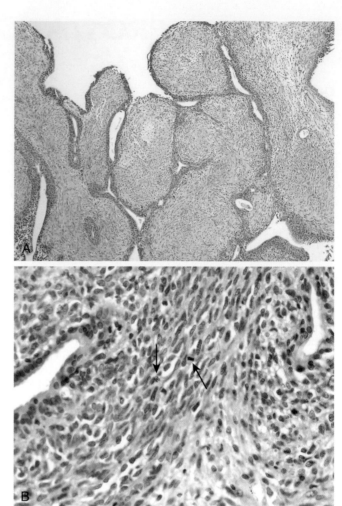

Fig 3. **A,** Malignant phyllodes tumor. **B,** High magnification shows markedly hypercellular mitotically active stroma beneath benign prostate gland.

Fig 4. **A,** Malignant phyllodes tumor. **B,** Markedly hypercellular stroma with mitoses *(arrows)* intermixed with benign prostate glands.

ATYPICAL GLANDS SUSPICIOUS FOR CARCINOMA

Definition
- Small focus of atypical glands suggestive of, but not diagnostic for, prostatic adenocarcinoma

Clinical features
Epidemiology
- Occurs in an average of 5% of prostate needle biopsies (range, 0.7% to 23%)

Presentation
- There is no specific presentation; as with all patients, prostate biopsy is typically done following increased PSA or abnormal findings on digital rectal examination.

Prognosis and treatment
- The mean risk of cancer on repeated biopsy following an atypical diagnosis is 40.2% (median 38.5%, range 17% to 70%).
- Only a handful of studies show the median time to repeated biopsy (mean, approximately 9 months).
- Nine of 10 studies examining whether serum PSA predicts cancer following an atypical needle biopsy diagnosis showed no correlation.
- Recommend repeated biopsy following a diagnosis of atypical glands, within 6 months.
- For repeated biopsy, extended sampling (two to three cores) of initial atypical site is recommended, along with adjacent ipsilateral and contralateral sites with routine biopsies of the remainder of the prostate.

Pathology
Histology
- There are small atypical glands that lack sufficient architectural or cytologic atypia for a definitive diagnosis of carcinoma or in which the quantity of glands is insufficient for a definitive diagnosis.
- Features qualifying as architectural atypia include small, crowded glands with straight luminal borders and glands that contain blue mucin, crystalloids, or dense secretions.
- Features of cytologic atypia include nuclear enlargement and hyperchromasia, typically with prominent nucleoli.
- Findings that may warrant a diagnosis of atypical glands, even in the presence of significant cytologic or architectural atypia, are:
  - Acute inflammation in or around glands
  - Atypical glands at outer edge of biopsy core where PIN cannot be excluded
  - Pale cytoplasm or papillary infoldings in some atypical glands
  - Adjacent PIN with only a few atypical glands
  - Atrophic cytoplasm
  - Insufficient quantity of atypical glands

Immunopathology
- High-molecular-weight keratin and p63 immunostaining may reveal patchy basal cells or absence of basal cells in atypical glands.
- Absence of basal cells in small atypical glands on immunostaining is not diagnostic of cancer by itself without appropriate histologic features.
- α-Methylacyl-CoA racemase may be negative or positive in atypical glands.

Main differential diagnosis
- Prostatic adenocarcinoma: quantity of atypical glands and cytologic and architectural atypia must be sufficient for this diagnosis.
- PIN typically occurs in larger glands, with papillary infoldings and nuclear atypia. The presence of small crowded glands is not typical of PIN.
- Adenosis is characterized by a fairly well-circumscribed collection of glands of different sizes. The diagnosis of adenosis rests of the nuclear and cytoplasmic similarity of the small crowded glands to admixed larger and more recognizably benign glands. There is typically a patchy basal cell layer on immunostaining.
- Partial atrophy shows minimal cytologic atypia and is typically lobular, with pale cytoplasm, undulating luminal surfaces with papillary infoldings. Cells are often wider than they are tall (i.e., nuclei reach full height of cytoplasm in some areas). There is typically has a patchy basal cell layer on immunostaining.
- Postatrophic hyperplasia is basophilic at low power because of a lack of cytoplasm and has a lobular appearance. Atypia may be mild to moderate. Always exercise extreme caution in diagnosing carcinoma when atypical glands are atrophic.

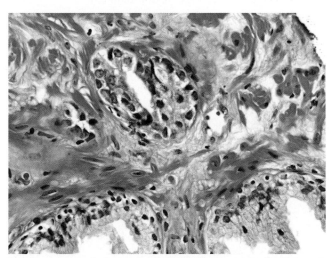

Fig 1. One atypical gland with prominent nucleoli. Although this may represent carcinoma, a tangential section from a high-grade prostatic intraepithelial neoplasia gland cannot be ruled out.

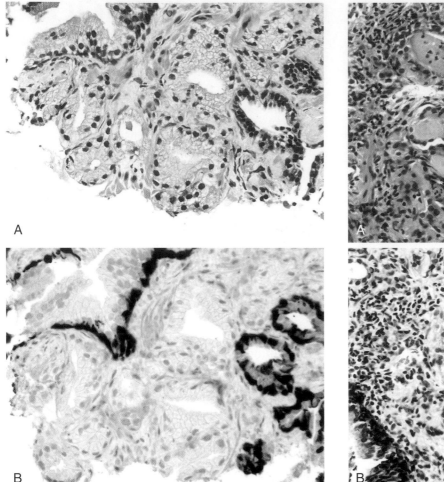

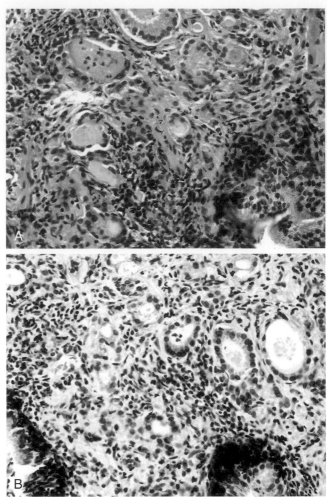

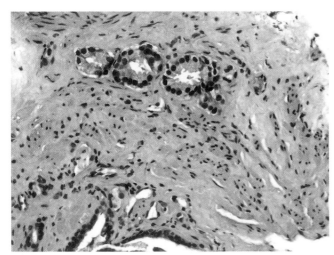

Fig 2. A, Crowded small glands suspicious for carcinoma. However, the glands have pale cytoplasm and lack nuclear atypia such that adenosis cannot be excluded despite negative stains for p63 and high-molecular-weight cytokeratin **(B).**

Fig 4. A, Although the crowded glands are suggestive of carcinoma, they are atrophic and inflamed. **B,** Negative stains for high-molecular-weight cytokeratin make the focus highly suggestive of carcinoma, but a definitive diagnosis of carcinoma is not recommended based on the appearance on hematoxylin and eosin staining.

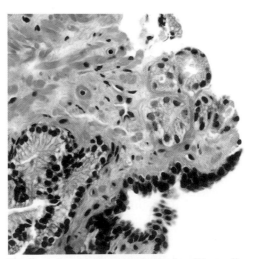

Fig 3. Three atypical glands with slightly hyperchromatic nuclei *(top).*

Fig 5. A few small atypical glands with small nucleoli are seen at the edge of the core. It is important to be more cautious diagnosing cancer on a few atypical glands at the edge because it is not possible to visualize the relationship to surrounding glands (e.g., whether there is adjacent high-grade prostatic intraepithelial neoplasia, adenosis).

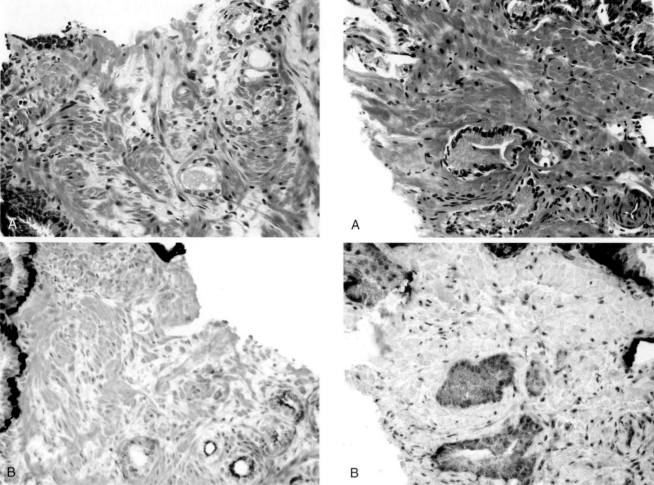

Fig 6. **A,** Small atrophic glands with pale cytoplasm and minimal nuclear atypia. **B,** The glands are positive for α-methylacyl–coenzyme A racemase and negative for basal cell markers. This focus is suggestive of carcinoma; however, a definitive diagnosis of cancer was not rendered because partial atrophy could stain similarly to cancer.

Fig 8. **A,** A few atypical glands with slightly more amphophilic cytoplasm, one with prominent nucleoli are seen *(bottom)*. **B,** Although most of the glands lack basal cells (p63, high-molecular-weight cytokeratin), one had a single basal cell such that a definitive diagnosis of cancer could not be made.

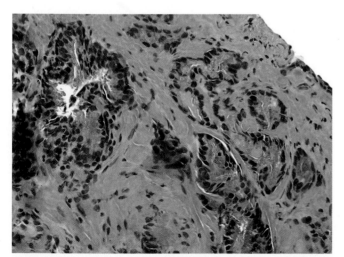

Fig 7. This small focus of atypical glands *(right)* is suggestive of carcinoma in a 46-year-old man. Carcinoma was not diagnosed because of poor cellular preservation and the patient's age.

HIGH-GRADE PROSTATIC INTRAEPITHELIAL NEOPLASIA WITH ADJACENT ATYPICAL GLANDS

Definition
- Focus of HGPIN with adjacent small atypical glands, suggestive of but not diagnostic for prostatic adenocarcinoma (PINATYP)

Clinical features
Epidemiology
- Similar to all men undergoing prostate biopsy

Presentation
- There is no specific presentation; as with all patients, prostate biopsy is typically done following increased PSA or abnormal findings on digital rectal examination.

Prognosis and treatment
- Rate of carcinoma diagnosed on subsequent biopsy is higher than that seen in patients with PIN alone (approximately 40%), although there are few large studies.

Pathology
Histology
- PINATYP consists of a focus of high-grade prostatic intraepithelial neoplasia (HGPIN), with a few small adjacent atypical glands
- These atypical glands may represent tangential sections off of PIN or adjacent infiltrating carcinoma.
- Atypical glands are small, with straight luminal borders, and may contain blue mucin.
- Nuclear atypia similar to or greater than adjacent PIN may be present in small glands, and nucleoli are often prominent.

Immunopathology
- High-molecular-weight keratin and p63 immunostaining may reveal patchy basal cells or the absence of basal cells in atypical glands.
- Absence of basal cells in small atypical glands is not diagnostic of cancer if adjacent PIN is present, because PIN often has a patchy basal cell layer compared with benign glands.
- α-Methylacyl-CoA racemase (p504S) may be negative or positive in atypical glands.

Main differential diagnosis
- PIN typically occurs in larger glands, with papillary infoldings and nuclear atypia. The presence of small atypical glands is not typical of PIN and is more consistent with PINATYP.
- Prostatic adenocarcinoma with adjacent PIN—a diagnosis of carcinoma can only be rendered if glands are too numerous or too far away from HGPIN to represent a tangential section of PIN. It can be extremely difficult to distinguish PINATYP from PIN with cancer, such that in the presence of atypical glands with adjacent PIN, it is recommended that immunohistochemistry for basal cell markers be performed. If there are numerous glands with an absent basal cell layer, a diagnosis of cancer can be rendered. If there are even only a few scattered glands with a patchy basal cell layer, then the diagnosis of PINATYP should be made.

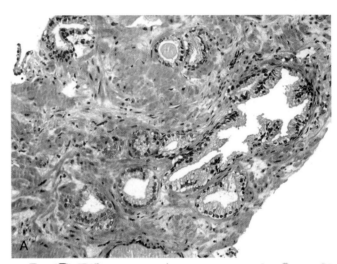

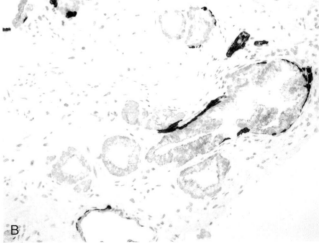

Fig 1. **A,** Prostatic intraepithelial neoplasia with adjacent atypical small glands. **B,** Immunostaining for high-molecular-weight keratin and p63 are negative in the atypical adjacent glands, and racemase is positive; however, their close proximity to prostatic intraepithelial neoplasia makes a definitive diagnosis of carcinoma impossible in this focus.

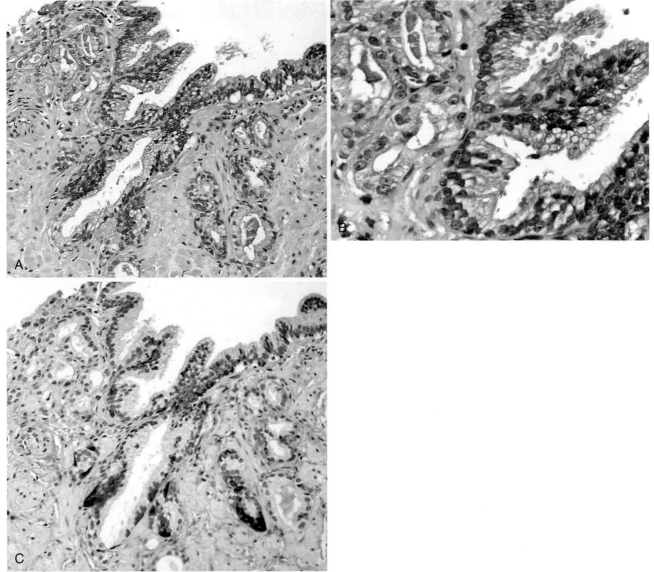

Fig 2. A, Larger gland of prostatic intraepithelial neoplasia, with smaller atypical glands on both sides. **B,** Small glands contain blue mucin and show prominent cytologic atypia with enlarged nucleoli in close proximity to prostatic intraepithelial neoplasia. **C,** Immunostaining for high-molecular-weight keratin and p63 reveals a patchy basal cell layer around the prostatic intraepithelial neoplasia and some adjacent small atypical glands, consistent with PINATYP.

Definition
- Primary effect of radiation therapy is the damage of endothelial cells, which causes ischemia that leads to atrophy.
- Radiation-induced changes on prostatic tissue are variable, more severe, and durable when delivered as interstitial seed implants (brachytherapy) than by external beam, and also vary with the dose and duration of the irradiation.
- Changes associated with radiation may persist for years after the final radiation treatment.

Clinical Features
Epidemiology
- Radiation therapy for prostate cancer may be applied in the form of external beam, interstitial implantation, or a combination of both.

Presentation
- Postradiation biopsies will most commonly be performed 18 to 24 months after the final radiation therapy treatment, because of the length of time required for histologic clearance of tumor.

Prognosis and treatment
- Changes associated with radiation therapy may persist for years after the final radiation treatment.
- Postradiation biopsy has been used as an independent predictor of outcome and of subsequent biochemical disease-free survival.
- Patients with persistent tumor without significant treatment affect after radiation therapy are more likely to demonstrate local disease progression, distant metastases, and die of disease than those with a negative biopsy.

Pathology
Histology
- Effect on benign prostatic tissue
  - Extensive glandular atrophy with stromal predominance (decreased ratio of acini to stroma) is present.
  - Glands retain their lobular architecture, although individual glands often assume irregular, angulated contours.
  - Secretory cells are flattened and atrophic.
  - Basal cells become hyperplastic and multilayered, with scattered markedly atypical nuclei that appear degenerated and occassional prominent nucleoli.
  - Basal cells may display vacuolated cytoplasm.
  - Stroma contains a sparse chronic inflammatory infiltrate.
  - Vascular changes include intimal thickening and medial fibrosis with luminal narrowing and fibrous obliteration.
  - Urothelial and squamous cell metaplasia are common radiation-associated changes.

- Effect on prostatic intraepithelial neoplasia and prostate cancer
  - The prevalence and extent of high-grade prostatic intraepithelial neoplasia is diminished in biopsies performed after radiotherapy.
  - Prostate cancer glands show variable appearance, from no or minimal radiation effect to significant radiation-induced changes.
  - The classic radiation-induced changes in prostate carcinoma are a decrease in number of cancer glands, poorly formed glands and single cancer cells, abundant vacuolated cytoplasm, nuclear pyknosis, and stromal fibrosis.
  - In contrast to irradiated benign glands, nuclear pleomorphism is not common in prostate cancer with therapy effect.
  - Architecturally, the key feature for recognizing the radiated cancer includes closely packed glands with a haphazard infiltrative growth pattern and the presence of infiltrating individual cancer cells.
- Effect on tumor grade
  - Radiation-treated prostate cancer should not be graded, unless prostate biopsy specimens show a minimal degree of treatment effect (Gleason score should be applied in such cases).
  - The degree of postradiation effects may provide important prognostic information in patients with a positive biopsy analysis, because cancers with severe treatment effect appear to have a favorable prognosis.

Immunopathology (including immunohistochemistry)
- Atrophic benign secretory cells and basal cells are positive for basal cell markers.
- Following radiotherapy, some prostate cancer glands can lose PSA expression.

Main differential diagnosis
- The most important differential diagnosis is between prostate cancer without treatment effects and benign prostate glands with radiation effects. Features favoring benign glands with treatment effects include: (1) architecturally normal with more widely spaced glands; (2) multilayered cells; (3) more pronounced atypia with variable-sized nuclei within a gland; (4) often degenerative nuclear atypia, although some radiated benign cells can have prominent nucleoli; (5) streaming of cells parallel to the basement membrane; and (6) positive results of immunohistochemical analysis for basal cell markers.

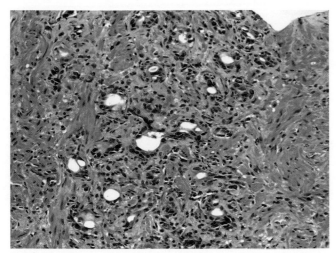

Fig 1. Benign prostatic glands retain their lobular architecture, although individual glands often assume irregular, angulated contours.

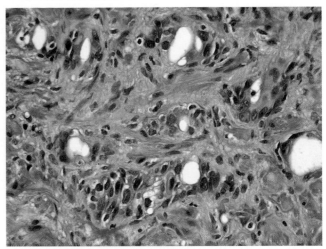

Fig 4. Benign prostatic glands with radiation atypia. Basal cells may display vacuolated cytoplasm.

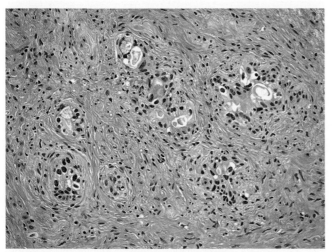

Fig 2. Benign prostatic glands with radiation atypia. Note the glandular atrophy, multilayering, and randomly atypical nuclei.

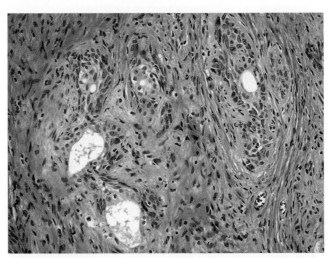

Fig 5. Benign prostatic glands with radiation atypia with prominent multilayering.

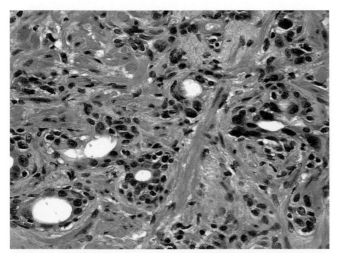

Fig 3. Benign prostatic glands with radiation atypia. Basal cells become hyperplastic and multilayered with scattered markedly atypical nuclei that appear degenerated and hyperchromatic, often without prominent nucleoli.

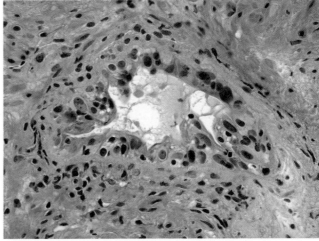

Fig 6. Benign atrophic prostatic glands with radiation atypia.

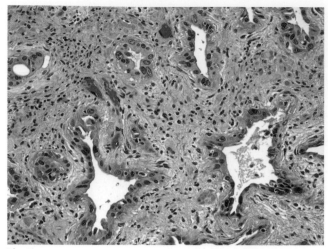

Fig 7. Benign prostatic glands with radiation atypia. The stroma frequently contains a sparse chronic inflammatory infiltrate.

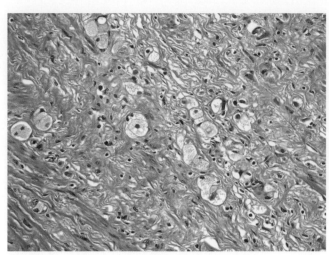

Fig 10. Prostate cancer glands showing significant radiation-induced changes with abundant vacuolated cytoplasm, nuclear pyknosis, and stromal fibrosis.

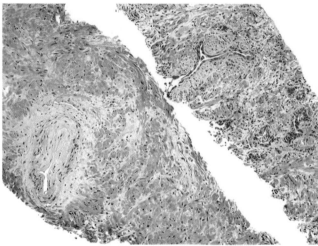

Fig 8. Intimal thickening with luminal narrowing are common vascular changes *(left)* associated with radiation therapy. Core on the right shows benign prostatic glands with radiation atypia.

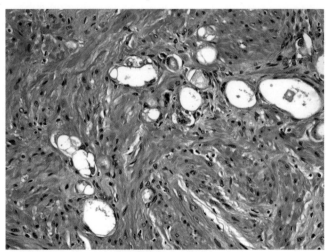

Fig 11. Prostate cancer glands showing significant radiation-induced changes. Note that the cancer glands are poorly formed and decreased in number.

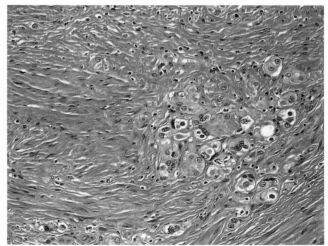

Fig 9. Prostate cancer with radiation-induced changes. Architecturally, the radiated cancer cells and glands are closely packed with a haphazard infiltrative growth pattern. Infiltrating individual cancer cells are noted in the *upper left corner* of the microphotograph.

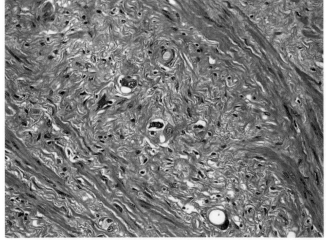

Fig 12. Nuclear pleomorphism is not common in prostate cancer with therapy effect, but can occasionally be seen.

HORMONAL ABLATION–INDUCED CHANGES

Definition
- Androgen deprivation therapy is one of the most popular forms of treatment of prostate cancer.
- Androgen deprivation can be achieved with multiple methods:
  - Orchiectomy
  - Estrogen
  - Gonadotrophin-releasing hormone antagonists (lutenizing hormone–releasing hormone [LH-RH] agonists)
  - Antiandrogen
  - 5α-Reductase inhibitors
- Agents are used for preoperative tumor shrinkage, symptomatic relief of metastases, cancer prophylaxis, and treatment of hyperplasia.

Clinical features
Epidemiology
- Androgen deprivation by surgical castration or pharmacologic blockade has become a common treatment modality for patients with locally advanced or metastatic prostate carcinoma.
- Preoperative (neoadjuvant) hormonal ablation is sometimes used for clinically localized prostate carcinoma to retard tumor growth before surgery if there is a delay between biopsy and definitive resection.

Presentation
- Typical side effects of androgen deprivation therapy include hot flashes, loss of libido, and impotence.

Prognosis and treatment
- Neoadjuvant hormonal therapy may be able to downstage the disease and decrease the positive margin rate, although the cure rate is not affected.
- Most studies have reported a decrease of extraprostatic extension between surgically and hormonally treated patients.

Pathology
Histology
- Effect on benign prostate glands
  - Decreased glandular elements are accompanied by increased, sometimes hypercellular stromal tissue with scattered lymphocytic infiltrates.
  - Prostatic acini are atrophic and collapsed, typically with prominent basal cell hyperplasia and squamous metaplasia and epithelial cell vacuolization.
  - Luminal secretory cells become atrophic and exhibit nuclear pyknosis, inconspicuous nucleoli, and cytoplasmic clearing.
- Effect on prostatic intraepithelial neoplasia and prostate cancer
  - Following hormone therapy, high-grade prostatic intraepithelial neoplasia may be significantly less extensive, and nucleolar prominence is much less evident.
  - The neoplastic glands tend to be smaller and atrophic with compressed or obliterated lumina.
  - Tumor cells develop pyknotic nuclei and abundant foamy or clear vacuolated cytoplasm.
  - Sometimes single tumor cells are widely scattered within the stroma resembling histiocytes.
  - Dissolution of tumor cells leaving empty clefts or mucin aggregates can also be seen (mucinous degeneration).
  - Ruptured malignant glands with mucin extravasation is common; the cells of neoplastic glands may be almost completely degenerated, leaving irregular, mucinous pools with rare cancerous cells.
  - Occasional cases display the "vanishing cancer phenomenon," in which no residual cancer is found in the radical prostatectomy specimen.
- Effect on tumor grade, stage, and surgical margins
  - Hormone-treated prostate cancer should not be graded.
  - Neoadjuvant hormonal therapy may be able to downstage the disease and decrease positive margin rate by shrinkage of the prostate gland.

Immunopathology (including immunohistochemistry)
- PSA, PSAP, and racemase expression can decline after long androgen blockade therapy.
- Prostate cancer cells after hormonal treatment are still positive for pan-cytokeratin and negative for HMWCK and p63.

Main differential diagnosis
- Atrophic and hyperplastic changes in benign glands
  - Clear cell cribriform hyperplasia
  - Sclerosing adenosis
  - Acinar atrophy
  - Postatrophic hyperplasia
  - Atypical adenomatous hyperplasia
  - Atypical basal cell hyperplasia
- Minute clusters of tumor cells
  - Lymphocytes
  - Fibroblasts

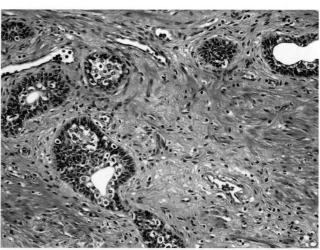

Fig 1. After androgen deprivation therapy, benign prostatic acini are atrophic and collapsed, typically with prominent basal cell hyperplasia and epithelial cell vacuolization.

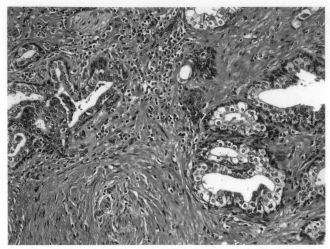

Fig 2. Benign prostatic tissue shows decreased glandular elements accompanied by increased, sometimes hypercellular stromal tissue with scattered lymphocytic infiltrate.

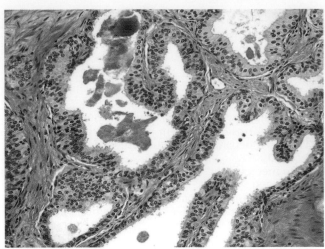

Fig 5. Following hormone therapy, high-grade prostatic intraepithelial neoplasia may be significantly less extensive, and nucleolar prominence is less evident.

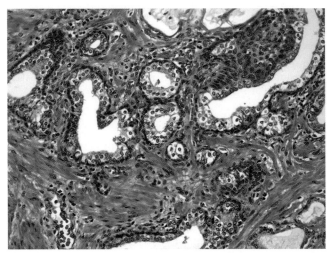

Fig 3. Benign prostatic luminal secretory cells become atrophic and exhibit nuclear pyknosis, inconspicuous nucleoli, and cytoplasmic clearing.

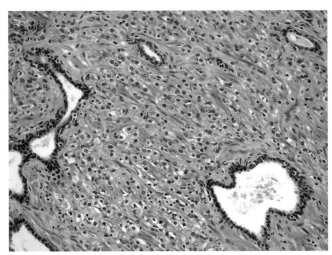

Fig 6. Prostatic adenocarcinoma with marked nuclear shrinkage and distortion (pyknotic nuclei).

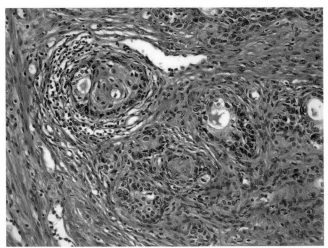

Fig 4. Benign atrophic prostatic acini may show squamous metaplasia.

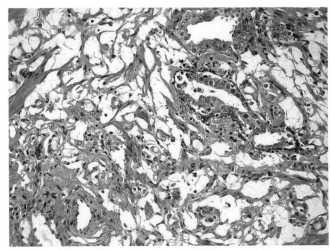

Fig 7. Prostatic adenocarcinoma with prominent dissolution of tumor cells leaving empty clefts. Note the entrapped gland high-grade prostatic intraepithelial neoplasia.

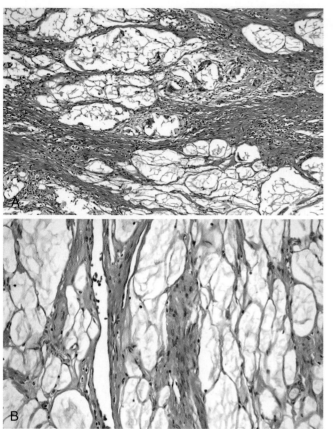

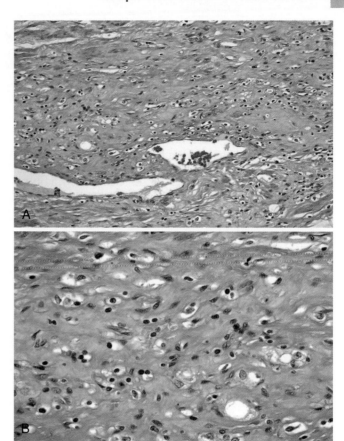

Fig 8. Prostatic adenocarcinoma with prominent mucin extravasation. **A,** When rupture of malignant glands occur, the cells of neoplastic glands may be almost completely degenerated, leaving irregular acid mucinous pools with rare cancerous cells. **B,** Note the rare cancer gland *(lower right).*

Fig 9. **A,** Sometimes, single tumor cells are widely scattered within the stroma resembling histiocytes. **B,** At higher magnification, the presence of nucleoli and the occasional lumen formation should raise the suspicion of residual adenocarcinoma with androgen deprivation therapy effect.

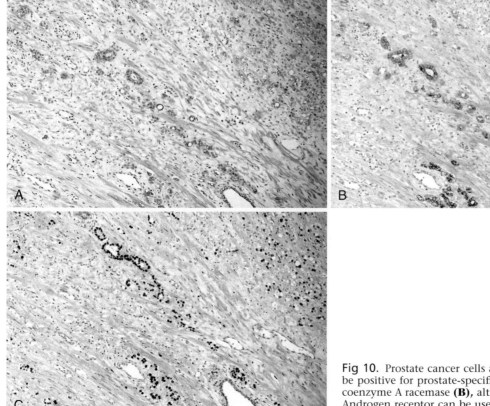

Fig 10. Prostate cancer cells after hormonal treatment can still be positive for prostate-specific antigen **(A),** and α-methylacyl–coenzyme A racemase **(B),** although the expression can decline. Androgen receptor can be useful in a subset of cases because its intensity of staining is less affected by treatment **(C).**

Definition
- *Cryosurgical ablation* refers to rapid deep freezing of the prostate gland.
- Multiple cryoprobe needles filled with circulating liquid nitrogen transform the prostate into an ice ball.
- Cryoablation results in substantial tissue destruction and death of benign and malignant cells.
- The flow of liquid nitrogen through the probes is adjusted to create the desired freezing pattern and extent of tissue destruction in the prostate.
- Liquid nitrogen does not come in contact with tissue.
- Given the focal nature of the treatment, the histologic changes are most likely to be confined to the targeted areas.

Clinical features
Epidemiology
- Cryotherapy of the prostate represents a potential treatment for localized recurrent prostate cancer after external beam radiotherapy.

Prognosis and treatment
- Several studies have reported salvage cryotherapy results with biopsy-proven local failure after external beam radiotherapy.
- The presence of residual or recurrent cancer in histopathologic evaluation after cryotherapy is a worrisome finding; it is considered evidence of inadequate cryotherapy and inadequate radiotherapy.

Pathology
Histology
- Effect on benign prostate glands and stroma
  - Features of repair include marked stromal fibrosis and hyalinization, basal cell hyperplasia with ductal and acinar regeneration, squamous and urothelial metaplasia, stromal hemorrhage, and hemosiderin deposition.
  - Coagulative necrosis is present between 6 and 30 weeks from therapy, but patchy chronic inflammation is more common afterward.
  - Focal granulomatous inflammation is associated with epithelial disruption resulting from corpora amylacea.
  - Dystrophic calcification is infrequent and usually appears in areas with the greatest reparative response.
  - As the postoperative interval increases, biopsy specimens are more likely to contain unaltered benign prostatic tissue.
- Effect on prostatic intraepithelial neoplasia and prostate cancer
  - Biopsy after cryosurgery may reveal no evidence of recurrent or residual carcinoma, even in some patients with elevated PSA.
  - In some cases, the cancer appears unchanged, with no change in grade or definite evidence of tissue or immune response, indicating a lack of inclusion of that area in the ablation killing zone.

- Effect on tumor grade
  - There is no consensus regarding grading after cryoablation therapy.
  - Most pathologists routinely report Gleason grade.

Immunopathology (including immunohistochemistry)
- HMWCK, p63, and racemase expression persist after cryoablation and are of diagnostic value in separating treated adenocarcinoma and its mimics.

Main differential diagnosis
- Prostatic infarct, yet diffuse nature of the necrosis along with the clinical history of cryotherapy, rules out an infarct.

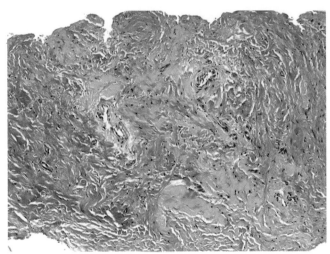

Fig 1. Prostate biopsy specimen after cryotherapy showing marked stromal fibrosis and hyalinization.

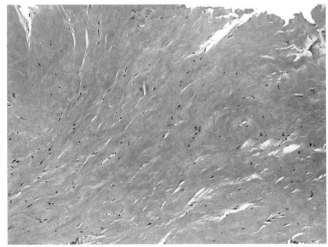

Fig 2. Prostate biopsy specimen after cryotherapy showing extensive dense stromal fibrosis.

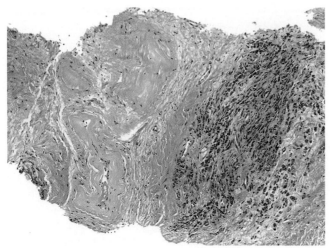

Fig 3. Prostate needle biopsy core specimen showing fibrosis, hyalinization, and hemosiderin deposition.

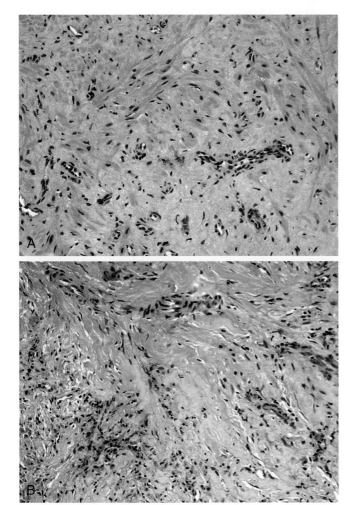

Fig 4. The amount of hemosiderin can vary from focal perivascular deposition (A) to more prominent perivascular and diffuse stromal deposition (B).

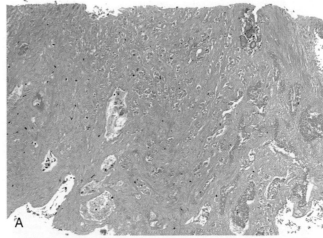

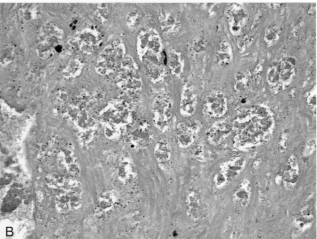

Fig 5. A, Coagulative necrosis may present between 6 and 30 weeks following cryotherapy. B, High-power view of an area of coagulative necrosis showing ghost tumor cells.

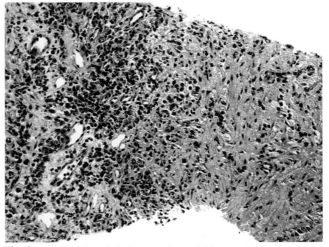

Fig 6. Patchy chronic inflammation within prostatic stroma is a common finding after cryoablation.

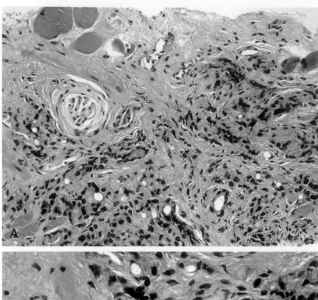

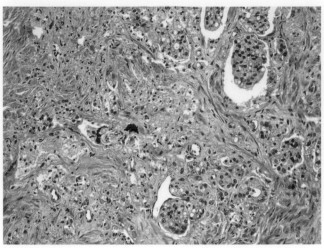

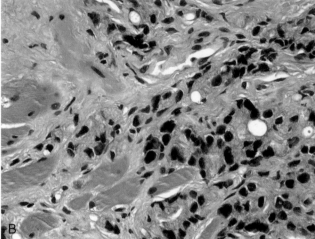

Fig 8. Residual, recurrent prostatic adenocarcinoma with focal evidence *(left)* of treatment effect. Occasional tumor cells show pyknotic nuclei and degenerated granular eosinophilic cytoplasm.

Fig 7. Residual, recurrent prostatic adenocarcinoma **(A)** with no change in grade or definite evidence of tissue or immune response indicating lack of treatment effect **(B)**.

IMMUNOHISTOCHEMICAL WORK-UP OF PROSTATE CARCINOMA

Pathology
Immunohistochemistry
- Guideline for using immunohistochemistry in the work-up of prostate biopsies
  - It applies to selected cases whose differential diagnosis includes prostate carcinoma (PCa) based on histologic evaluation.
  - Immunostain must be performed and interpreted in the context of H&E morphology.
    - Clearly define benign and atypical glands on H&E slide.
    - Define the nature of atypical glands: favors PCa versus benign.
    - Use immunostain results to corroborate H&E diagnosis.
- Commonly used immunohistochemical markers for differential diagnosis of prostate carcinoma
  - Markers to distinguish prostate carcinoma from its mimics
    - Basal cell markers
      - HMWCK
      - p63
    - AMACR (p504S)
    - ETS gene fusion product ERG
  - Markers to distinguish prostate carcinoma from nonprostatic malignancy secondarily involving prostate
    - Cytokeratin 7 and 20
    - Prostate basal cell markers
      - HMWCK
      - p63
    - Prostate-specific markers
      - PSA
      - PAP
      - PSMA
      - p501S
    - Other tissue-specific lineage markers
      - TTF-1
      - CDX2
- Basal cell markers
  - HMWCK: cytoplasmic antigen detected by several antibody preparations (34βE12, CK5/6, CK14)
  - p63: nuclear antigen
  - Basal cell cocktail (34βE12 plus p63)
  - Prostate carcinoma lacks basal cells and staining for basal cell markers
  - Adenosis, partial atrophy, and HGPIN possibly having discontinuous or absent basal cell lining
- AMACR (p504S)
  - Positive in 80% of prostate carcinomas in needle biopsy specimens
  - Lower positive rate in several prostate carcinoma histologic variants (foamy gland, atrophic and pseudohyperplastic)
  - Positive in more than 90% of HGPINs, 20% of adenosis, some partial atrophy, occasional morphologic benign glands
- Basal cell marker plus an AMACR cocktail
  - Combine both basal cell marker (HMWCK or p63, or both) and AMACR in the same staining reaction
  - Staining sensitivity and specificity similar to each antibody used separately
  - Useful on prostate biopsy specimen containing small focus of cancer
- ETS gene fusion product ERG
  - ERG immunostaining highly specific for TMPRSS2-ERG gene fusion
  - Positive in 40% to 50% of prostate cancers and in 20% of HGPINs that intermingle with PCa
  - Positive staining exceedingly rare in other noncancerous glands distant from PCa

Main differential diagnosis
- Prostate carcinoma: pan-cytokeratin positive, basal cell marker negative, AMACR positive, prostate-specific marker positive
- Prostate carcinoma with treatment effect: pan-cytokeratin positive, basal cell marker negative, AMACR positive (may be reduced), prostate-specific marker positive (may be reduced)
- Normal prostate or nonprostatic structures
  - SEVD: pan-cytokeratin positive, basal cell marker positive, AMACR negative, prostate-specific marker negative, MUC6 positive
  - Verumontanum mucosal gland hyperplasia: pan-cytokeratin positive, basal cell marker positive, AMACR negative, prostate-specific marker positive
  - Cowper glands: pan-cytokeratin positive, basal cell marker positive, AMACR negative, prostate-specific marker negative (variable PSA staining), mucicarmine positive, PAS-D positive, Alcian blue positive
  - Paraganglia: pan-cytokeratin negative, basal cell marker negative, AMACR negative, prostate-specific marker negative, neuroendocrine markers positive
  - Mesonephric remnants: pan-cytokeratin positive, basal cell marker variable, AMACR negative, prostate-specific marker negative
- Benign prostatic lesion
  - Partial atrophy: pan-cytokeratin positive, basal cell marker variable, AMACR variable, prostate-specific marker positive
  - Postatrophic hyperplasia: pan-cytokeratin positive, basal cell marker positive, AMACR negative, prostate-specific marker positive
  - Urothelial metaplasia: pan-cytokeratin positive, basal cell marker positive, AMACR negative, prostate-specific marker negative
  - Squamous metaplasia: pan-cytokeratin positive, basal cell marker positive, AMACR negative, prostate-specific marker negative
  - Basal cell hyperplasia: pan-cytokeratin positive, basal cell marker positive, AMACR negative, prostate-specific marker variable
  - Adenosis: pan-cytokeratin positive, basal cell marker variable, AMACR variable, prostate-specific marker positive
  - Sclerosing adenosis: pan-cytokeratin positive, basal cell marker positive, AMACR negative prostate-specific marker positive, SMA positive, S100 positive

- Nonspecific granulomatous prostatitis: pan-cytokeratin negative, basal cell marker negative, AMACR negative, prostate-specific marker negative, CD68+
- BPH: pan-cytokeratin positive, basal cell marker positive, AMACR negative, prostate-specific marker positive

- HGPIN: pan-cytokeratin positive, basal cell marker variable, AMACR positive, prostate-specific marker positive
- Intraductal carcinoma of the prostate: pan-cytokeratin positive, basal cell marker positive, AMACR positive, prostate-specific marker positive

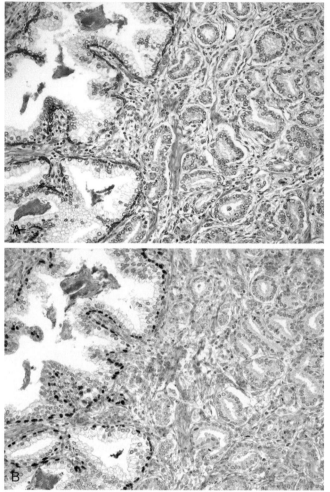

Fig 1. Prostate cancer lacks basal cell marker high-molecular-weight cytokeratin **(A)** and p63 **(B).**

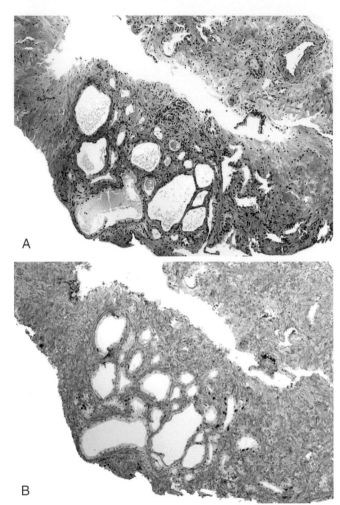

Fig 3. Partial atrophy **(A)** is focally positive for basal cell marker p63 **(B).** A few glands are entirely negative for p63.

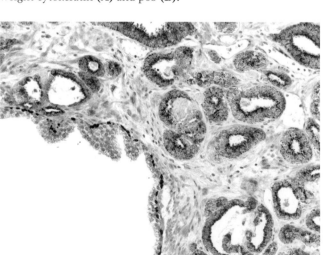

Fig 2. Cancer glands stained with an antibody cocktail containing both p63 and α-methylacyl–coenzyme A racemase (AMACR) antibodies. Cancer glands are negative for p63. The AMACR staining appears granular predominantly in the apical portion of cancer glands. An adjacent benign gland is focally and weakly positive for AMACR.

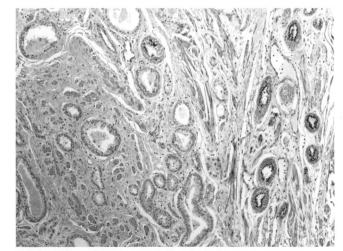

Fig 4. Heterogeneous α-methylacyl–coenzyme A racemase staining in cancer glands. The staining is strong in some cancer glands and weak or negative in others.

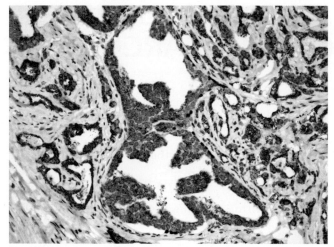

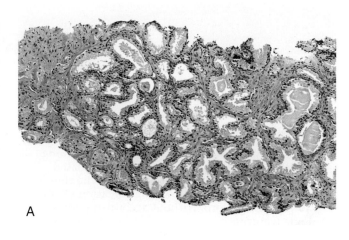

A

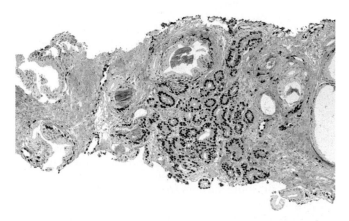

Fig 5. Prostate cancer stained with a cocktail of α-methylacyl–coenzyme A racemase (AMACR) and basal cell markers (high-molecular-weight cytokeratin and p63). The cancer glands are positive for AMACR (red signal) and negative for basal cell markers (brown signal), whereas benign glands are negative for AMACR but positive for basal cell markers.

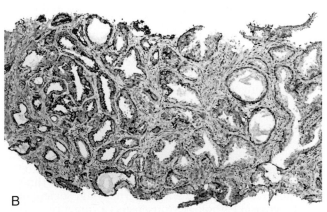

B

Fig 7. α-Methylacyl–coenzyme A racemase (AMACR) expression in adenosis. **A,** Adenosis comprises closely packed, variably sized glands. **B,** The basal cell marker high-molecular-weight cytokeratin is positive in a patchy fashion. These glands are moderately to strongly positive for AMACR.

Fig 6. Prostate cancer stained with antibody cocktail for both basal cell marker p63 (brown nuclear staining) and ERG (red nuclear staining). Cancer glands are positive for ERG and negative for p63, whereas benign glands are positive for p63 and negative for ERG.

GLEASON GRADING OF PROSTATE CARCINOMA

Definition

- Original Gleason grading system
  - The Gleason grading system is the most commonly used grading scheme for prostate cancer worldwide.
  - The Gleason system is relatively unique among pathologic grading systems in that it is based solely on the architectural pattern of the tumor evaluated at relatively low magnification (4× or 10× magnification), without accounting for cytologic features.
  - The grade of the tumor is defined as the sum of the two most common architectural patterns and is reported as the *Gleason score*.
  - Different growth patterns are consolidated into five basic grade patterns, in which patterns 1 to 3 represent prostate tumors closely resembling normal prostatic glands, and patterns 4 and 5 tumors show increasingly abnormal glandular architecture.
  - The five grade patterns are used to generate a histologic score, which can range from 2 to 10, by adding the primary (or predominant) grade pattern and the secondary (second most common) grade pattern.
  - Gleason's original description of each grade pattern has undergone significant modification over time, most recently at the 2005 International Society of Urological Pathology Consensus Conference.
- Modified Gleason grading system
  - With the use of immunoperoxidase staining for basal cell markers, many of the original Gleason score 2 (1 + 1) carcinomas would currently be regarded as adenosis (atypical adenomatous hyperplasia).
  - The diagnosis of Gleason score 2 to 4 based on a needle biopsy specimen should be made rarely if ever. At TURP, which samples the transition zone, cancer with a Gleason score of 2 to 4 may still be diagnosed, but it is uncommon.
  - Many of the tumors originally diagnosed as cribriform Gleason pattern 3 would currently be diagnosed as either cribriform high-grade prostatic intraepithelial neoplasia or intraductal carcinoma if labeled with basal cell markers.
  - Tumor glands with cribriform pattern should be diagnosed as Gleason pattern 4.
  - Individual tumor cells and ill-defined glands with poorly formed glandular lumina warrant the diagnosis of Gleason pattern 4.
  - True comedonecrosis within solid nests and cribriform masses should be regarded as Gleason pattern 5.
- Grading variants of prostate cancer
  - Tumors with vacuoles should be graded as if the vacuoles were not present, by only evaluating the underlying architectural pattern.
  - Most cases of foamy gland carcinoma would be graded as Gleason score 3 + 3 = 6, although higher-grade foamy gland carcinoma exists.

- Ductal adenocarcinoma of the prostate should be graded as Gleason score 4 + 4 = 8, with the exception of PIN-like ductal adenocarcinoma, which is graded as 3 + 3 = 6.
- Small cell carcinoma of the prostate should not be assigned a Gleason grade.
- Reporting limited secondary pattern of lower and higher grade
  - In the setting of high-grade cancer, lower-grade patterns should be ignored if they occupy less than 5% of the tumor area.
  - A high-grade tumor of any quantity on a needle biopsy specimen, identified at low to medium magnification, should be included within the Gleason score.
- Tertiary Gleason patterns
  - Biopsy
    - In the rare case in which there are three different patterns on needle biopsy, but the third pattern is lower grade, the lower-grade pattern should be ignored.
    - Tumors with patterns 3, 4, and 5 on a needle biopsy specimen should be classified overall as high grade (Gleason score, 8 to 10); for these tumors, both the primary pattern and the highest grade should be recorded.
  - Radical prostatectomy
    - The presence of a third component of a Gleason pattern higher than the primary and secondary grades, visually estimated to be less than 5% of the whole tumor, is considered a tertiary pattern; when the third most common component is the highest grade and occupies greater than 5% of the tumor, some authors would record it as secondary pattern.
    - On radical prostatectomy, assigning a separate Gleason score to each dominant tumor nodule is recommended.
  - Needle biopsy specimens with different cores showing different grades
    - Individual Gleason scores should be assigned to separates cores as long as the cores are submitted separately.
- Effects of modified Gleason grading system
  - A consequence of narrowing the definition of Gleason pattern 3 and expanding the definition of pattern 4 has been Gleason grade migration or upgrading: Gleason score 6 prostate cancer, once the most common pattern on needle biopsy, has become less common than Gleason score 7.
  - After the modified Gleason grading, the agreement of Gleason score between needle core biopsy and radical prostatectomy specimens for Gleason score 7 has improved (from 45% to more than 85%).
  - The interobserver reproducibility among pathologists using the modified Gleason system has improved compared with the old conventional Gleason grading (from 60% to 80%).

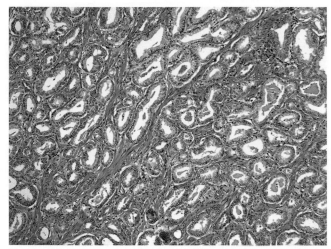

Fig 1. Adenocarcinoma of the prostate Gleason pattern 3. The tumor consists of small to medium-sized single glands of irregular shape and spacing, with elongated and angular forms.

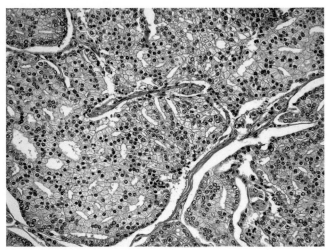

Fig 4. Adenocarcinoma of the prostate Gleason pattern 4 with cribriform architecture.

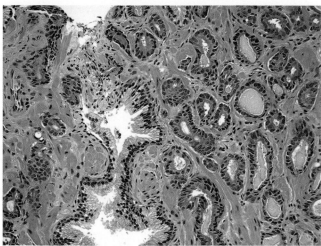

Fig 2. Adenocarcinoma of the prostate, Gleason pattern 3. The tumor has infiltrating edges and shows irregular extension into stroma with neoplastic glands on both sides of a benign gland.

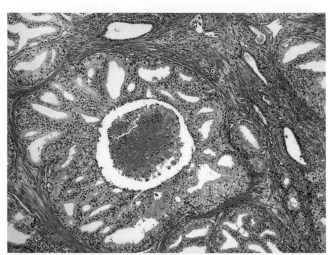

Fig 5. Adenocarcinoma of the prostate Gleason pattern 5; cribriform glands with central necrosis (comedonecrosis).

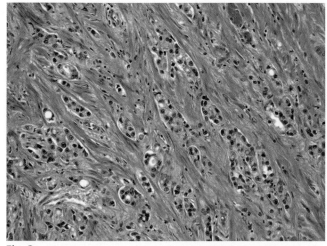

Fig 3. Adenocarcinoma of the prostate, Gleason pattern 4. The glands are fused and poorly formed with microacinar formation.

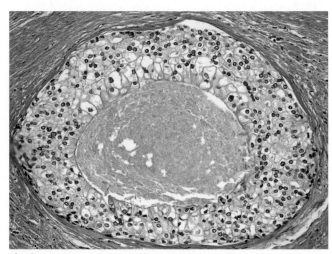

Fig 6. Adenocarcinoma of the prostate Gleason pattern 5; solid gland with central necrosis (comedonecrosis).

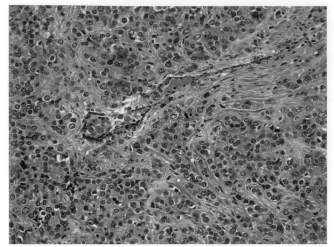

Fig 7. Adenocarcinoma of the prostate Gleason pattern 5, composed of sheets of tumor cells.

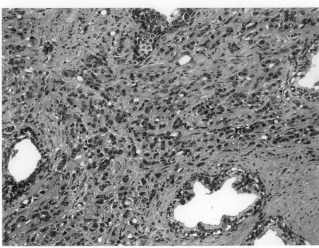

Fig 9. Adenocarcinoma of the prostate Gleason pattern 5; diffusely infiltrative sheets and individual tumor cells.

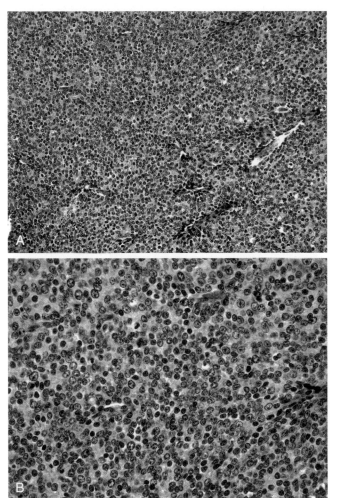

Fig 8. **A,** Adenocarcinoma of the prostate Gleason pattern 5; expansile mass of tumor cells. **B,** The tumor is still pattern 5, despite a lack of prominent pleomorphism.

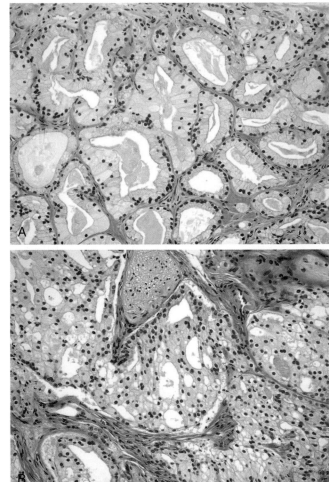

Fig 10. Foamy gland adenocarcinoma of the prostate. Most cases of foamy gland carcinoma would be graded as Gleason score 3 + 3 = 6 **(A),** although Gleason pattern 4 foamy gland carcinoma exists **(B).**

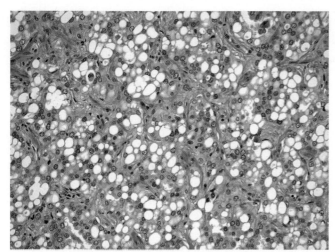

Fig 11. Adenocarcinoma of the prostate with vacuoles should be graded as though the vacuoles were not present, by only evaluating the underlying architectural pattern. This specific case would be graded as Gleason pattern 4.

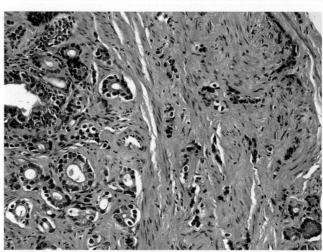

Fig 13. Adenocarcinoma of the prostate with Gleason pattern 3 *(left)* and Gleason pattern 5 *(right)*.

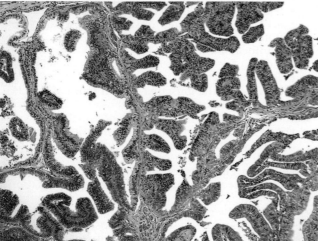

Fig 12. Ductal adenocarcinoma of the prostate (except prostatic intraepithelial neoplasia–like ductal variant) should be graded as Gleason score 4 + 4 = 8.

PROSTATE CANCER STAGING IN RADICAL PROSTATECTOMY

Definition

- The objective of staging is to group malignancies with a similar prognosis and therapeutic approach to be able to compare clinicopathologic data on a homogeneous patient population.
- Staging involves determining the anatomic extent or spread of prostate cancer at the time of diagnosis based on clinical and pathologic criteria.
- The TNM staging is the most widely used system for prostate cancer staging and assesses the extent of primary tumor (T stage), the absence or presence of regional lymph node involvement (N stage), and the absence or presence of distant metastases (M stage).
- Pathologic classification of the radical prostatectomy specimen after surgery provides important prognostic information.

Clinical features

Prognosis and treatment

- Reporting pathologic staging parameters in radical prostatectomy specimens is essential not only in determining the most appropriate treatment of individual patients, but also in predicting the likelihood of local and distant disease recurrence.
- Seminal vesicle invasion, extraprostatic extension (EPE), lymph node status, and positive surgical margins are significant predictors of clinical and biochemical recurrence.

Pathology

- Pathologic staging (pTNM) is based on gross and microscopic examination of the prostate gland and is performed after surgical resection of the primary tumor (radical prostatectomy).

Histology

- Pathologic stage T2
  - pT2a: involvement of less than half of one side of the prostate (unilateral disease)
  - pT2b: involvement of more than half of one side of the gland (unilateral disease)
  - pT2c: involvement of both sides of the prostate gland (bilateral disease)
  - Although the AJCC recommends this substaging, it is without merit because (1) pT2b virtually does not exist, as tumors that are this large almost always are bilateral and (2) there are no prognostic differences between the substages of pT2 disease. It is more valid to merely report pT2 disease without substaging.
- Pathologic stage T3
- Extraprostatic extension (EPE) in any location (pT3a)
  - Presence of prostate cancer beyond the confines of the prostate
  - Recognition of EPE variable depending on the anatomic site
    - Posterior and posterolateral—EPE is diagnosed: (1) the tumor is admixed or at the same plane with periprostatic fat; (2) there is a distinct tumor nodule within desmoplastic stroma bulging beyond the normal rounded contour of the gland; or (3) the tumor extends beyond the compact dense smooth muscle of the prostate to involve loose connective periprostatic tissue.
    - Anterior: there is no well-defined edge at this site, and EPE is diagnosed with the tumor in or at the same plane of adipose tissue.
    - Apex: the boundaries of the prostate are poor with normal prostate glands admixed with skeletal muscle. If the tumor is within skeletal muscle but yet not at the inked margin, the consensus is to diagnose as organ confined. If tumor at the apex is at the ink, it is diagnosed as pT2+ (pT2x) because it cannot be determined whether the margin is positive in an area of intraprostatic incision or EPE owing to the ambiguous boundaries of the prostate at this site.
    - Bladder neck: EPE is diagnosed when a tumor is seen in thick muscle bundles in the absence of associated benign prostatic glands. Prostatic adenocarcinoma microscopically infiltrating among thick smooth muscle bundles of the coned bladder neck is equivalent to pT3a.
  - Extraprostatic extension is subdivided as follows:
    - Focal: few neoplastic glands outside the prostate (<1 high-power field on two or fewer separate sections)
    - Nonfocal: more than a few glands
  - Presence of seminal vesicle invasion is by definition EPE (pT3b)
    - Invasion of the muscular wall of seminal vesicle by prostate cancer
- Pathologic stage T4
  - Direct invasion of rectum, gross invasion of urinary bladder, external sphincter, levator muscles, or pelvic wall, with or without fixation
- Surgical margin of resection status
  - Positive resection margin on pathologic evaluation is defined as cancer cells touching the inked surgical margin of the radical prostatectomy specimen.
  - Surgical margin of resection is considered negative as along as cancer cells or glands do not reach the inked surface of the specimen, despite microscopically close distances (<0.1 mm).
- Lymphovascular invasion
  - Lymphovascular invasion is the unequivocal existence of tumor cells within endothelial-lined spaces with no underlying muscular walls or as the presence of tumor emboli in small intraprostatic vessels.
- Regional lymph nodes (N)
  - For prostate cancer, the regional lymph nodes are the nodes of the true pelvis, located below the bifurcation of the common iliac arteries.
- Metastases
  - Involvement of lymph nodes lying outside the boundaries of the true pelvis is classified as M1a disease.
  - Bone lesions (osteoblastic metastases) are classified as M1b disease.
  - Lung and liver metastases are classified as M1c disease.

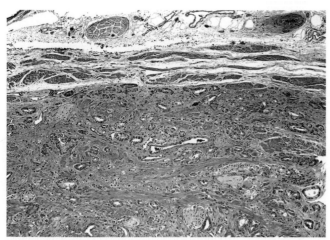

Fig 1. Organ-confined prostate cancer. The tumor docs not extend beyond the condensed smooth muscle that defines the edge of the prostate posteriorly and posterolaterally.

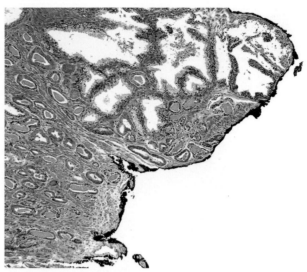

Fig 4. Pt2+ (pT2x) resulting from a positive margin in an area of intraprostatic incision (note benign glands adjacent to cancer at the margin). Because the edge of the prostate has been left in the patient, the tumor cannot be staged in this area.

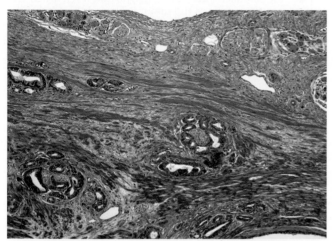

Fig 2. Prostate cancer is within the condensed muscle and is organ confined. The presence of perineural invasion does not affect staging, because it can be seen within and outside the prostate.

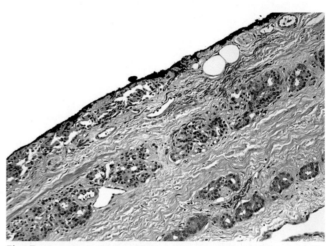

Fig 5. Positive resection margin in an area of extraprostatic extension adjacent to adipose tissue.

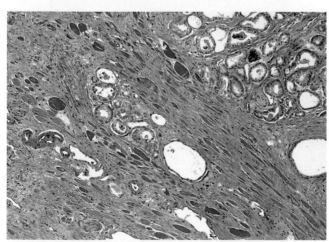

Fig 3. At the apex, the edge of the prostate is ill defined where benign prostate glands are admixed with skeletal muscle fibers. The consensus is that if the tumor does not extend to the ink, it is considered organ confined. If it extends to the ink at the apex, the tumor is staged as pT2+ or pT2x (i.e., cannot determine whether the margin is positive in an area that would have been organ confined if not incised or positive in an area of extraprostatic extension) because of the ambiguities of the edge of the prostate at this site.

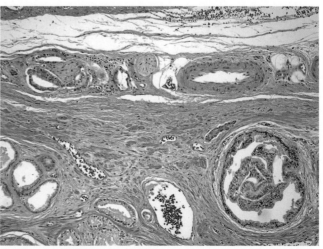

Fig 6. Focal extraprostatic extension. Only a few cancer glands (<1 high-power field) are noted outside the confines of the prostate, at the same level of periprostatic fat.

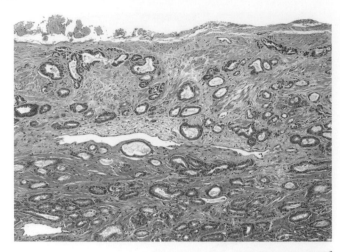

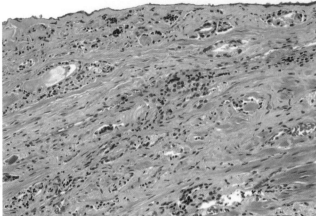

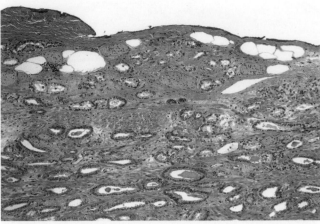

Fig 9. Nonfocal extraprostatic extension (EPE) in which prostatic adenocarcinoma extends beyond the condensed smooth muscle of the edge of the prostate to involve periprostatic fat. The tumor is associated with a desmoplastic reaction that can obscure the fat, such that EPE is diagnosable even when not seen next to fat as long as the tumor is beyond the edge of the prostate.

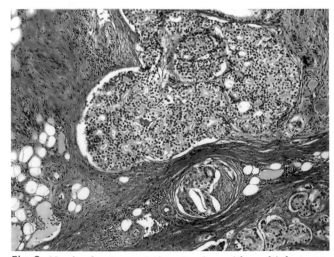

Fig 7. Negative resection margin. Despite being microscopically close to the inked surface of the specimen, the cancer glands do not reach the ink and the tumor is organ confined within the dense smooth muscle of the prostate.

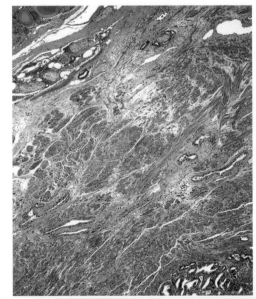

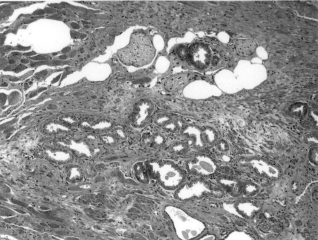

Fig 8. Nonfocal extraprostatic extension with multiple tumor glands admixed with periprostatic fat.

Fig 10. Extraprostatic anterior extension. Adenocarcinoma glands are present beyond the contour of the prostate with infiltration of the anterior periprostatic fat.

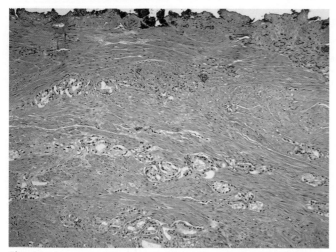

Fig 11. Prostatic adenocarcinoma microscopically infiltrating among thick muscle bundles of the coned bladder neck in the absence of benign prostatic glandular tissue, consistent with extraprostatic extension.

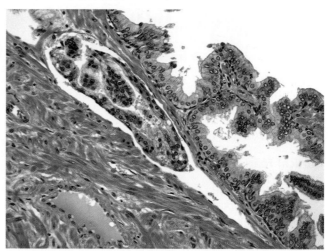

Fig 13. Lymphovascular invasion. Tumor cells are present within an intraprostatic endothelium-lined space with no underlying muscular wall.

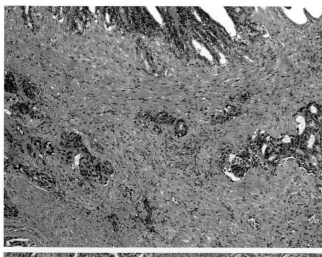

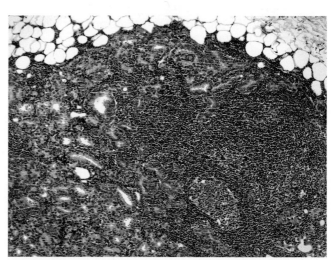

Fig 14. Metastatic prostate cancer involving a regional lymph node (pathologic stage N1).

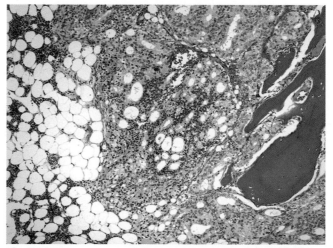

Fig 12. Invasion of the muscular wall of the seminal vesicle by prostate cancer is equivalent to stage pT3b.

Fig 15. Metastatic prostate cancer involving femoral head bone (M1b disease).

WORK-UP OF "VANISHING" CANCER IN RADICAL PROSTATECTOMY

Definition
- Inability to identify residual cancer in the final surgical specimen despite complete sampling in patients undergoing radical prostatectomy for biopsy-confirmed prostate carcinoma

Clinical features
Epidemiology
- The phenomenon is attributed to a wrong diagnosis on biopsy, pathologic technique (i.e., not fully sampling the prostate or cancer in unsampled areas of paraffin blocks), or being induced by therapy (i.e., hormonal therapy).
- Most cases of "vanishing cancer" in radical prostatectomy specimens reflect a chance sampling of a minute cancer on biopsy and not a switch in specimens.

Presentation
- Patient undergoing radical prostatectomy for biopsy-confirmed prostate cancer
- No residual cancer in the final specimen despite careful sampling

Prognosis and treatment
- Vigilant screening of men for prostate cancer seems to be associated with an increase in tumors with little or no residual cancer at radical prostatectomy.
- The prognosis is excellent, indicating that there is no clinical significance to microscopic foci of cancer that remain undetected after reasonably complete pathologic sampling.

Pathology
- A work-up of vanishing cancer in radical prostatectomy includes:
  - Review of the diagnostic needle biopsy specimen to confirm the presence of prostate cancer
  - Complete radical prostatectomy sampling
  - Exclusion of prior therapy with a luteinizing hormone–releasing hormone agonist
  - Levels threefold and potentially immunohistochemical stains of areas with atypical glands and or high-grade prostatic intraepithelial neoplasia
  - Levels threefold for posterior blocks in sextant and adjacent site of positive biopsy; if no cancer, flip these blocks and level threefold
  - In cases in which high-grade or a lot of cancer is present on the prostate biopsy specimen with no or minimal cancer in the radical prostatectomy specimen, the prostate for patient identity (PCR-based microsatellite marker analysis) should be evaluated to exclude mislabeling of the specimen.

Immunopathology (including immunohistochemistry)
- HMWCK or p63, or both, may be helpful in the evaluation of atypical glands.

NONPROSTATIC ADENOCARCINOMA INVOLVING THE PROSTATE

Definition
- Metastatic adenocarcinomas to the prostate are secondary adenocarcinomas that have spread to the prostate gland via angiolymphatic invasion.
- More commonly, adenocarcinomas from contiguous organs directly invade the prostate.

Clinical features
Epidemiology
- Distant metastases to the prostate from adenocarcinomas arising in noncontiguous organs (e.g., the lung) are exceptionally rare in clinical specimens.
- They are typically noted only with disseminated disease at autopsy (5% of cases in some series).
- The most common adenocarcinomas that directly invade to the prostate are from the urinary bladder, colon/rectum, or urethral in origin.

Presentation
- Patients may be asymptomatic.
- Presenting features include primary tumor, including bladder mass, colorectal mass, urethral mass, and hematuria.

Pathology
Gross pathology
- Examination might not show significant gross features.
- Pelvic exenteration and cystoprostatectomy may show primary bladder, colorectal, or urethral mass.

Histology
- Metastatic tumor typically similar to primary tumor
- Desmoplastic or inflammatory stromal reaction (unlike most primary prostatic adenocarcinomas)
- May demonstrate perineural invasion (mimicking primary prostatic adenocarcinoma)
- May demonstrate angiolymphatic invasion

- True mucin-positive signet ring cell adenocarcinomas exceedingly rare for prostate adenocarcinoma and most likely representing spread from gastrointestinal or bladder adenocarcinoma
- Mucinous lakes lined by columnar mucinous adenocarcinoma typical of gastrointestinal or bladder adenocarcinoma

Immunopathology (including immunohistochemistry)
- Negative: PSA, PSAP, p501S, PSMA
- Identical immunoprofile as primary tumor (i.e., colorectal: positive CDX2 and CK20, negative CK7)

Molecular diagnostics
- None

Main differential diagnosis
- Primary prostatic adenocarcinoma: high-grade adenocarcinoma of the prostate typically has relatively uniform cytology compared with adenocarcinoma of the bladder or colon.

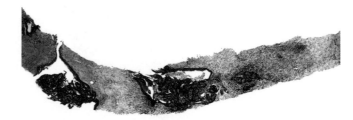

Fig 1. Prostate needle core biopsy specimen with involvement by colonic adenocarcinoma.

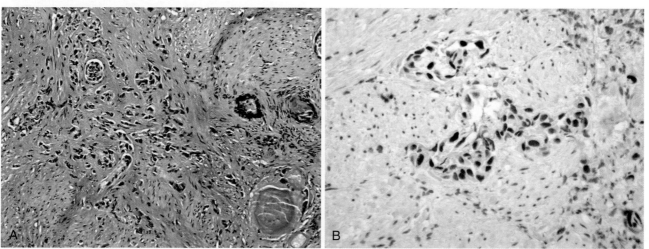

Fig 2. **A,** Poorly differentiated carcinoma involving the prostate in a man with a history of adenocarcinoma of the lung. **B,** The tumor was positive for TTF-1 (shown) and negative for prostate markers (not shown), which is consistent with metastatic lung carcinoma to the prostate.

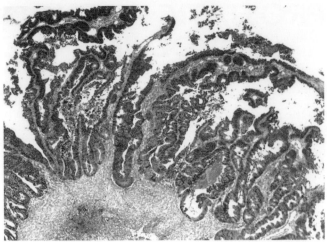

Fig 3. Colonic adenocarcinoma in the prostate involving the prostatic urethra and mimicking prostatic duct adenocarcinoma.

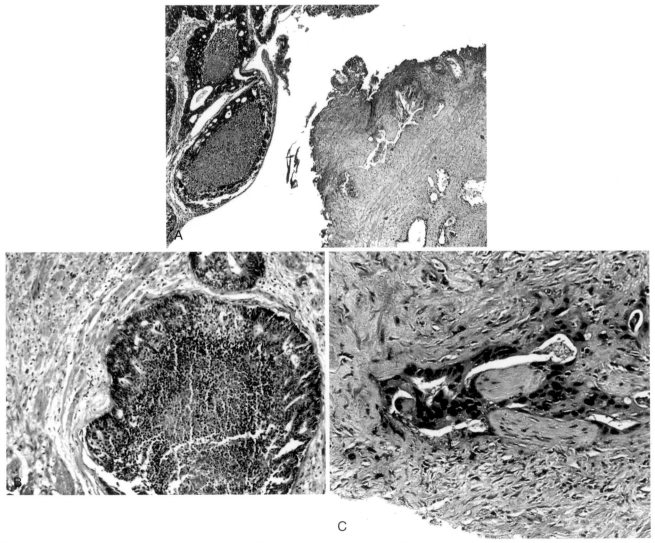

Fig 4. A, Transurethral resection of the prostate with colonic adenocarcinoma. **B,** Colonic adenocarcinoma involving the prostate mimicking prostatic adenocarcinoma, Gleason pattern 5. **C,** Colonic adenocarcinoma in the prostate with perineural invasion, mimicking prostatic adenocarcinoma.

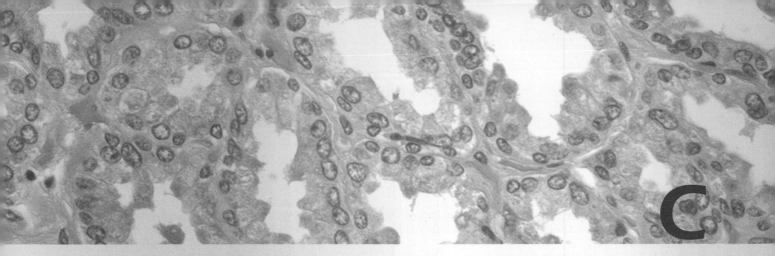

SEMINAL VESICLES

ANATOMY AND HISTOLOGY OF SEMINAL VESICLES

Definition

- Paired male accessory sex glands produce an alkaline secretion known to constitute the bulk of the ejaculate, promote sperm function, and provide an assortment of potent antibacterial factors to the male genital tract.
- Seminal vesicles develop as outpouchings of the lower mesonephric ducts.
- Coiled tubular structures are located along the posterolateral aspect of the external surface of the base of the urinary bladder, superior to the posterior surface of the prostate.
- In adult males, seminal vesicles average approximately 6 cm in length and 2 cm in width.
- The ducts of the seminal vesicles merge with the ampullary portion of the vasa deferentia on each side to form the ejaculatory ducts, which then enter the central zone of the prostate and converge at either side of the verumontanum in the prostatic sinus of the prostatic urethra.

Pathology

Histology

- The muscular wall of the seminal vesicles consists of a thick, circumferential coat of smooth muscle that contracts during ejaculation.
- Unlike the seminal vesicles, the ejaculatory ducts lack a thick muscular wall and are surrounded by a collagenous stroma.
- With puberty, the ductal structures develop elaborate mucosal folds resulting in complex structures and irregular convoluted lumina on cross-section.
- Glands are lined by a layer of pseudostratified, nonciliated, tall columnar to cuboidal secretory cells and basal cells.
- The cells are predominantly secretory and contain microvesicular lipid droplets and characteristic lipofuscin pigment granules.
- The pigment is golden brown and refractile; it increases in amount with age; similar pigment can be seen in the prostatic epithelium, but it lacks the honey color and globular nature of seminal vesicle lipofuscin.
- The tall columnar cells lining the mucosa in young men are replaced over time by flattened cuboidal cells.
- Flattening of the epithelium is accompanied by striking nuclear abnormalities and highly atypical cells with large irregular hyperchromatic nuclei, coarse chromatin, and prominent nucleoli. Multinucleated cells are also present, as are giant ring-shaped nuclei with large intranuclear cytoplasmic inclusions. Mitotic figures are absent.
- Nuclear abnormalities, not observed in young men, are probably degenerative changes reflecting hormonal influences.
- With advancing age, the stroma of the seminal vesicles becomes hyalinized and fibrotic.

Immunopathology

- In contrast to the prostate, the secretory cells of the seminal vesicles stain negative for prostate-specific antigen, prostate-specific acid phosphatase, and α-methylacyl–coenzyme A racemase; the basal cells stain for high-molecular-weight cytokeratin and show a distinct p63 nuclear staining.
- Nuclear PAX2 immunoreactivity in the epithelium of seminal vesicle and ejaculatory duct supports the proposed embryogenesis of the prostatic central zone, seminal vesicle, and ejaculatory ducts from the wolffian system.

Main differential diagnosis

- Tangential sampling of the seminal vesicle epithelium may be a potential source of diagnostic confusion and could be mistaken for adenocarcinoma. The presence of characteristic lipofuscin and random cells with marked yet degenerative atypia rules out prostate cancer. Positive labeling of basal cells in seminal vesicles with p63 and high-molecular-weight cytokeratin along with negative stains for PSA is definitive if there is diagnostic uncertainty on hematoxylin and eosin–stained slides.

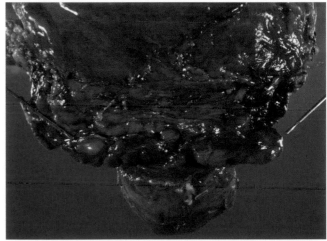

Fig 1. Seminal vesicles are located along the posterolateral aspect of the external surface of the base of the urinary bladder, superior to the posterior surface of the prostate.

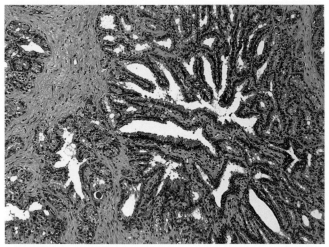

Fig 2. Normal adult seminal vesicle with slitlike glandular pattern with few papillae.

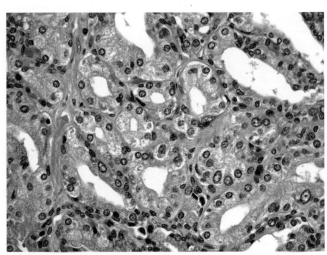

Fig 5. Secretory cells contain microvesicular lipid droplets and characteristic lipofuscin pigment granules.

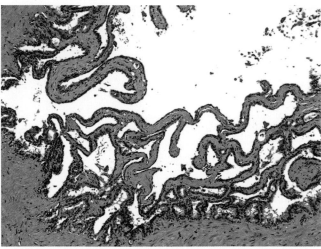

Fig 3. Normal adult seminal vesicle with central lumina surrounded by outpouching of small glands.

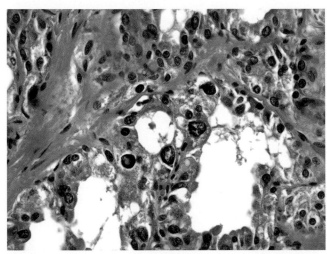

Fig 6. Flattening of the epithelium is accompanied by highly atypical cells with large irregular hyperchromatic nuclei and coarse chromatin. Most of the nuclei have degenerative atypia but occasionally prominent nucleoli are visible.

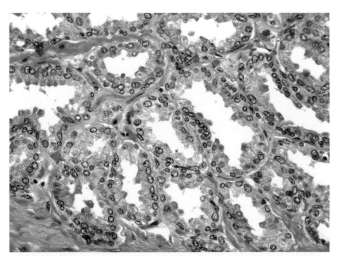

Fig 4. Glands are lined by a layer of pseudostratified, nonciliated, cuboidal secretory cells and basal cells.

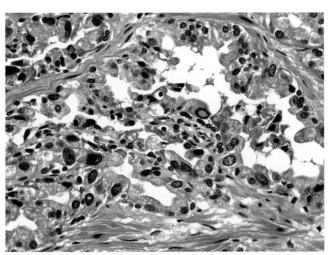

Fig 7. Marked degenerative nuclear atypia with large intranuclear cytoplasmic inclusions.

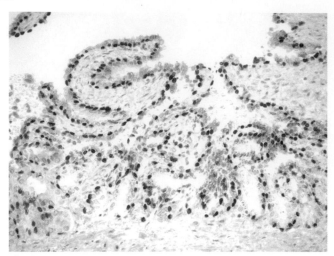

Fig 8. Seminal vesicle showing distinct p63 nuclear staining in the basal cells.

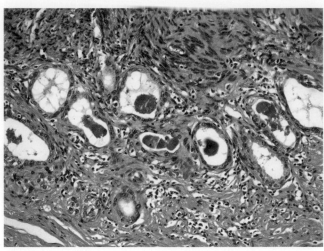

Fig 9. Tangential sampling of seminal vesicle epithelium mimicking adenocarcinoma.

Definition
- Bilateral localized and isolated amyloid deposits in the subepithelial region of the seminal vesicles and ejaculatory systems (senile seminal vesicle amyloid)

Clinical features
Epidemiology
- Senile seminal vesicle amyloid is one of the most common forms of localized amyloidosis.
- It is identified at autopsy in 9% to 16% of men, and in 1% to 5% of prostatectomy specimens removed for clinically localized prostate cancer.
- Frequency increases with age (21% to 34% of men older than 75 years).
- It is usually an incidental finding, although it may be associated with hematospermia.
- Most cases are not associated with systemic amyloidosis, although localized and systemic amyloidosis can coexist.
- Rarely, amyloid in the seminal vesicles reflects systemic involvement by AA amyloid.

Presentation
- Usually asymptomatic
- May cause hematospermia and chronic perineal pain

Prognosis and treatment
- The condition is benign and is associated with the male aging process.
- Localized amyloidosis of seminal vesicles may be derived from a secretory exocrine product of the lining epithelium of the ejaculatory duct system. As shown by mass spectrometric analysis, amyloid fibrils comprise mainly polypeptide fragments identical to the sequence of the N-terminal portion of semenogelin I, the major secretory product of the seminal vesicles.

Pathology
Histology
- The deposits of amyloid tend to be nodular and affect the subepithelial region of seminal vesicles, vasa deferentia, and ejaculatory ducts, spreading to include the wall of these organs.
- Localized amyloidosis in the seminal vesicles is always associated with amyloid deposition in the vasa deferentia and ejaculatory ducts.
- Amyloid deposition is associated with thickening of the walls of the ejaculatory system and secondary narrowing of the lumina.
- Localized amyloidosis of ejaculatory system involves only subepithelial tissue, sparing blood vessels or muscular wall of ejaculatory system, prostatic parenchyma, and adjacent fibroadipose tissue.

Immunopathology (including immunohistochemistry)
- Congo red stain demonstrates amorphous light red deposits and typical apple-green birefringence under polarization.
- Amyloid deposition in the ejaculatory system is permanganate sensitive and positive for lactoferrin and amyloid P components, but is negative for amyloid A protein, λ and κ chains, and β2-microglobulin.

Main differential diagnosis
- Systemic amyloidosis affecting the seminal vesicles (amyloid deposits involve vascular walls, smooth muscle, and stroma)

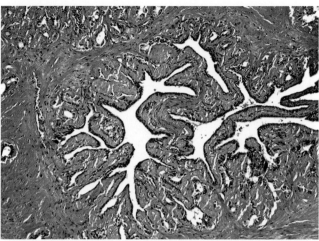

Fig 1. Diffuse amyloid deposition is noted in the seminal vesicle.

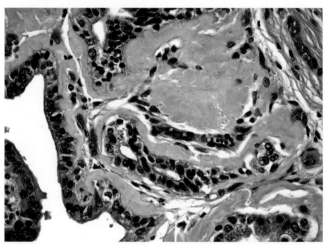

Fig 2. The deposits of amyloid tend to be nodular and are associated with thickening of the walls of the ejaculatory system.

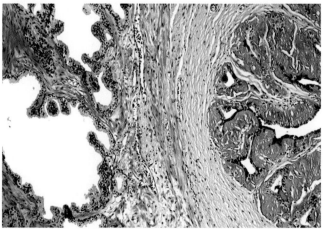

Fig 3. Localized amyloid deposition in subepithelial tissue of the ejaculatory duct with no prostatic parenchyma involvement.

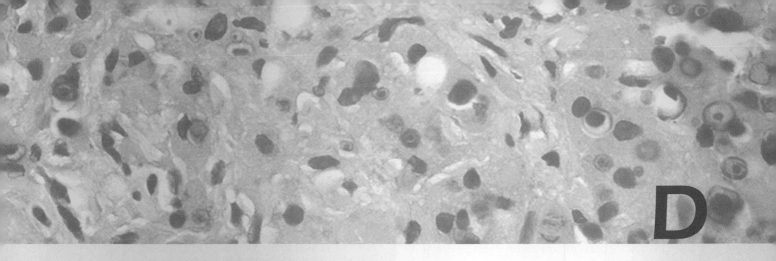

D

NONNEOPLASTIC DISEASE OF THE URINARY BLADDER

ANATOMY AND HISTOLOGY OF THE URINARY BLADDER

Definition

- The normal bladder is a hollow pelvic organ that temporarily stores and excretes urine.
- It develops during the 4th to 7th weeks of gestation.
- It is derived from the urogenital sinus.
- It has a pyramidal shape that distends with filling.
- It is covered by peritoneum along the superior and posterior aspects.
- Ureters enter the bladder posteriorly at the base.
- In males, the bladder neck sits in association with the prostate gland.
- In females, the bladder neck rests on the urogenital sinus.
- The bladder is held in place by the pelvic fascia and peritoneum that anchor the organ to the anterior abdominal wall, pubis, and lateral pelvis.
- The obliterated urachus–median umbilical ligament connects the superior aspect of the bladder to the umbilicus.
- The main blood supply is via the superior and inferior vesical arteries, which derive from the anterior trunk of the iliac artery.
- Venous drainage occurs via the vesical venous plexus.
- The bladder is innervated via the autonomic nervous system with fibers that arise from the pelvic plexus.

Pathology

Histology

- Histologic layers including urothelium, lamina propria, muscularis propria (detrusor muscle), and perivesical fat
- Urothelium
  - The urothelium (formerly *transitional epithelium*) forms an impermeable barrier to urine.
  - Generally, it is 4 to 7 cell layers thick.
  - Umbrella cells form a single layer along the luminal aspect of the urothelium and are cytokeratin 20 positive.
  - Cells are polarized to the luminal surface.
  - Nuclei are relatively uniform, are generally the size of a lymphocyte, and have smooth, open chromatin with occasional pinpoint nucleoli.
  - Reactive atypia may be present, which is most commonly seen in the setting of inflammation and is characterized by modest nuclear enlargement and small nucleoli.
  - It is separated from the lamina propria by a basement membrane.
  - Urothelial cells show immunoreactivity for cytokeratin 7, p63, and full-thickness CD44 positivity.
- Lamina propria
  - There is loose connective tissue below the urothelium.
  - Blood vessels (intermediate size venules and arteries) can be used as a landmark on transurethral resection of bladder (TURB) specimens.
  - Fibers of muscularis mucosae are present and have a wispy, disorganized appearance, although they may be hypertrophic.
  - Inflammatory cells are frequently present in this layer.
  - Stromal cells may appear multinucleated.

- Muscularis propria
  - Clinically, often referred to as *detrusor muscle*
  - Thick bundles of smooth muscle fibers that give structure to the bladder and aid in bladder emptying
  - Often demonstrates diffuse smoothelin expression
- Perivesical fat
  - Outermost layer of bladder wall
  - Often demonstrates a somewhat irregular interface with the muscularis propria
  - Consists primarily of fat cells with interspersed blood vessels and nerves

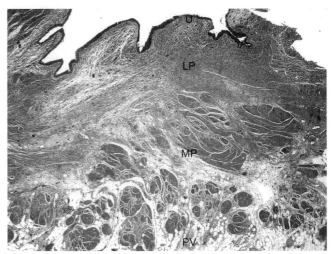

Fig 1. Low-magnification view of the bladder reveals four layers that include the urothelium *(U)*, lamina propria *(LP)*, muscularis propria *(MP)*, and perivesical fat *(PV)*.

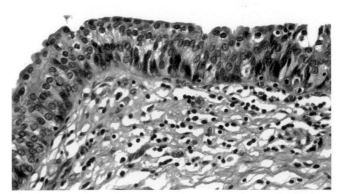

Fig 2. Normal urothelium is polarized to the urothelial surface and consists of four to seven cell layers with an outermost umbrella cell layer.

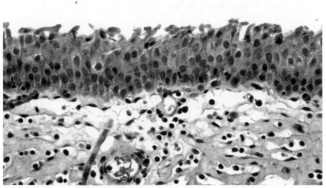

Fig 3. Reactive urothelium demonstrates mild disorganization, slight nuclear enlargement, and pinpoint nucleoli and is often associated with an inflammatory infiltrate.

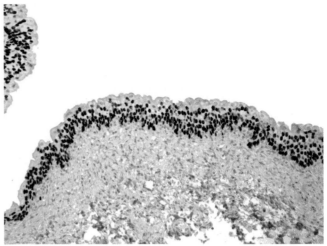

Fig 6. p63 immunostain highlights urothelial cells.

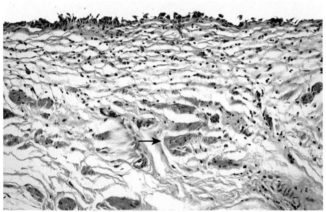

Fig 4. Muscularis mucosae are composed of thin, wispy smooth muscle fibers *(arrow)* that are present within the lamina propria.

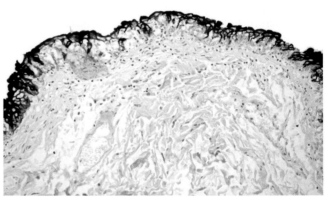

Fig 7. Cytokeratin 20 expression is limited to the umbrella cell layer in normal urothelium.

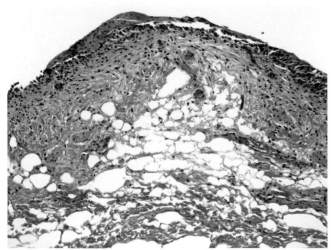

Fig 5. Adipose tissue may be present within the lamina propria.

Definition
- Solid urothelial nests budding beneath the urothelium, seen along the entire urinary tract, considered as a variant normal urothelial histology; may also occur as a result of local inflammation and reactive proliferative change

Clinical features
Epidemiology
- One of the most common nonneoplastic urothelial proliferations
- Present in up to 85% of urinary bladders in autopsy series

Presentation
- Typically asymptomatic and found incidentally
- Less than 5 mm in diameter mostly; not visible to the naked eye
- Most commonly located in the trigone area

Prognosis and treatment
- Not a risk factor for malignancy
- No treatment is necessary

Pathology
Histology
- Small, well-defined solid nests composed of normal urothelial cells within lamina propria, formed by invaginated urothelium
- Round, smooth contours
- Evenly spaced and often in clusters
- Usually located in the superficial mucosa
- In the ureter and renal pelvis, smaller individual nests possibly observed, usually with more irregular contours
- Sharp, linear border at the deeper aspect of the proliferation
- Subject to the same changes that affect the surface urothelium, such as hyperplasia, reactive atypia and carcinoma in situ

Immunopathology (including immunohistochemistry)
- Not contributory

Molecular diagnostics
- Not contributory

Main differential diagnosis
- Inverted papilloma
- Nested variant of urothelial carcinoma
- Papillary urothelial neoplasm of low malignant potential with inverted growth pattern

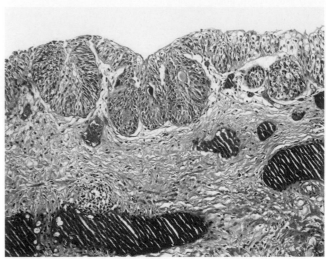

Fig 1. von Brunn nests formed by invaginations of the urothelium.

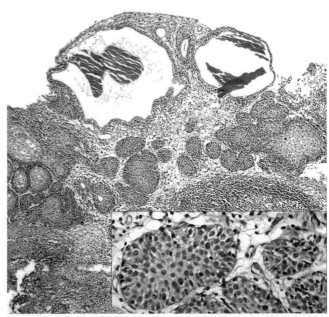

Fig 2. von Brunn nests with cystitis cystica-like changes. The base of the proliferation is broad and well-defined. *Inset,* No atypias are noted in urothelial cells.

Definition
- Proliferative or reactive changes occurring in von Brunn nests, which become cystically dilated and acquire a luminal space (cystitis cystica) or undergo further glandular metaplasia (cystitis glandularis)

Clinical features
Epidemiology
- Extremely common, especially in association with von Brunn nests
- Frequently associated with chronic cystitis or other causes of mucosal irritation

Presentation
- May appear as a papillary or polypoid mass
- Incidental finding in cystoscopy done for other reasons

Prognosis and treatment
- No treatment required; may regress if the cause of bladder irritation is removed
- No increased risk of developing urothelial carcinoma

Pathology
Histology
- Nests of urothelium in superficial lamina propria, some of which have cystically dilated lumen either without glandular lining cells (cystitis cystica), or with glandular lining cells (cystitis glandularis)
- Often with a vaguely lobular distribution and a non-infiltrative pattern of growth at the base, with variable connection to the surface
- von Brunn nests and cystitis cystica et glandularis often coexist in the same case; the latter possibly showing intestinal metaplasia and occasional extravasated mucin
- Degenerative atypia occasionally present

Immunopathology (including immunohistochemistry)
- Not contributory

Main differential diagnosis
- Inverted urothelial papilloma
- Invasive urothelial carcinoma, nested variant
- Carcinoma in situ involving von Brunn nests or cystitis cystica et glandularis
- Invasive enteric-type bladder adenocarcinoma

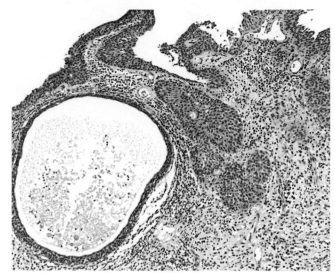

Fig 1. Cystitis cystica with cystic space lined by flattened urothelial cells, adjacent von Brunn nests, and stromal chronic inflammation.

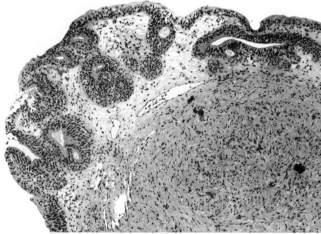

Fig 2. Cystitis glandularis showing luminal spaces lined by cuboidal, columnar cells.

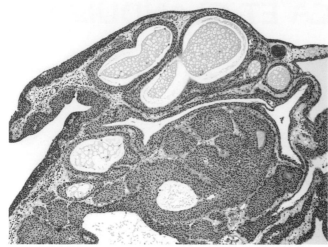

Fig 3. Cystitis cystica et glandularis with coexisting von Brunn nests.

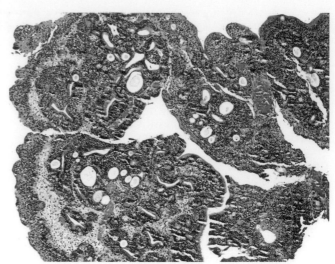

Fig 6. Florid cystitis cystica et glandularis, mimicking invasive carcinoma.

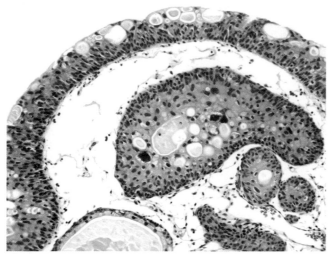

Fig 4. Cystitis cystica with degenerative atypia in the umbrella cells.

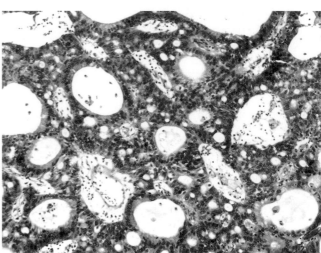

Fig 7. Florid cystitis cystica et glandularis with a cribriform pattern of growth, mimicking adenocarcinoma or carcinoid tumor.

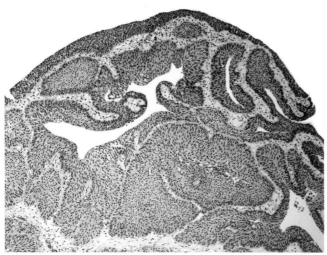

Fig 5. Cystitis cystica with prominent endophytic growth pattern, mimicking inverted papilloma.

Definition
- Metaplastic process in which the normal urothelium is replaced by either keratinizing or nonkeratinizing stratified squamous epithelium

Clinical features
Epidemiology
- Squamous metaplasia of the bladder is fourfold more common in women than men; however, women tend to present nonkeratinizing squamous metaplasia while keratinizing squamous metaplasia is more frequent in men.
- It typically affects older adults.
- It is often seen as response to urothelial injury (e.g., chronic infection, indwelling catheter, calculi, neurogenic bladder, *Schistosoma* spp. infection).
- Nonkeratinizing, glycogenated, squamous metaplasia of the trigone is seen in up to 90% of adult women and is considered a variant of normal histology; it is also seen occasionally in men receiving antiandrogen or estrogen therapy, or both.

Presentation
- Most commonly with hematuria (gross or microscopic) or urinary frequency or urgency
- Less frequently with abdominal pain or urinary retention

Prognosis and treatment
- Nonkeratinizing squamous metaplasia has not been associated with an increased risk of developing future urothelial neoplasms or squamous cell carcinoma of the bladder and does not requires specific treatment.
- Keratinizing squamous metaplasia, however, is associated with an increased risk of squamous cell carcinoma and should be followed closely with urine cytologic and cystoscopic examination.
- Identification of the cause of squamous metaplasia in a patient may be important for treatment (e.g., *Schistosoma* spp. infection).
- Some cases of squamous metaplasia may lead to bladder contracture or ureteral obstruction requiring surgical intervention.

Pathology
Histology
- Nonkeratinizing glycogenated squamous metaplasia resembles vaginal epithelium, with keratinocytes having small, dark nuclei, abundant clear cytoplasm, prominent cell borders, and no stratum corneum.
- Nonkeratinizing squamous metaplasia elsewhere shows keratinocytes with dense eosinophilic cytoplasm, intercellular bridges, occasional small nucleoli, and no keratin formation.
- Keratinizing squamous metaplasia has similar features as nonkeratinizing squamous metaplasia, except for the formation of a keratin layer showing parakeratosis, hyperkeratosis, or both.

Immunopathology (including immunohistochemistry)
- Noncontributory

Molecular diagnostics
- Noncontributory

Main differential diagnosis
- Squamous cell carcinoma in situ
- Squamous cell dysplasia

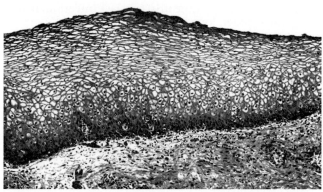

Fig 1. Nonkeratinizing glycogenated squamous metaplasia is most frequently seen in women and, in the trigone, is considered a variant of normal histology.

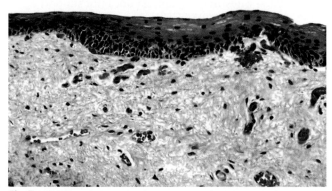

Fig 2. Nonkeratinizing squamous metaplasia, in contrast to glycogenated squamous metaplasia, does not have glycogenated, clear cytoplasm but dense, eosinophilic cytoplasm.

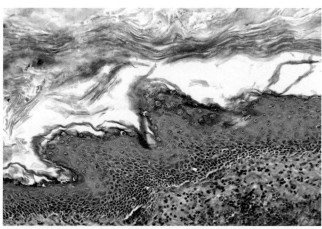

Fig 3. Keratinizing squamous metaplasia is associated with an increased risk of subsequent carcinoma. Hyperkeratosis, and occasionally parakeratosis, is present. Many cases have a granular cell layer as seen in this image.

Definition
- Replacement of the urothelium, either in the surface or in the glandular elements of cystitis glandularis, by colonic-type mucosa (goblet cells)

Clinical features
Epidemiology
- Associated with chronic irritation of the bladder (urinary stones, chronic urinary tract infection, neurogenic bladder, long-term catheterization)
- Associated with bladder exstrophy

Presentation
- Incidental finding on a biopsy specimen or as a mucosal or submucosal nodule on cystoscopic examination
- Florid cases possibly associated with irritative symptoms, hematuria, and occasionally hydronephrosis if located at the bladder neck or trigone

Prognosis and treatment
- Relationship with bladder adenocarcinoma is controversial.
- A recent large study shows frequent coincidental association with bladder carcinoma (urothelial carcinoma and adenocarcinoma), but long-term follow-up of isolated intestinal metaplasia does not support a preneoplastic nature of these lesions.

Pathology
Histology
- Mucin-producing goblet cells (similar to those found in the colonic mucosa) replacing the urothelial lining; Paneth cells rarely present
- In florid cases, possible focal and superficial involvement of muscularis propria by glands with intestinal metaplasia
- Focal cell-free mucin extravasation
- Reactive cytologic atypia, usually minimal
- Low mitotic activity

Immunohistochemistry
- Positive staining for CDX2 and CK20
- Negative staining for CK7 and p63

Main differential diagnosis
- Well-differentiated adenocarcinoma, intestinal type
- Glandular dysplasia, intestinal type

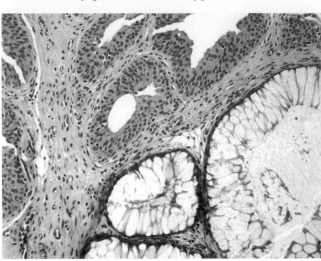

Fig 2. Intestinal metaplasia in which the lining of the glands of cystitis glandularis is replaced by mucin-producing goblet cells resembling colonic mucosa. Note the associated cystitis cystica proliferation.

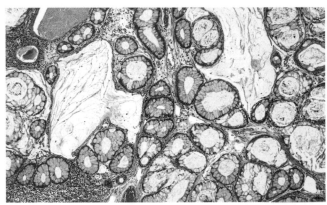

Fig 3. Acellular mucin extravasation, usually as isolated foci, is rarely observed in intestinal metaplasia acellular. In contrast, invasive mucinous carcinoma has large dissecting pools of mucin containing strips or glands composed of malignant cells.

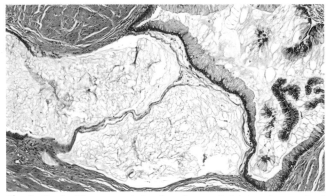

Fig 1. In florid cases, minimal and superficial involvement of muscularis propria by glands might be noted.

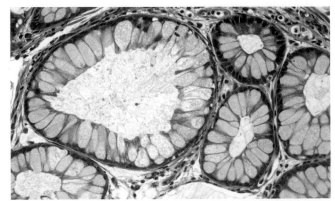

Fig 4. The glands are lined by benign goblet cells. Minimal reactive cytologic atypia may be observed, but the presence of moderate to severe atypia warns against the diagnosis of intestinal metaplasia.

NEPHROGENIC METAPLASIA/ADENOMA

Definition
- Benign proliferation of glandlike structures, most frequently found in the urinary bladder, which are thought to derive from implantation of shed renal tubular epithelium or from metaplasia of the urothelium, or both

Clinical features
Epidemiology
- Male predominance, approximately 2:1 to 3:1
- Most commonly found in patients 40 to 49 years old (range, 20 to 80 years)
- History of urothelial injury such as urinary stones, instrumentation, radiation, intravesical instillations, infection, or trauma
- Immunosuppressed patients following renal transplantation

Presentation
- Irritative voiding symptoms; hematuria
- Cystoscopic finding of polypoid, fungating, velvety, or flat lesions, single or multifocal; typically small (<1 cm), but can grow up to 7 cm

Prognosis and treatment
- There is a variable reported recurrence rate of 0.5% to 88%.
- The treatment of choice is transurethral resection with regular follow-up.

Pathology
Histology
- Typically, nephrogenic adenoma is composed of tubules lined by cuboidal to low columnar epithelium with eosinophilic cytoplasm; a peritubular hyaline rim of collagen is a common finding.
- Other patterns include:
  - Cystically dilated glands lined with flattened or hobnail cells resembling vessels
  - Atrophic tubules containing eosinophilic colloid-like material mimicking thyroid follicles and mesonephric hyperplasia
  - Small, mucin-containing tubules resembling signet ring cells
  - Exophytic papillae with or without true fibrovascular cores
  - A rare fibromyxoid variant with compressed spindle cells, and rare cords and atrophic tubules embedded in a fibromyxoid background, typically found in patients after radiotherapy
- There may be enlarged nuclei, prominent nucleoli, and degenerative atypia.
- Rarely, foci of solid growth pattern and clear cell changes might also be seen.
- Stroma may be inflammatory and edematous, but without desmoplasia.
- May involve the superficial aspects of muscularis propria.
- Features that should not be seen in nephrogenic adenomas include conspicuous solid growth patterns, diffuse clear cell changes, prominent cytologic atypia, and brisk mitotic activity.

Immunopathology (including immunohistochemistry)
- Positive for PAX2, PAX8, α-methylacyl–coenzyme A racemase, CD10, and CK7
- Can be weakly positive for prostate-specific antigen and prostate-specific acid phosphatase
- Negative for high-molecular-weight cytokeratin; usually negative for p63
- Low Ki-67 rate (<5%)

Main differential diagnosis
- Adenocarcinoma of the prostate, particularly the atrophic variant
- Müllerian clear cell adenocarcinoma (in female patients)
- Clear cell adenocarcinoma of bladder
- Signet ring cell carcinoma
- High-grade papillary urothelial carcinoma
- Infiltrating mucinous adenocarcinoma

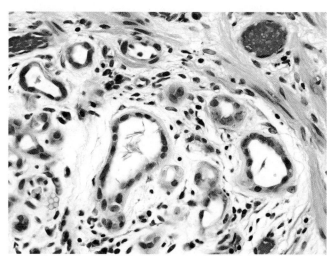

Fig 1. Classic pattern of nephrogenic adenoma showing tubules lined by flat to cuboidal eosinophilic cells, with occasional peritubular hyaline rim.

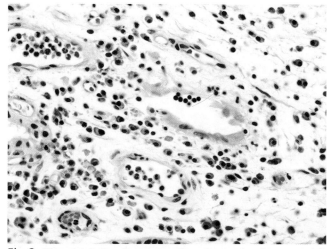

Fig 2. Vascular hobnail pattern of nephrogenic adenoma with chronic inflammation in the stroma.

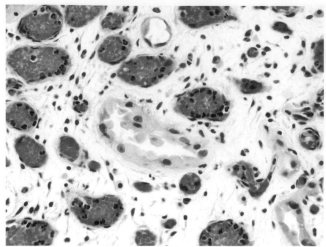

Fig 3. Vascular hobnail pattern of nephrogenic adenoma growing between muscle bundles of the muscularis mucosae.

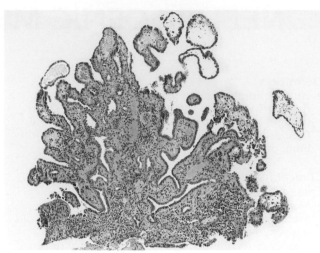

Fig 6. Low-power view of a nephrogenic adenoma with an exophytic papillary pattern of growth.

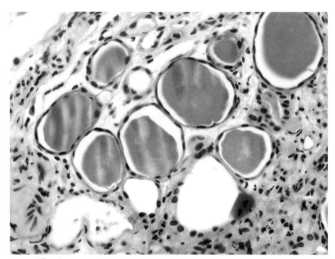

Fig 4. Thyroid-like pattern of nephrogenic adenoma.

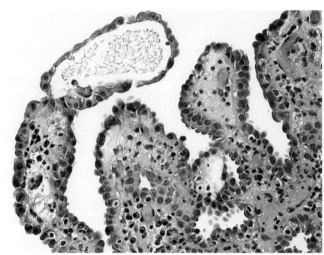

Fig 7. Papillary nephrogenic adenoma lined by a cuboid to columnar single-cell epithelium.

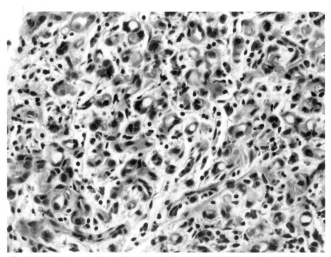

Fig 5. Nephrogenic adenoma with small tubules mimicking signet ring cells.

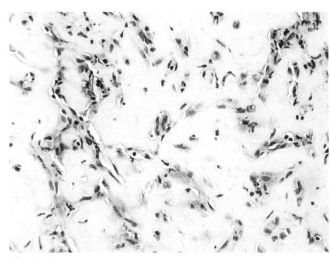

Fig 8. Fibromyxoid variant of nephrogenic adenoma composed of spindle cells forming clefts.

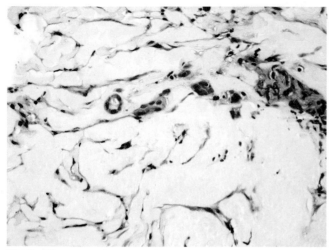

Fig 9. Fibromyxoid variant of nephrogenic adenoma with focal, uncompressed tubules.

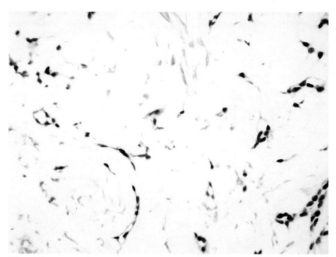

Fig 10. The identification of PAX8-positive cells aids in the diagnosis of the fibromyxoid variant of nephrogenic adenoma.

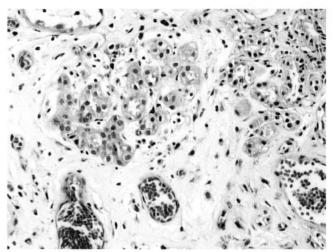

Fig 11. Nephrogenic adenoma with focal clear cell changes. Tubules are cytologically bland.

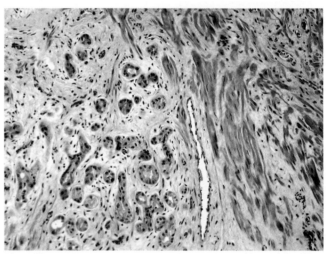

Fig 12. Nephrogenic adenoma with extensive downward growth and involvement of the bladder muscularis propria.

Definition
- Exophytic reactive lesion forming a broad-based polypoid or fingerlike papillary structure

Clinical features
Epidemiology
- Patient age ranges from 20 months to 79 years.

Presentation
- Can result from any inflammatory insult to the urinary mucosa
- Prevalent in patients with indwelling catheters (up to 80%)
- Often seen in patients with bladder fistulas
- Cystoscopically, friable broad-based or fingerlike exophytic lesion in an inflammatory background
- Variable size, but usually small lesions (up to 5 mm)

Prognosis and treatment
- No increased risk for development of urothelial carcinoma
- Usually disappears with the removal of the irritating agent

Pathology
Histology
- There is a normal or reactive urothelium overlying congested, inflamed, and edematous fibrovascular cores.
- Depending of the degree of edema in the fibrovascular cores, the lesion ranges from bullous cystitis to polypoid or papillary cystitis.
- Some authors distinguish polypoid from papillary cystitis based on the width of the fibrovascular cores (broader in the former) and the presence of fibrosis (more marked in the latter), but the distinction lacks clinical significance.
- In older lesions, the fibrovascular cores might become less edematous and replaced by dense fibrosis, often associated with chronic inflammation.
- Diagnosis should be based on the examination of the entire lesion and not on the features of single, isolated papillae.
- Because it is easy to appreciate the inflammatory nature of polypoid and papillary cystitis on cystoscopic examination, the diagnosis of urothelial carcinoma should be reconsidered when the cystoscopic clinical impression strongly favors an inflammatory or reactive lesion.

Immunopathology (including immunohistochemistry)
- Not contributory

Main differential diagnosis
- Papillary urothelial neoplasms

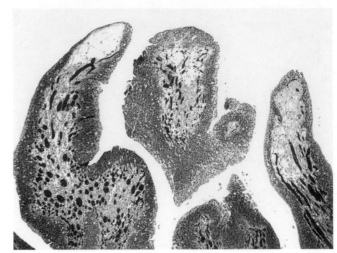

Fig 1. Polypoid cystitis showing broad-based exophytic structures with congestion and edema in lamina propria.

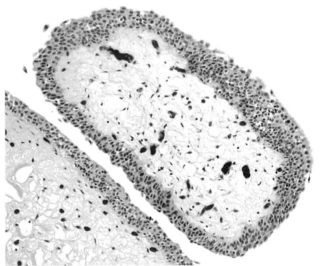

Fig 2. Polypoid cystitis showing normal urothelium lining the edematous fibrovascular core.

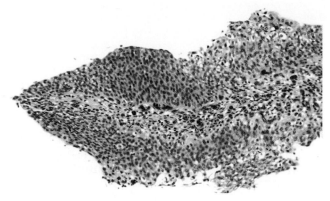

Fig 4. Papillary cystitis forming a fingerlike frond with no apparent edema in the fibrovascular core, mimicking a papillary urothelial carcinoma. Other areas showed the typical aspect of polypoid cystitis.

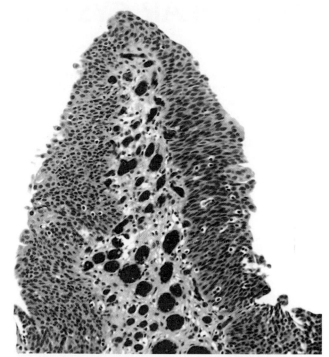

Fig 3. Papillary cystitis showing a hyperplastic urothelium lining the congested fibrovascular core.

Definition
- Inflammatory cystitis characterized by the presence of lymphoid follicles with germinal center formation.

Clinical features
Epidemiology
- Children affected more commonly than adults
- May be associated with a concurrent urothelial malignancy or urinary tract infection

Presentation
- Often nonspecific signs and symptoms including dysuria, frequency, urgency, and hematuria
- May be found coincidentally on evaluation for bladder cancer
- Cystoscopically, may demonstrate a nodular white-gray appearance on a background of erythematous mucosa

Prognosis and treatment
- Treatment of the underlying urinary tract infection often will resolve the condition.

Pathology
Histology
- Numerous lymphoid follicles are present in the lamina propria.
- Germinal centers are prominent.
- Associated acute and chronic inflammation often accompanies lesions.
- Urothelial lining might show reactive changes, but frank epithelial atypia is absent.

Immunopathology (including immunohistochemistry)
- Immunohistochemical stains or molecular diagnostics may be used to rule out a diagnosis of low-grade lymphoma, such as follicular lymphoma.

Main differential diagnosis
- Malignant lymphoma, low grade (e.g., follicular B cell lymphoma, mantle zone lymphoma)

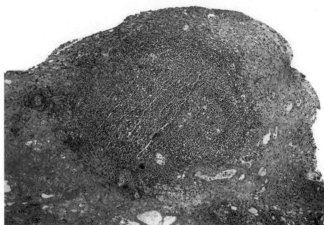

Fig 2. Denudation and accompanying inflammation of the bladder is common in follicular cystitis.

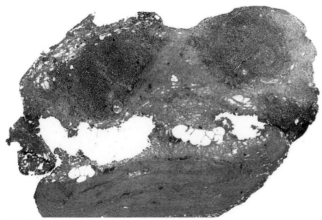

Fig 1. Low-power view of follicular cystitis showing multiple lymphoid follicles within lamina propria.

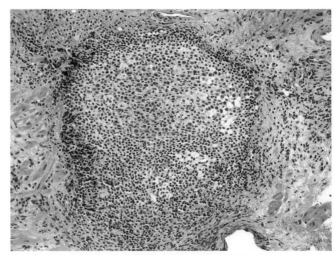

Fig 3. The lymphoid follicles observed in follicular cystitis frequently contain germinal centers that are normal in appearance.

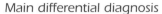

Definition
- The presence of atypical stroma cells in an otherwise unremarkable bladder

Clinical features
Presentation
- Not a clinical entity
- Similar cells sometimes seen in patients treated with chemotherapeutic agents and radiation

Prognosis and treatment
- Benign changes
- No treatment required

Pathology
Histology
- Normal histologic finding; commonly seen in bladder biopsy specimens taken for unrelated conditions
- Presence of atypical stroma cells in the lamina propria showing enlarged, hyperchromatic, multilobulated nuclei (i.e., degenerative atypia) and low or null mitotic rate

Immunopathology (including immunohistochemistry)
- Not required

Main differential diagnosis
- Radiation- or chemotherapy-related atypia
- Sarcomatoid urothelial carcinoma
- Primary bladder sarcoma

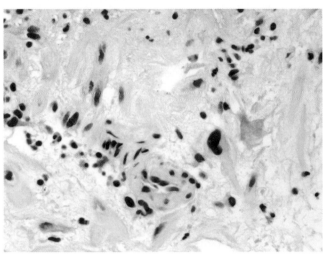

Fig 2. Atypical stromal cells in a case of giant cell cystitis. Other inflammatory cells are also seen.

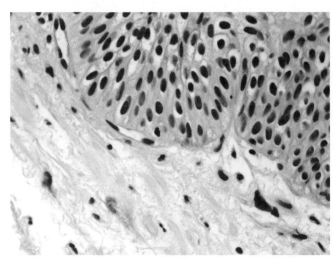

Fig 1. Giant cell cystitis is characterized by the presence of isolated atypical stromal cells in the lamina propria of the urinary bladder. The urothelium is unremarkable.

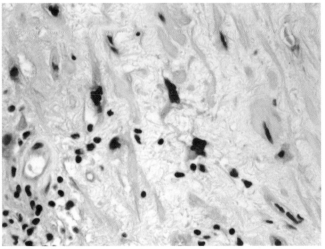

Fig 3. Atypical stromal cells with hyperchromatic, multilobulated nuclei.

INTERSTITIAL CYSTITIS/PAINFUL BLADDER SYNDROME

Definition
- Clinical pelvic pain syndrome characterized by bladder pain or urinary urgency (or both), glomerulations or Hunner ulcers visualized at cystoscopy with hydrodistention, and absence of other pathologies (diagnosis of exclusion)

Clinical features
Epidemiology
- Typically occurs in middle-aged females, with a female-to-male predominance as high as 10:1

Presentation
- The clinical picture is variable, often with insidious onset and being undiagnosed for years.
- Symptoms include suprapubic pain on bladder filling, nocturia, urinary urgency, and frequency with flares and remissions.
- Exacerbations before menstruation and with sexual activity are common.
- On cystoscopic examination, Hunner ulcers (erythematous patches of sloughed urothelium) and glomerulations (pinpoint petechial hemorrhages) are common.

Prognosis and treatment
- Prognosis is variable.
- Oral therapy with tricyclic agents (amitriptyline), antihistamines, intravesicular therapies, judicious use of analgesics, and surgical urinary diversion are used if all conservative therapies fail.

Pathology
Histology
- The primary role of histologic examination of bladder biopsy specimens is to rule out other bladder pathologies that can mimic interstitial cystitis.
- Common findings include denuded urothelium, ulceration, and submucosal inflammation.
- Findings may be divided into nonulcerative (punctuate hemorrhages under mucosa, multiple mucosal ruptures) and ulcerative (wedge-shaped ulcers with granulation tissue, fibrin and necrosis).
- Mast cells (in urothelium, lamina propria and muscularis propria) have been reported to be associated with interstitial cystitis; however, their presence is not specific for this disease and they are increased in urothelial carcinomas as well. Mast cell counts are no longer performed to diagnose interstitial cystitis.

Immunopathology (including immunohistochemistry)
- Not contributory

Main differential diagnosis
- Urothelial carcinoma in situ
- Eosinophilic cystitis

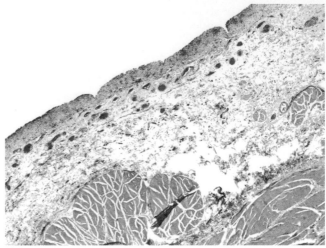

Fig 1. Focally denuded urothelium with edematous lamina propria. Denudation may also be associated with urothelial carcinoma in situ.

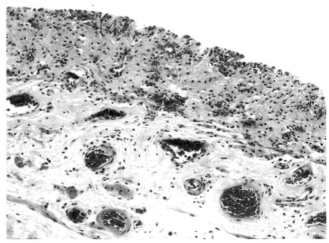

Fig 2. Punctate hemorrhage and extravasated red blood cells are visible in the lamina propria, with scattered chronic inflammatory cells and overlying urothelial denudation.

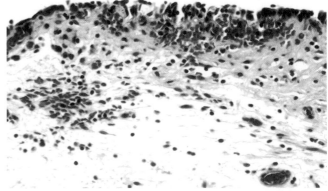

Fig 3. Focally, reactive-appearing urothelium is present. Because the cystoscopic findings of interstitial cystitis and carcinoma in situ may be similar, cystoscopy with biopsy specimens are necessary to rule out malignancy.

Definition
- Inflammatory condition of the bladder that can be idiopathic, but also associated with a variety of systemic triggers, such as food allergens, systemic allergic conditions like asthma or allergic gastroenteritis, topical insults with chemicals, parasites, systemic drugs, local trauma, and prior transurethral resection or catheterization

Clinical features
Epidemiology
- It has been reported at all ages, and approximately one fifth of cases occur in children.
- Overall female-to-male ratio is approximately 2:1.

Presentation
- The most common reported symptom is urinary frequency, followed by dysuria, gross hematuria, and suprapubic pain during urination.
- Other less frequent manifestations include microscopic hematuria, urinary retention, gastrointestinal symptoms, urgency, and incontinence.
- On cystoscopic examination, the appearance is variable with ulcers, exudates, edematous bullae, or polyps.
- On computed tomography or ultrasound examination, thickening of the wall is the main finding.

Prognosis and treatment
- Nonsteroidal antiinflammatory agents and antihistamines are usually the first-line agents.
- Steroids, cyclosporine, and azathioprine are second-line considerations.
- Cystectomy may be necessary if medical management fails.

Pathology
Histology
- There is edematous lamina propria with a mixed inflammatory infiltrate with a predominance of eosinophils.
- The overlying mucosa may show reactive atypia and exophytic formations typical of polypoid cystitis.
- Squamous metaplasia and prominent cystitis cystica are sometimes observed.
- Overt atypia is absent, as well as abundant mitotic figures.
- Intense inflammation with foci of necrosis has been reported.

Immunopathology (including immunohistochemistry)
- Not contributory

Main differential diagnosis
- Papillary or polypoid cystitis
- Systemic vasculitis (e.g., Churg-Strauss syndrome)
- Postsurgical (transurethral resection–associated) granulomas
- Radiation cystitis

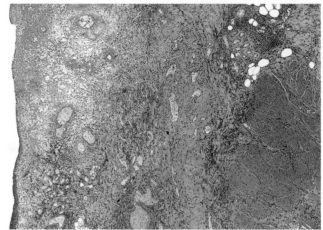

Fig 1. Low magnification of the bladder, transurethral resection specimen. There is denudation of the epithelium *(left)* with striking edema of the lamina propria associated with sheets of inflammatory cells infiltrating all layers, including muscularis propria.

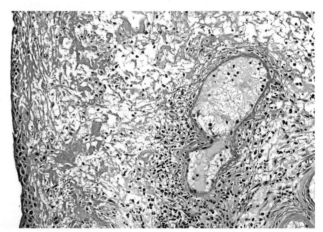

Fig 2. At higher magnification, there is a mixed inflammatory infiltrate in the lamina propria, composed mostly of eosinophils. Interstitial edema is pronounced.

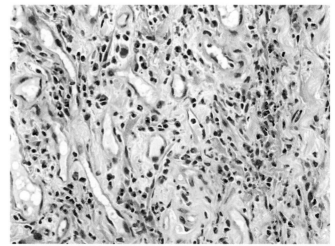

Fig 3. The inflammatory infiltrate is composed mainly of eosinophils infiltrating lamina propria.

Definition
- Infectious disease of urinary bladder owing to invasion by microorganisms (bacteria, viruses, fungi, or parasites)

Clinical features
Epidemiology
- Bacterial cystitis is caused mainly by coliform bacteria, is the most common cause of cystitis, and is much more common in women because of their shorter urethra. Predisposing conditions include structural abnormalities of the genitourinary tract (e.g., exstrophy, urethral malformations, fistulae with other organs, diverticula), bladder calculi, urine stasis, alkaline urine or systemic diseases such as diabetes, chronic renal disease, and immunosuppression.
- Tuberculous cystitis is almost always caused by mycobacterium tuberculosis, usually following renal tuberculosis, and rarely as a primary infection; it accounts for 7% of extrapulmonary tuberculosis cases.
- Viral cystitis is usually observed in immunosuppressed patients after bone marrow or kidney transplantation. The most common causative agents include adenoviruses types 11 and 21, papovavirus and rarely herpes simplex type 2, herpes zoster, or cytomegalovirus.
- Fungal cystitis is mainly caused by *Candida albicans* and rarely by *Aspergillus* spp. or other fungi; it affects mostly women, debilitated patients, patients with diabetes, or patients receiving antibiotic therapy.
- Schistosomal cystitis is more prevalent in the Middle East and in most African countries.

Presentation
- Complaints of dysuria, urinary frequency, urgency
- Possible hematuria
- Suprapubic or lower abdominal pain
- On cystoscopic examination, edematous bladder mucosa with areas of erythema, sometimes hemorrhage, diffusely or focally, and fibrinous exudates with mucosal ulceration

Prognosis and treatment
- Urine cultures to isolate the organism and appropriate antimicrobial therapy
- May recur if there are predisposing conditions
- May lead to gangrene of the bladder as a serious complication in the cases of circulatory compromise, vascular insufficiency, debilitating systemic diseases, or instillation of corrosive chemicals
- Increased risk for development of bladder malignancy in schistosomal cystitis, most frequently squamous cell carcinoma, with fewer cases of urothelial carcinoma, adenocarcinoma, and verrucous carcinoma

Pathology
Histology
- Bacterial cystitis: ulcerated bladder mucosa is covered by fibrinous exudates, mixed with bacterial colonies. There is neutrophilic infiltration in lamina propria, sometimes with abscess formation.
- The urothelium can be hyperplastic or metaplastic and may show reactive atypia. Granulation tissue and bladder wall fibrosis might be seen in late lesions.

- Tuberculous cystitis begins around ureteral orifices with superficial ulceration, acute and chronic inflammation, and marked mucosal congestion, initially with small noncaseating granulomas.
- Later, larger coalescent caseating granulomas with Langerhans giant cells, lymphocytes, and plasma cells can be observed.
- Viral cystitis: inflammation and hemorrhage (hemorrhagic cystitis) with adenovirus or herpes simplex virus type II. Intranuclear inclusions in urine cytology samples may be seen in cases caused by human polyomavirus.
- Fungal cystitis: ulceration and inflammation is seen in lamina propria with hyphae and yeast forms.
- Schistosomiasis: intense granulomatous inflammation with numerous eosinophils in response to schistosomal eggs in active stages. In late stages, destroyed and calcified schistosomal eggs, fibrosis, atrophy, and metaplastic changes in urothelial mucosa (keratinizing squamous metaplasia and intestinal metaplasia) and faded inflammation are seen.

Immunohistochemistry and special studies
- Histochemical stains: Ziehl-Neelsen stains for *Mycobacterium tuberculosis,* and egg shells of *Schistosoma hematobium, S. japonicum,* and *S. intercalatum*, PAS and GMS for fungal organisms
- Electron microscopy to demonstrate viral particles
- Immunohistochemical stains to show specific viruses

Molecular diagnostics
- Polymerase chain reaction–based techniques to show genetic material of the microorganism for viruses or mycobacterium

Main differential diagnosis
- Interstitial cystitis
- Nonspecific cystitis (polypoid cystitis, follicular cystitis, giant cell cystitis, hemorrhagic cystitis)
- Urothelial carcinoma in situ when prominent viral cytopathic changes are misinterpreted as a neoplastic process

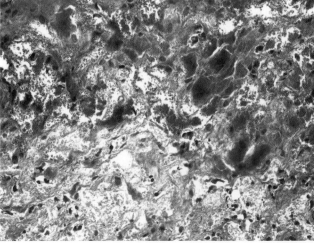

Fig 1. Bacterial ulcerative cystitis. Fibrinous exudate containing numerous bacterial colonies.

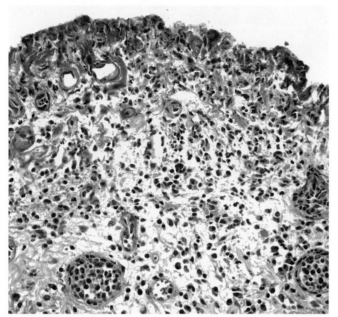

Fig 2. Acute bacterial cystitis. Leukocyte margination in congested vessels, along with neutrophils, plasma cells, and edema in lamina propria, and eroded urothelium are common findings.

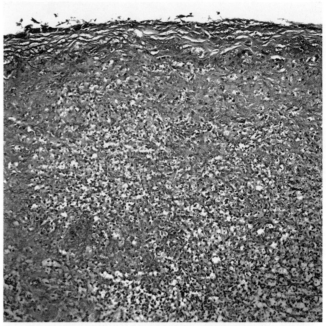

Fig 4. Gangrenous cystitis characterized by the necrosis of the bladder wall and suppurative inflammation.

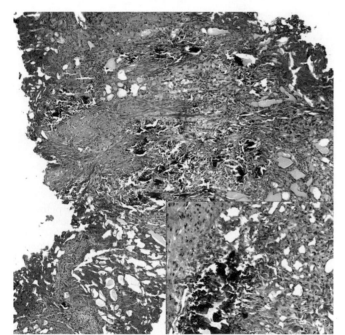

Fig 3. Encrusted cystitis. Large deposits of calcium salts are seen in bladder mucosa as the consequence of alkalization of urine by gram-negative urea splitting bacteria and deposition of inorganic salts including calcium *(inset)* in damaged mucosa.

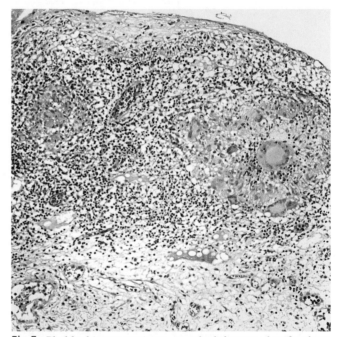

Fig 5. Bladder biopsy specimen near the left ureteral orifice from a 19-year-old female with renal tuberculosis. Two small tuberculoid granulomas with typical Langhans multinucleated giant cells and a peripheral mantle of lymphocytes are seen.

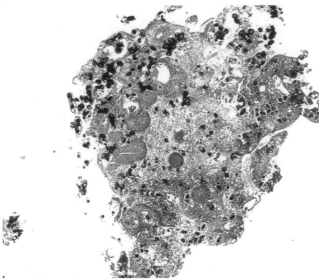

Fig 6. Schistosomiasis. Numerous ova in bladder mucosa, most of which are calcified.

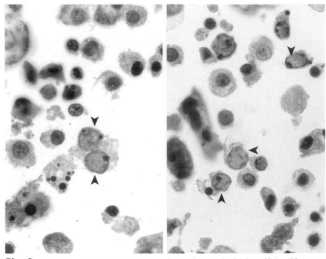

Fig 9. Decoy cells (BK virus infected urothelial cells). Characteristic basophilic homogenous, ground-glass intranuclear inclusions are noted.

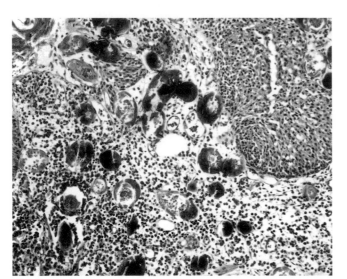

Fig 7. Active schistosomiasis. Eggs of *Schistosoma hematobium* surrounded by eosinophils and other inflammatory cells.

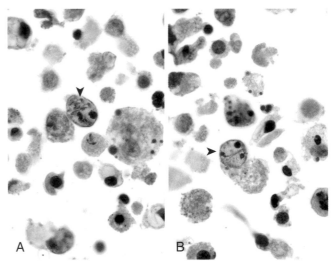

Fig 10. Urine cytology from a patient with renal transplant and BKV nephropathy. Different types of BKV-induced nuclear alterations are seen. **A,** The *arrow* shows a vesicular nucleus with the peculiar network of coarsely granular and clumped chromatin. **B,** The *arrow* depicts the nucleus with granular inclusions and incomplete halo surrounding them.

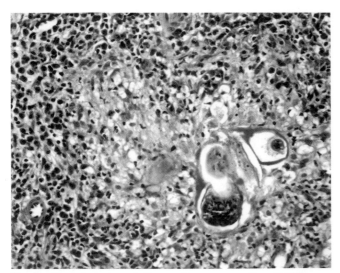

Fig 8. Granulomatous inflammation surrounding *Schistosoma* eggs.

Definition
- Relatively uncommon lesion caused by defects in phagocytic or degradative functions of histiocytes in response to bacteria (gram-negative coliforms)

Clinical features
Epidemiology
- More common in women (4:1), older patients, and immunosuppressed patients (HIV-positive and renal transplant recipients)
- Wide age range, typically 50 to 70 years

Presentation
- Most commonly involves the trigone bladder; may involve other sites including other genitourinary organs, gastrointestinal tract, lymph nodes, lungs, and bone
- Typically, symptoms of urinary tract infection
- Rarely associated with renal failure
- Cytoscopically characterized by multiple, soft, yellow-brown plaques (3 to 4 mm)
- Nodular thickenings of the bladder wall adjacent to the trigone

Prognosis and treatment
- Antibiotics that concentrate in macrophages (quinolones or trimethoprim-sulfamethoxazole)
- Discontinuation of immunosuppressive drug therapy

Pathology
Histology
- Foamy epithelioid histiocytes with granular eosinophilic cytoplasm in lamina propria (von Hansemann histiocytes), some lymphocytes, and occasional giant cells
- Histiocytes with an increased number of phagosomes containing undigested bacteria (usually *Escherichia coli* or *Proteus* spp.).
- Iron-containing, laminated mineralized concretions in the cytoplasm of histiocytes (Michaelis-Gutmann bodies)
- Development of fibrosis and scarring over time

Immunopathology (including immunohistochemistry)
- Histiocytic markers: CD68 and CD163
- PAS-positive Michaelis-Gutmann bodies
- Calcium in the early stages detected with von Kossa stain

Main differential diagnosis
- Xanthogranulomatous inflammation
- Granulomatous cystitis of other etiologies
- Langerhans cell histiocytosis

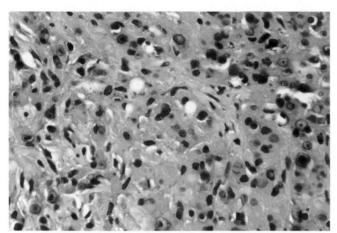

Fig 1. Michaelis-Gutmann bodies are easily found.

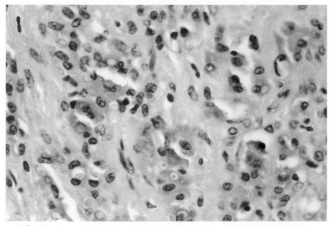

Fig 2. Iron stain highlighting Michaelis-Gutmann bodies.

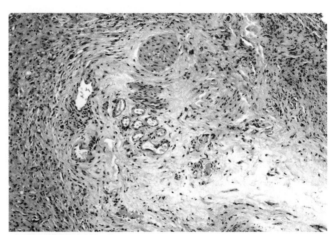

Fig 3. Medium-sized view of a case of malakoplakia showing a tumorlike lesion composed of abundant epithelioid cells with eosinophilic cytoplasm and ill-defined borders.

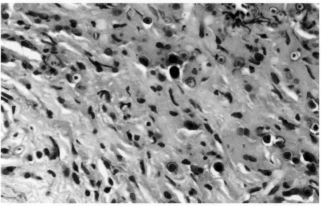

Fig 4. Abundant Michaelis-Gutmann bodies in a case of malakoplakia.

GRANULOMATOUS CYSTITIS AFTER BACILLUS CALMETTE-GUÉRIN THERAPY

Definition
- Granulomatous inflammation ensuing intravesical therapy with bacillus Calmette-Guérin (BCG) for superficial urothelial carcinoma

Clinical features
Presentation
- No specific clinical manifestations
- Erythematous or polypoid inflammation on cystoscopic examination

Prognosis and treatment
- No treatment required
- May cause tuberculous inflammation of the urinary tract in extremely rare cases

Pathology
Histology
- Caseating or noncaseating granulomatous inflammation with epithelioid histiocytes and multinucleated giant cells in the lamina propria of the bladder
- Superficial urothelium possibly showing ulceration or reactive atypia

Immunopathology (including immunohistochemistry)
- Ziehl-Neelsen stains might show some bacilli, but are seldom required for diagnosis.

Main differential diagnosis
- Tuberculous cystitis
- Postsurgical necrobiotic granuloma

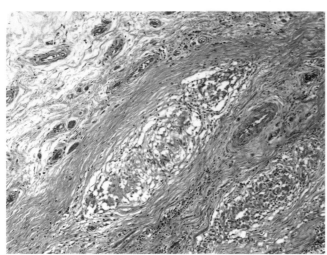

Fig 1. Granuloma in lamina propria of the bladder composed of epithelioid histiocytes and surrounding fibrosis and chronic inflammation.

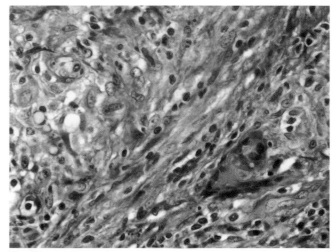

Fig 3. Multinucleated giant cells, epithelioid histiocytes, and lymphocytes forming a granuloma.

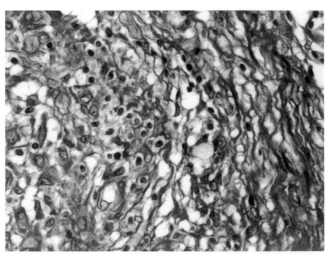

Fig 2. Granulomas are composed of epithelioid histiocytes with eosinophilic cytoplasm and ill-defined borders.

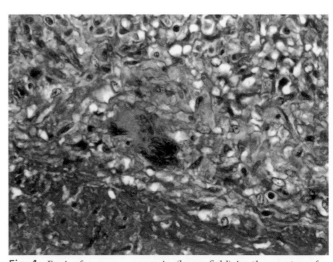

Fig 4. Foci of caseous necrosis *(lower field)* in the center of a granuloma composed of epithelioid histiocytes and a multinucleated giant cell.

Definition
- Radiation cystitis is characterized by a bladder lesion caused by irradiation of a pelvic organ for urothelial or nonurothelial malignancies. These lesions are dose- and time-dependent, and their spectrum can range from an inflammatory response to complete bladder retraction.

Clinical features
Epidemiology
- Frequency of chronic lesions is estimated to be 5% to 10% of patients receiving pelvic radiotherapy.

Presentation
- Acute radiation cystitis may appear 4 to 6 weeks after radiation treatment and is characterized by hematuria associated with frequency and urgency.
- Late radiation cystitis can develop from 6 months to 20 years after radiation therapy.

Prognosis and treatment
- It is not associated with increased risk of developing bladder cancer.
- Acute radiation cystitis is usually self-limiting and is generally managed conservatively.

Pathology
Histology
- Cells with high nuclear-to-cytoplasmic ratios with prominent, hyperchromatic nuclei, mild to moderate nuclear pleomorphism, and null to minimal mitotic activity; reactive cells are typically more bizarre than carcinoma in situ cells.
- Edema, vascular congestion and hemorrhage in lamina propria, with acute and chronic inflammation and hemosiderin deposits. Ulceration, hemorrhage, fibrin deposition, fibrin thrombi, fibrosis, thickened vessels, and vascular changes are commonly found.
- In pseudocarcinomatous hyperplasia, pseudoinvasive urothelial nests wrap around the vessels associated with fibrin deposition composed of cells with eosinophilic cytoplasm or squamous differentiation, or both. It can mimic carcinoma in situ or invasive cancer within the lamina propria.

Immunopathology (including immunohistochemistry)
- Immunohistochemistry using CK20, p53, and Ki-67 are helpful in distinguishing reactive changes of radiation cystitis from urothelial neoplasia.

Main differential diagnosis
- Invasive urothelial carcinomas

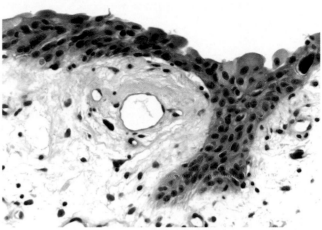

Fig 1. Radiation cystitis with isolated urothelial cells with marked atypia and nuclear hyperchromasia that mimics urothelial carcinoma in situ. Note the marked edema within the lamina propria.

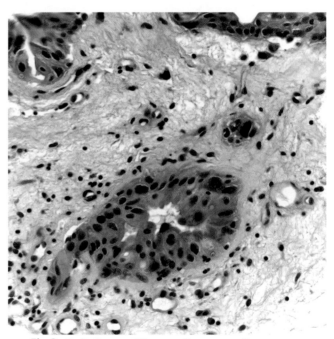

Fig 2. Radiation cystitis extending to von Brunn nests.

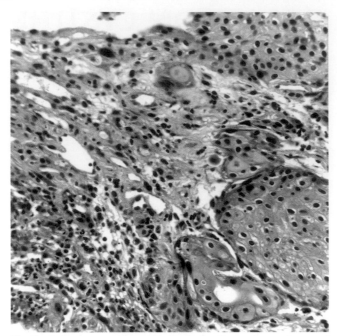

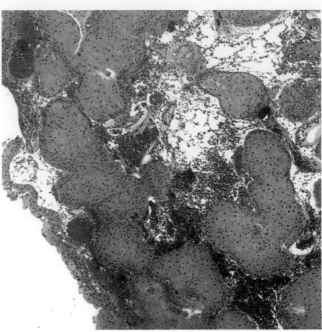

Fig 3. Radiation cystitis with atypical cells in the surface and within von Brunn's nests. Note the stromal edema and the presence of eosinophils and other inflammatory cells.

Fig 4. Radiation cystitis with pseudocarcinomatous hyperplasia: pseudoinvasive urothelial nests wrapping around the vessels associated with fibrin deposition. Note the edema, hemorrhage, and ecstatic vessels with fibrin.

CHEMOTHERAPY-INDUCED CYSTITIS

Definition
- Hemorrhagic inflammation of the bladder resulting from systemic chemotherapeutic agents or intravesical instillation of chemotherapy for superficial bladder cancer

Clinical features
Epidemiology
- Associated with the use of systemic chemotherapeutic agents owing to topical effects of excreted metabolites on the bladder
- Affects 8% of patients receiving cyclophosphamide; other systemic agents (e.g., gefitinib, gemtuzumab, ozogamicin, bortezomib, dacarbazine) and intravesical chemotherapeutic agents (e.g., mitomycin-C, busulfan) also associated with chemotherapy-induced cystitis

Presentation
- Hematuria, sometimes severe and uncontrollable
- Urinary frequency, urgency
- Cystoscopically, small capacity with erythematous lesions throughout the bladder mucosa

Prognosis and treatment
- Potentially life threatening
- Some cases with severe hematuria necessitate cystectomy
- Continuous bladder irrigation can be effective to stop severe hematuria.

Pathology
Histology
- Ulcerated or denuded mucosa with extensive edema
- Atypical reactive cells similar to those observed in radiation-induced cystitis with minimal mitotic activity
- Increased vascularity, hemorrhage, and neutrophilic infiltration in lamina propria
- Attenuated residual urothelium in early stages, but thickens and becomes hyperplastic in the later regenerative phase

Immunopathology (including immunohistochemistry)
- Not contributory

Main differential diagnosis
- Infectious cystitis
- Urothelial carcinoma in situ
- Urothelial dysplasia

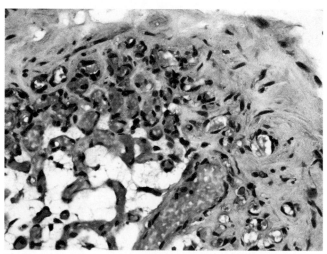

Fig 2. Chemotherapy-induced cystitis with markedly increased vascularity.

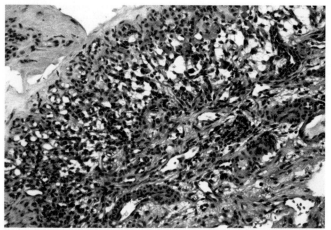

Fig 1. Chemotherapy-induced cystitis showing ulcerated mucosa with granulation tissue.

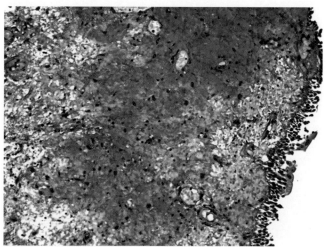

Fig 3. Chemotherapy-induced cystitis with extensive suburothelial hemorrhage.

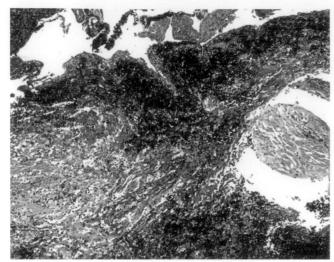

Fig 4. Ulceration with fibrinohemorrhagic exudate.

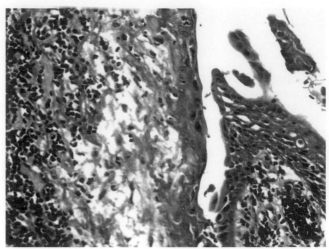

Fig 7. In early stages, residual urothelium is attenuated and atypical.

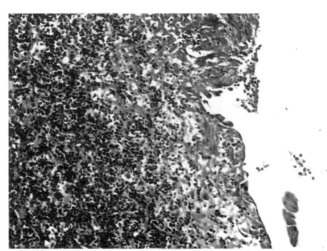

Fig 5. Fibrinohemorrhagic exudate with neutrophils.

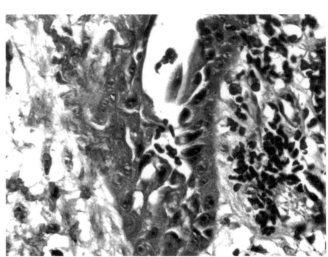

Fig 8. At higher magnification the urothelium shows atypical changes.

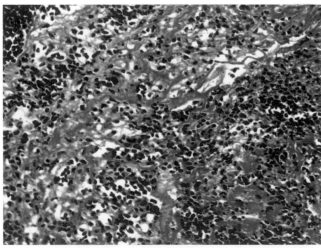

Fig 6. Chemotherapy-induced cystitis with extensive suburothelial hemorrhage and ulceration.

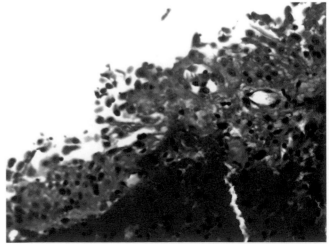

Fig 9. In chemotherapy-induced cystitis, the urothelium can be thickened or of normal thickness and display some atypical changes.

ENDOMETRIOSIS OF THE BLADDER

Definition
- Ectopic endometrial tissue consisting of endometrial-type glands, with or without accompanying endometrial stroma, within the bladder wall

Clinical features
Epidemiology
- Constitutes 1% to 2% of all endometriotic lesions in women
- Affects adult women in the reproductive age group, often with a history of prior pelvic surgery
- Can be found in postmenopausal women receiving estrogen therapy
- Rare in men, but reported in prostate cancer patients treated with estrogen

Presentation
- May be asymptomatic
- Pelvic pain and dysmenorrhea, dyspareunia
- Persistent cystitis with dysuria, frequency, hematuria
- Catamenial exacerbation of urinary symptoms
- Rarely with a pelvic mass
- Severity of symptoms possibly related to location and size of endometriotic lesions, with those at the base and larger lesions leading to more significant symptoms
- Cystoscopic examination showing congested edematous mucosa with underlying blue, blue-black to red cysts, or a hemorrhagic mass protruding into the bladder cavity

Prognosis and treatment
- Treatment includes medical hormonal administration or surgical resection, which can be accomplished by transurethral or laparoscopic methods.
- Symptoms may persist if the lesion is not resected.
- Rare reports of clear cell and endometrioid adenocarcinoma as well as endometrial stromal sarcoma have been documented as arising from bladder endometriosis.

Pathology
Histology
- Endometrial glands cuffed by endometrial stroma are found in the bladder wall, located in any layer of the bladder wall; mucosal erosions can be seen.
- When the endometriotic focus is discovered within the muscularis propria, the urothelial mucosa may be normal.
- There can be accompanying hemorrhage with siderophages and fibrosis in the vicinity of the endometriotic foci.
- Arias-Stella reaction can be seen in the endometrial glands under the influence of hormones, such as during pregnancy, and can pose a diagnostic pitfall.

Immunopathology (including immunohistochemistry)
- Epithelial cells lining the endometriotic glands are CK7+ and CK20+.

Main differential diagnosis
- Cystitis cystica et glandularis
- Endocervicosis
- Müllerianosis
- Adenocarcinoma

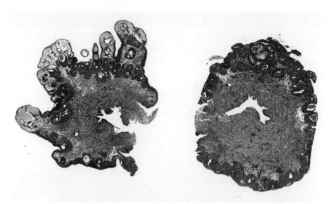

Fig 1. Bladder mucosa with irregularly dilated glands of endometriosis rimmed by accentuated stroma. Note the presence of broad edematous fronds in keeping with polypoid cystitis, cystitis cystica et glandularis, and colonic metaplasia.

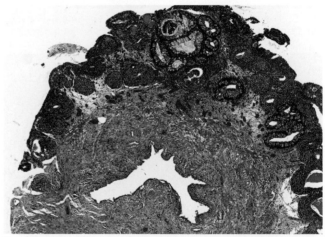

Fig 2. Medium magnification of the endometriotic gland, colonic metaplasia, and cystitis cystica et glandularis.

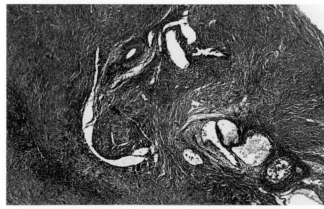

Fig 3. Several irregularly shaped endometrial glands with stroma.

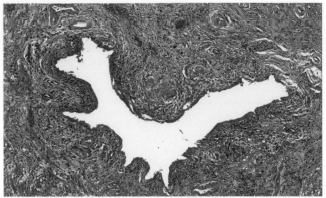

Fig 4. High magnification of the endometriotic gland lined by cuboidal to flattened epithelium harboring pink cytoplasm and vesicular nuclei and surrounded by plump stroma.

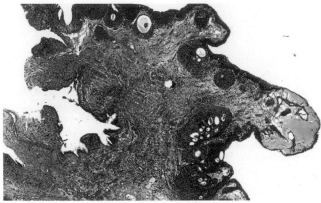

Fig 5. Polypoid cystitis and underlying endometrial glands amid smooth muscle fibers.

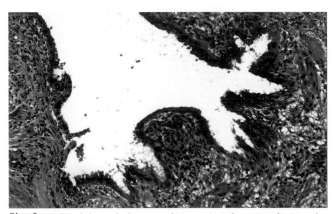

Fig 6. Cuboidal epithelium with occasional snouts lining the endometriotic gland and rimmed by a more cellular stroma.

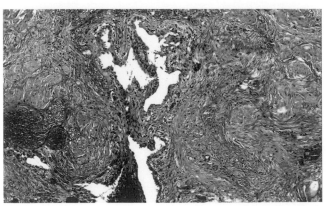

Fig 7. Another case with endometrial glands and stroma embedded within the muscle bundles of the muscularis propria.

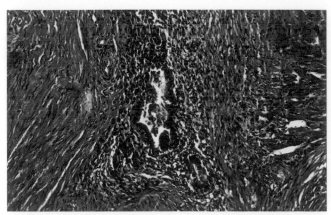

Fig 8. Endometrial glands with accompanying stroma within the bladder muscular wall.

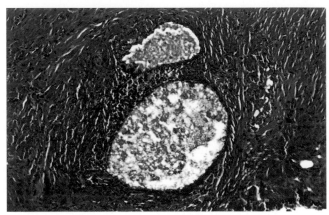

Fig 9. Glands lined by flattened epithelium with luminal eosinophilic, proteinaceous material.

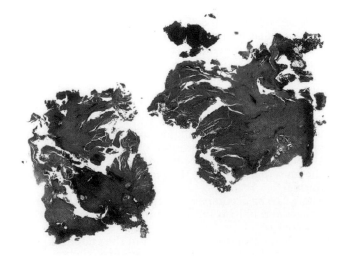

Fig 10. Bladder dome lesion composed mostly of fibromuscular stroma with a few glandular structures.

Definition
- Rare benign proliferation of prominent endocervical-type glands in the wall of bladder, especially within the bundles of muscularis propria, or at other sites of the genitourinary tract

Clinical features
Epidemiology
- Incidence is low, occurring mostly in women of childbearing age.
- There is an association with prior cesarean section.
- The lesion has been reported in males receiving estrogen therapy for prostate cancer.

Presentation
- Suprapubic pain, frequency, and dysuria
- Incidental finding of a bladder mass, usually located in the dome or posterior wall
- Also found incidentally in transurethral resection specimens for other causes

Prognosis and treatment
- Well-defined masses are usually resected by transurethral resection. No further therapy is necessary.

Pathology
Histology
- There is proliferation of irregularly shaped glands usually within the muscularis propria, but also involving the adventitia and mucosa of the bladder.
- The epithelium is columnar with pale cytoplasm and abundant mucin production.
- Scattered ciliated cells can be found easily.
- Gland rupture with mucin extravasation and stromal reaction is observed frequently.
- The architecture is haphazard, mimicking invasion into muscularis propria bundles.

Immunopathology (including immunohistochemistry)
- Positivity for HBME-1, estrogen receptor (ER), and progesterone receptor (PR), is common.
- The common cytokeratin profiles are CK7⁺ and CK20⁻.
- Ki-67 proliferative index is approximately 15%.

Main differential diagnosis
- Invasive adenocarcinoma
- Endosalpingiosis

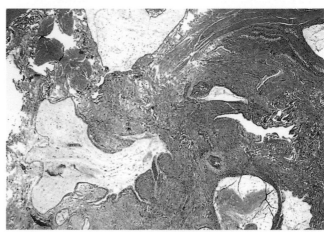

Fig 2. At low magnification, endocervicosis can mimic invasive adenocarcinoma, with a complex architecture of glands within the wall of the bladder. Note the presence of mucin extravasation and associated chronic inflammation.

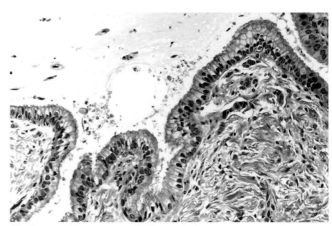

Fig 3. The lining of the glands resembles the one observed at the uterine cervix, with tall columnar cells, eccentric nuclei, and apical mucin. Nuclear grooves can also be seen. Nucleoli are small.

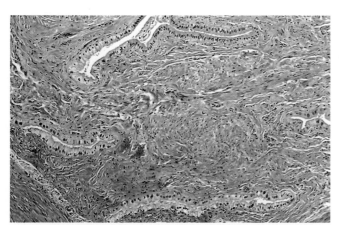

Fig 1. The glands of endocervicosis are commonly located within the bundles of the detrusor muscle (muscularis propria), mimicking invasive adenocarcinoma.

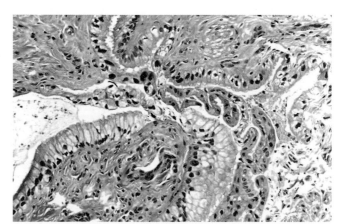

Fig 4. Occasionally, reactive nuclear atypia (hyperchromasia, loss of polarity, and increase in nuclear size) can be seen, but mitoses are rare and the other benign features are helpful on the correct diagnosis.

Definition
- Congenital anomaly in which the abdominal wall fails to close, allowing a portion of the bladder to protrude onto the surface of the abdomen

Clinical features
Epidemiology
- Rare; approximately 1 case per 50,000 live births
- Male-to-female ratio of 2.3:1
- May occur in the same family, with a risk of 1:100

Presentation
- Lower abdominal wall defect with bladder present on exterior of body
- May occur as part of the exstrophy-epispadias complex that includes undescended testicles and epispadias in males and a bifid clitoris in females

Prognosis and treatment
- Treatment involves surgical reconstruction.
- Patients are at risk for the development of bladder adenocarcinoma, as well as recurrent urinary tract infections and incontinence.

Pathology
Histology
- Grossly, the bladder is everted through the lower abdominal wall.
- Histology of the bladder is unaffected, although inflammation may be prominent.

Immunopathology (including immunohistochemistry)
- Not contributory

Main differential diagnosis
- Cloacal exstrophy

Definition
- Malformation of the urachus that includes a patent urachus, umbilical-urachus sinus, urachal diverticulum, and urachal cyst

Clinical features
Epidemiology
- Often diagnosed in infancy or childhood
- Occasionally identified on prenatal ultrasound

Presentation
- Often asymptomatic and found incidentally
- Possibly as an abdominal mass or discharge from the umbilicus if infection occurs
- Occasional urinary tract infections as sign of a urachal diverticulum

Prognosis and treatment
- Surgical reconstruction

Pathology
Histology
- The urachus connects the umbilicus and the apex of the bladder and undergoes atrophy and fibrosis after birth.
- Patent urachus is characterized by the peristant presence of a communication between the bladder and the umbilicus, with occasional periumbilical swelling and redness if inflamed.
- Umbilical-urachus sinus derives from a long-standing patent urachus that is often associated with purulent discharge, redness, and granulation tissue formation at the umbilicus.
- Urachal diverticulum represents an outpouching of the urothelium at the bladder apex caused by incomplete urachal closure.
- Urachal cysts are fluid-filled or mucinous cysts located between the umbilicus and the dome of the bladder, which are prone to infection by *Staphylococcus aureus;* they rarely may develop an adenocarcinoma.

- On histologic examination, urachal structures demonstrate pseudostratified columnar epithelium with surrounding concentric bundles of smooth muscle and are generally located deep within the bladder wall.
- Inflammation and granulation tissue may be prominent in inflamed structures.

Immunopathology (including immunohistochemistry)
- Urachal remnants are positive for CK7 and negative for CK20.

Main differential diagnosis
- Urachal adenocarcinoma
- Metastatic adenocarcinoma of extravesical origin

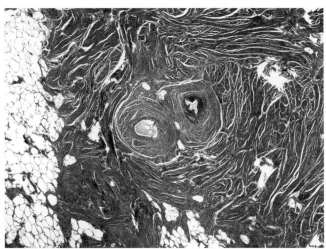

Fig 2. Urachal remnants occur in up to one third of adults and are generally located deep in the bladder wall of the apex, demonstrated here within the deep muscularis propria.

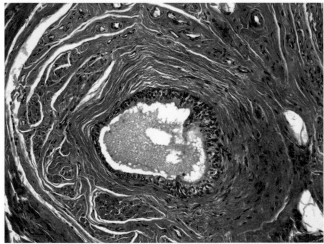

Fig 1. Urachal remnants contain pseudostratified columnar epithelium surrounded by a concentric muscle layer.

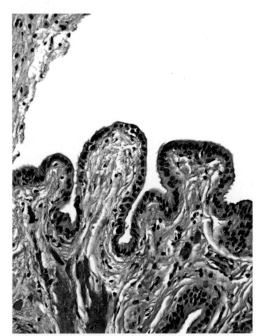

Fig 3. Urachal cysts may be mucinous or fluid-filled and show a compressed urachal lining.

Definition
- Outpouching of the urothelial lining of the bladder through the muscular wall of the bladder

Clinical features
Epidemiology
- It is diagnosed primarily in adult patients, especially middle-aged to older males, but can affect any age group.
- Congenital diverticula are more common in male patients and may be associated with urinary retention and vesicoureteral reflux.
- Acquired diverticula can result from neurogenic bladder or bladder outlet obstruction and also appear to have a male predominance.

Presentation
- Often asymptomatic, incidentally found
- Possible inflammatory symptoms, bladder stones, or urinary retention
- Can occur at any location of the bladder wall, ranging in size from 1 to 18 cm; rarely larger; single or multiple
- Rarely with a primary malignancy located within the diverticulum

Prognosis and treatment
- Treatment is primarily surgical for symptomatic patients.
- Although most diverticula have benign features, a bladder carcinoma may occasionally be present that will affect the prognosis.

Pathology
Histology
- Diverticula lack a muscularis propria; rather, a dense band of fibroconnective tissue is often present at the junction between lamina propria and perivesical fat.
- The urothelial lining is frequently inflamed and denuded with abundant acute and chronic inflammatory cells in the lamina propria.
- Granulation tissue, squamous metaplasia, and florid cystitis cystica et glandularis may be present.
- Neoplasms arising in diverticula include noninvasive papillary urothelial carcinoma, invasive urothelial carcinoma, squamous cell carcinoma, and small cell carcinoma.
- Staging of diverticular carcinomas may be challenging, especially as the distinction between lamina propria and perivesical fat is often poorly defined.

Immunopathology (including immunohistochemistry)
- Not contributory

Main differential diagnosis
- Associated cyst arising from adjacent location, including urachal cyst

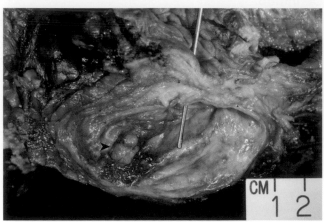

Fig 1. This large diverticulum connects to the urothelial lining of the bladder via a small, probe-patent opening. An associated urothelial carcinoma *(arrow)* is present within the diverticulum.

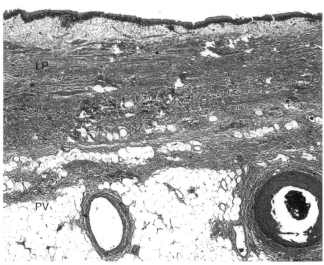

Fig 2. Bladder diverticula are characterized by a lack of the muscularis propria layer. The transition between lamina propria *(LP)* and perivesical fat *(PV)* is irregular and contains a significant amount of fibroconnective tissue.

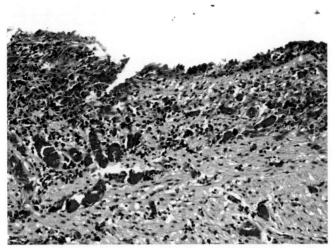

Fig 3. Diverticula frequently contain marked acute and chronic inflammation, shown here with ulceration of the surface urothelium.

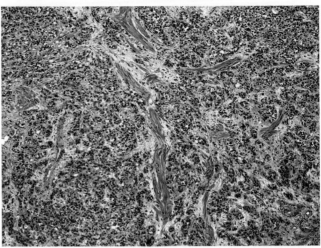

Fig 5. Invasive bladder carcinoma occurs in a subset of diverticula. Although urothelial carcinoma is common, other, less common subtypes of bladder cancer may also occur in these locations.

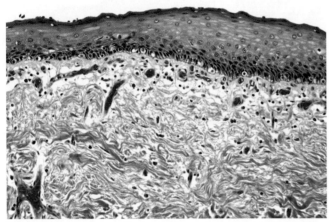

Fig 4. Squamous metaplasia is also commonly found in bladder diverticula.

Definition
- Benign prostatic glands and stroma forming a polypoid or papillary mass within the bladder

Clinical features
Epidemiology
- Often younger adult men (20 to 40 years old), but reported in a wide range of adult males

Presentation
- Gross or microscopic hematuria is most common, followed by voiding symptoms (urgency, hesitancy).
- Prostatic ectopic tissue is typically found in the bladder neck, trigone, or interureteral ridge.

Prognosis and treatment
- Transurethral resection is usually curative.

Pathology
Histology
- A polypoid or papillary lesion is typically composed of broad-based papillae, but occasionally of fingerlike villous projections.
- The surface is lined by benign urothelial cells or benign prostatic epithelial cells, or both, with underlying benign prostatic glands and stroma.
- Submucosal prostatic glands may contain corpora amylacea.

Immunopathology (including immunohistochemistry)
- Positive staining for prostate markers (e.g., prostate-specific antigen, prostate-specific membrane antigen) in the secretory cells

Main differential diagnosis
- Prostatic-type urethral polyp (only difference is location)
- Prostatic ductal adenocarcinoma
- Papillary urothelial neoplasm
- Benign prostatic hyperplasia
- Nephrogenic adenoma
- Adenocarcinoma of the bladder or urachus, or metastatic adenocarcinoma

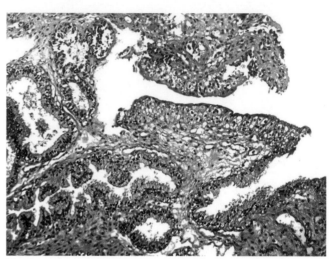

Fig 2. Ectopic prostate tissue appearing as a polypoid lesion, with the prostatic glandular tissue underlying the normal urothelial mucosa.

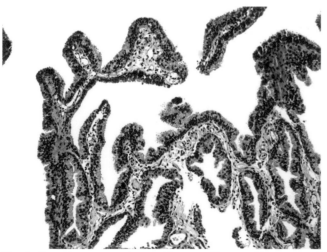

Fig 1. Ectopic prostate tissue with a papillary architecture and lined entirely by prostatic epithelium.

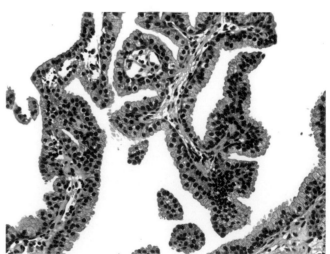

Fig 3. High-power image demonstrating papillary fronds lined by benign prostatic secretory cells.

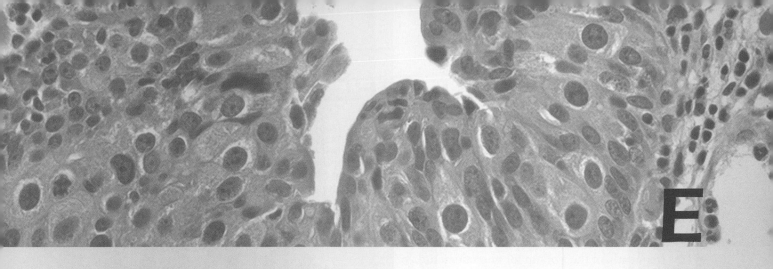

E

NEOPLASTIC DISEASE OF THE URINARY BLADDER

PAPILLARY UROTHELIAL HYPERPLASIA

Definition
- Undulating mucosal papillary folds lined by benign urothelium thicker than normal

Clinical features
Presentation
- Often identified as focally elevated lesion on routine follow-up cystoscopy for papillary urothelial neoplasms
- Less frequently in the workup for microhematuria or other urinary symptoms

Prognosis and treatment
- De novo urothelial hyperplasia is associated with an increased risk yet variable progression to low-grade papillary neoplasm.
- In patients with a prior history of papillary urothelial neoplasm, occurrence of papillary urothelial hyperplasia indicates early recurrence.
- Patients should be monitored more closely than the general population.

Pathology
Histology
- There are undulating papillary mucosal folds without true branching papillary fronds.
- The papillary folds are thicker than, but cytologically indistinguishable from, normal urothelium.
- Tangential section of papillary folds can focally mimic papillary fronds, but these structures are of limited quantity and contain more stroma than the delicate fibrovascular stalks in low-grade papillary neoplasms.
- Although reactive or degenerative atypia is allowed, if atypia reached the level of dysplasia or carcinoma in situ (CIS), the lesions should be diagnosed as dysplasia or CIS with early papillary formation.

Immunopathology (including immunohistochemistry)
- Similar to normal urothelium, positive for CK903, CK7, and p63

Main differential diagnosis
- Urothelial papilloma
- Papillary urothelial neoplasm of low malignant potential (PUNLMP)
- Polypoid cystitis

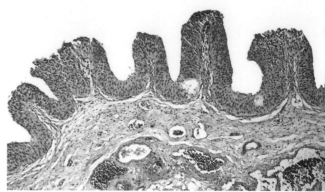

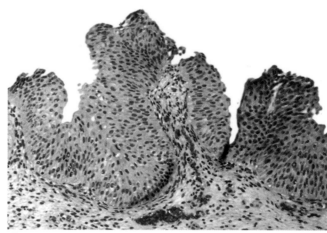

Fig 2. Papillary hyperplasia with tent-shaped, slightly broader folds. Note the absence of edema and inflammation typical of polypoid cystitis.

Fig 3. Urothelium in papillary hyperplasia is thicker than normal.

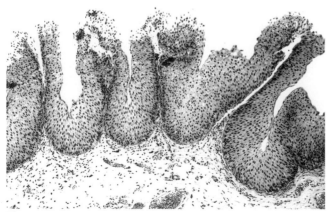

Fig 1. Papillary hyperplasia consists of undulating urothelium arranged in narrow papillary folds of varying height.

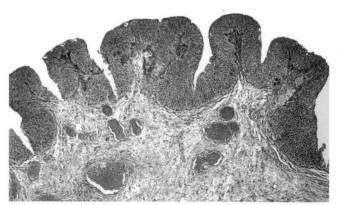

Fig 4. Lesion displays an architectural pattern of papillary hyperplasia at low-power examination.

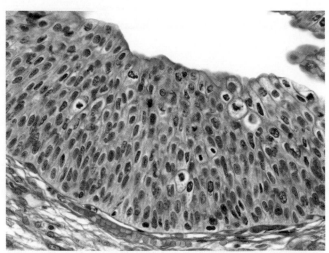

Fig 5. When atypias and mitoses are identified in an otherwise papillary hyperplasia, the lesion is better classified as *dysplasia/ marked atypia with early papillary formation.*

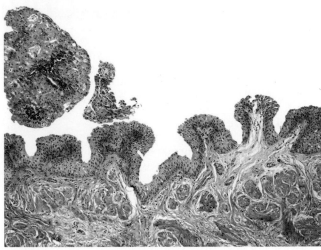

Fig 6. Transition from papillary hyperplasia *(right)* to urothelial papilloma *(left).*

Definition

- Benign epithelial changes, predominantly nuclear, seen in response to a secondary stimulus; reactive or regenerative urothelial changes

Clinical features

Epidemiology

- History of infection, urinary calculi, prior instrumentation, indwelling catheter, cystitis, or previous therapy
- Seen in men and women of all ages

Presentation

- Signs and symptoms owing to the underlying causative agent (e.g., stones, infection)

Prognosis and treatment

- Reactive atypia by itself is benign and requires no treatment; however, the source of the reactive atypia should be addressed.

Pathology

Histology

- Mild nucleomegaly (no more than twofold to threefold the size of a lymphocyte nucleus) is present.
- There are finely dispersed chromatin and pinpoint nucleoli (usually single, but may be multiple).
- Polarity perpendicular to the basement membrane is maintained.
- Cells may become rounded rather than elongate or fusiform.
- Pleomorphism is absent.
- Mitotic figures can be frequent and occasionally present in the upper layers of the urothelium; however, atypical mitotic figures should not be seen.
- Acute or chronic inflammation, or both, within the urothelium is often present.

Immunopathology (including immunohistochemistry)

- Negative or only surface umbrella cell staining with CK20
- Negative or only patchy and weak staining for p53
- Full-thickness or nearly full-thickness (superficial cells may be negative) staining for CD44 typical of reactive lesions

Main differential diagnosis

- Urothelial dysplasia (low-grade intraurothelial neoplasia)
- Urothelial CIS
- Urothelial atypia of uncertain significance (i.e., cannot definitively distinguish between reactive atypia and dysplasia/CIS)

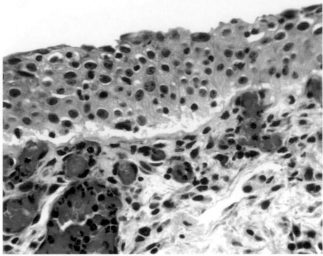

Fig 1. Reactive urothelial atypia is characterized by mild nucleomegaly, occasionally prominent nucleoli, fine chromatin, and nuclear rounding. Pleomorphism and detachment or loss of polarity are absent. Intraepithelial lymphocytes are present.

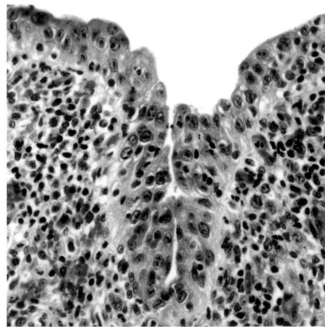

Fig 2. Nuclei in reactive atypia may be up to threefold the size of a stromal lymphocyte, and nucleoli may be prominent, as shown here. However, the nuclear chromatin pattern is still fine, and the urothelial cells show relative monotony. Again, intraepithelial neutrophils and lymphocytes are seen.

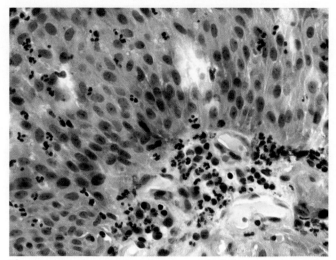

Fig 3. Numerous intraepithelial neutrophils are present. The urothelial cells have one or more pinpoint nucleoli in a background finely dispersed chromatin. Polarity perpendicular to the basement membrane is maintained.

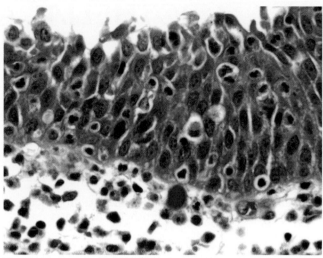

Fig 4. Nucleomegaly (twofold to threefold the size of lymphocyte nucleus) and variable nucleoli are evident in the reactive urothelial cells above. Mild, nuclear enlargement is common, particularly when marked intraurothelial inflammation is present. Clumped chromatin, hyperchromasia, and loss of polarity or cellular detachment are absent in this case and should not be seen in reactive processes.

UROTHELIAL ATYPIA OF UNKNOWN SIGNIFICANCE

Definition
- A descriptive category that was recently introduced to describe flat urothelial lesions in which the pathologist is uncertain whether changes are reactive or neoplastic

Clinical features
Epidemiology
- Often seen in biopsy specimens taken from patients with a previous history of urothelial neoplasia

Prognosis and treatment
- The term was originally introduced to convey the need for follow-up biopsy.
- The utility of creating this category is questionable.

Pathology
Histology
- Flat urothelial lesion with inflammation in which the severity of atypia appears to be out of proportion to the extent of inflammation, such that dysplasia cannot be confidently excluded
- Urothelium usually of normal thickness but can be thickened
- Acute or chronic inflammation, or both, in the lamina propria and urothelium often present
- Usually maintained cellular polarity
- Scattered mitotic activity

Main differential diagnosis
- Urothelial dysplasia
- Urothelial CIS

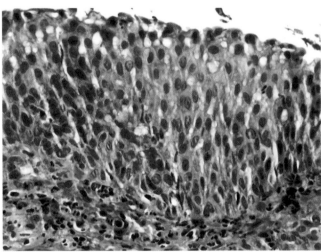

Fig 1. Severely inflamed urothelium in which the urothelial cells show mild loss of polarity, enlarged nuclei, hyperchromasia, and mild pleomorphism such that it is difficult to distinguish reactive from neoplastic cellular atypias.

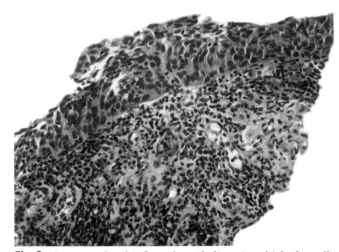

Fig 2. An example of inflamed urothelium in which the cells show mild loss of polarity and occasional large hyperchromatic nuclei with nuclear atypia somewhat out of proportion to the extent of inflammation, where it is difficult to determine whether those are reactive or neoplastic in nature.

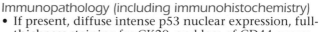

Definition
- Presence of distinct atypical changes in the urothelium falling short of the diagnosis of CIS

Clinical features
Epidemiology
- Predominantly middle-aged men

Presentation
- Usually found in patients with previous or concurrent urothelial cancer
- In de novo dysplasia, irritable bladder symptoms with or without hematuria
- Cystoscopically silent or mildly erythematous patch

Prognosis and treatment
- Dysplasia in patients with noninvasive papillary urothelial neoplasia is an indicator of urothelial instability and increased risk of disease progression (recurrence or invasion).
- It requires close follow-up with urine cytology for patients with de novo dysplasia, which progresses to urothelial neoplasia in 5% to 19% of patients.

Pathology
Histology
- Urothelium in normal thickness, but can be decreased or increased
- Loss of polarity and nuclei crowding
- Appreciable nuclear enlargement and hyperchromasia, noticeable at ×10 magnification field; nuclear enlargement falling short of the size of CIS nuclei (at least fivefold the size of a lymphocyte)
- Usually inconspicuous nucleoli (diffusely prominent nucleoli favor reactive atypia or CIS)
- Increased mitotic figures, occasionally in the upper layers
- Occurs in absence of inflammation, or the atypia appears disproportionate to the degree of inflammation
- May have early papillary formation and neovasculature at base
- Extensive denudation with clinging atypical cells not common

Immunopathology (including immunohistochemistry)
- If present, diffuse intense p53 nuclear expression, full-thickness staining for CK20, and loss of CD44 expression can be supportive.

Main differential diagnosis
- Normal urothelium
- Reactive urothelial changes to inflammation or therapy
- CIS

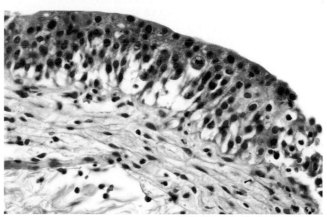

Fig 2. Urothelial dysplasia showing enlarged, hyperchromatic nuclei and mitotic figures in the upper layers.

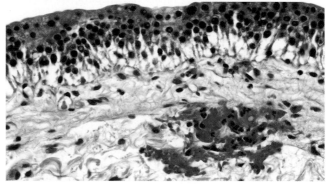

Fig 3. Urothelial dysplasia with abundant mitoses.

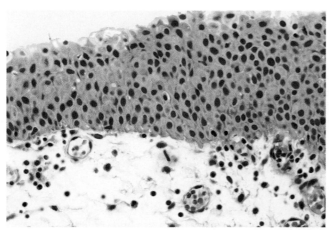

Fig 1. Urothelial dysplasia showing loss of polarity, nuclei crowding, and enlarged nuclei with hyperchromasia.

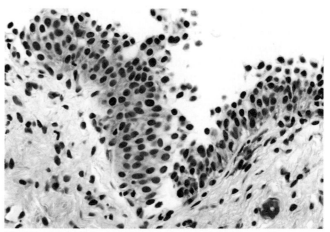

Fig 4. Urothelial dysplasia with discohesiveness and partial detachment.

173

Definition
- High-grade urothelial carcinoma confined to the urothelium that is flat (nonpapillary) in appearance

Clinical features
Epidemiology
- Similar distribution to invasive urothelial carcinomas
- Risk factors including tobacco smoke and exposure to industrial compounds such as aromatic amines
- Most common in the sixth to seventh decades, although may be seen in patients as young as 30 years
- Males more commonly affected

Presentation
- Generally identified in association with invasive urothelial carcinoma
- Possibly with nonspecific urinary symptoms such as hematuria, dysuria, or urgency
- Cystoscopically, urothelium often appearing erythematous but possibly normal
- Frequently multifocal

Prognosis and treatment
- Approximately half of all patients will develop invasive urothelial carcinoma.
- Bacillus Calmette-Guérin (BCG) therapy for initial presentation
- Cystectomy should be considered for patients with concurrent invasive urothelial carcinoma into the muscularis propria or patients with refractory CIS disease who did respond to repeated attempts of intravesical therapy.

Pathology
Histology
- Atypia ranges from subtle, enlarged nuclei to marked anaplasia.
- Nuclear enlargement is often greater than fivefold the size of a lymphocyte, with hyperchromasia and loss of polarity and disorganized appearance to the urothelium.
- Apoptotic debris are commonly observed.
- Frequent mitoses, including atypical mitoses, extend throughout the urothelium.
- Cell adhesion is lost, occasionally resulting in prominent denudation.
- Subtypes include micropapillary, clinging, and pagetoid variants.
- It may involve von Brunn nests and spread into prostatic ducts when the prostatic urethra is colonized.

Immunopathology (including immunohistochemistry)
- CK20 demonstrates full-thickness immunoreactivity, in contrast to an umbrella cell–only pattern in normal and reactive conditions.
- There is increased p53 immunoreactivity.
- CD44 immunostaining is limited to basal layers of the urothelium or absent.

Main differential diagnosis
- Reactive or inflammatory urothelial atypia
- Radiation urothelial atypia

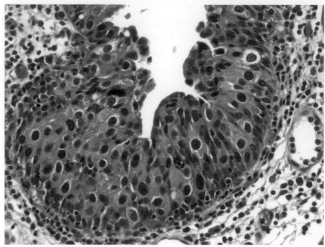

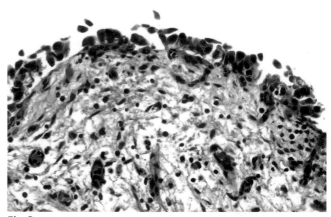

Fig 1. Flat CIS is characterized by enlarged, hyperchromatic nuclei with variable atypia and frequent mitoses, including atypical mitoses. Nuclei are frequently greater than fourfold to fivefold the size of a lymphocyte. Loss of polarity is common.

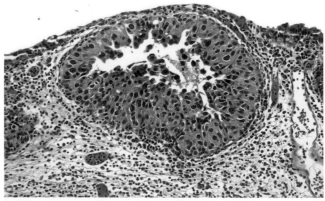

Fig 2. Flat CIS can vary in thickness and may be relatively thin, as demonstrated here. Occasionally, individual CIS cells may be present along a denuded surface in the case of clinging CIS.

Fig 3. Extension of carcinoma in situ into von Brunn nests.

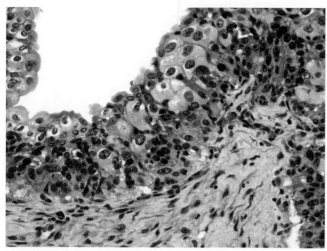

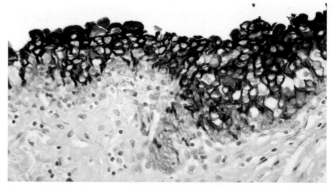

Fig 7. Full-thickness CK20 is common in carcinoma in situ. In contrast, normal urothelium demonstrates CK20 only in the umbrella-cell layer.

Fig 4. Carcinoma in situ with a pagetoid pattern of growth. Note the large, balloonlike cells that interdigitate between normal urothelial cells.

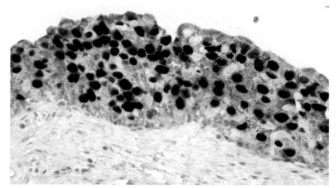

Fig 8. Full-thickness, intense nuclear p53 staining is frequently observed in CIS and occurs in association with p53 mutation.

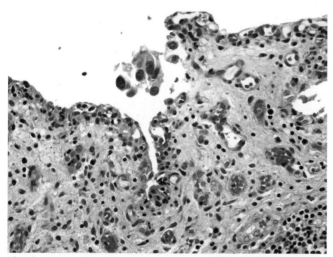

Fig 5. Occasionally, small detached clusters of CIS in a background of extensive denudation may be the only indicator of disease.

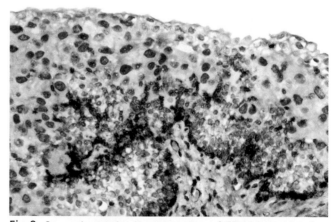

Fig 9. In carcinoma in situ, expression of CD44 is restricted to the basal layers of the urothelium or may be entirely absent.

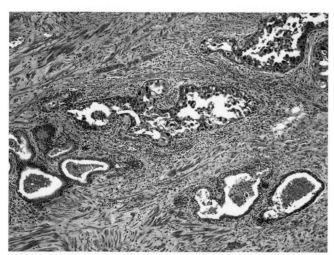

Fig 6. In cases of carcinoma in situ involving the prostatic urethra, it can spread within prostatic ducts (intraductal spread).

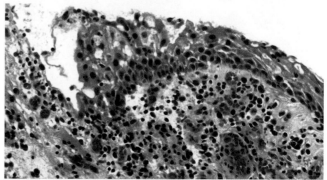

Fig 10. Reactive atypia can be distinguished by associated inflammation, pinpoint nucleoli, and occasional squamous changes.

Definition
- Benign exophytic urothelial neoplasm characterized by simple, usually nonbranching papillary fronds lined by normal-appearing urothelium

Clinical features
Epidemiology
- Accounts for 1% to 4% of bladder tumors
- Male-to-female ratio, 0.9:1
- Usually occurs in young patients
- Can be seen in children

Presentation
- Hematuria
- Cystoscopic appearance similar to other low-grade papillary urothelial neoplasms

Prognosis and treatment
- Clinical course is typically favorable, although rarely patients may experience recurrence and progression to higher-grade disease.

Pathology
Histology
- Papillary fronds are lined by normal-appearing urothelium lacking atypia.
- Most papillomas have slender fibrovascular stalks.
- Superficial umbrella cells are often prominent with vacuolization of the cytoplasm and eosinophilic changes.
- Urothelial atypia, other than that in umbrella cells, excludes the diagnosis of papilloma.
- Mitoses are rare or absent.

Immunopathology (including immunohistochemistry)
- CK20 expression is confined to the umbrella cells, similar to normal urothelium.

Main differential diagnosis
- PUNLMP
- Low-grade urothelial carcinoma

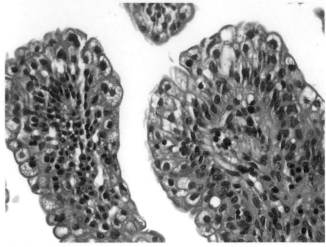

Fig 2. At high-power view the papillary fronds are lined by cytologically and architecturally normal-appearing urothelium.

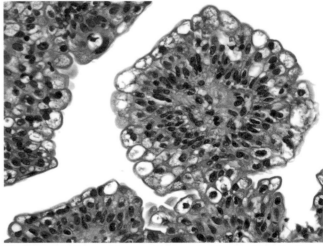

Fig 3. Urothelial papilloma with superficial umbrella cells showing prominent vacuolization and eosinophilic cytoplasm.

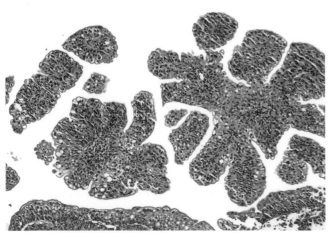

Fig 1. Low-power view of urothelial papilloma with slender, delicate fibrovascular stalks.

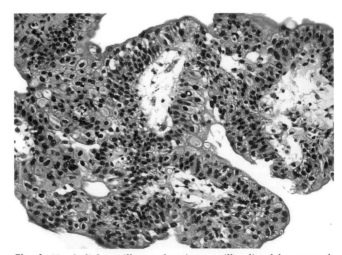

Fig 4. Urothelial papilloma showing papillae lined by normal-appearing urothelium.

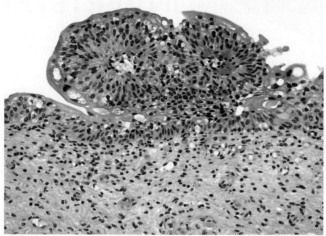

Fig 5. Urothelial papilloma with prominent umbrella cells.

Definition
- Benign urothelial neoplasm with a predominant endophytic pattern of growth

Clinical features
Epidemiology
- Unusual lesion, accounting for less than 1% of all bladder urothelial neoplasms
- Male predominance with a broad range of age

Presentation
- Gross or microscopic hematuria
- Slightly raised or polypoid lesions at cystoscopy, most common at trigone and bladder neck, measuring usually less than 3 cm

Prognosis and treatment
- Complete transurethral resection
- Recurrence in less than 1% of cases

Pathology
Histology
- Endophytic proliferation of thin interconnecting cords and trabeculae is formed by urothelial cells with no cytologic atypia and showing peripheral palisading, smooth borders, and no stromal reaction.
- Nonkeratinizing squamous metaplasia and cystitis cystica et glandularis–like changes are common.
- Mitotic activity is null to minimal and restricted to the basal layer.
- Surface is normal and nonpapillomatous.

Immunopathology (including immunohistochemistry)
- Not required

Main differential diagnosis
- Noninvasive urothelial neoplasms with inverted growth pattern (e.g., inverted PUNLMP)
- Invasive nested urothelial carcinoma
- Paraganglioma
- Florid von Brunn nests
- Cystitis cystica et glandularis
- Carcinoid tumor

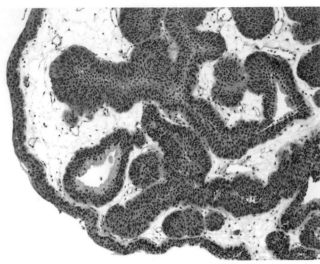

Fig 2. Inverted papilloma with thin, anastomosing trabeculae. Note the unremarkable urothelial surface.

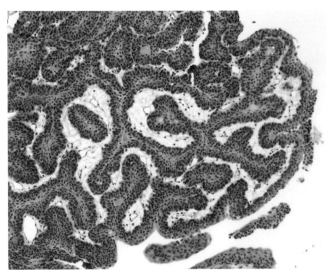

Fig 1. Inverted papilloma composed of endophytic nests forming anastomosing cords and trabeculae.

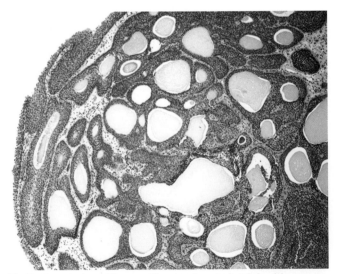

Fig 3. Inverted papilloma with prominent glandular-like spaces.

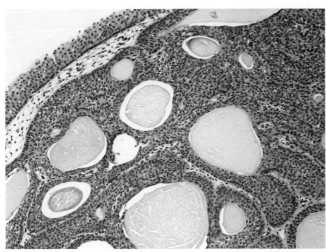

Fig 4. Inverted papilloma with cystitis cystica–like changes. Note the normal overlying urothelium.

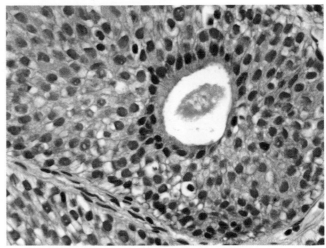

Fig 7. Inverted papilloma with cystitis glandularis–like metaplasia.

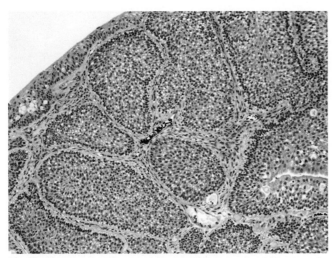

Fig 5. Inverted papilloma with round nests and evident peripheral palisading.

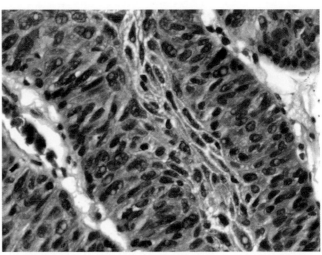

Fig 8. Inverted papilloma with squamous metaplasia (spindle-shaped cells with distinctive cellular borders and intercellular bridges) at the center of the tumor nest.

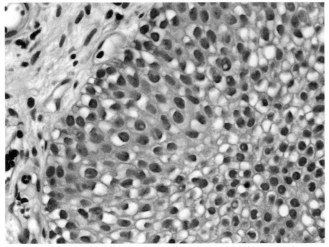

Fig 6. Inverted papilloma with vacuolization. Note the absence of atypias in the tumor cells.

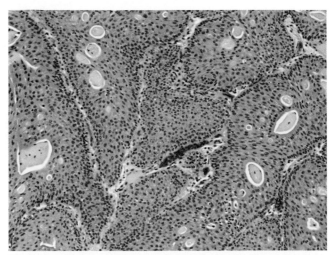

Fig 9. Inverted papilloma composed of tumor cells with prominent eosinophilic cytoplasm and glandular metaplasia. Borders are slightly irregular, but there is evident peripheral palisading and no atypias.

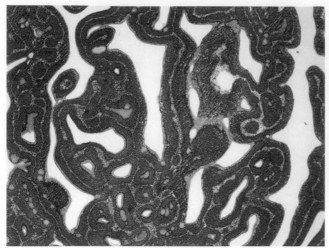

Fig 10. Inverted papilloma with prominent glandular metaplasia.

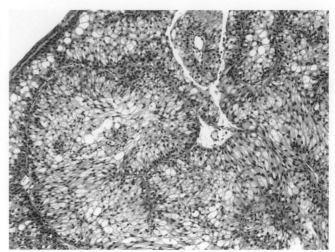

Fig 12. Inverted papilloma composed of tumor cells with foamy cytoplasm.

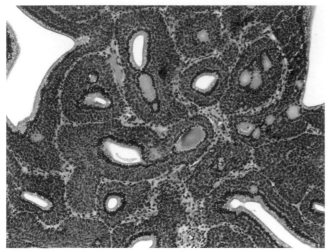

Fig 11. Inverted papilloma with cystitis glandularis–like changes.

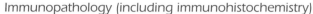

PAPILLARY UROTHELIAL NEOPLASM OF LOW MALIGNANT POTENTIAL

Definition
- Papillary urothelial tumor with abnormally thick urothelium, but lacking cytologic atypia

Clinical features
Epidemiology
- Three in 100,000 individuals per year
- Average age, approximately 65 years
- Predominance of males; male-to-female ratio, 5:1
- Comprise approximately 15% of all noninvasive urothelial neoplasms

Presentation
- Gross or microscopic hematuria
- Typically negative urine cytology
- On cystoscopy, a papillary tumor typically measuring less than 2 cm

Prognosis and therapy
- Complete transurethral resection (therapy of choice)
- Recurrence in 18% to 47%
- Progression in less than 2%
- No deaths reported

Pathology
Histology
- Papillae lined by thickened urothelium (more than seven cell layers) with a monotonous population of cells, often in a parallel arrangement
- Urothelial polarity preserved, with intact umbrella cells
- Absence of cytologic atypia
- Mitoses rare and restricted to basal layer

Immunopathology (including immunohistochemistry)
- Not contributory

Main differential diagnosis
- Noninvasive low-grade urothelial carcinoma
- Urothelial papilloma

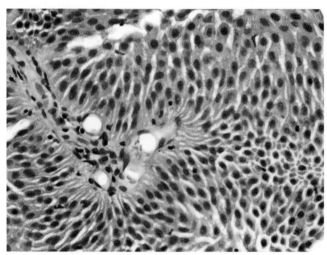

Fig 2. Polarized urothelial cells without atypia or mitoses.

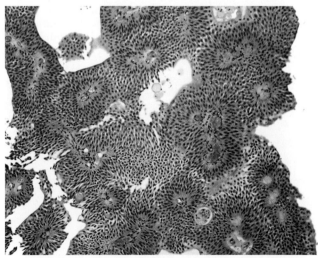

Fig 1. Papillary tumor with thickened urothelium.

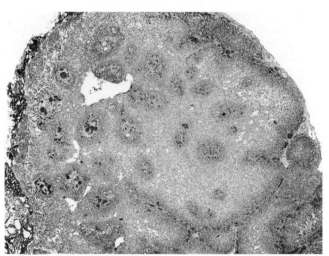

Fig 3. Low-power view shows thickened papillae. This tumor has an inverted growth pattern.

LOW-GRADE PAPILLARY UROTHELIAL CARCINOMA

Definition
- Papillary neoplasm lined by urothelium with easily recognizable variation in cytologic features and characterized by an overall orderly appearance of the urothelium lining papillary fronds

Clinical features
Epidemiology
- It is slightly more common in men.
- Age at diagnosis ranges from 28 to 90 years.
- Tumors are usually solitary, but two or more lesions can be present.

Presentation
- Usually with gross or microscopic hematuria

Prognosis and treatment
- Recurrence is common and occurs in approximately 50% to 70% of patients.
- Progression to invasion and cancer deaths occurs in less than 5% of cases.
- Transurethral resection is the treatment of choice.
- Multifocal or recurrent disease is sometimes treated with intravesical immunotherapy.

Pathology
Histology
- Slender papillary fronds show frequent branching and minimal fusion.
- Architectural appearance is orderly with easily recognizable variations in cytologic features.
- Nuclei are uniformly enlarged with mild differences in shape, contour, and chromatin distribution,
- Inconspicuous nucleoli may be present.
- Mitoses can occur at any level of the urothelium.
- If a tumor contains a high-grade component of more than 5%, the lesion should be classified as high-grade papillary urothelial carcinoma.
- In cases with a high-grade component of less than 5%, the lesion can be diagnosed as low-grade papillary urothelial carcinoma with a comment indicating the presence of focal high-grade tumor; the significance of such categorization remains unknown.

Immunopathology (including immunohistochemistry)
- Generally noncontributory: immunohistochemical p53 and Ki-67 expression is less intense than in high-grade urothelial carcinoma.

Main differential diagnosis
- Papillary urothelial neoplasm of low malignant potential
- High-grade papillary urothelial carcinoma

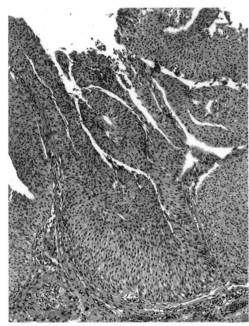

Fig 2. Low-grade papillary urothelial carcinoma with slender papillary fronds showing minimal fusion.

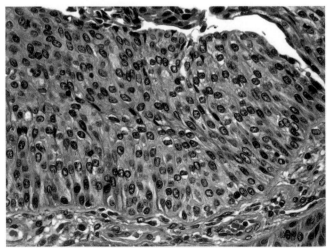

Fig 3. At high-power view the lesion shows an orderly architectural appearance with easily recognizable variations in cytologic features. The nuclei are uniformly enlarged with mild differences in shape, contour, and chromatin distribution.

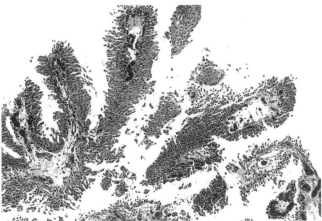

Fig 1. Low-grade papillary urothelial carcinoma with slender papillae and vascular congestion.

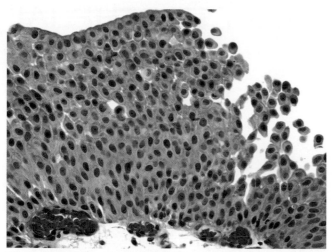

Fig 4. At high-power view the lesion shows enlarged nuclei with some contour irregularity and small nucleoli.

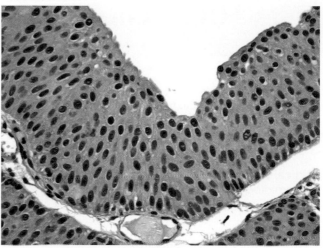

Fig 6. Low-grade papillary urothelial carcinoma with minimal architectural disorganization and mild cytologic atypia.

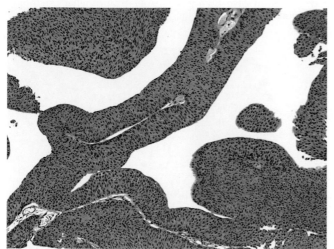

Fig 5. Low-grade papillary urothelial carcinoma with slender papillae.

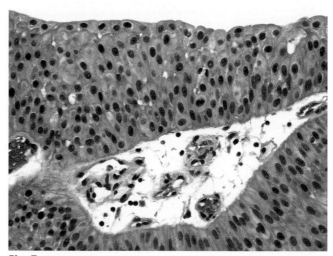

Fig 7. Low-grade papillary urothelial carcinoma with mitotic figures above the basal layer.

HIGH-GRADE PAPILLARY UROTHELIAL CARCINOMA

Definition
- Urothelial neoplasm exhibiting papillary fronds, which shows a significantly disordered architectural and cytologic pattern with moderate cytologic atypia

Clinical features
Epidemiology
- Predominantly male, older than 50 years

Presentation
- Gross or microscopic hematuria
- Cystoscopic findings varying from papillary to solid sessile lesions, single or multiple

Prognosis and treatment
- Progression to invasive cancer in 15% to 40% of patients
- Transurethral resection and fulguration, followed by regular cystoscopy and urine cytology
- Intravesical BCG immunotherapy
- Intravesical chemotherapy (mitomycin-C, doxorubicin, Gemcitabine, and thiotepa), interferon-α therapy, or photodynamic therapy
- Cystectomy considered rarely in refractory, multifocal, and large lesions

Pathology
Histology
- Architectural features include: frequently fused papillae, variable urothelial thickness, cellular disorganization, and loss of polarity.
- Cytologic features include: moderate to marked pleomorphism, frequent mitotic figures throughout the urothelium, enlarged nuclei with variation in size, irregular nuclear contour, clumped chromatin, and prominent and occasionally multiple nucleoli.
- Urothelium is more likely to be denuded with prominent cellular detachment.
- There may be a variable degree of squamous differentiation.
- There may be focal glandular differentiation.
- When coexisting with low-grade papillary urothelial carcinoma, the histologic grade should be given according to the highest grade.
- Occasionally, a tumor may be graded as low grade with a minor component (<5%) of high-grade tumor if the high-grade component is focal.

Immunopathology (including immunohistochemistry)
- Diffuse intense p53 nuclear expression, full-thickness staining for CK20, and loss of CD44 expression is observed in two thirds of the cases.

Main differential diagnosis
- Low-grade papillary urothelial carcinoma
- Invasive papillary urothelial carcinoma

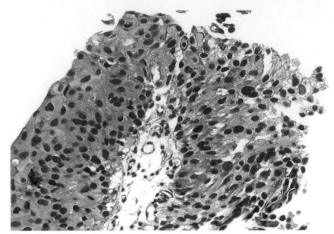

Fig 1. Noninvasive high-grade papillary urothelial carcinoma with moderate pleomorphism.

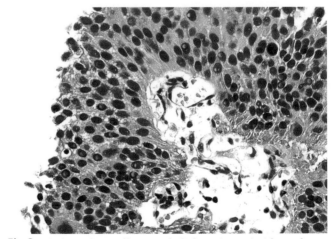

Fig 2. High-grade papillary urothelial carcinoma with moderate architectural disorganization.

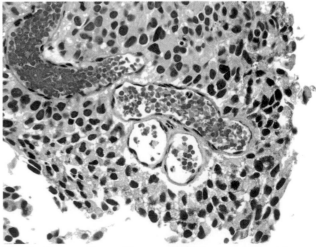

Fig 3. High-grade papillary urothelial carcinoma with more marked architectural disorganization and nuclear pleomorphism.

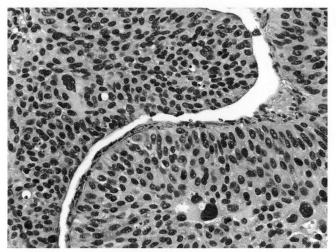

Fig 4. High-grade papillary urothelial carcinoma with giant cells and moderate architectural disorganization.

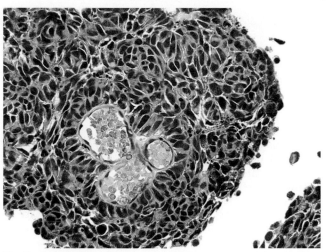

Fig 7. High-grade papillary urothelial carcinoma with spindling and whirling pattern of growth.

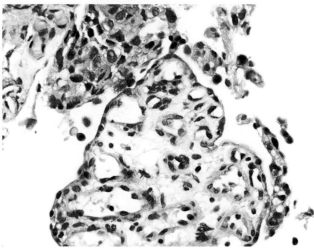

Fig 5. High-grade papillary urothelial carcinoma with extensive denudation.

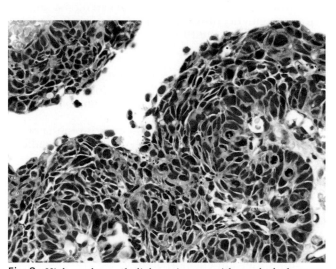

Fig 8. High-grade urothelial carcinoma with marked pleomorphism and spindle-shaped cells.

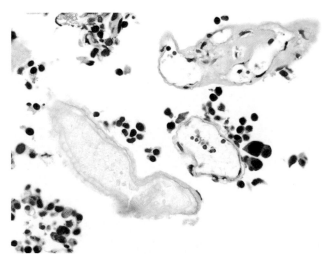

Fig 6. High-grade urothelial carcinoma with naked papillae owing to extensive cellular detachment.

Definition

- Carcinoma derived from the urothelial lining the urinary tract that invades into the underlying tissues

Clinical features

Epidemiology

- It is the seventh most common cancer worldwide.
- It is the most common form of bladder cancer in the United States.
- Males are affected threefold to fourfold more frequently than females.
- Smoking and exposure to industrial compounds are significant risk factors.

Presentation

- Hematuria and nonspecific urinary symptoms are common but may be an incidental finding.
- Cystoscopically, invasive urothelial carcinoma ranges from exophytic, fungating tumors to ulcerated lesions, either solitary or multifocal.

Prognosis and treatment

- Carcinoma confined to the lamina propria is treated with BCG intravesical therapy. Occasionally other intravesical therapies, such as mitomycin, may be used.
- For tumors invading into the muscularis propria or beyond, radical cystectomy with or without neoadjuvant chemotherapy should be considered.
- Prognosis is associated with pathologic stage or depth of invasion. Recent modifications to staging criteria require muscularis propria to be present on a biopsy specimen and transurethral resection specimens for accurate staging.
- Lymph node metastases may be identified in up to one third of patients at radical cystectomy and requires adjuvant chemotherapy.

Pathology

Histology

- Invasion may be present as single cells or as urothelial nests.
- Retraction artifact and paradoxical differentiation are common.
- The overwhelming majority of invasive carcinomas are high grade.
- Nuclear atypia and mitotic activity may be variable.
- Divergent urothelial carcinoma variants are described separately.

Immunopathology (including immunohistochemistry)

- Frequently positive for cytokeratin 7, high-molecular-weight cytokeratin (CK903), and p63
- CK20 immunoreactivity often focally observed
- Less commonly used urothelial markers: uroplakin, thrombomodulin, GATA3, and S100p
- Nuclear p53 accumulation is commonly seen and usually reflects a mutation in the p53 tumor suppressor gene.

Molecular diagnostics

- Mutations in p53 occur in approximately 80% of cases.

Main differential diagnosis

- Benign urothelial proliferations (florid proliferation of von Brunn nests, cystitis cystica, and pseudocarcinomatous hyperplasia)
- Paraganglioma
- In males, secondary bladder involvement by Gleason pattern 5 prostate carcinoma (prostate-specific antigen [PSA], p501s, prostate-specific membrane antigen, or prostein positivity is helpful in this differential)

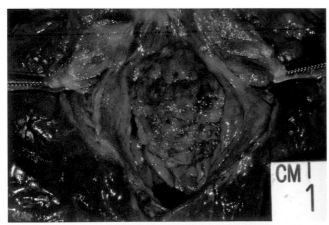

Fig 1. High-grade papillary urothelial carcinoma that fills the bladder lumen and shows underlying invasion into the muscularis propria.

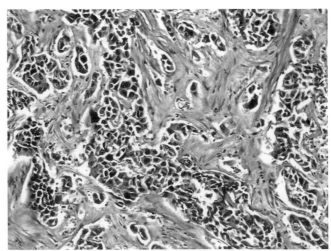

Fig 2. Conventional urothelial carcinoma often shows nests of invasive tumor cells with variable nuclear atypia, which may be striking.

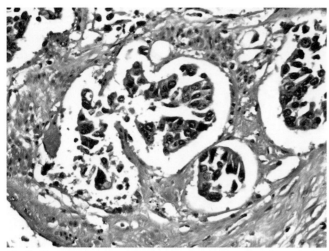

Fig 3. Retraction artifact is commonly associated with urothelial carcinoma and may mimic angiolymphatic invasion.

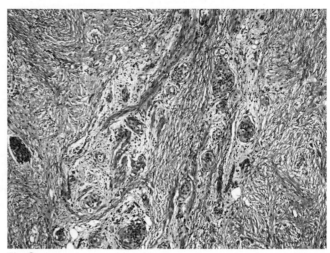

Fig 6. Invasion into the lamina propria may involve small bundles of muscularis mucosae. This finding should not be confused with muscularis propria invasion. Note the prominent desmoplasia associated with this carcinoma.

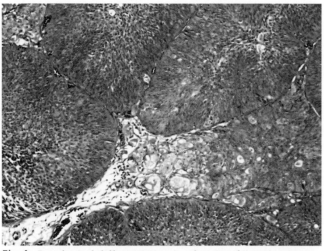

Fig 4. Paradoxical differentiation is a feature of invasion in urothelial carcinoma and appears as small clusters of eosinophilic cells with more abundant cytoplasm, often located at the point of early invasion.

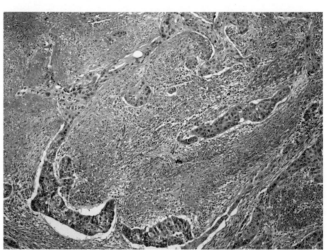

Fig 7. True muscularis propria invasion shows tumor cells at the level of the muscle, occasionally present between or within muscle bundles.

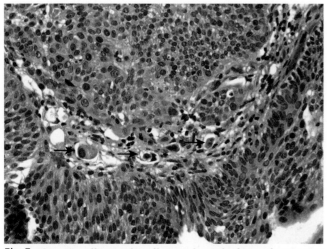

Fig 5. Occasionally, single cells invade at the base of an in situ lesion *(arrows)* and may be missed.

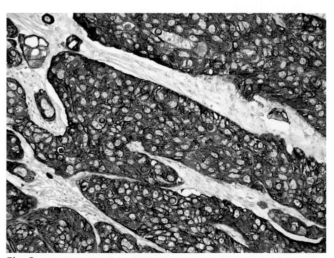

Fig 8. Cytokeratin 7 is diffusely positive in a case of invasive urothelial carcinoma.

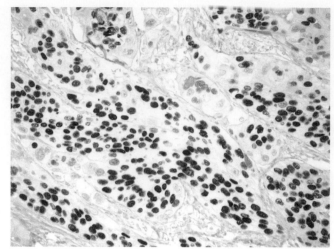

Fig 9. Invasive urothelial carcinomas with diffuse p63 immunoreactivity.

UROTHELIAL CARCINOMA WITH INVERTED GROWTH PATTERN

Definition
- Noninvasive low- or high-grade urothelial carcinoma showing an inverted–endophytic pattern of growth; may have a coexisting exophytic papillary component

Clinical features
Epidemiology
- Relatively uncommon

Presentation
- Hematuria
- Variable cystoscopy aspect, more prominent if there is a coexisting exophytic component

Prognosis and treatment
- Prognosis is similar to noninvasive urothelial carcinoma.

Pathology
Histology
- Two patterns: inverted papilloma-like growth pattern and broad-based verrucous carcinoma-like growth pattern
- Large tumor nests in the lamina propria, with rounded borders, smooth basement membrane with no retraction artifact, inflammatory or desmoplastic stromal reaction
- No angiolymphatic or perineural invasion and no muscularis propria (detrusor muscle) invasion

Immunopathology (including immunohistochemistry)
- Neoplastic cells are positive to CK7, thrombomodulin, and uroplakin.

Main differential diagnosis
- Invasive urothelial carcinoma
- Inverted urothelial papilloma

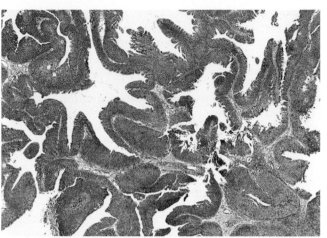

Fig 2. Noninvasive low-grade papillary urothelial carcinoma with inverted growth pattern. Note prominent umbrella cells.

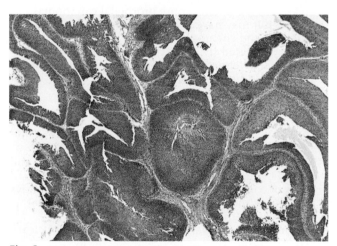

Fig 3. Noninvasive low-grade papillary urothelial carcinoma with inverted growth pattern and focal cystic change.

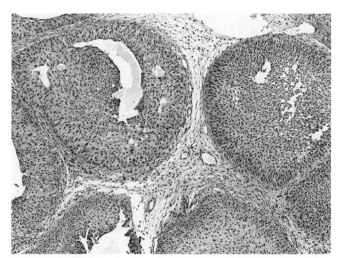

Fig 1. Noninvasive low-grade papillary urothelial carcinoma with inverted growth pattern and focal cystic change. Note broad nests with pushing borders in the lamina propria.

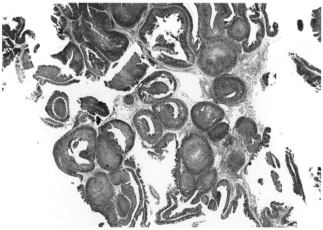

Fig 4. Superficial detached fragments of noninvasive low-grade papillary urothelial carcinoma with inverted growth pattern.

UROTHELIAL CARCINOMA WITH SQUAMOUS DIFFERENTIATION

Definition
- Urothelial carcinoma showing focal areas of keratinization or intercellular bridge formation

Clinical features
Epidemiology
- The most common divergent differentiation in urothelial carcinoma
- Present in 21% of urothelial carcinomas of the bladder and 44% of urothelial carcinomas of the renal pelvis
- Patient age similar to pure urothelial carcinomas (mean age, seventh decade of life)
- Incidence increased in higher-grade or higher-stage lesions and with patient's age

Presentation
- Presentation similar to pure urothelial carcinomas, such as hematuria, dysuria, and urinary obstruction

Prognosis and treatment
- Treatment is similar to pure urothelial carcinomas, although it may have a less favorable response to radiation and chemotherapy.
- When compared stage by stage with conventional urothelial carcinoma, the clinical significance of focal squamous differentiation is unclear.

Pathology
Histology
- Squamous differentiation is characterized by keratinization and presence of intercellular bridges.
- The percentage of squamous differentiation varies and should be included in the pathology report.
- Areas of conventional urothelial carcinoma are always present, although in some cases the only urothelial component is in the form of a CIS.
- Squamous differentiation may show basaloid or clear cell features.

Immunopathology (including immunohistochemistry)
- Neoplastic cells with squamous differentiation are positive for CK14, L1 antigen, and caveolin-1 and negative for uroplakin.

Main differential diagnosis
- Invasive squamous cell carcinoma of the bladder (pure form)

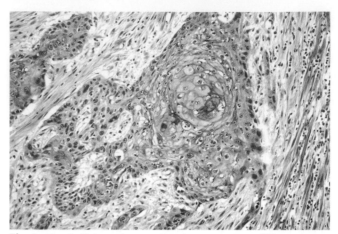

Fig 1. Urothelial carcinoma showing squamous differentiation with distinct cell borders.

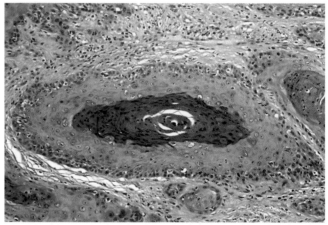

Fig 2. Urothelial carcinoma showing squamous differentiation with keratin pearl formation.

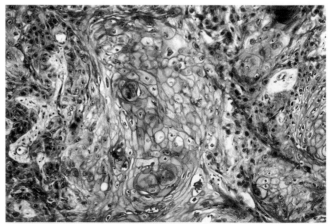

Fig 3. Urothelial carcinoma showing squamous differentiation with focal clear cell features.

UROTHELIAL CARCINOMA WITH VILLOGLANDULAR DIFFERENTIATION

Definition
- Urothelial carcinoma intimately admixed with both villous and glandular components

Clinical features
Epidemiology
- Relatively uncommon variant
- Male predominance (5:1)
- Mean patient age of 70 years (range, 46 to 84 years)

Presentation
- Hematuria
- Mucosuria (rare)
- Cystoscopically, tumor characterized by papillary and villiform projections

Prognosis and treatment
- Poorer prognosis compared with conventional urothelial carcinoma

Pathology
Histology
- Superficial fingerlike processes lined by epithelium having true glandular lumina
- Glands intimately admixed with areas of high-grade urothelial carcinoma
- Glands with cribriform features and lined by non–mucin-producing cuboidal to columnar cells
- Variably sized and shaped glands with some being small and slitlike and others being large and adenoma-like, occasionally with intraluminal mucin
- Variable quantities of intraluminal dirty necrosis, apoptotic bodies, and eosinophilic secretions
- Other aggressive variants of urothelial carcinoma possibly present, including micropapillary, plasmacytoid, and small cell carcinoma

Immunopathology (including immunohistochemistry)
- Neoplastic cells positive for CK7, thrombomodulin, uroplakin, CDX2 (variable), and β-catenin (variable)

Main differential diagnosis
- Urachal carcinoma
- Secondary spread from colorectal adenocarcinoma
- Prostatic duct adenocarcinoma

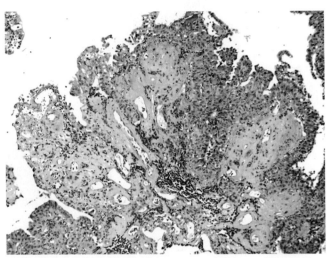

Fig 2. Urothelial carcinoma with villoglandular differentiation and focally denuded papillae.

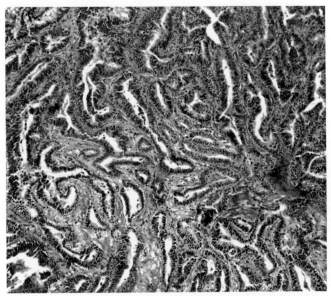

Fig 1. Invasive urothelial carcinoma with villoglandular differentiation and foci of intraluminal necrosis.

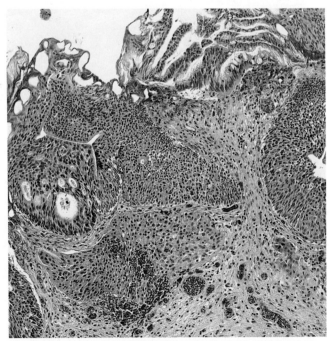

Fig 3. Urothelial carcinoma with villoglandular differentiation composed of invasive high-grade urothelial carcinoma intimately admixed with villous and glandular components.

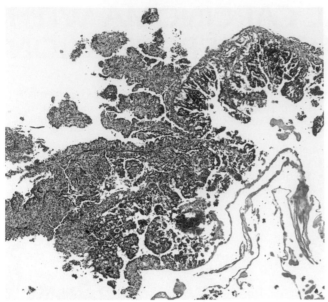

Fig 4. Detached fragments of urothelial carcinoma with villoglandular differentiation.

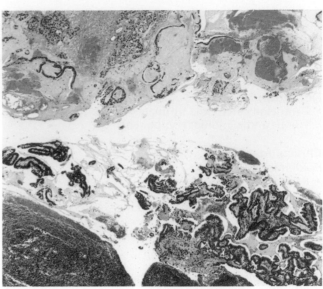

Fig 6. Detached fragments of predominantly villoglandular components with adjacent mucinous features.

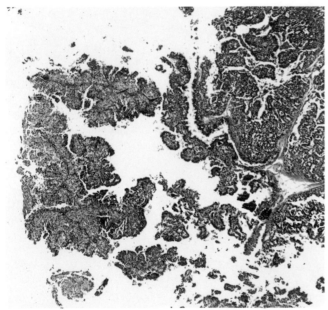

Fig 5. Detached fragments of urothelial carcinoma with villoglandular differentiation.

UROTHELIAL CARCINOMA, MICROPAPILLARY VARIANT

Definition
- Morphologically distinct variant of invasive urothelial carcinoma

Clinical features
Epidemiology
- Incidence less than 1% to 6% of all invasive urothelial carcinomas
- Most common in the sixth decade (range, 45 to 82 years)
- Males more frequently affected (male-to-female ratio, 5:1 to 10:1)

Presentation
- Gross or microscopic hematuria
- Rarely, dysuria, recurrent urinary tract infections, and urinary obstruction

Prognosis and treatment
- It is often present at an advanced stage.
- Compared with conventional urothelial carcinoma, disease-specific survival is significantly worse.
- The presence of a minor proportion of micropapillary component can affect survival and adversely affects outcome in urothelial carcinoma.
- Radical cystectomy recommended even for pT1 disease. Radiotherapy, BCG and currently used combinations of chemotherapy for conventional urothelial carcinoma, seems to be ineffective in micropapillary urothelial carcinoma.

Pathology
Histology
- Surface micropapillary carcinoma exhibits small papillary tufts and delicate filiform processes, with or without central fibrovascular cores.
- Invasive micropapillary carcinoma exhibits small, tight nests of cells often seen within tissue retraction spaces.
- Tumor cells have a high nuclear-to-cytoplasmic ratio.
- Small irregular nuclei with uneven coarse chromatin may have prominent nucleoli.
- Mitoses can be numerous.
- Lymphovascular invasion is common.
- It is almost always associated with a component of conventional urothelial carcinoma including CIS.
- It is invariability high grade.
- Metastatic micropapillary urothelial carcinoma is morphologically similar to the primary tumor.

Immunopathology (including immunohistochemistry)
- Positive for ethelial membrane antigen (EMA), CK7, CK20, and Leu-M1
- Most cases positive for CEA, 34βE12, and p63
- α-Methylacyl–coenzyme A racemase possibly positive
- Some cases positive for CA 125, B72.3, PLAP, S100 protein, uroplakin-III, and thrombomodulin

Molecular genetics
- Nondiploid indices with higher DNA indices than conventional urothelial carcinoma
- Point mutations in *p53* and *H-ras*

Main differential diagnosis
- Nephrogenic adenoma
- Metastatic or secondary spread of micropapillary carcinoma from ovary, endometrium, lungs, breasts, salivary glands, or gastrointestinal tract

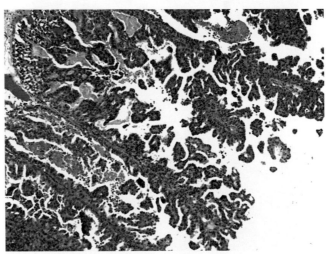

Fig 1. Radical cystectomy specimen showing extensive bladder wall infiltration by micropapillary urothelial carcinoma.

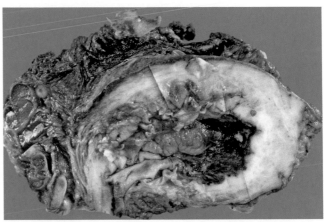

Fig 2. Surface micropapillary urothelial carcinoma showing small papillary tufts and delicate filiform processes.

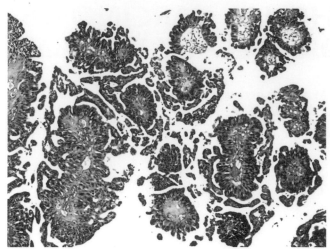

Fig 3. Surface micropapillary urothelial carcinoma with small papillary tufts and delicate filiform processes in a filigree pattern.

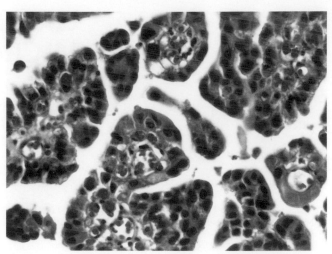

Fig 6. Surface micropapillary urothelial carcinoma composed of tumor cells with more cytoplasm and larger nuclei.

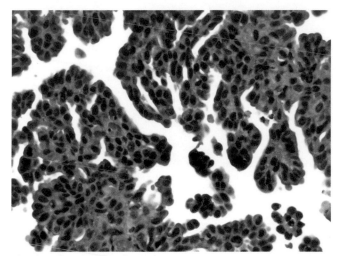

Fig 4. Micropapillary urothelial carcinoma showing papillae without central fibrovascular cores.

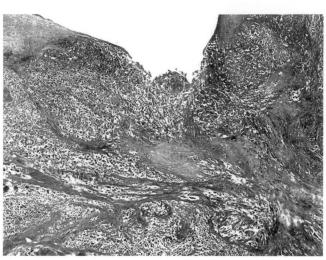

Fig 7. Invasive micropapillary urothelial carcinoma invading into muscularis propria.

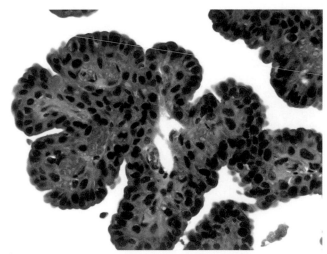

Fig 5. Surface micropapillary urothelial carcinoma composed of cells with high nuclear-to-cytoplasmic ratio and small irregular nuclei with uneven coarse chromatin.

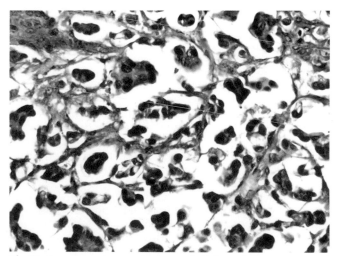

Fig 8. Invasive micropapillary urothelial carcinoma composed of small, tight nests of cells within tissue retraction spaces.

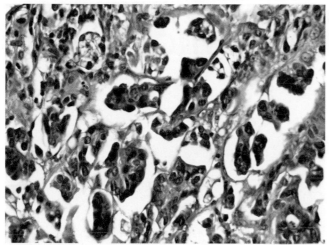

Fig 9. Invasive micropapillary urothelial carcinoma with tumor cells showing small irregular nuclei and a high nuclear-to-cytoplasmic ratio.

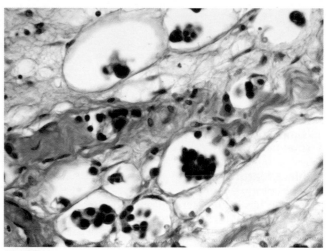

Fig 12. Metastatic micropapillary urothelial carcinoma in the abdominal wall.

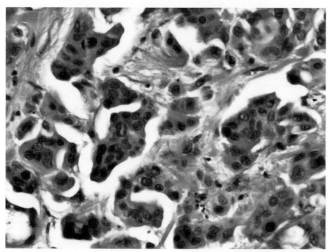

Fig 10. Invasive micropapillary urothelial carcinoma composed of tumor cells with larger irregular nuclei and more cytoplasm.

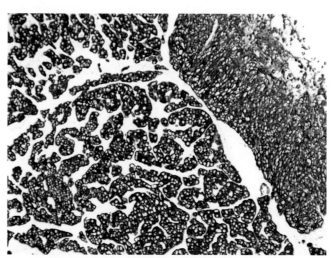

Fig 13. Micropapillary urothelial carcinoma displaying strong diffuse positivity for CK7.

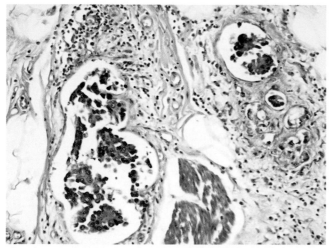

Fig 11. Micropapillary urothelial carcinoma displaying lymphovascular invasion.

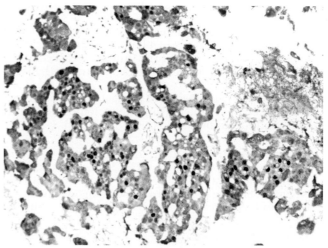

Fig 14. Micropapillary urothelial carcinoma displaying positivity for α-methylacyl–coenzyme A racemase and p63.

Definition
- Also known as *urothelial carcinoma with glandlike lumens,* it is a rare variant of urothelial carcinoma comprising cysts and tubules as part of the architectural pattern.

Clinical features
Epidemiology
- So far it has been described only in the bladder.
- Epidemiology is that of urothelial bladder carcinoma, with a male-to-female predominance of 2:1 to 5:1.
- Risk factors are smoking and exposure to aniline dyes and aromatic amines.
- Analgesic use, urinary tract infections, and chemotherapeutic agents are possible predisposing causes.

Presentation
- Gross and microscopic hematuria is present.
- Irritative urinary symptoms of urgency, frequency, and dysuria are present.
- Cystoscopy shows mucosal lesions that can be papillary or flat.
- Multifocal lesions may be encountered.

Prognosis and treatment
- May be potentially more aggressive

Pathology
Histology
- Some authors advocate that at least 25% of the urothelial carcinoma contain microcysts for this diagnosis.
- Cysts range in size from a few millimeters to 2 cm in diameter and may be empty, contain necrotic debris, granular eosinophilic material, or mucin; cyst walls may be calcified.
- Cysts and tubules within the lamina propria and muscularis propria, often merging with conventional areas of urothelial carcinoma with a nested appearance, may show a deeply infiltrative growth pattern.
- Lining of cysts comprise neoplastic urothelial cells, which may be cytologically bland to more atypical depending on the grade of the tumor. Stroma can be cellular to scant inbetween the neoplastic urothelial cysts.
- Luminal secretions may have a targetoid appearance and may be highlighted using the periodic acid-Schiff (PAS) and Alcian blue stains.

Immunopathology (including immunohistochemistry)
- Positive staining to 34βE12, p63, CK7, uroplakin, and thrombomodulin
- Negative staining to α-methyl–coenzyme A racemase
- Ki-67 and p53 overexpressed in high-grade cancers

Main differential diagnosis
- Florid cystitis cystica et glandularis
- Nephrogenic adenoma
- Adenocarcinoma

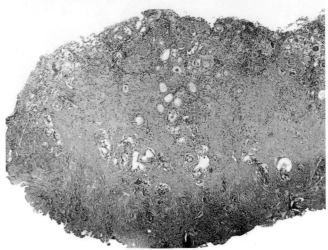

Fig 1. Low-power view of a microcystic carcinoma showing the presence of cysts invading through the bladder wall.

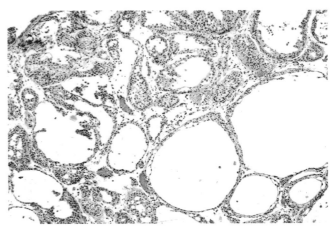

Fig 2. Microcystic carcinoma composed of cysts of different sizes infiltrating the bladder lamina propria. Lining cells display bland nuclear features.

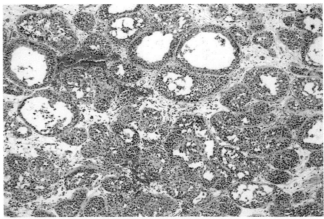

Fig 3. Microcystic carcinoma with middle-sized cysts showing more atypias. Note the merging with more typical areas of usual urothelial carcinoma *(bottom field)*.

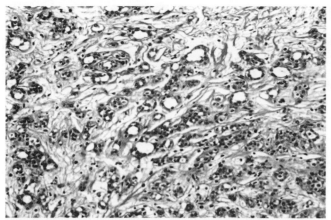

Fig 4. Microcystic carcinoma composed of small-sized cysts infiltrating the bladder wall.

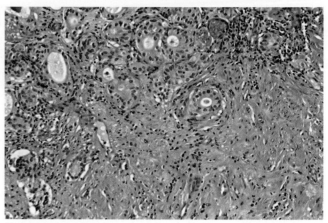

Fig 6. Microcystic carcinoma composed of infiltrative small cysts with mild to moderate atypias.

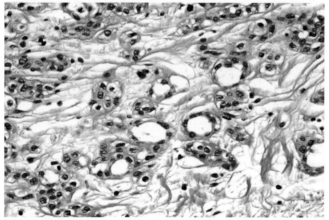

Fig 5. Microcystic carcinoma showing small-sized cysts with moderate nuclear atypias.

UROTHELIAL CARCINOMA, LYMPHOEPITHELIOMA-LIKE CARCINOMA VARIANT

Definition
- Undifferentiated carcinoma of the urinary bladder with a prominent lymphocytic stroma and morphologic resemblance to the undifferentiated nasopharyngeal carcinoma variant

Clinical features
Epidemiology
- Male-to-female ratio is 2:1.
- Most patients are in late adulthood, with a mean age at diagnosis of 70 years.
- Usual stage at presentation is T2-T3.

Presentation
- Hematuria

Prognosis and treatment
- Pure forms were originally thought to be more responsive to systemic therapy. Later studies failed to confirm a favorable response.
- Transurethral resection of the bladder, adjuvant chemotherapy, or radical cystectomy cisplatin-based chemotherapy and radiotherapy

Pathology
Histology
- A syncytial, sheetlike, or trabecular growth pattern is composed of neoplastic cells containing vesicular nuclei, prominent nucleoli, indistinctive cellular borders, and numerous mitoses. A prominent lymphoid infiltrate is present, with a prominence of T cells; a mixed population of plasma cells and eosinophils may also be observed.
- Overlying urothelium may show dysplasia or urothelial CIS.
- Tumors can be pure (100%), predominant (>50%), or focal lymphoepithelioma-like carcinomas (<50%).
- Tumor can have concurrent adenocarcinoma and squamous cell carcinoma.

Immunopathology (including immunohistochemistry)
- Positive for cytokeratin and EMA
- Negative for leukocyte common antigen, vimentin, and desmin
- Predominance of CD3-positive T cells
- No association with Epstein-Barr virus infection

Molecular diagnostics
- In situ hybridization to Epstein-Barr virus–encoded RNA is negative.

Main differential diagnosis
- Malignant lymphoma
- Marked chronic cystitis or intense chronic inflammation
- Small cell carcinoma

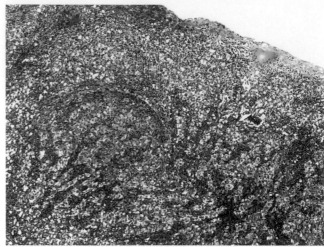

Fig 1. Low magnification of a case of lymphoepithelioma-like carcinoma with solid growth of undifferentiated tumor cells, medium to large, admixed with a dense inflammatory component. The low-power appearance is that of a dense inflammatory process or even a lymphoproliferative process such as a B cell lymphoma.

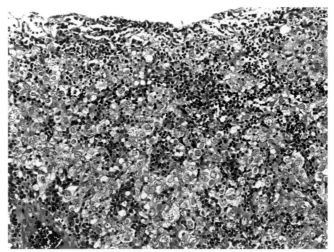

Fig 2. The neoplastic cells of lymphoepithelioma-like carcinoma are larger and have a syncytial growth pattern and are easily distinguishable from the inflammatory cells surrounding them. The inflammatory infiltrate can obscure the carcinoma cells and consists primarily of mature lymphocytes (T and B), plasma cells, and histiocytes (variable) and rarely may contain neutrophils, or eosinophils.

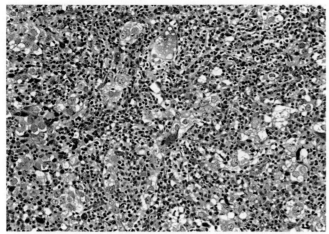

Fig 3. Neoplastic cells are highly pleomorphic, some with bizarre atypia and multinucleation. There are numerous mitoses, some of which have an atypical appearance.

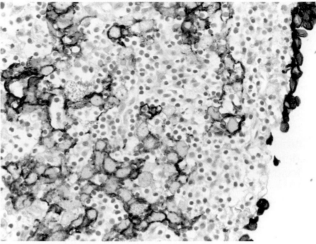

Fig 5. Lymphoepithelioma-like urothelial carcinoma demonstrating cytokeratin-positive neoplastic cells in a background of dense inflammation.

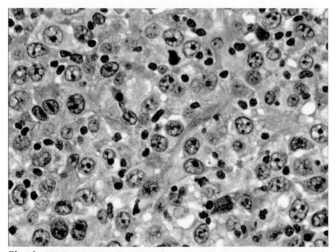

Fig 4. Higher magnification showing the neoplastic cells with indistinct cell borders and with moderate clear to eosinophilic cytoplasm, large vesicular nuclei, coarse chromatin, and prominent nucleoli.

UROTHELIAL CARCINOMA, CLEAR CELL (GLYCOGEN-RICH) VARIANT

Definition
- Urothelial carcinoma showing clear cell pattern with glycogen-rich cytoplasm

Clinical features

Epidemiology
- Occurs usually in adults, but within a wide age range (17 to 82 years; mean, 53 years)
- Occurs predominantly in females

Presentation
- Same as conventional urothelial carcinoma

Treatment and prognosis
- Treatment: surgery, chemotherapy, and radiotherapy.
- Prognosis: same as conventional urothelial carcinoma.

Pathology

Histology
- Histologic findings consist predominantly or exclusively of tumor cells with abundant clear cytoplasm.
- Typically, nuclei show high-grade features (enlarged nuclei, hyperchromatic, irregular nuclear contour, and brisk mitotic activity).
- PAS stain highlights the presence of glycogen in the cytoplasm.
- There is usually a lack of a well-developed alveolar or nested pattern, and a lack of nuclear hobnailing that can be encountered in clear cell (mesonephric) adenocarcinoma of the bladder and in Müllerian clear cell carcinoma counterpart.

Immunopathology (including immunohistochemistry)
- Positive to CK7, CK20, high-molecular-weight cytokeratin, p63, and thrombomodulin
- Negative to RCC marker, PAX2, vimentin PSA, p501S, and prostate-specific membrane antigen

Main differential diagnosis
- Secondary spread from Müllerian clear cell adenocarcinoma
- Metastatic clear cell renal cell carcinoma
- Secondary spread from prostate carcinoma

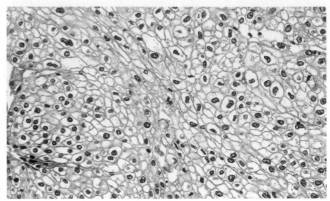

Fig 2. Urothelial carcinoma with clear cytoplasm. The tumor shows a sheetlike growth pattern with few fibrovascular cores. These features are keys to differentiate from clear renal cell carcinoma and prostate adenocarcinoma.

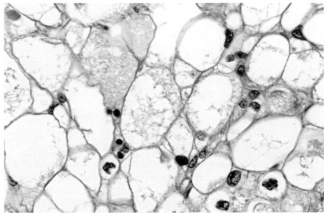

Fig 3. Urothelial carcinoma with clear cytoplasm. Tumor cells of clear cell variant usually have large clear cytoplasm. Although the tumor cells show a low nuclear-to-cytoplasmic ratio, their nuclei are usually enlarged.

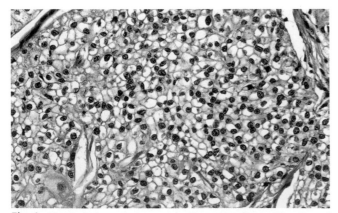

Fig 1. Urothelial carcinoma with clear cytoplasm. The size of tumor cells clear cell varies by location or by case.

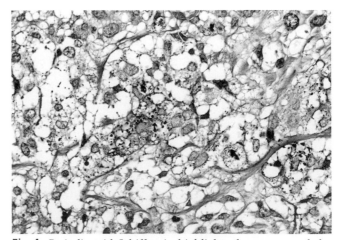

Fig 4. Periodic acid–Schiff stain highlights the presence of glycogen in the cytoplasm.

UROTHELIAL CARCINOMA, LIPOID CELL VARIANT

Definition
- A rare variant of urothelial carcinoma, characterized by the presence of lipoblast-like epithelial tumor cells, also known as *lipidoid variant of urothelial carcinoma*

Clinical features
Epidemiology
- Rare variant, with only a few reported cases reported

Presentation
- Most common symptoms are macroscopic hematuria.
- Other symptoms of urothelial carcinoma can be seen.

Prognosis and treatment
- Aggressive behavior, probably related to the association with high-stage and high-grade conventional urothelial carcinoma

Pathology
Histology
- Associated with conventional high-grade urothelial carcinoma and comprising at least 10% of the tumor. No cases of pure lipoid variant have been reported to date.

- Tumor is composed of solid sheets or infiltrating nests of large malignant epithelial cells with irregular, hyperchromatic, and eccentrically placed nuclei, and abundant, vacuolated cytoplasm resembling lipoblasts.
- Electron microcopy analysis confirms the presence of lipid content in tumor cells.

Immunopathology (including immunohistochemistry)
- Positive for CK7, CK20, 34βE12, AE1/AE3, and CAM 5.2
- Negative for thrombomodulin; vimentin, S100 protein, and mucin stains (PAS, Alcian Blue)

Main differential diagnosis
- Liposarcoma
- Sarcomatoid carcinoma
- Signet ring cell carcinoma

UROTHELIAL CARCINOMA WITH SYNCYTIOTROPHOBLASTIC GIANT CELLS

Definition
- Unusual form of divergent differentiation in urothelial carcinoma characterized by the presence of human chorionic gonadotrophin (hCG) positive syncytiotrophoblastic giant cells or by a choriocarcinoma component

Clinical features
Epidemiology
- Presence of syncytiotrophoblastic giant cells admixed with urothelial carcinoma is rare.
- Urothelial carcinoma associated with choriocarcinoma is exceedingly uncommon.

Presentation
- Asymptomatic macroscopic hematuria
- Tumor mass on cystoscopy
- Elevation of serum hCG and urinary hCG
- Gynecomastia owing to elevated hCG in some cases

Prognosis and treatment
- Prognosis is worse than typical high-grade urothelial carcinoma, even for those with syncytiotrophoblastic cells.
- In most cases, survival is less than 1 year.
- Treatment includes cystectomy and combination chemotherapy.

Pathology
Histology
- Invasive high-grade urothelial carcinoma with scattered syncytiotrophoblastic giant cells
- Invasive high-grade urothelial carcinoma with associated choriocarcinoma in which there is an admixture of syncytiotrophoblastic, cytotrophoblastic, and intermediate trophoblastic tissue in a hemorrhagic background
- Highly vascular with prominent necrosis
- Frequent mitoses including atypical mitoses

Immunopathology (including immunohistochemistry)
- hCG positivity in syncytiotrophoblastic giant cells

Main differential diagnosis
- Urothelial carcinoma displaying osteoclast-like giant cells
- Pleomorphic giant cell carcinoma
- High-grade urothelial carcinoma displaying hCG positivity
- Secondary bladder involvement by gestational choriocarcinoma

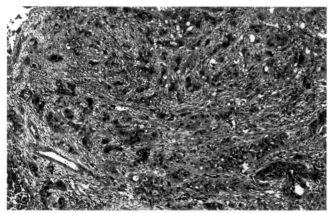

Fig 1. Invasive high-grade urothelial carcinoma with numerous scattered syncytiotrophoblastic giant cells.

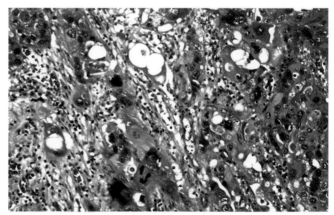

Fig 3. Invasive high-grade urothelial carcinoma with syncytiotrophoblastic malignant giant cells.

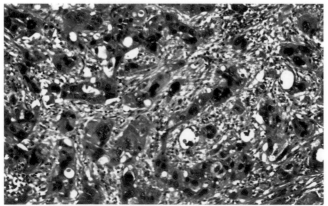

Fig 2. Invasive high-grade urothelial carcinoma with numerous syncytiotrophoblastic malignant giant cells.

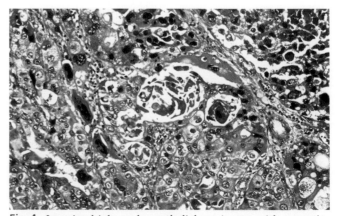

Fig 4. Invasive high-grade urothelial carcinoma with syncytiotrophoblastic malignant giant cells.

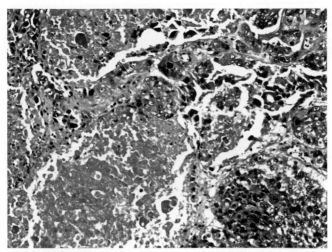

Fig 5. High-grade urothelial carcinoma with syncytiotrophoblastic malignant giant cells displaying necrosis.

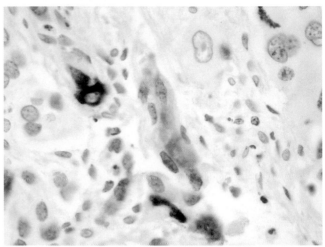

Fig 8. High-grade urothelial carcinoma with hCG-positive syncytiotrophoblastic malignant giant cells.

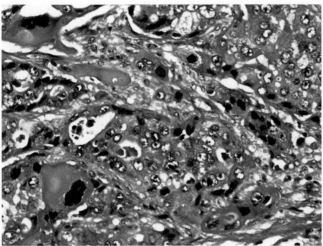

Fig 6. High-grade urothelial carcinoma with syncytiotrophoblastic malignant giant cells.

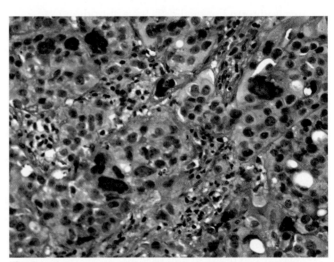

Fig 9. Pleomorphic giant cell carcinoma showing a high-grade urothelial carcinoma with pleomorphic malignant giant cells.

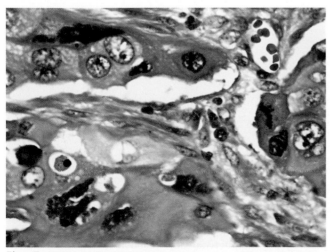

Fig 7. High-grade urothelial carcinoma with syncytiotrophoblastic malignant giant cells. Atypical mitotic figures are observed.

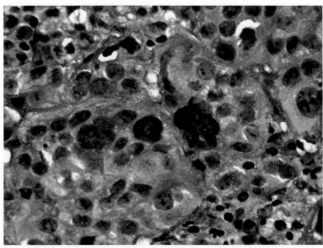

Fig 10. Pleomorphic giant cell carcinoma. High-grade urothelial carcinoma with pleomorphic malignant giant cells.

UROTHELIAL CARCINOMA WITH RHABDOID DIFFERENTIATION

Definition
- Unusual variant of urothelial carcinoma characterized by presence of cells with prominent rhabdoid features

Clinical features
Epidemiology
- Wide age range (2 to 84 years old)

Presentation
- Hematuria

Prognosis and treatment
- Poor outcome and an aggressive clinical course

Pathology
Histology
- Large and round or oval cells have abundant cytoplasm, containing a brightly eosinophilic body eccentrically displacing a vesicular nuclei and a prominent nucleolus (rhabdoid cells).
- Eosinophilic cytoplasmic inclusions are composed of intermediate filaments.
- Rhabdoid component range from 40% to 100%.
- Rhabdoid cells are discohesive and are present singly, in clusters, or in large sheets.
- Most cases have associated conventional urothelial carcinoma, at least focally.
- Concurrent flat CIS is often present.

Immunopathology (including immunohistochemistry)
- Immunohistochemical stains for cytokeratin show either dotlike positivity or diffuse cytoplasmic staining in the rhabdoid component of the tumors.
- Immunohistochemical analysis usually demonstrates reactivity to vimentin and desmin.

Main differential diagnosis
- Malignant extrarenal rhabdoid tumor
- Inflammatory myofibroblastic tumors
- Urothelial carcinoma, plasmacytoid variant

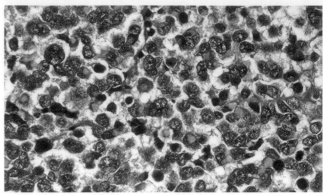

Fig 2. Higher magnification of the case illustrated in Fig 1 highlighting the characteristic large rhabdoid cells with abundant cytoplasm containing a brightly eosinophilic body, vesicular nuclei, and a prominent nucleolus in a myxoid background.

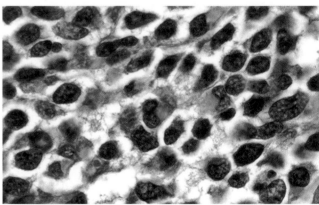

Fig 3. Invasive urothelial carcinoma with rhabdoid features highlighting the rhabdoid cells with large round and oval rhabdoid cells with prominent nucleoli. Note the vesicular chromatin and irregular nuclear contours. The eosinophilic inclusions within the cells are composed of intermediate filaments, demonstrable by electron microscopy.

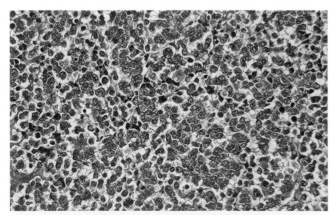

Fig 1. Low-power view of an invasive urothelial carcinoma with rhabdoid features showing abundant rhabdoid neoplastic cells, some of which are discohesive and present singly, in clusters, or in large sheets.

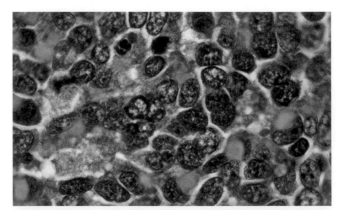

Fig 4. Higher magnification of the case illustrated in Fig 3, highlighting the characteristic large rhabdoid cells with abundant cytoplasm. Immunohistochemical stains for cytokeratin shows either dotlike positivity or diffuse cytoplasmic staining in the rhabdoid component of the urothelial tumors.

UROTHELIAL CARCINOMA SIMILAR TO GIANT CELL TUMOR OF BONE

Definition
- Urothelial carcinoma variant resembling giant cell tumor of the bone

Clinical features
Epidemiology
- Rare variant of invasive urothelial carcinoma
- Male predominance
- Elderly age (majority in seventh decade or older)

Presentation
- Gross hematuria
- Dysuria
- Flank pain or renal colic if located in renal pelvis
- Passage of tissue fragments with urine

Prognosis and treatment
- Highly malignant disease with advanced stage at the time of diagnosis
- Similar to urothelial carcinomas in the same stage

Pathology
Histology
- There is biphasic mixture of oval to plump mononuclear cells with mild to moderate pleomorphism and cytologically bland multinucleated osteoclast-like giant cells.
- Neoplastic cells form sheets and nodules.
- Mononuclear cells may acquire a spindle cell morphology.
- A concentration of giant cells around hemorrhagic foci exhibits phagocytosis.
- Richly vascularized stroma have frequent areas of erythrocyte extravasation and occasional large, blood-filled lakes.
- Prevalent mitoses are among mononuclear cells but not the giant cell population.
- Large areas of necrosis are present.
- A tonguelike infiltrative growth pattern is present.
- Associated papillary or in situ urothelial carcinomas, or both, are present.

Immunopathology (including immunohistochemistry)
- Giant cells are immunoreactive for CD68, vimentin, tartrate-resistant acid phosphatase, α1-antitrypsin, leukocyte common antigen, and osteoclast markers CD51 and CD56, and are negative to epithelial markers.
- Mononuclear cells express CD68, smooth muscle actin, S100, focal staining to epithelial markers, and p53 in half of the cases.

Main differential diagnosis
- Pleomorphic giant-cell urothelial carcinoma
- Syncytiotrophoblastic giant cells in high-grade infiltrating urothelial carcinoma
- Choriocarcinoma of the bladder
- Metastatic true giant cell tumors of bone and soft tissues
- Granulomatous inflammation

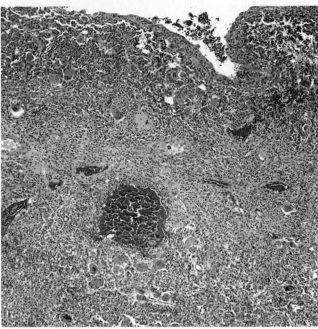

Fig 1. Hypercellular tumor diffusely infiltrating bladder wall. Note the urothelium in the upper field.

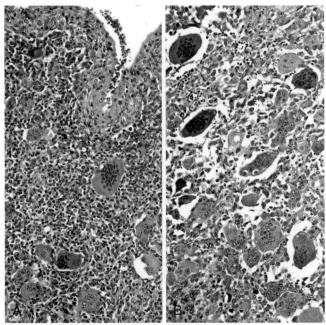

Fig 2. Biphasic neoplasm composed of oval to plump mononuclear cells with mild to moderate pleomorphism and numerous multinucleated osteoclast-like giant cells.

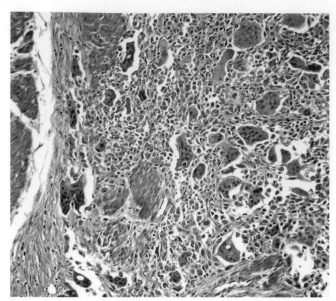

Fig 3. Tumor invading muscularis propria. Note the presence of abundant multinucleated osteoclast-like giant cells.

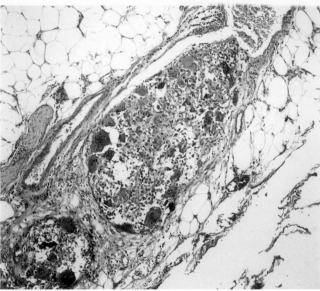

Fig 4. Giant cell urothelial carcinoma showing vascular invasion in the adipose tissue surrounding the bladder.

Definition
- High-grade bladder carcinoma with "oat cell" morphology and neuroendocrine differentiation

Clinical features
Epidemiology
- Demographics similar to other forms of bladder cancer
- More common in males
- Middle-aged to elderly patients most commonly affected

Presentation
- Often associated with a concurrent urothelial carcinoma, adenocarcinoma, or squamous cell carcinoma of the bladder
- Possibly with widespread metastases

Prognosis and treatment
- The tumor is highly aggressive with a poor prognosis.
- Distant metastases are common.
- Treatment often involves a platinum-based regimen.
- The presence of even a small focus of small cell carcinoma will affect prognosis and should be described in the final report.

Pathology
Histology
- Sheets and nests of small epithelial neuroendocrine cells ("blue cells")
- High nuclear-to-cytoplasmic ratio
- Prominent necrosis and brisk mitotic activity
- Crush artifact readily identified
- Nuclear molding
- Finely stippled chromatin
- Lack of prominent nucleoli

Immunopathology (including immunohistochemistry)
- Positivity for neuroendocrine markers, including synaptophysin, chromogranin, CD56, and neuron-specific enolase
- CK7 often positive
- TTF-1 possibly expressed

Main differential diagnosis
- Malignant lymphoma
- Primitive neurectodermal tumor (PNET)–Ewing sarcoma
- Embryonal rhabdomyosarcoma
- Metastatic or secondary spread of small cell carcinoma of other primary site

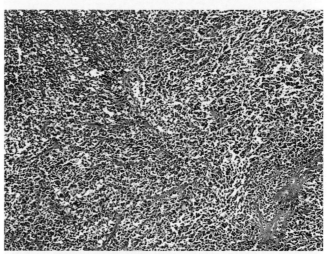

Fig 1. Low magnification reveals sheets of blue cells with minimal cytoplasm.

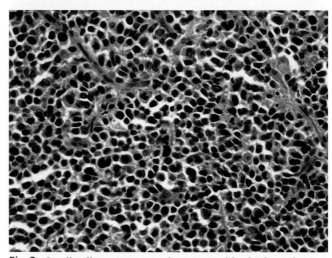

Fig 2. Small cell carcinoma is characterized by high nuclear-to-cytoplasmic ratio, brisk mitotic activity, necrosis, and nuclei with finely stippled chromatin.

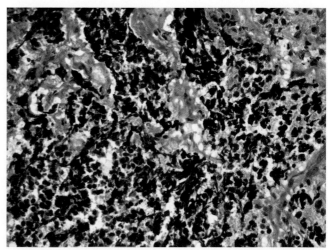

Fig 3. Crush artifact is common in small cell carcinoma.

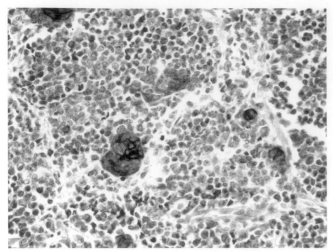

Fig 4. Cytokeratin is often focally positive.

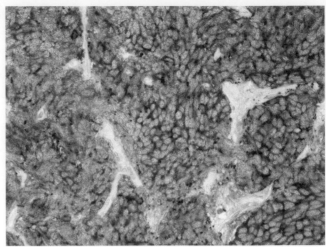

Fig 6. Neuron-specific enolase can also be used to demonstrate neuroendocrine differentiation.

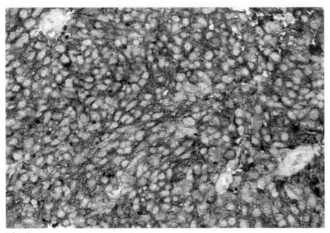

Fig 5. Neuroendocrine markers such as synaptophysin are often strongly and diffusely positive.

LARGE CELL UNDIFFERENTIATED CARCINOMA

Definition
- Carcinoma is composed of poorly differentiated neoplastic cells that cannot be otherwise classified. These tumors are analogous to the large cell undifferentiated carcinoma of the lung.

Clinical features
Epidemiology
- There is limited information about these extremely rare tumors.
- These tumors have typically been considered by other authors as poorly differentiated urothelial carcinoma, as it is the most common carcinoma in the urinary bladder.

Presentation
- Similar to other carcinomas involving the bladder
- Previous history of papillary urothelial tumors absent in most cases

Prognosis and treatment
- Aggressive variant with dismal prognosis even when treated with aggressive surgery, radiation, or chemotherapy
- Outcome is generally worse than comparably staged and treated conventional high-grade urothelial carcinoma.
- Most patients have lymph node metastases at the time of surgery.
- Most patients die of their disease within 2 years of diagnosis.

Pathology
Histology
- Solid, nodular or transmural diffuse growth can be observed with frequent tumoral necrosis.
- There are sheets of large polygonal or round cells with moderate to abundant cytoplasm and distinct cell borders.
- Invasion patterns vary from infiltrating tumor to solid expansible nests with focal detached growth pattern.
- Most cases lack any associated identifiable urothelial, squamous, or glandular differentiation.
- Lymphovascular invasion is usually extensive.
- Tumors with neuroendocrine features should be classified in a distinct category (large cell neuroendocrine carcinoma).

Immunopathology (including immunohistochemistry)
- Large cell undifferentiated carcinoma is positive for cytokeratins AE1/AE3 and CK7. Most cases are also positive with CAM 5.2 and p53.
- Variable positivity is seen with CK20, thrombomodulin, and uroplakin III.
- Ki-67 labeling index is high (50% to 90%).
- Neuroendocrine markers are negative in addition to other markers performed in the differential diagnosis of other variants.

Main differential diagnosis
- Secondary spread from high-grade prostate cancer or other sites
- Large cell neuroendocrine carcinoma

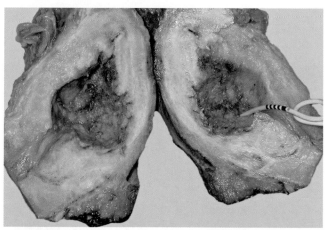

Fig 1. Urinary bladder after fixation showing a large ulcerative lesion deeply infiltrating the bladder wall with extension in the perivesical fat.

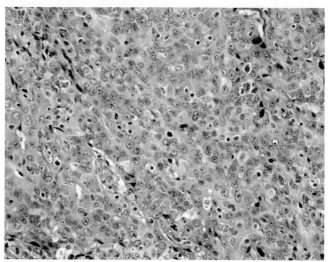

Fig 2. Poorly differentiated carcinoma characterized by a solid growth pattern, frequent mitotic figures, and apoptotic bodies. Focally, rare intratumoral lymphocytes are observed but, this is insufficient for the diagnosis of a lymphoepithelioma-like variant.

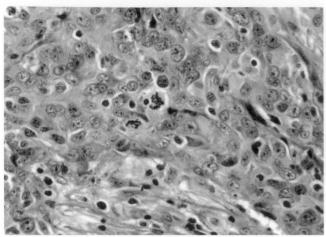

Fig 3. High-power view showing large malignant cells with abundant eosinophilic cytoplasm and prominent nucleoli.

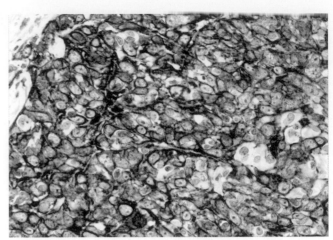

Fig 5. Strong and diffuse immunoreactivity with CK7 antibody in tumor cells.

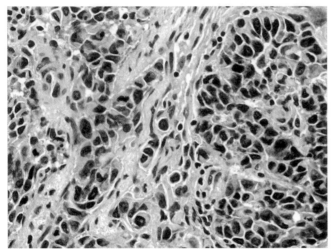

Fig 4. Infiltrative nests and cords of a poorly differentiated carcinoma. Nuclei are large and hyperchromatic. Mitotic figures are frequent. Neuroendocrine stains were all negative.

UROTHELIAL CARCINOMA WITH UNUSUAL STROMAL REACTIONS

Definition
- Primary or metastatic urothelial carcinoma showing in the stroma a pseudosarcomatous response, osseous or cartilaginous metaplasia, osteoclast-type giant cells, or a prominent lymphoid infiltrate

Clinical features
Epidemiology
- Rare urothelial carcinoma variant

Presentation
- Hematuria

Prognosis and treatment
- No influence on prognosis or treatment

Pathology
Histology
- Pseudosarcomatous stroma: myofibroblastic reaction in the stroma surrounding the invasive areas of urothelial carcinoma, background varying from edematous or myxoid to collagenous with sclerosing features. There are atypical mesenchymal cells in stroma, which are similar to those seen in giant cell cystitis. Abundant eosinophilic cytoplasm and degenerative-type pleomorphic nuclei in atypical stromal cells can also be found, with normal-appearing mitotic figures when present, and no expansible growth in the spindle cell component. There is also a lack of morphologic transition between spindle cells and carcinoma cells.
- Osseous or cartilaginous metaplasia is characterized by histologically benign mature bone or cartilage islands in the stroma without atypia in the stroma of carcinoma, no evidence of sarcomatous component, and absence of mesenchymal cell proliferation.
- Osteoclast-type giant cells are present in tumor stroma without nuclear pleomorphism.
- Prominent lymphoid infiltrate is characterized by intense lymphocytic infiltrate in the stroma adjacent to invasive urothelial carcinoma, with variable admixture of plasma cells, and occasionally neutrophilic or eosinophilic component.

Immunopathology (including immunohistochemistry)
- Stromal cells positive for vimentin and negative for cytokeratins
- Immunoreactivity in giant cells for vimentin and CD68 and negative staining for cytokeratins and epithelial membrane antigen

Main differential diagnosis
- Sarcomatoid urothelial carcinoma with heterologous differentiation
- Primary sarcoma of bladder

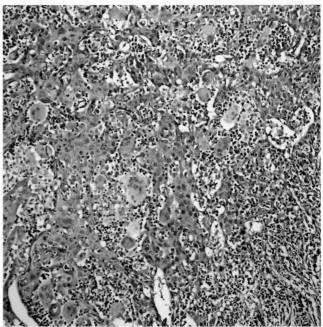

Fig 1. Urothelial carcinoma containing osteoclast-type multinucleated giant cells in the stroma in addition to a lymphocyte and eosinophil-rich infiltrate.

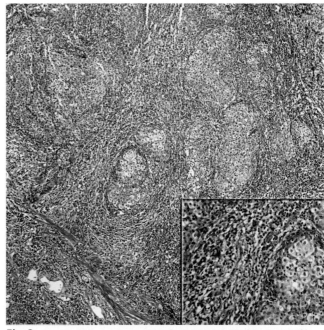

Fig 2. Urothelial carcinoma with intense lymphocytic infiltration in the stroma surrounding invasive tumor islands.

UROTHELIAL CARCINOMA WITH SARCOMATOID DIFFERENTIATION

Definition
- Biphasic malignant neoplasms with morphologic or immunohistochemical evidence of epithelial and mesenchymal differentiation; common clonal origin for the carcinomatous and sarcomatous components is presumed.

Clinical features
Epidemiology
- It is rare but more common than primary (true mesenchymal) sarcoma of the urinary bladder.
- A history of radiation and intravesical cyclophosphamide chemotherapy has been associated with sarcomatoid carcinoma.

Presentation
- Likely present at a more advanced stage than high-grade conventional urothelial carcinoma

Prognosis and treatment
- Heterologous differentiation may be present but has no definite prognostic significance.
- Outcome data are inconclusive when compared with high-grade urothelial carcinoma, although some evidence suggests a greater risk for death even after adjusting for stage at clinical presentation.
- Treatment is similar to high-grade urothelial carcinoma. Neoadjuvant chemotherapy has been suggested.

Pathology
Histology
- The sarcomatous component is usually a high-grade spindle cell neoplasm with nondescript architecture, resembling malignant fibrous histiocytoma.
- The epithelial component can be in the form of invasive urothelial carcinoma, squamous cell carcinoma, adenocarcinoma, small cell carcinoma, or overlying CIS.
- Heterologous differentiation (sometimes termed *carcinosarcoma*) often includes rhabdomyosarcomatous, osteosarcomatous, chondrosarcomatous, or a mixture of these as well as other forms of sarcomatous components.
- Even in the absence of an obvious epithelial component, a history of urothelial neoplasia or strong and relatively diffuse cytokeratin immunoreactivity will favor the diagnosis of sarcomatoid carcinoma over a primary sarcoma.
- A subset of cases display prominent myxoid stroma, mimicking inflammatory myofibroblastic tumors.
- Sarcomatous component often show prominent nuclear atypia and pleomorphism.
- A transition between epithelial cells and spindle cells sometimes can be appreciated.

Immunopathology (including immunohistochemistry)
- Positive for pancytokeratin, HMCK (34βE12), p63, CK5/6, but reactivity possibly focal or only limited to the epithelial component
- Variable reactivity for smooth muscle actin and desmin
- Negative for ALK-1

Main differential diagnosis
- Inflammatory myofibroblastic tumors (pseudosarcomatous myofibroblastic proliferations)
- Primary bladder sarcoma
- Urothelial carcinoma with focal metaplasia in the stroma
- Urothelial carcinoma with unusual stromal reaction (pseudosarcomatous stroma)

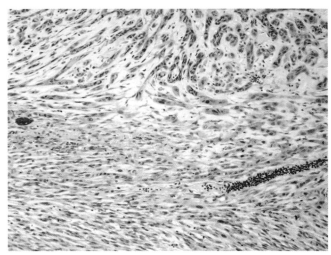

Fig 1. Transition of an invasive urothelial carcinoma *(top)* into malignant spindle cell proliferation *(bottom)* is characteristic of sarcomatoid carcinoma or urothelial carcinoma with sarcomatoid differentiation.

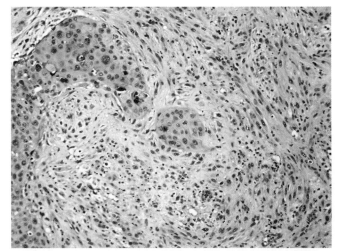

Fig 2. Foci of squamous carcinoma (epithelial component) surrounded by spindle cells with scattered nuclear atypia and pleomorphism (mesenchymal component).

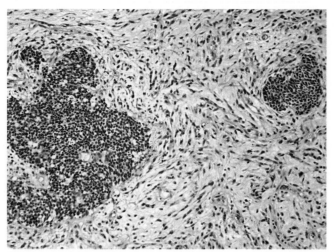

Fig 3. Small cell carcinoma associated with a myxoid malignant spindle cell sarcomatous component.

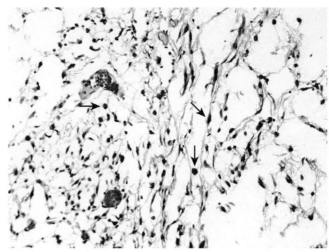

Fig 6. Some myxoid sarcomatoid carcinomas display only limited atypia and closely mimic inflammatory myofibroblastic tumors. Scattered enlarged hyperchromatic nuclei are the clues to a correct diagnosis.

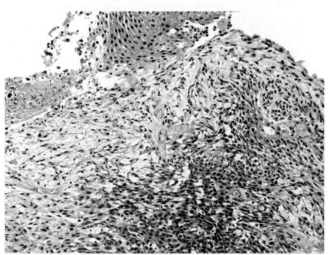

Fig 4. Occasionally sarcomatoid differentiation can be seen in association with a low-grade urothelial carcinoma.

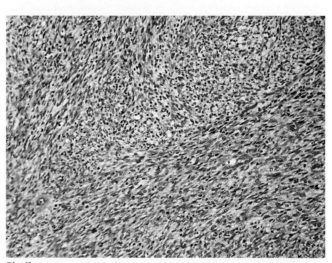

Fig 7. Sarcomatoid carcinoma mostly composed of undifferentiated spindle cells.

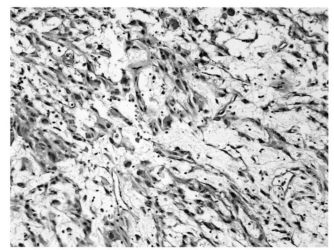

Fig 5. A subset of sarcomatoid carcinomas has prominent myxoid stroma. The epithelioid spindle cells in this case have apparent nuclear pleomorphism and atypia.

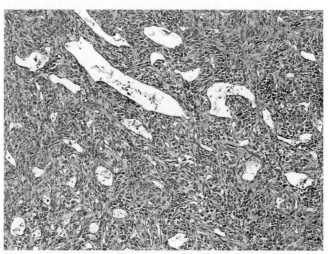

Fig 8. Hemangiopericytoma-like vascular pattern can be seen in the sarcomatoid component.

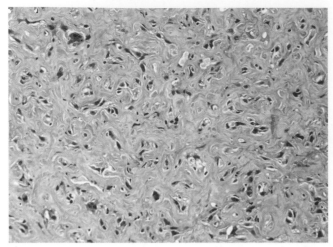

Fig 9. Sarcomatoid carcinoma shows epithelioid spindle cells in a markedly sclerotic stroma.

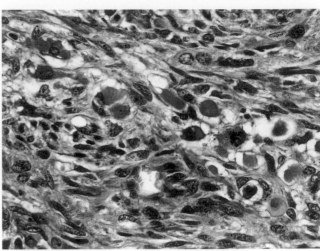

Fig 12. Sarcomatoid carcinoma with rhabdomyosarcomatous differentiation.

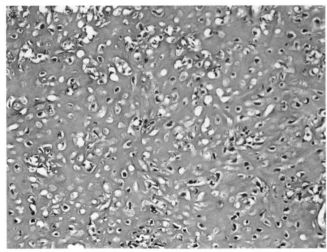

Fig 10. Sarcomatoid carcinoma showing heterologous osteoid differentiation.

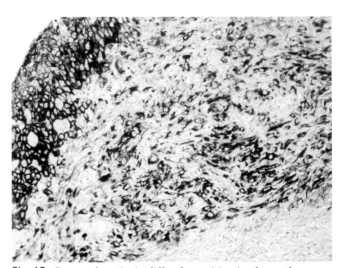

Fig 13. Pancytokeratin is diffusely positive in the surface urothelial carcinoma *(upper left)*, focally positive in the transitional area *(center)*, and entirely negative in the sarcomatoid component *(lower right)*.

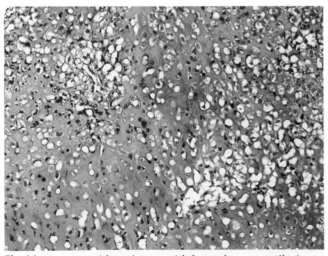

Fig 11. Sarcomatoid carcinoma with heterologous cartilaginous differentiation.

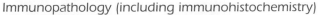

VILLOUS ADENOMA

Definition
- Benign glandular neoplasm of the bladder, typically with a papillary–villiform growth pattern, that is histologically indistinguishable from similar neoplasms of the colon and rectum

Clinical features
Epidemiology
- Rare
- Typically older patients (mean age, 65 years)
- Male predominance

Presentation
- Hematuria and irritative bladder symptoms are most common.
- Mucosuria is a rare finding.
- It is usually located within the dome and trigone of the bladder, as well as the urachus.
- Cystoscopically, it mimics papillary urothelial neoplasm.

Prognosis and treatment
- Benign neoplasm: complete resection is curative.
- Treatment can progress to invasive adenocarcinoma in up to one third of cases.

Pathology
Histology
- Microscopic appearance is similar to villous adenoma of the colon and rectum.
- Papillary–villiform architecture with fingerlike projections are present.
- Epithelium is columnar with intracellular acid mucin.
- Nuclear crowding, stratification, and hyperchromasia are typical.
- Prominent nucleoli may occasionally be seen.
- Areas of high-grade dysplasia–adenocarcinoma in situ should be identified and reported when present.
- Specimen should be submitted in its entirety to exclude invasion.

Immunopathology (including immunohistochemistry)
- As with their enteric counterparts, it is almost always CK20 positive and frequently positive for CEA.
- CK7 positivity is seen in about half of cases.
- CDX2 positivity may be seen in villous adenomatous lesions and should not be used to distinguish enteric-type bladder neoplasms from colorectal adenocarcinomas.

Main differential diagnosis
- In situ or invasive adenocarcinoma of urinary bladder
- Invasive adenocarcinoma from secondary site (e.g., direct extension from colorectal cancer or an adenocarcinoma from the gynecologic tract)
- Papillary urothelial carcinoma with glandular differentiation
- Florid cystitis cystica et glandularis with intestinal metaplasia

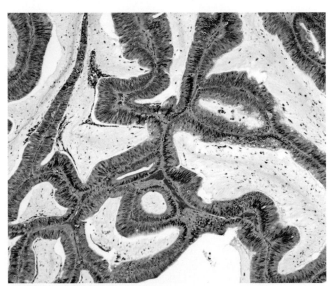

Fig 2. In some cases extracellular mucin may be abundant, although goblet cells are inconspicuous at low power.

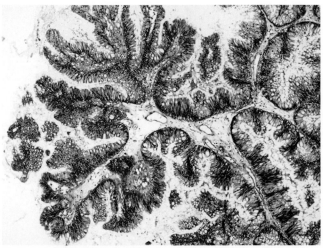

Fig 1. Even at low magnification, intracellular mucin (goblet cells) can be appreciated, and the arborizing growth pattern is typical of villous adenoma of the bladder.

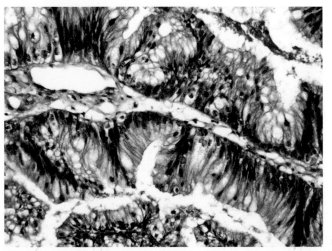

Fig 3. High-power examination shows pseudostratified columnar cells with variable amounts of intracytoplasmic mucin. Nucleoli are variable.

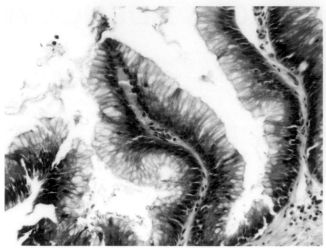

Fig 4. Abundant apical intracytoplasmic mucin is seen in this case. Nuclei are small and hyperchromatic without prominent nucleoli.

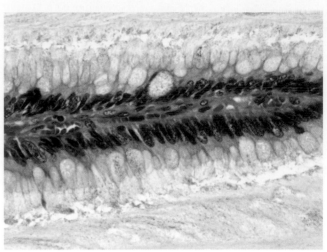

Fig 5. Cytologically, the cells of villous adenoma of the bladder are indistinguishable from those of similar lesions occurring in the colon and rectum. Careful examination, including complete submission of the specimen, is necessary to exclude foci of high-grade dysplasia or invasive adenocarcinoma.

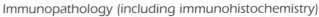
Definition
- Malignant neoplasm showing pure glandular phenotype

Clinical features
Epidemiology
- 0.5% to 2% of malignant bladder tumors
- Male predominance
- Peak incidence in the sixth decade
- Higher frequency in bladder carcinoma associated with exstrophy and nonfunctioning bladder

Presentation
- Hematuria most common symptom followed by dysuria and mucosuria

Prognosis and treatment
- Prognosis is poor but depends on stage.
- Management includes surgery, chemotherapy, and radiation therapy depending on the tumor's stage.

Pathology
Histology
- Composed purely of malignant glands or mucin-producing cells
- Classified according to histologic appearance, by order of frequency, into: not otherwise specified, mucinous (colloid), enteric (colonic), signet ring, and mixed
- Mucinous: small cell clusters or individual tumor cells floating in pools of mucin
- Enteric: resembles adenocarcinoma of the colon
- Signet ring: diffuse infiltration by single cells with eccentric nuclei and single large cytoplasmic vacuoles filled with mucin

Immunopathology (including immunohistochemistry)
- Variable immunoprofile but generally resembles that of colonic adenocarcinoma: positivity for CK20, p63 and CK5/6; variable positivity for CK7 and CDX2; and negative for nuclear β-catenin

Main differential diagnosis
- High-grade prostatic adenocarcinoma, metastasis, or direct extension
- Colonic adenocarcinoma, metastasis, or direct extension
- Florid cystitis glandularis, intestinal metaplasia
- Endometriosis, endocervicosis

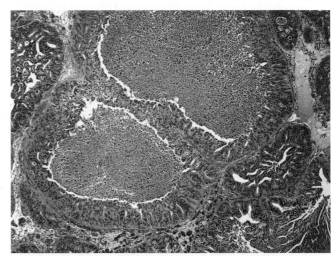

Fig 2. Bladder adenocarcinoma, enteric type, growing as large complex malignant glandular structures with confluent intraluminal areas of necrosis.

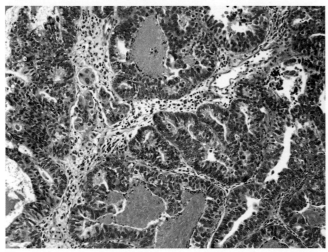

Fig 1. Bladder adenocarcinoma, enteric type, resembling colonic adenocarcinoma with malignant glands and central dirty necrosis.

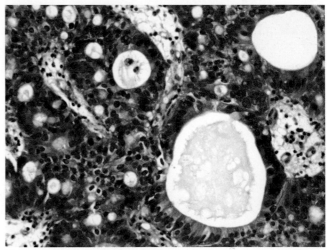

Fig 3. Bladder adenocarcinoma, not otherwise specified, showing nonspecific glandular growth without the associated necrosis that is typical of colonic-type adenocarcinoma.

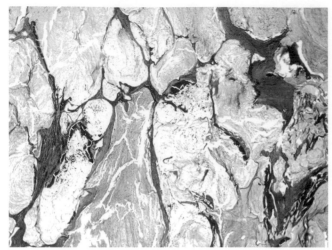

Fig 4. Bladder mucinous (colloid) adenocarcinoma showing large pools of mucin dissecting the bladder wall and clusters of malignant cells lining the mucin pools. In other examples, single cells (rather than strips of cells or glands) are seen floating in the mucin pools.

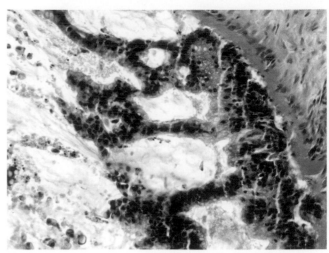

Fig 6. High magnification of bladder mucinous (colloid) adeno-carcinoma showing that the cells lining the mucin pools have obvious malignant cytologic features. In comparison when mucin extravasation is encountered in florid cases of intestinal metaplasia, it is a focal finding and the associated glandular cells do not show marked nuclear atypia.

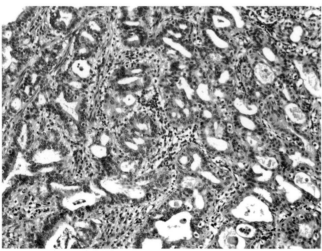

Fig 5. Bladder adenocarcinoma, not otherwise specified.

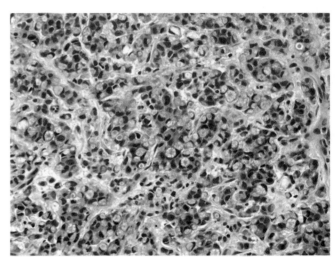

Fig 7. Bladder signet ring adenocarcinoma in which the bladder wall is diffusely infiltrated by single cells with eccentric hyper-chromatic nuclei and single, large cytoplasmic vacuoles filled with mucin.

Definition
- Also named *mesonephric adenocarcinoma,* is a distinct variant of bladder adenocarcinoma characterized by the presence of neoplastic cells with clear, eosinophilic cytoplasm

Clinical features
Epidemiology
- Exceedingly unusual
- Female predominance, with a broad range of age

Presentation
- Gross or microscopic hematuria
- Dysuria

Prognosis and treatment
- Tumors at advanced stage are associated with a high mortality rate while noninvasive or superficially invasive tumors are less aggressive.

Pathology
Histology
- Papillary or polypoid tumors exhibit a tubulocystic, papillary, or diffuse pattern of growth and composed of neoplastic cells with moderate to severe atypia, clear or eosinophilic cytoplasm, and high mitotic rate, showing overt stromal invasion.
- Hobnail configuration of the tumor cells is not unusual.
- Myxoid stromal changes are frequently seen.

Immunopathology (including immunohistochemistry)
- Positive for CK7, CEA, CA125, PAX2, PAX8, AMACR, p53, and sometimes CK20
- Negative for PSA, ER, and PR

Main differential diagnosis
- Nephrogenic adenoma
- Urothelial carcinoma with clear cell changes (glycogen rich)
- Metastatic renal cell carcinoma

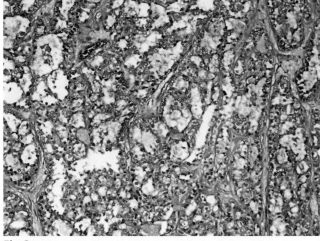

Fig 2. Clear cell adenocarcinoma with a tubulocystic pattern of growth.

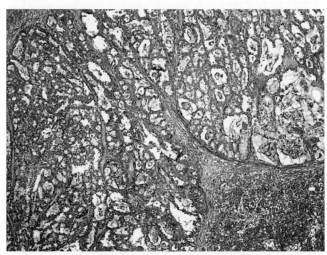

Fig 3. Clear cell adenocarcinoma with a predominant cystic pattern of growth and foci of necrosis *(lower right field).*

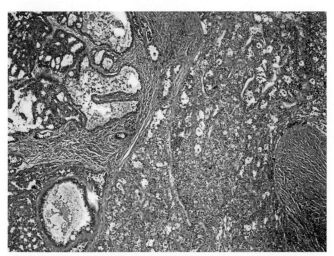

Fig 1. Clear cell carcinoma showing cystic and tubulocystic patterns of growth.

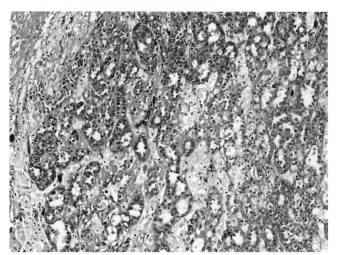

Fig 4. Clear cell adenocarcinoma composed of small tubules and cysts.

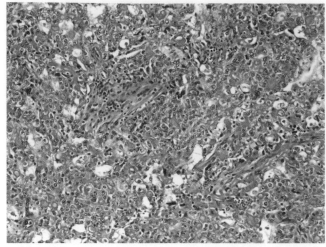

Fig 5. Clear cell adenocarcinoma with a solid pattern of growth mixed with small tubules.

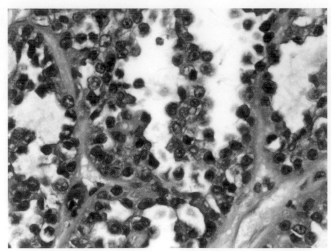

Fig 7. Clear cell adenocarcinoma with neoplastic cells depicting a hobnail configuration and lining tubulocystic structures.

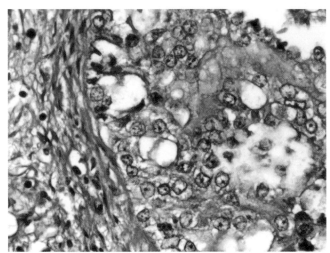

Fig 6. Clear cell adenocarcinoma showing neoplastic cells with ample, eosinophilic cytoplasm and evident atypias.

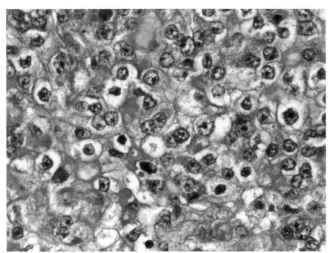

Fig 8. Solid clear cell adenocarcinoma showing tumor cells with ample, clear, eosinophilic cytoplasm and overt nuclear atypias.

Definition
- Malignant bladder neoplasm with glandular features arising from the urachus

Clinical features
Epidemiology
- Twice as common in males as females
- Peak incidence in fifth and sixth decades

Presentation
- Located at dome of bladder
- Nonspecific urinary tract signs and symptoms, including hematuria, urgency, frequency, and dysuria
- Mucosuria in a subset of cases

Prognosis and treatment
- Prognosis is poor: worse when signet ring differentiation is present.
- Five-year survival is 25% to 50%.
- Surgical resection in the form of partial or radical cystectomy with resection of the umbilicus is the primary treatment modality.
- Utility for chemotherapy is limited.

Pathology
Histology
- Grossly, it is located in the dome of the bladder.
- The majority are high-grade glandular lesions.
- Subtypes include enteric, mucinous, and signet ring cell.
- Low-grade mucinous neoplasms have been described that mimic those found in the appendix.
- Urachal remnants may be identified in a subset of cases.
- Background (nonurachal) bladder lacks in situ carcinoma and glandular differentiation.
- Cytology is generally of high grade.
- Extravasated mucin may predominate.

Immunopathology (including immunohistochemistry)
- Demonstrates immunoreactivity for CK20 and CK7
- May have CDX2 nuclear expression
- Often lack nuclear β-catenin expression
- Special stains for mucin include mucicarmine and PAS

Main differential diagnosis
- Secondary spread from colorectal adenocarcinoma
- Secondary extension from nonurachal primary adenocarcinoma of bladder

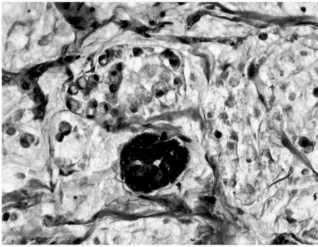

Fig 2. Higher magnification reveals marked nuclear atypia in adenocarcinoma containing glandular and signet ring features.

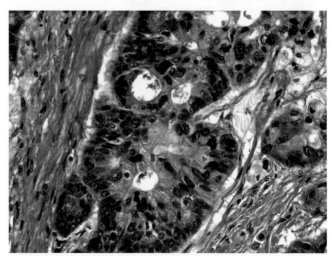

Fig 3. Colonic-type glands may be present occasionally and raise the differential diagnosis of a colonic primary adenocarcinoma.

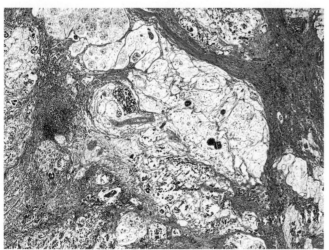

Fig 1. A large proportion of urachal adenocarcinomas demonstrate mucinous features and may appear as cells floating in pools of extravasated mucin.

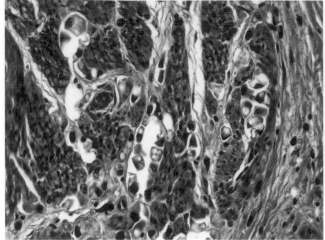

Fig 4. Signet ring cells may be identified in a subset of cases and generally confer a worse prognosis.

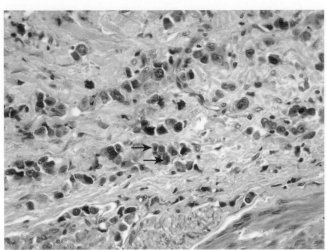

Fig 6. Mucicarmine stains may help in the identification of intracellular mucin *(arrows)*.

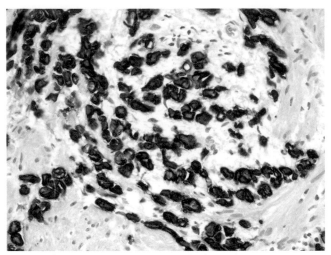

Fig 5. CK20 is positive in the majority of cases.

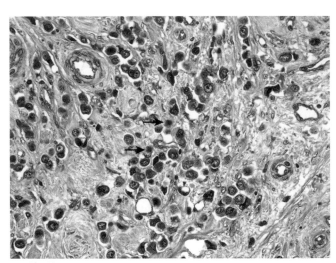

Fig 7. PAS may also be used to highlight mucin *(arrows)*.

Definition
- Malignant bladder neoplasm consisting of a purely squamous invasive component

Clinical features
Epidemiology
- Males are more commonly affected.
- Incidence is most common in the sixth to seventh decades, which is similar to urothelial carcinoma.
- In parts of the Middle East and Africa, there may be an association with *Schistosoma hematobium* and *Schistosoma mansonii* infection.
- Noninfectious causes include tobacco smoke and chronic inflammation of the bladder as caused by chronic indwelling catheters, neurogenic bladder, and bladder stones.
- Bladder exstrophy is a risk factor.

Presentation
- Nonspecific urinary tract signs and symptoms including dysuria and hematuria

Prognosis and treatment
- Prognosis is dependent on pathologic stage.
- Five-year progression-free probability is approximately 45%.
- Treatment is primarily via radical cystectomy.
- The benefits of adjuvant chemotherapy are unclear.
- Verrucous carcinoma subtype has a significantly more favorable prognosis.

Pathology
Histology
- Grossly appears as a white, flaky, and often exophytic mass
- Characterized microscopically as well, moderately, or poorly differentiated
- Analogous to squamous cell carcinoma at other sites, including the formation of keratin pearls and the presence of irregular nests of atypical squamous cells
- Lacks any urothelial carcinoma component within the invasive carcinoma
- Associated features including prominent desmoplasia and a giant cell reaction to keratin
- Associated with a variety of in situ lesions, including keratinizing squamous metaplasia, squamous dysplasia, squamous CIS, verrucous squamous hyperplasia, and rarely condylomata and urothelial CIS
- Verrucous carcinoma subtype demonstrating a bland cytologic appearance with minimal atypia and characterized by broad-based, pushing invasive borders; often associated with schistosomal infection

Immunopathology (including immunohistochemistry)
- Similar to squamous cell carcinoma at other sites, including immunoreactivity for cytokeratin 5/6 and p63
- No reliable immunohistochemical marker to distinguish invasive squamous cell carcinoma from urothelial carcinoma with extensive squamous differentiation

Main differential diagnosis
- Invasive urothelial carcinoma with squamous differentiation

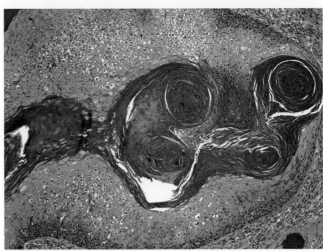

Fig 1. Well-differentiated squamous cell carcinoma demonstrating minimal atypia and abundant keratinization.

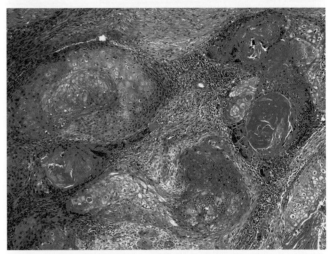

Fig 2. Keratin formation is still apparent in this moderately differentiated squamous cell carcinoma.

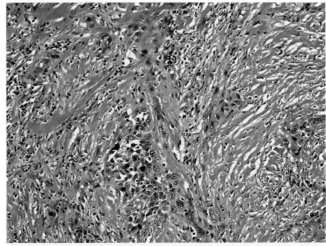

Fig 3. Poorly differentiated squamous cell carcinoma showing more prominent atypia and only rare squamous differentiation.

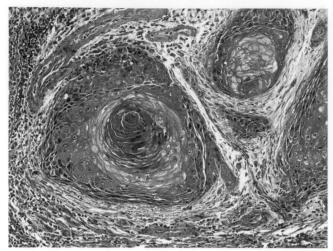

Fig 4. Keratin pearls are a classic feature of squamous cell carcinoma.

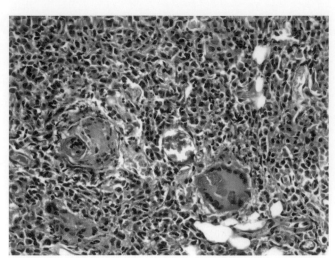

Fig 7. In areas in which schistosomal infection is prevalent, bladders may demonstrate calcified parasitic eggs and organisms associated with a giant cell reaction and marked inflammatory infiltrate rich in eosinophils.

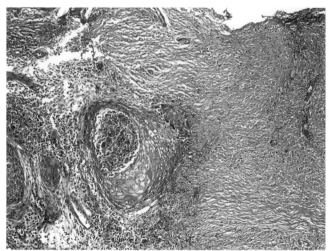

Fig 5. Desmoplasia is commonly found surrounding nests of invasive squamous cell carcinoma.

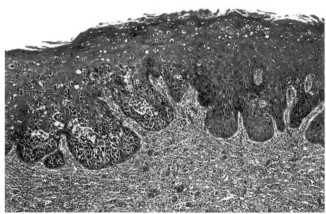

Fig 8. In situ squamous cell carcinoma is frequently found in association with invasive carcinoma.

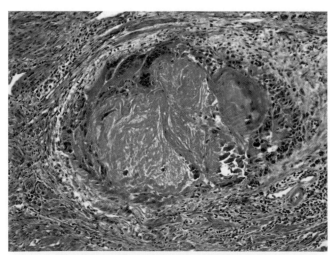

Fig 6. Giant cell reactions to keratin are frequently found in these lesions and may be a predominant feature.

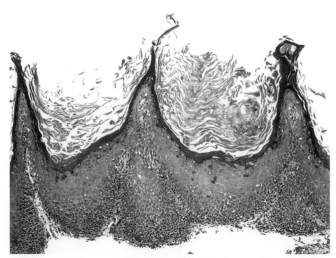

Fig 9. Verrucous squamous hyperplasia is another precursor lesion defined as repetitive, church-spire–like upward tenting of the urothelial surface associated with prominent hyperkeratosis.

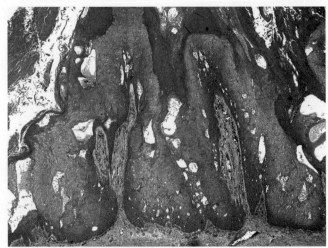

Fig 10. Verrucous carcinoma is an uncommon form of bladder squamous carcinoma and is characterized by well-differentiated, hyperkeratotic squamous epithelium and a broad pushing base.

Definition
- Neoplasm derived from the paraganglial cells in the bladder wall

Clinical features
Epidemiology
- Rare (<0.1% of all bladder tumors)
- Wide age range (10 to 88 years)
- Slight female predominance (male-to-female ratio, 2:3)

Presentation
- Hypertension in two thirds of patients
- Symptoms associated with sympathetic stimulation (headache, palpation, blurred vision and sweating) in half of all patients
- Hematuria in half of all patients

Prognosis and treatment
- Biologic behavior not reliably predictable based on histologic findings
- 10% to 15% malignant
- Localized tumor treated with transurethral, wedge, or partial resection
- Malignant tumor treated with radical cystectomy and metastasectomy

Pathology
Histology
- May occur in any part and level of the bladder wall
- Most commonly centered in the muscularis propria
- Nests of cells in Zellballen or diffuse growth pattern
- Prominent thin-walled vascular network
- Round cells with clear, eosinophilic, amphophilic cytoplasm, and ovoid nuclei
- Variable nuclear pleomorphism and mitosis
- Can invade deeply into muscularis propria and show vascular invasion

Immunopathology (including immunohistochemistry)
- Negative for epithelial markers
- Positive for neuroendocrine markers (chromogranin, synaptophysin, NSE)
- Sustentacular cells positive for S100

Main differential diagnosis
- Urothelial carcinoma
- Metastatic melanoma
- Malignant PEComa

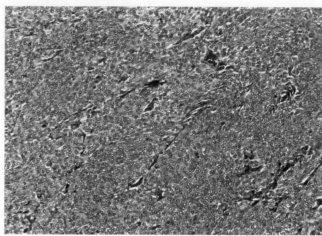

Fig 2. Bladder paraganglioma with a diffuse pattern of growth.

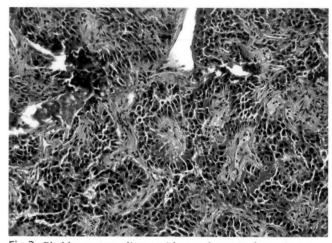

Fig 3. Bladder paraganglioma with pseudorosette formation.

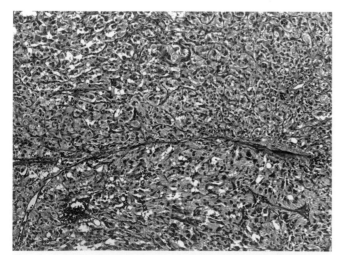

Fig 1. Bladder paraganglioma with a Zellballen pattern of growth.

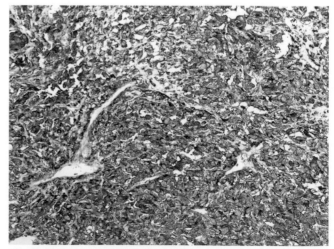

Fig 4. Bladder paraganglioma with tumor cells positive for neuroendocrine marker chromogranin.

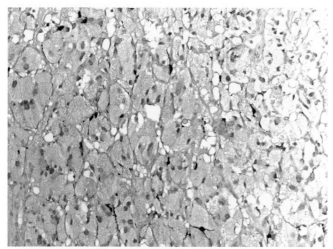

Fig 5. Bladder paraganglioma with S100 staining the sustentacular cells.

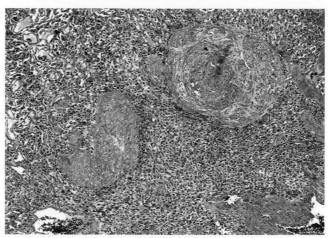

Fig 7. Paraganglioma cells enveloping thick muscularis propria muscle bundles without eliciting a desmoplastic response.

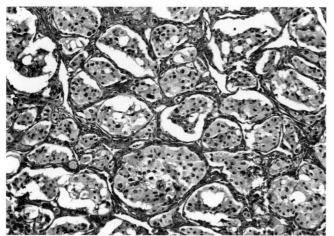

Fig 6. Characteristically, tumor cells have abundant granular cytoplasm and uniform nuclei. Occasionally, pleomorphic nuclei are present.

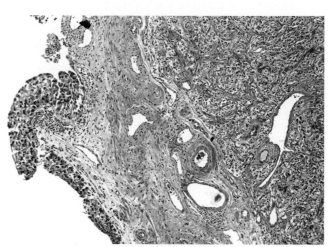

Fig 8. Urothelium involved by carcinoma in situ with paraganglioma situated in the lamina propria.

Definition

- Biopsy and transurethral resection (TUR)
  - A staging requirement of bladder cancer on biopsy and the reporting of the presence or absence of muscularis propria, absence of muscularis propria in invasive carcinoma will require a repeated procedure to ascertain depth of invasion.
  - In instances in which the distinction between invasion into the muscularis propria and into the muscularis mucosae is indeterminate, a statement to this regard should be made.
  - Although no commonly accepted markers to distinguish muscularis propria and muscularis mucosae are available, recent research suggests that strong, diffuse smoothelin immunoreactivity may be indicative of muscularis propria.
  - Biopsy and TUR cannot be used to distinguish invasion into the perivesical fat, as fat may be present at all layers of the bladder wall.
  - Caution should be exercised to identify single-cell invasion at the base of a flat urothelial CIS or high-grade papillary urothelial carcinoma.
  - Although the majority of papillary lesions that invade are high-grade carcinomas, some low-grade carcinomas may rarely demonstrate invasion.
  - Invasion into the papillary stalk of an exophytic lesion is considered lamina propria invasion.
- Radical cystectomy and cystoprostatectomy
  - TNM criteria include the presence of multiple tumors (m), recurrent tumors (r), and whether the tumor is posttreatment (y).
  - Depth of invasion into the lamina propria, muscularis propria, perivesical fat or adjacent organs such as prostate and vagina are reported as American Joint Committee on Cancer (AJCC) tumor criteria:
    - pT0: no primary tumor identified
    - pTa: noninvasive papillary carcinoma
    - pTis: flat urothelial CIS
    - pT1: invasion into the lamina propria
    - pT2: invasion into the muscularis propria (detrusor muscle)
      - pT2a: superficial muscularis propria (inner half)
      - pT2b: deep muscularis propria (outer half)
    - pT3: invasion into the perivesical fat
      - pT3a: microscopically
      - pT4a: macroscopically
    - pT4: invasion into the prostatic stroma, seminal vesicles, uterus, vagina, pelvic wall, or abdominal wall
      - pT4a: invasion into prostatic stroma, uterus, or vagina
      - pT4b: invasion into the pelvic or abdominal wall
  - AJCC lymph node criteria have been recently revised and no longer require size restrictions:
    - pNX: no lymph nodes for assessment
    - pN0: no lymph node metastases
    - pN1: single regional lymph node metastasis in the true pelvis, including hypogastric, obturator, external iliac, or presacral lymph nodes
    - pN2: multiple regional lymph node metastases in the true pelvis (locations as above)
    - pN3: lymph node metastases to the common iliac lymph nodes
  - Distant metastases are staged as either not applicable or pM1 (distant metastases). In general, a greater burden of metastatic disease in lymph nodes corresponds with reduced survival.
  - Margins include the ureteral margins, urethral margins, soft tissue resection margins, and vaginal cuff, when present. The presence of invasive or in situ carcinoma at a margin should be distinguished.
- Partial cystectomy
  - Tumor and lymph node staging is as described for radical cystectomy.
  - Margins of resection include the soft tissue resection margins and circumferential bladder mucosal margins.
- Prostatic urethra
  - Involvement of the prostatic urethra by urothelial carcinoma should be staged following new criteria:
    - pT0: no evidence of carcinoma
    - pTa: noninvasive papillary carcinoma
    - pTis: flat urothelial CIS
    - pT1: superficial invasion into the subepithelial connective tissue from the surface urothelium of the prostatic urethra
    - pT2: invasion into the prostatic stroma either from the surface urothelium or from prostatic ducts colonized by urothelial carcinoma
    - pT3: invasion beyond the prostatic capsule

SECONDARY SPREAD OF PROSTATE CARCINOMA TO THE BLADDER

Definition
- Secondary involvement of the urinary bladder by prostatic carcinoma, most often by direct extension

Clinical features
Epidemiology
- Metastatic tumors to the bladder may comprise up to 10% of malignant tumors in this location.
- Up to 20% of all metastatic tumors to the bladder are prostatic in origin.

Presentation
- Hematuria
- Increased serum PSA

Prognosis and treatment
- Poor because of typically high-grade and high-stage tumors
- Treatment with hormonal therapy: androgen ablation
- Second-line hormonal therapies and palliative radiotherapy
- Surgery to relieve obstructive symptoms

Pathology
Histology
- Poorly differentiated tumor cells growing in sheets, typically with minimal pleomorphism or mitotic activity as compared with urothelial carcinoma
- May have focal lumen formation
- Typically, prostatic carcinoma growing with infiltrating cords of cells or focal cribriform architecture
- Round nuclei with prominent nucleoli, possibly with more than one nucleoli
- Prostate carcinomas with minimal variability in nuclear sizes and shapes
- Lacks urothelial dysplasia or flat CIS on the surface or the presence of a concurrent papillary urothelial neoplasm
- May show involvement only of the muscularis propria

Immunopathology (including immunohistochemistry)
- Positive for PSA, PSMA, Prostein and NKX3.1
- Negative for high-molecular-weight cytokeratin, p63, uroplakin, and thrombomodulin

Main differential diagnosis
- Urothelial carcinoma with or without glandular differentiation
- Primary adenocarcinoma of the bladder
- Metastatic carcinoma from other sites such as lung or gastrointestinal tract

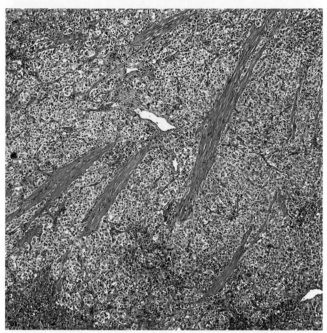

Fig 1. Low-power view of prostate carcinoma, metastatic to the urinary bladder with poorly differentiated tumor cells growing in sheets, with minimal pleomorphism or mitotic activity as compared with urothelial carcinomas. Note the monotonous appearance of the tumor cells.

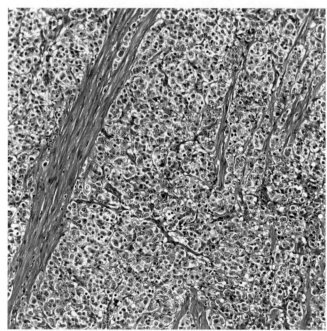

Fig 2. A typical metastatic prostatic carcinoma growing with infiltrating cords of cells with focal lumen formation and the involvement of the muscularis propria. Note the solid sheets of neoplastic cells with a monomorphic appearance, more characteristic of prostatic adenocarcinoma, compared with urothelial carcinoma.

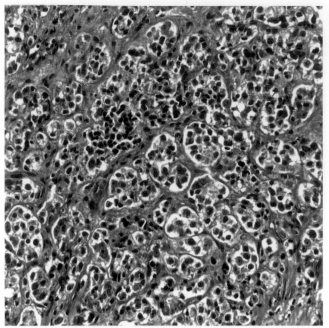

Fig 3. Higher magnification of the case illustrated in Fig 2 highlighting the round nuclei with prominent nucleoli. Some of the nuclei have more than one nucleolus. Note the minimal variability in nuclear size and shape.

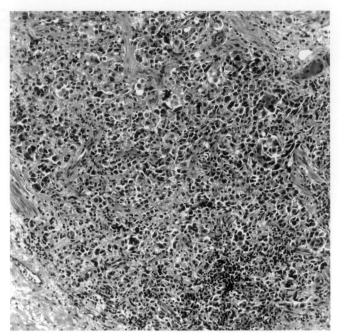

Fig 5. Poorly differentiated prostatic adenocarcinoma extending into the urinary bladder. The neoplastic cells appear more pleomorphic and lack typical features of prostatic adenocarcinoma, raising the possibility that this represents a high-grade urothelial carcinoma. There is no urothelial dysplasia or flat carcinoma in situ on the surface or the presence of a concurrent papillary urothelial neoplasm in this case.

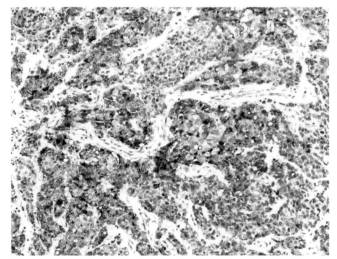

Fig 4. Diffuse positivity for prostate specific antigen in the neoplastic cells from the case illustrated in Fig 5, confirming the diagnosis of metastatic prostatic adenocarcinoma.

SECONDARY ADENOCARCINOMA INVOLVING THE BLADDER, OTHER THAN PROSTATIC CARCINOMA

Definition
- Adenocarcinoma originating in other organs with secondary involvement of the bladder through direct extension or via lymphatic or vascular spread

Clinical features
Epidemiology
- The most frequent primary sites of adenocarcinoma secondarily involving the bladder are the colon and rectum, accounting for about 33% of cases.
- Other sites reported, excluding the prostate, are the lung, uterine cervix, stomach, esophagus, kidney, breast, skin and appendix, accounting for 40% of bladder metastases.

Presentation
- Usually asymptomatic
- Hematuria
- Bladder tumor on cystoscopy
- Bladder wall mass on radiologic assessment

Prognosis and treatment
- Prognosis depends on the type of primary tumor.
- Surgical resection can be considered for localized metastases.

Pathology
Histology
- There is typically but not always outer bladder wall involvement that is more prominent than mucosal involvement.
- There is no associated papillary, invasive, or in situ urothelial carcinoma. Although in situ adenocarcinoma is usually lacking, colonization of surface mucosa could be misinterpreted as such. Usually, intestinal metaplasia or cystitis cystica et glandularis is also lacking.

Immunopathology (including immunohistochemistry)
- CK20, CDX2 (nuclear), and β-catenin (membranous) are positive while CK7 is usually negative in colorectal metastases.
- CK7, CDX2 (nuclear), and β-catenin (membranous) are positive, while CK20 is usually negative in gastric metastases.
- CK7 and estrogen receptor are positive, while CK20 is negative in breast carcinoma metastases.
- CK7, CK20, 34βE12, p63, uroplakin, thrombomodulin, and CDX2 are positive, while estrogen receptor–progesterone receptors are usually negative in primary bladder adenocarcinoma. WT1, β-catenin, and TTF1 are also negative.

Main differential diagnosis
- Urothelial carcinoma with glandular differentiation
- Urothelial carcinoma with abundant myxoid stroma
- Micropapillary urothelial carcinoma
- Plasmacytoid urothelial carcinoma
- Primary bladder adenocarcinoma, urachal or nonurachal including clear cell adenocarcinoma and signet ring cell adenocarcinoma of the urinary bladder

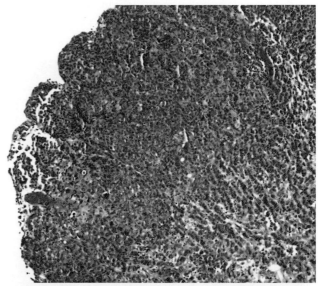

Fig 1. Metastatic breast carcinoma to urinary bladder.

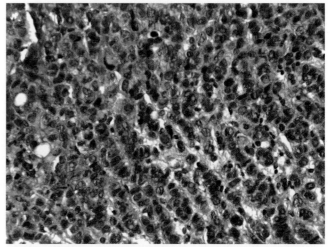

Fig 2. Metastatic breast carcinoma to urinary bladder at higher magnification.

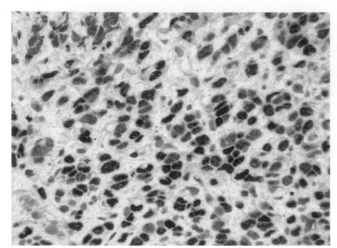

Fig 3. Metastatic breast carcinoma to urinary bladder, estrogen receptor positive.

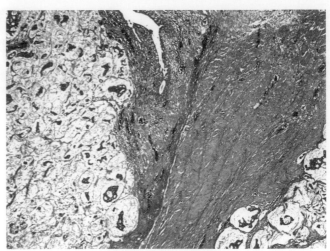

Fig 6. Metastatic mucinous adenocarcinoma to urinary bladder from an appendiceal primary.

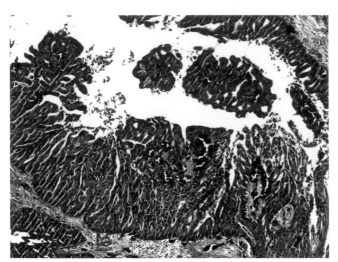

Fig 4. Metastatic colonic adenocarcinoma to urinary bladder.

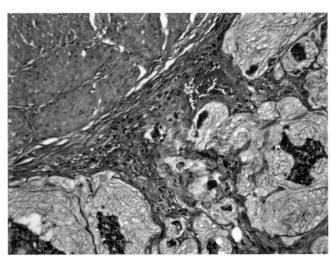

Fig 7. Metastatic mucinous adenocarcinoma to urinary bladder from an appendiceal primary.

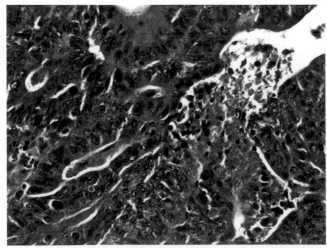

Fig 5. Metastatic colonic adenocarcinoma to urinary bladder with evident dirty necrosis.

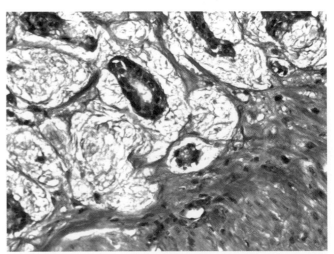

Fig 8. Metastatic mucinous adenocarcinoma to urinary bladder from an appendiceal primary at higher magnification.

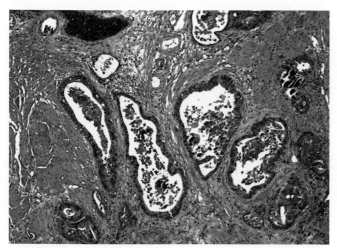

Fig 9. Metastatic rectal adenocarcinoma to urinary bladder.

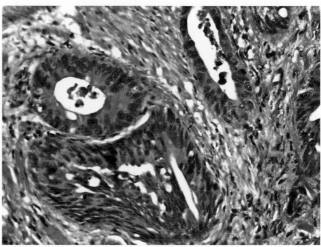

Fig 10. Metastatic rectal adenocarcinoma to urinary bladder.

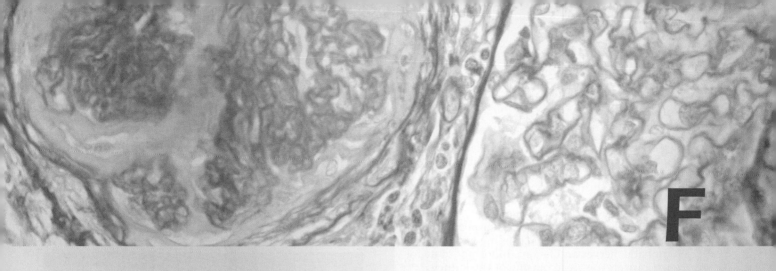

F

NONNEOPLASTIC DISEASE OF THE KIDNEY

- Gross anatomy
  - Retroperitoneal organ invested in a layer of peri-nephric fat and covered anteriorly with Gerota's fascia (a landmark for staging renal cancers)
  - Renal hilum: slitlike space on medial border through which runs the ureter, branches of arteries and veins, nerves, and lymphatics
  - Renal sinus: space on the medical aspect of the kidney that contains renal colleting system, vessels, lymphatic, nerves and fat; an important route for renal cancers to spread outside of the kidney
- Renal capsule
  - Covers the convex portion of the renal cortex
  - Cortex in contact with the renal sinus lacks capsule, therefore allowing tumor access to the renal sinus
- Cortex
  - One-centimeter layer beneath the renal capsule and extending down between the renal pyramids (columns of Bertin)
- Medulla
  - Divided into outer medulla and inner medulla (papilla)
  - At the tips of papillae, the epithelium of collecting ducts transforms into the urothelium.
- Vasculature
  - The renal artery branches into segmental arteries in renal hilum.
  - Segmental arteries enter the kidney and become interlobar arteries that branch farther into arcuate arteries, traversing the renal parenchyma near the corticomedullary junction.
  - Arcuate arteries give rise to interlobular arteries and subsequently afferent arterioles that course into the glomerular capillary tufts.
  - Venous return follows the arterial tributary pattern in reverse.
- Lymphatic system
  - A dual lymphatic system is present.
  - Major lymphatic drainage follows the vasculature from parenchyma to the sinus and terminates in lateral paraaortic lymph nodes.
  - Minor capsular lymphatic drainage from the super-ficial cortex courses along the capsule to the hilum to join the major lymphatic drainage.

- Collecting system
  - Nine to 11 funnel-shaped minor calyces surround the papillary tips.
  - Minor calyces converge into major calyces, which unite to form pelvis and ureter.
  - A continuous layer of smooth muscle originates from minor calyces and continues along the major calyces, pelvis, and ureter.

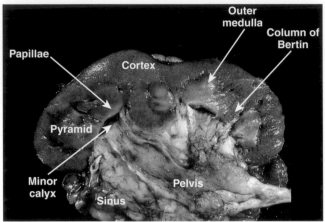

Fig 2. A kidney resected for pelvic urothelial carcinoma demonstrates the renal cortex and columns of Bertin situated between the renal pyramids. The latter consists of an outer medulla and an inner medulla or papilla. The sinus adipose tissue separates the kidney from the collecting system and also contains numerous nerves and lymphatics.

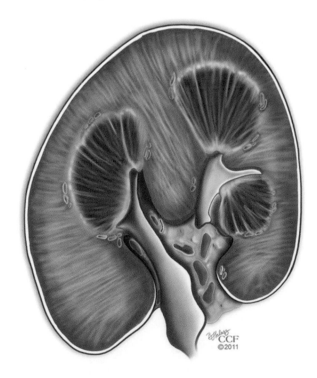

Fig 3. A kidney in cross section. The renal sinus contains the collecting system, large vessels, lymphatics, and nerves. The renal capsule, shown as white line, surrounds the convex surface of the kidney but is absent from the cortical surface that is in contact with the sinus.

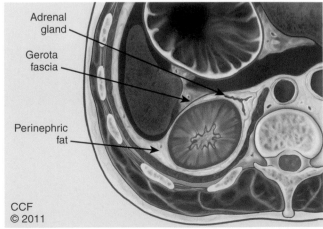

Fig 1. The retroperitoneal location of the kidney, perinephric fat, and Gerota fascia. (Copyright 2011, Cleveland Clinic Foundation.)

Definition
- A congenital developmental renal malformation resulting from abnormal nephrogenesis because of the inability of the ureteric bud to communicate with the metanephric blastema

Clinical features
Epidemiology
- Relatively common, affecting 1 in 1000 to 4000 of the general population
- Most often sporadic, but family history of renal and urinary tract malformations in 10% of cases
- Two phenotypes described with urinary tract abnormality: multicystic dysplasia and obstructive

Presentation
- Bilateral severe disease: maternal oligohydramnios, neonatal pulmonary, and renal failure
- Unilateral kidney mass
- Chronic renal failure in childhood
- Diagnosis can be made on antenatal ultrasonography, including small renal size, subcortical cysts, patchy contrast enhancement, architectural disarray, distorted pelvicalyceal system
- May be associated with multiple malformation syndromes

Prognosis and treatment
- Worse prognosis in bilateral diseases, diminished functional renal mass, lower urinary tract obstruction, anhydramnios, or severe polyhydramnios
- Decreasing renal dimensions, declining amniotic fluid during sequential antenatal assessment indicating a worse prognosis
- Treatment options: observation, prophylactic antibiotics, or surgery

Pathology
Gross pathology
- Range from small and solid to large and partially or completely cystic, depending on the type and degree of the dysplastic changes

Histology
- Range from rudimentary to well-developed renal architecture
- Primitive or malformed glomeruli and tubules lacking proper organization
- Dysplastic ducts lined by columnar epithelium and rimmed by spindle cell collars
- Fetal cartilage

Immunopathology (immunohistochemistry)
- PAX2, BCl2, and galectin-3 are expressed by dysplastic epithelium.

Molecular diagnostics
- Genetic abnormalities include mutations in individual genes such as TCF2/hepatocyte nuclear factor 1ss, PAX2, and uroplakins.
- Compound heterozygote mutations are also described in genes involved in renal and urinary tract development.

Main differential diagnosis
- Autosomal recessive polycystic kidney disease: bilateral cystic kidney disease and congenital hepatic fibrosis; manifest at birth or childhood, radial cysts in cortex and medulla on imaging; normal-appearing nephrons in the cystic septa; no fetal cartilage
- Autosomal dominant polycystic kidney disease: onset in third to fourth decades; normal-appearing nephrons in the cystic septa; no fetal cartilage
- Acquired renal cystic disease: history of renal failure from another cause unrelated to the cystic renal disease
- Cystic renal neoplasm: fibrous capsule separating the cystic lesion and normal kidney; no nephronic structures in the cystic septa

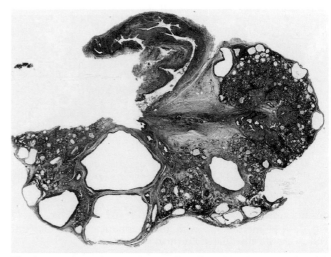

Fig 1. Dysplastic kidney from a female infant (4.5 months old) showing multiple cysts, reduced normal renal parenchyma, and depressed renal cortex.

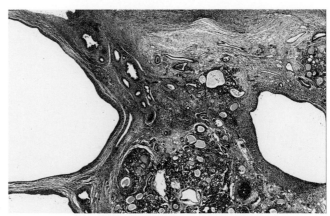

Fig 2. The cysts are lined by flattened and attenuated epithelium. Glomerular cysts, dilated tubules, and cysts contain thin pink secretions.

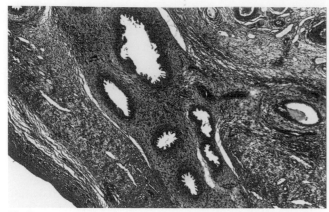

Fig 3. Primitive tubules lined by cuboidal epithelium with some degree of stratification and tufting into the lumens, cuffed by spindle cells forming whorls around the tubular walls.

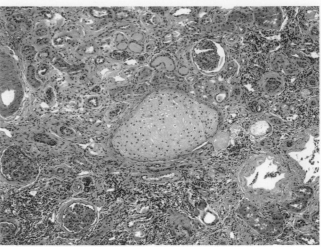

Fig 5. Fetal cartilage in renal dysplasia.

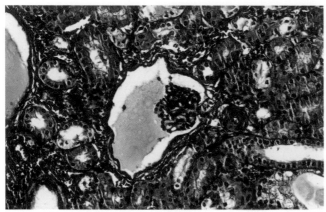

Fig 4. A glomerulocyst, with the diminutive glomerular tuft within a cystically dilated Bowman space.

AUTOSOMAL RECESSIVE POLYCYSTIC KIDNEY DISEASE

Definition
- Rare, early onset, autosomal recessive inherited polycystic kidney disease
- Associated with single gene (*PKHD1*) mutation on chromosome 6p21-23
- *PKHD1* gene encodes polyductin or fibrocystin

Clinical features
Epidemiology
- Found in 1/10,000 to 1/50,000 live births

Presentation
- Massively enlarged kidneys
- Can usually be detected before birth or in the neonatal period; minority of cases diagnosed later in childhood
- Associated with congenital hepatic fibrosis in patients who survive infancy
- Lungs possibly poorly developed and hypoplastic owing to compression of the thoracic organs

Prognosis and treatment
- Usually results in stillbirth or early neonatal death
- Fatal in 75% of cases

Pathology
Gross pathology
- Bilateral massive enlargement of kidneys with smooth external surface is observed.
- Bivalved kidney shows reniform shape with diffuse, relatively uniform cysts involving the cortex and medulla.

Histology
- Renal parenchyma shows numerous small cysts involving cortical and medullary collecting ducts.
- Cysts are radially arranged and are oriented perpendicular to the renal capsule.
- Dilated collecting ducts are lined by a single layer of uniform cuboidal cells.
- Cyst content may be proteinaceous and contain calcific deposits.
- Normal-appearing nephrons are seen between cysts.

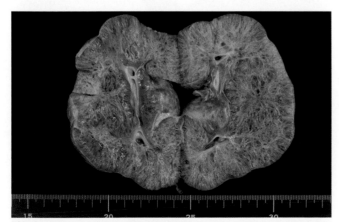

Fig 1. A bivalved kidney involved by autosomal recessive polycystic kidney disease shows an enlarged, reniform shape. The cortex and medulla are replaced by numerous, uniform, elongated cysts that are perpendicular to the surface.

Main differential diagnosis
- Dysplastic kidney: aberrantly formed nephronic structures; primitive tubules surrounded by spindle cells; characteristic fetal cartilage
- Medullary cystic disease: autosomal dominant; cysts located at the corticomedullary junction
- Medullary sponge kidney: no evidence of genetic transmission; cystic changes involving one or more renal papillae

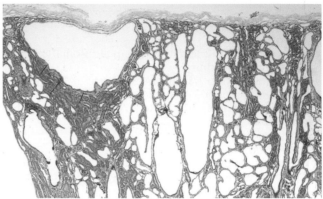

Fig 2. Cysts are radially arranged and perpendicular to the renal capsule and involve cortical and medullary collecting ducts.

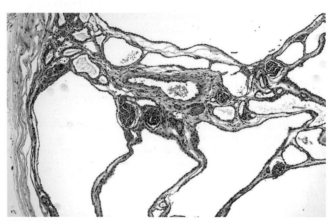

Fig 3. Dilated collecting ducts are lined with one layer of uniform cuboidal epithelium. Nephrons between cysts appear normal.

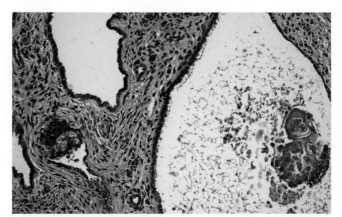

Fig 4. Cysts may contain proteinaceous calcified secretions.

AUTOSOMAL DOMINANT POLYCYSTIC KIDNEY DISEASE

Definition
- A late-onset, autosomal dominant disorder character-ized by the progressive development of innumerable cysts in the kidney, leading to renal insufficiency
- Associated with mutations in the *PKD1* gene on chromosome 16 (16q13.3) in 85% of patients, or the *PKD2* gene on chromosome 4 (4q21-23) in approximately 15% of cases
  - *PKD1* encodes the protein polycystin 1
  - *PKD2* encodes the protein polycystin 2

Clinical features
Epidemiology
- More common but less severe than autosomal reces-sive polycystic kidney
- Found in 1/400 to 1/1000 live births
- Found in 5% to 10% of all patients receiving dialysis
- Family history in approximately 70% to 75% of affected patients

Presentation
- It typically appears in the fourth to fifth decades after sufficient renal parenchyma destruction has occurred and renal failure has developed.
- It usually occurs with hematuria or proteinuria, or both.
- Chronic flank pain is common.
- Patients often develop urinary tract infections (UTIs).
- Extrarenal manifestations include intracranial berry aneurysms, hypertension, colonic diverticula, extrarenal cysts (pancreatic, hepatic), and cardiac valve abnormalities including mitral valve prolapse.

Prognosis and treatment
- It is one of the leading causes of end-stage renal disease in adults.
- End-stage kidney disease is found in approximately 50% of patients by 60 years of age.
- Renal transplant is curative when the patient develops end-stage kidney disease.

Pathology
Gross pathology
- At the early stage, kidneys are of normal size with few cysts in cortex and medulla.
- Progression of disease leads to marked bilateral kidney enlargement with an increase in size and number of cysts.
- Kidneys have irregular contour because of numerous peripheral cysts.

Histology
- Cysts range in size from a few millimeters to several centimeters.
- Cysts contain hemorrhagic or clear yellow protein-aceous fluid; calcified deposits are often seen.
- Cysts are lined by a single layer of flattened to cuboidal epithelium; small papillary projections may be seen.
- Intervening kidney tissue typically shows interstitial fibrosis, lymphocytic infiltrate, tubular atrophy, and glomerular and vascular sclerosis.
- Renal cell carcinomas can occur.

Main differential diagnosis
- Acquired cystic disease: patients receiving dialysis because of chronic renal failure as the result of nonhe-reditary kidney disease such as diabetes or hyperten-sion; kidney often reduced in size

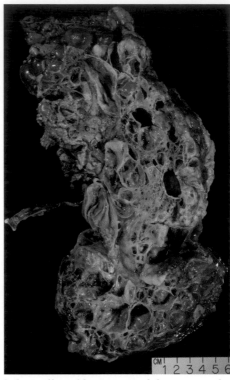

Fig 1. A kidney affected by autosomal dominant polycystic kidney disease is markedly enlarged with numerous cysts of different size. Note the irregular contour of the kidney resulting from numerous peripheral cysts.

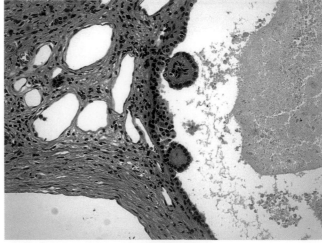

Fig 2. Small papillary epithelial hyperplasia may be seen in the cystic lining.

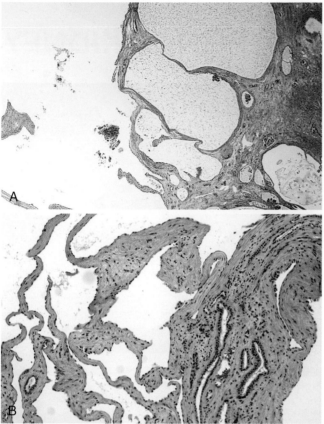

Fig 3. **A,** Cysts range in size from a few millimeters to several centimeters. **B,** Cysts are lined by a single layer of flattened to cuboidal epithelium.

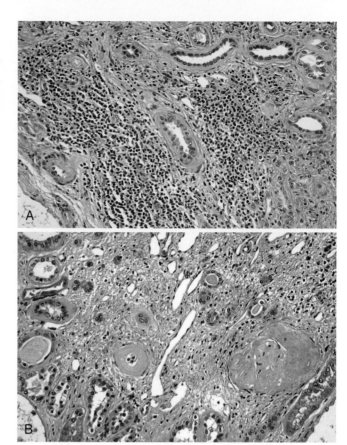

Fig 5. Kidney parenchyma between cysts shows interstitial fibrosis, lymphocytic infiltrate **(A),** tubular atrophy, and glomerular and vascular sclerosis **(B).**

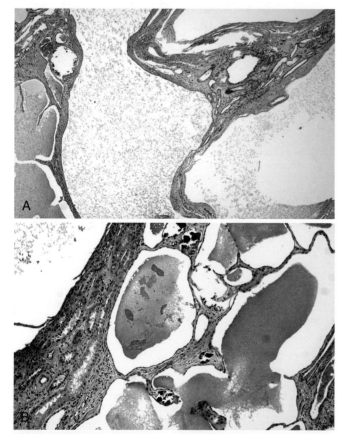

Fig 4. Cysts may contain proteinaceous fluid **(A)** or hemorrhagic fluid **(B).** Calcium oxalate crystals are often seen **(B).**

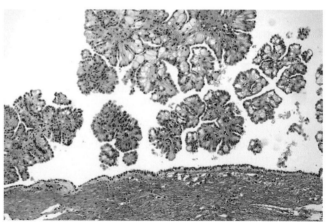

Fig 6. Papillary renal cell carcinomas arising in autosomal dominant polycystic kidney disease.

Definition
- Cystic dilatation of papillary collecting ducts of one or more renal pyramids

Clinical features
Epidemiology
- Cause unknown but without evidence of genetic transmission
- Significant number of asymptomatic patients; condition never diagnosed
- 0.5% in large pyelogram series and 14% to 21% in patients with nephrolithiasis in radiology literature
- Age, fourth to sixth decades
- Male predominance
- Bilateral in 80% of cases

Presentation
- Renal colic (50% to 60%)
- Urinary tract infection (20% to 33%)
- Gross hematuria (10% to 18%)
- Hypercalcemia (33% to 50%)
- Radiologic findings: multiple small calculi within the renal papillae, dilated collecting ducts with the appearance of "bristles on a brush"

Prognosis and treatment
- Treatment focuses on complications of medullary spongy kidney (calculi formation and infection).
- Less than 10% of symptomatic patients have a poor long-term outcome.

Pathology
Gross pathology
- Multiple small cysts (1 to 5 mm) involving the tip of renal papillae; one or multiple papillae possibly involved
- Microcalculi in the dilated collecting ducts; possible lithiasis in the calyceal system

Histology
- Dilated collecting ducts lined with cuboidal or flattened epithelium
- Inflammation in the interstitium

Main differential diagnosis
- Medullary cystic disease: autosomal dominant; cysts located at the corticomedullary junction
- Infantile polycystic kidney disease: autosomal recessive affecting infants and young children; uniform cysts involving cortex and medulla in a distinctive radiating pattern

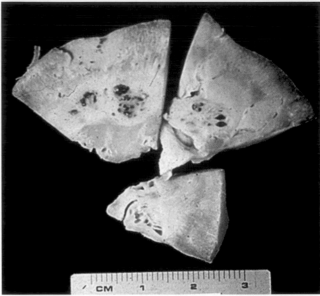

Fig 1. Multiple small cysts involve the tip of several renal papillae in a case of medullary spongy kidney. (Courtesy Howard Levin, Cleveland, Ohio.)

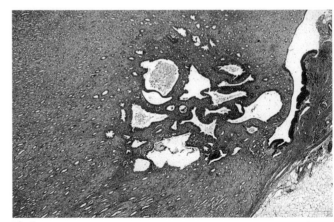

Fig 2. Medullary spongy kidney showing marked dilatation of papillary collecting ducts. (Courtesy Howard Levin, Cleveland, Ohio.)

ACQUIRED CYSTIC KIDNEY DISEASE

Definition
- Development of bilateral and multiple renal cysts in patients whose chronic renal failure can not be attributed to a hereditary etiology

Clinical features
Epidemiology
- Cysts are present in 8% of patients when dialysis is initiated.
- Incidence, number, and size of cysts increase with the duration of dialysis (50% and 90% of patients developed cysts after 3 to 5 years and 10 years of dialysis, respectively).
- Renal tumors develop in 5% to 20% cases.

Presentation
- Patient receiving dialysis for end-stage kidney disease owing to various nongenetic etiologies
- Usually asymptomatic; development of cysts detected on imaging studies
- Flank pain because of cyst expansion or hemorrhage
- Symptoms uncommonly because of the development of a renal tumor

Prognosis and treatment
- Longer dialysis duration leads to higher incidence of cyst formation.
- Complications include intracystic or retroperitoneal bleeding, infection, and development of renal cell carcinomas.
- Renal cell carcinoma appears to have a better prognosis when associated with acquired renal cystic disease compared with those without this disease.

Pathology
Gross pathology
- Bilateral involvement
- Kidney size reduced or modestly enlarged (more common in patients receiving dialysis longer than 3 years)
- Multiple cysts of variable sizes (up to 2 cm) initially affecting cortex, medulla, and entire kidney at advanced stage

Histology
- Cysts lined with flattened epithelium and possibly containing proteinaceous and serosanguineous fluid
- Foci of epithelial hyperplasia common
- Noncystic kidney with end-stage changes

Main differential diagnosis
- Hereditary polycystic kidney disease: autosomal dominant or recessive transmission; affected kidney markedly enlarged
- Cystic renal dysplasia: usually unilateral involvement; malformed glomeruli; immature tubules rimmed with spindle cells and cartilage

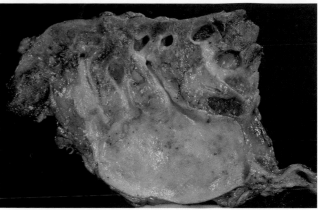

Fig 1. Acquired cystic kidney disease. The parenchyma is atrophic with several cysts. Renal sinus fat is prominent. The pelvis is markedly dilated.

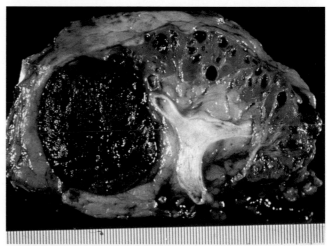

Fig 2. Acquired cystic kidney disease with a secondary tumor. The kidney is atrophic with numerous variably sized cysts. Renal sinus fat is prominent. A large renal tumor arose at one of the poles. (Courtesy Dr. Howard Levin, Cleveland, Ohio.)

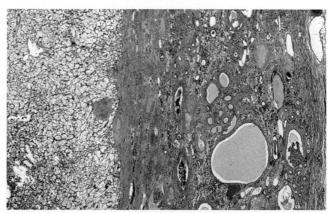

Fig 3. Acquired cystic kidney disease. The kidney has an end-stage appearance with cysts, atrophic tubules, and interstitial inflammation. A clear cell renal cell carcinoma arose in this kidney. (Courtesy Howard Levin, Cleveland, Ohio.)

Definition
- An acquired cystic lesion with fluid collection in the kidney, probably originating from diverticula of the distal renal tubules or collecting ducts

Clinical features
Epidemiology
- The most common cystic lesion in the kidney
- Rare before the age of 40 years
- Present in more than 20% of individuals older than 50 years
- Increased incidence in older age groups
- Multiple and large cysts in older patients

Presentation
- Usually asymptomatic
- Usually found incidentally on radiographic imaging
- Cystic renal lesions graded on radiographic imaging using the Bosniak classification system

Prognosis and treatment
- Benign lesion; no treatment required
- Occasional complications: hemorrhage or infection

Pathology
Gross pathology
- Within the kidney parenchyma or on its surface
- Can be single or multiple, usually less than 5 cm
- Usually discrete oval to round unilocular cyst with a smooth inner surface and containing clear or straw-colored fluid

Histology
- Inner surface lined with flat epithelial cells or denuded
- Cyst wall possibly calcified, mimicking malignancy on radiographic imaging

Main differential diagnosis
- Cystic clear cell renal cell carcinoma: cystic wall lined with two or more layers of clear cells, clear cells in the stroma, or clear cells with high nuclear grade (Fuhrman nuclear grade 3 or 4)
- Polycystic kidney disease: affecting children or young adults; bilateral and multifocal
- Pelvic diverticulum: cystic wall lined with urothelium

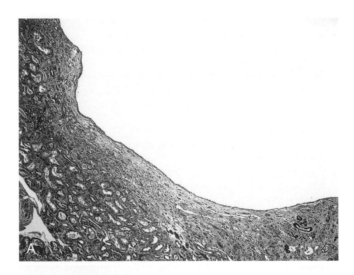

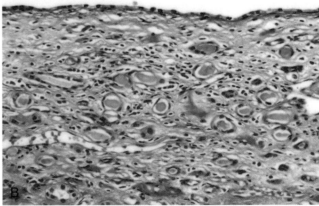

Fig 2. The inner lining of a simple renal cyst consists of a single layer of flat epithelial cells (**A**) with inconspicuous nuclei (**B**).

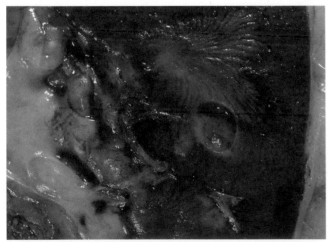

Fig 1. A unilocular simple renal cyst in the renal cortex.

Definition
- Acute suppurative inflammation of the kidney caused by bacterial infection, due most commonly to ascent from a lower urinary tract infection and less commonly to hematogenous spread in septic patients

Clinical features
Epidemiology
- Twelve to 13 cases per 10,000 population in women and 3 to 4 cases per 10,000 in men annually
- Dramatically increased incidence in women older than 19 years (28 cases per 10,000 in 18- to 49-year-old women in the United States)
- Predisposing conditions
  - Urinary obstruction, congenital or acquired
  - Instrumentation of urinary tract
  - Vesicoureteral reflux
  - Pregnancy
  - Preexisting renal lesions
  - Diabetes mellitus
  - Immunosuppression and immunodeficiency

Presentation
- Acute-onset fever, flank pain, and tenderness
- Dysuria and frequent micturition
- Peripheral blood leukocytosis
- Pyuria and leukocyte casts in urine
- Positive urine cultures, most commonly coliform bacteria
  - *Escherichia coli* is the most commonly identified organism.
  - *Streptococcus faecalis*, *Klebsiella*, *Proteus*, *Pseudomonas*, *Serratia*, and *Alcaligenes* species are rarely implicated, but are more common in repeated infections or hospital-acquired infections.
- Renal insufficiency in patients with bilateral and severe involvement with papillary necrosis

Prognosis and treatment
- Antibiotics are the treatment of choice.
- Nephrectomy is indicated if complications such as nephric and perinephric abscess or pyonephrosis develop.
- Course is benign for uncomplicated cases; symptoms disappear within several days after appropriate antibiotic therapy.
- More serious disease leads to repeated septicemic episodes in the presence of unrelieved urinary obstruction, diabetes mellitus, and immune deficiencies.
- Renal function can be compromised and progress to chronic pyelonephritis with repeated episodes.

Pathology
Gross pathology
- Abscess formation involving part of or the entire kidney
- Miliary pattern of small cortical abscesses in hematogenous acute pyelonephritis
- Perinephric abscess and pyonephrosis in severe cases

Histology
- Dense neutrophil aggregates, sometimes with bacteria, in tubular and collecting duct lumina in early phase
- Spill of suppurative inflammation into interstitium
- Acute inflammation in calyceal and pelvic urothelium with occasional mucosal ulceration
- Parenchymal destruction and abscess formations in severe disease
- Ascending acute pyelonephritis
  - More severe inflammation in renal papillae
  - Glomeruli and vessels spared initially
- Hematogenous acute pyelonephritis
  - Cortical miliary microabscesses with little involvement of papillary collecting duct
  - Abscesses more numerous in cortex than medulla
- Emphysematous pyelonephritis
  - Empty spaces lacking epithelial cell lining, distorting parenchyma
  - Vascular thrombosis, ischemic necrosis, suppurative inflammation in adjacent parenchyma
  - Widespread abscesses with papillary necrosis and cortical infarcts

Main differential diagnosis
- Acute tubulointerstitial nephritis with neutrophils: history of allergic reaction to various stimuli; neutrophils far less numerous and preferentially interstitial rather than intratubular; negative urine culture results
- Acute rejection in transplanted kidneys: history of kidney transplantation; neutrophils far less numerous and preferentially interstitial rather than intratubular; negative urine culture results

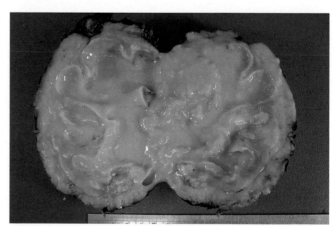

Fig 1. A case of acute pyelonephritis with hydropyonephrosis.

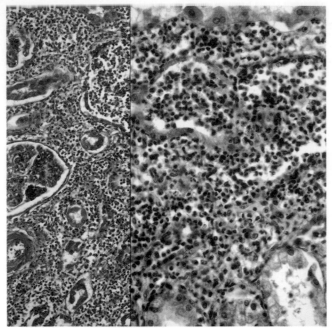

Fig 2. Acute pyelonephritis with intense neutrophilic infiltrate of interstitium and tubules.

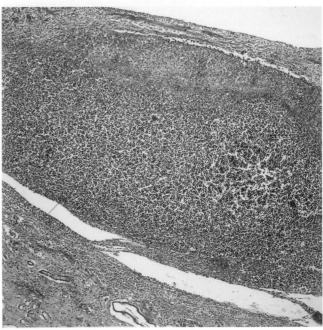

Fig 3. Abscess formation in the peripelvic tissue as a complication of acute pyelonephritis.

Definition
- Pathologic changes observed in the kidney as the result of vesicoureteral reflux (VUR), intrarenal reflux, and repeated UTIs; also termed *reflux nephropathy*

Clinical features
Epidemiology
- VUR occurs in approximately 1% of children and is found in 30% to 50% of children investigated for UTIs.
- Siblings of children affected with VUR are at higher risk.
- Of patients receiving dialysis, 11% to 20% have a diagnosis of chronic pyelonephritis not otherwise specified.

Presentation
- Clinical presentation is dependent on age and presence of prior diagnoses of UTIs and VUR.
- Patients can develop impaired renal function with or without hypertension and proteinuria.
- Radiologic findings show scars at the upper and lower poles of the kidney and dilatation of the pelvis.

Prognosis and treatment
- Progression to chronic renal insufficiency is more often seen when hypertension or significant proteinuria, or both, are present.
- Prevention of recurrent UTIs and surgical correction of severe VUR in children can decrease the incidence of renal scarring.

Pathology
Gross pathology
- Single or multiple, large, broad, U-shaped scars well demarcated from the normal parenchyma are present. Deformed calyces (flattened) and papillae are found beneath the scars.
- Calyces away from scars are normal.

Histology
- Scars consist of a demarcated zone of atrophy and loss of tubules, fibrosis of the interstitium, diffuse global glomerulosclerosis, and interstitial inflammation (mostly lymphocytes and plasma cells).
- Scars are deep and involve medullary areas (upper and lower poles).
- Thyroidization of the renal tubules is characteristic but not pathognomonic.
- Inflammation with lymphoid follicles beneath the urothelial lining of the pelvis suggests chronic infection.
- Arteriosclerosis and hyaline arteriolosclerosis are frequent when hypertension is present.
- Secondary focal segmental glomerulosclerosis and segmental renal dysplasia can be seen.

Immunopathology and electron microscopy
- Findings are nonspecific with no significant deposits of immunoglobulin or complement.
- Special stains or immunohistochemistry can help to exclude a specific infectious agent.

Main differential diagnosis
- Chronic interstitial nephritis can mimic chronic nonobstructive pyelonephritis. However, upper or lower pole scars with deformed calyces and a clinical history of VUR favor a diagnosis of chronic nonobstructive pyelonephritis.
- Hypertension and vascular diseases can cause scars, tubular atrophy, chronic inflammation, and interstitial fibrosis. In contrast to chronic nonobstructive pyelonephritis, medullary regions are less involved and deformations of the calyces are not seen (V-shaped scars in ischemia).
- Chronic primary glomerulonephritis has tubular and interstitial damages that can mimic chronic pyelonephritis; however, glomeruli will show, at least focally, changes that are suggestive of glomerular disease. Immunofluorescence highlights residual immune complex deposits.
- Infectious interstitial nephritis can also mimic chronic nonobstructive pyelonephritis. Radiologic findings, clinical history, and special stains can help to establish the correct diagnosis. Necrosis and granulomatous inflammation are not seen in chronic nonobstructive pyelonephritis.

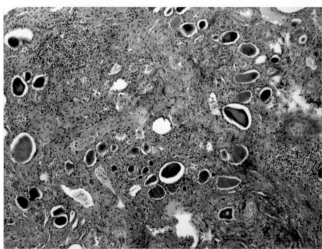

Fig 1. Chronic nonobstructive pyelonephritis (reflux nephropathy) with fibrosis, tubular atrophy, and chronic inflammation (hematoxylin-phloxine-saffron [HPS] stain).

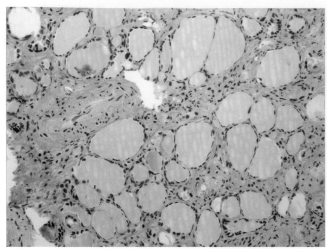

Fig 2. Renal parenchyma with severe tubular atrophy (thyroidization of the renal tubules, one of the three forms of tubular atrophy with classic and pseudo-endocrine forms; HPS stain).

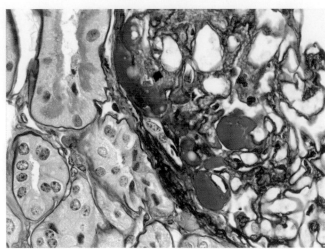

Fig 4. Focal segmental glomerulosclerosis lesion with subendothelial deposition of hyaline material and flocculocapsular synechia (periodic acid–Schiff stain).

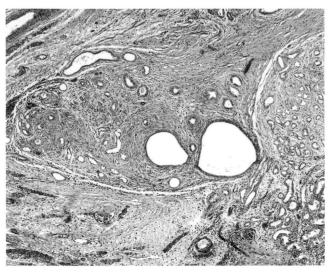

Fig 3. Renal dysplasia in reflux nephropathy.

Definition
- Pathologic changes secondary to chronic obstruction of the urinary outflow

Clinical features
Epidemiology
- Obstruction is more common in males during childhood (ureteropelvic obstruction, posterior urethral valves, and other congenital anomalies), in females during adulthood (gynecologic diseases), and in males at an older age (prostatic diseases).
- Increased pressure, reflux of urine with leakage into the interstitium, and ischemia of the inner medulla are key factors promoting atrophy and fibrosis of the renal parenchyma.

Etiology
- Nephrolithiasis
- Ureteropelvic junction obstruction
- Fibroepithelial polyps
- Ureteral valves
- Posterior urethral valves
- Acquired ureteral strictures (instrumentation, radiation, inflammation)
- Acquired urethral strictures (instrumentation, radiation, inflammation)
- Urinary tract tumors
- Benign prostatic hyperplasia
- Prostatic tumors
- Retroperitoneal fibrosis
- Extrinsic masses

Presentation
- Clinical presentation is highly variable and depends on the cause of the obstruction.
- Imaging findings demonstrate generalized atrophy of the kidney and dilatation of all portions of the pelvis.

Prognosis and treatment
- Treatment and prognosis depend on the cause, degree, and chronicity of the obstruction.

Pathology
Gross pathology
- Diffuse dilatation of the collecting system with occasional stones in the pelvis and calices
- Coarse scars on the cortical surface, severe parenchymal thinning, and deformed calices

Histology
- Diffuse atrophy of the parenchyma with scars; global glomerulosclerosis, atrophy, and loss of tubules, fibrosis and interstitial inflammation (with a richer neutrophilic inflammation, more severe than reflux nephropathy)
- Thyroidization less well developed compared with reflux nephropathy
- Inflammation with lymphoid follicles and neutrophils beneath the pelvic urothelial lining

- Renal dysplasia not found in obstruction that has developed in adulthood
- Arteriosclerosis and hyaline arteriolosclerosis frequently found when hypertension is present
- Secondary focal segmental glomerulosclerosis sometimes observed

Immunopathology and electron microscopy
- Findings are nonspecific with no significant deposits of immunoglobulin or complement.
- Special stains or immunohistochemistry can help to exclude a specific infectious etiology.

Main differential diagnosis
- Chronic interstitial nephritis can histologically mimic chronic obstructive pyelonephritis; however, diffuse dilatations of the pelvis and calyces and a clinical history of urinary obstruction favor a diagnosis of chronic obstructive pyelonephritis.
- Hypertension and vascular diseases can cause scars, tubular atrophy, chronic inflammation, and interstitial fibrosis. In contrast to chronic obstructive pyelonephritis, medullary regions are less involved, and diffuse dilatations of the calyces and pelvis are not seen (V-shaped scars in ischemia).
- Chronic primary glomerulonephritis has tubular and interstitial damages that can mimic chronic pyelonephritis; however, glomeruli will show, at least focally, changes that are suggestive of glomerular disease. Immunofluorescence can highlight residual immune complex deposits.

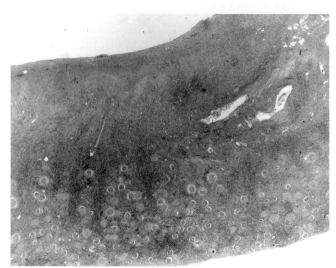

Fig 1. Low-power view of severe atrophy of the renal parenchyma, inflammation, and dilatation of the pyelocaliceal cavities (HPS stain).

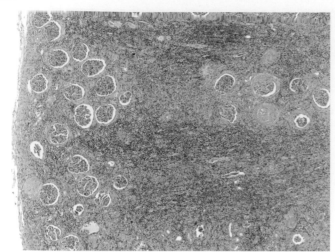

Fig 2. Clustering of glomeruli and interstitial inflammation. Glomeruli are close to each other because of the loss of intervening renal parenchyma (HPS stain).

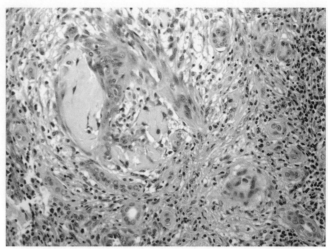

Fig 4. A ruptured tubule with accumulation of Tamm-Horsfall protein (HPS stain).

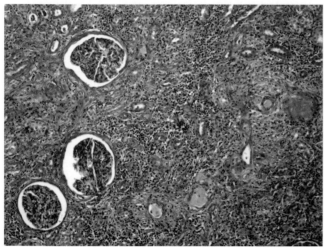

Fig 3. Marked chronic inflammation in the renal parenchyma and chronic tubulointerstitial damages (HPS stain).

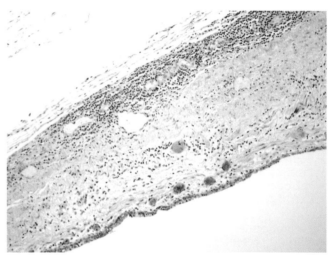

Fig 5. Chronic inflammation beneath the pelvic lining suggestive of chronic infection (HPS stain).

Definition
- A destructive granulomatous inflammatory process of renal parenchyma as the result of long-term urinary tract obstruction and infection

Clinical features
Epidemiology
- Seventy percent of patients are female.
- Ages ranges widely, from newborn to elderly.
- Urine cultures most frequently show *Escherichia coli* and *Proteus mirabilis*.

Presentation
- Flank or abdominal pain and mass
- Lower urinary tract symptoms with gross hematuria and pyuria

Prognosis and treatment
- Nephrectomy is curative for diffuse or advanced-stage disease.

Pathology
Gross pathology
- The kidney is typically enlarged with hydronephrosis, renal pelvic calculi with characteristic "staghorn" appearance, or some other evidence of obstruction.
- Single or multiple yellow to orange nodules may mimic tumor nodules.

Histology
- Xanthogranulomatous inflammation includes mixed histiocytes with foamy cytoplasm, neutrophils, lymphocytes, plasma cells, and multinucleated giant cells.
- Xanthogranulomatous nodules can have a zonal pattern with a central zone of neutrophils and necrosis rimmed by foamy macrophages and fibroblastic response at the periphery.
- The changes include variable degree of renal tubular atrophy, tubular dilatation, squamous metaplasia of the urothelium, microabscesses, and lymphoid follicle formation.

Immunohistochemistry and special studies
- The xanthomatous cells show positive cytoplasmic staining for α1-antitrypsin and lysozyme and positive for CD68.
- Epithelial markers may be used if renal cell carcinoma is included in the differential diagnosis.

Main differential diagnosis
- Clear cell renal cell carcinoma can be mistaken for lipid-laden xanthomatous cells, but has "water-clear" cytoplasm, and is positive for cytokeratin and negative for CD68.
- Sarcomatoid renal cell carcinoma can be mistaken for xanthogranulomatous pyelonephritis with prominent spindle cell proliferation or significant cytologic atypia in spindle cells; other epithelial component may be present.
- Sheets of eosinophilic histiocytes with Michaelis-Gutmann bodies might be suggestive of malakoplakia.

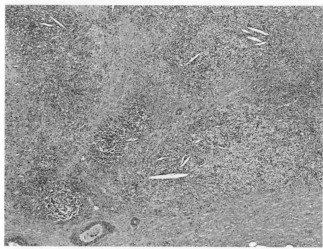

Fig 1. Xanthogranulomatous pyelonephritis is characterized by mixed inflammatory infiltrates with fibrosis and cholesterol clefts in the background.

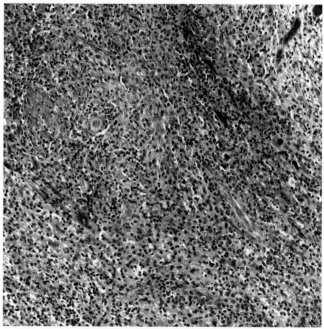

Fig 2. A xanthogranulomatous nodule with a zonal pattern consisting of central areas of neutrophils and peripheral diffuse sheets of foamy macrophages. Note the hemosiderin-laden macrophages.

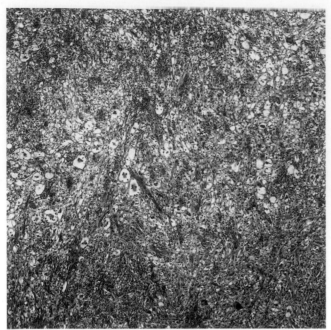

Fig 3. The mixed inflammatory infiltrate composed of a variable number of xanthomatous histiocytes with foamy cytoplasm, neutrophils, lymphocytes, plasma cells, and occasionally multi-nucleated giant cells.

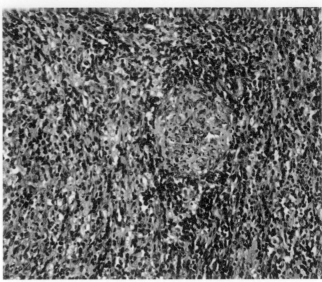

Fig 4. A central area of necrosis and neutrophils is surrounded by foamy macrophages. The most peripheral region has a florid fibroblastic response with more spindle-shaped fibroblastic cells.

Definition
- Coagulative necrosis involving papillae of renal medulla, classically associated with a number of underlying conditions, all of which predispose the patient to renal medullary ischemia

Clinical features
Epidemiology
- Most cases have one or more underlying predisposition: chronic analgesic ingestion (acetaminophen, phenacetin, COX2 inhibitors), diabetes, sickle cell disease, obstruction/infection, vasculitis, tuberculosis, renal allograft, and liver failure.
- Epidemiology varies by underlying cause: female predominance in cases caused by analgesic ingestion and diabetes, male predominance in cases caused by obstruction.
- Ninety percent of patients are older than 40 years.

Presentation
- Polyuria owing to an inability to concentrate urine
- Renal failure in extreme cases
- Hematuria, renal colic, and obstruction resulting from renal papillae sloughing
- Urinary tract infection

Prognosis and treatment
- Clinical course varies depending on underlying condition and number of affected papillae.
- Recovery can be complete with early management of focal lesions.

Pathology
Gross pathology
- Visibly necrotic medullary pyramids
- Features of obstruction possible present
- Fragments of sloughed papillae possibly visible in calyces

Histology
- Papillae showing geographic necrosis with ghosts of tubules visible
- Overlying cortical atrophy, interstitial fibrosis, and chronic inflammation
- Focality and chronicity of lesions varies by underlying cause:
  - In analgesic abuse, variably sized foci of geographic necrosis in various stages of chronicity (dystrophic calcification, sloughing) are present.
  - In cases with underlying *diabetes*, all papillae are at the same stage of acute necrosis and calcification is rare.
  - In sickle cell disease (or trait), only a few papillae may be focally affected and calcification is rare.
  - In cases of infection or obstruction, acute inflammation may indicate an underlying infection.

Main differential diagnosis
- Renal infarction: renal infarcts are wedge shaped and involve cortex and medulla, whereas papillary necrosis is limited to the medulla.

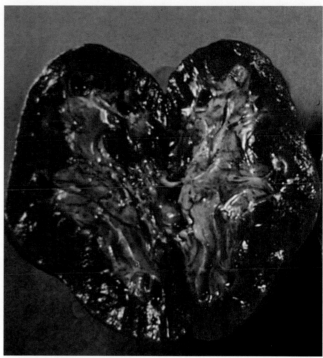

Fig 1. A bivalved kidney shows necrotic and cavitary changes involving the tips of renal papillae. (Courtesy Howard Levin, Cleveland, Ohio.)

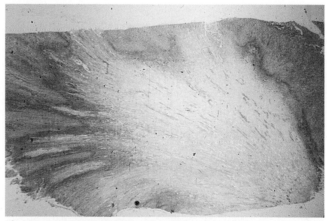

Fig 2. A necrotic papillae showing geographic necrosis with ghosts of tubules. (Courtesy Howard Levin, Cleveland, Ohio.)

Definition
- Pathologic changes in the kidney secondary to chronic mild to moderate hypertension

Clinical features
Epidemiology
- Hypertension affects 20% to 40% of the population in Western society.
- Vascular diseases of the kidneys can be both a cause and a consequence of hypertension.
- Hypertensive nephrosclerosis is fourfold more common in blacks than in whites.

Presentation
- Benign hypertension is usually asymptomatic until complications of the kidney and other organs occur.

Prognosis and treatment
- End-stage renal disease occurs in 25% to 30% of patients with chronic hypertension.
- Normalization of the blood pressure is the only way to slow the progression of benign nephrosclerosis.

Pathology
Gross pathology
- The kidneys may be reduced in size and weight.
- The capsular surface is usually granular with some deep triangular scars.
- The cortex is thinned and simple cysts may also be present.

Histology
- Focal global glomerulosclerosis, tubular atrophy, and interstitial fibrosis are invariably observed with some degree of chronic inflammation in the sclerotic areas.
- Arteries show intimal fibrosis, smooth muscle hyperplasia, and reduction of lumen size (arteriosclerosis). The internal elastic lamina becomes multilayered on elastic stains.
- Afferent arterioles and small arteries show subendothelial deposition of homogenous eosinophilic material (hyaline arteriolosclerosis).

Immunopathology and electron microscopy
- Immunoglobulin (Ig) M and C3 is frequently present within the hyaline layers of arterioles.
- Immunofluorescence staining is otherwise negative or minimal.
- Electron microscopy may show thickening or wrinkling of the glomerular capillary basement membranes.

Main differential diagnosis
- Chronic pyelonephritis can cause scars, tubular atrophy, and interstitial fibrosis similar to vascular diseases. Arteriosclerosis and hyaline arteriolosclerosis can be seen in this context. However, in contrast to chronic pyelonephritis, medullary regions are less involved, and deformations or dilatations of the calyces are not seen in benign nephrosclerosis.
- Chronic primary glomerular disease also shows tubular and interstitial damages and arteriosclerosis; however, glomeruli will show, at least in a focal distribution, some changes suggestive of a glomerular disease.

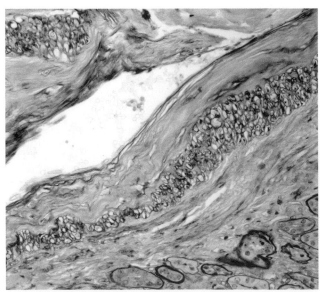

Fig 2. In benign nephrosclerosis, the surface of the kidney is finely granular because of depressions (scars).

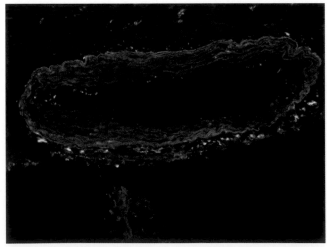

Fig 1. Benign nephrosclerosis. A characteristic feature of hypertensive arteriosclerosis is the reduplication or multiplication of the internal elastic lamina, which can be observed with elastic stains or at the time of the immunofluorescence studies.

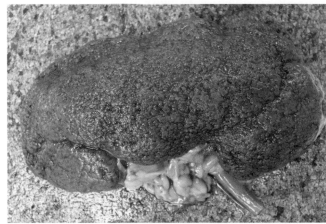

Fig 3. Benign nephrosclerosis. Periodic acid–Schiff stain showing arterial intimal thickening and atrophy of the media in a larger artery, another characteristic change in benign nephrosclerosis.

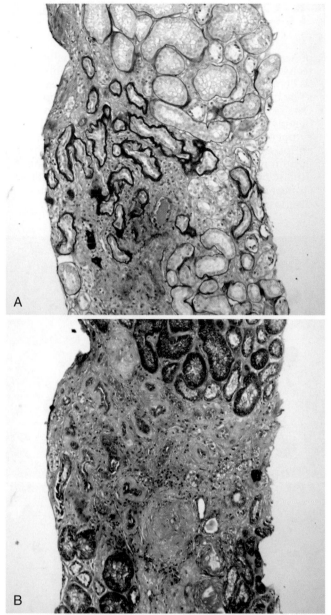

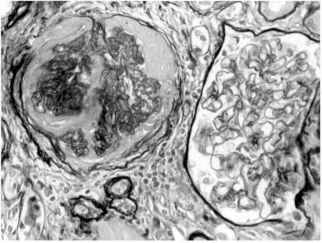

Fig 5. Benign nephrosclerosis. Periodic acid–Schiff stain showing the typical appearance of global glomerulosclerosis induced by chronic hypertension. The glomerular tuft is still visible.

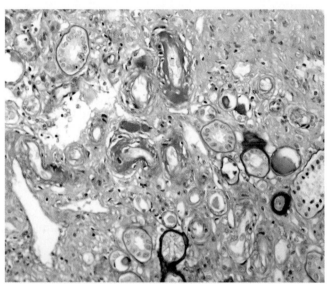

Fig 6. Benign nephrosclerosis. The characteristic change in benign nephrosclerosis is hyaline arteriolosclerosis. The eosinophilic deposits within the arteriolar wall represent insudation of plasma proteins in small vessels.

Fig 4. Benign nephrosclerosis. **A,** Periodic acid–Schiff stain shows an area of tubular atrophy with thickening of the tubular basement membrane. **B,** Trichrome stain shows an area with severe interstitial fibrosis and two globally sclerotic glomeruli.

Definition
- A form of thrombotic microangiopathy secondary to malignant hypertension (systolic pressure greater than 220 mm Hg or diastolic pressure greater than 120 mm Hg)

Clinical features
Epidemiology
- The average age at diagnosis is 40 years, and men are affected more often than women.
- Cigarette smokers, blacks, and patients with underlying chronic renal disease are at higher risk.
- Fifty percent have a history of benign nephrosclerosis.

Presentation
- Malignant hypertension is characterized by severe headache, blurred vision, neurologic symptoms, papilledema, congestive heart failure, and acute renal failure.
- Microangiopathic hemolytic anemia and thrombocytopenia can occur.

Prognosis and treatment
- The 5-year survival rate with appropriate treatment is close to 80%.
- The therapeutic goal is a gradual reduction of mean arterial pressure with intravenous vasodilators.

Pathology
Gross pathology
- Kidneys may show signs of benign nephrosclerosis.
- Petechial hemorrhages may be present.

Histology
- Interlobular arteries have intimal edematous (mucoid) thickening with occasional erythrocytes or erythrocytes fragments in the intima. The lumen is greatly reduced and may be occluded by fibrin thrombi.
- The wall of the arterioles is replaced by intensely eosinophilic material (fibrinoid necrosis).
- Glomeruli may have fibrinoid necrosis, segmental or global consolidation, and in the late phase, thickening and replication of the basement membrane.
- Focal acute tubular necrosis and small cortical infarcts may be present.

Immunopathology and electron microscopy
- Staining for fibrinogen, IgM, and C3 may be found in arterioles, small arteries, and glomerular capillaries.
- Electron microscopy shows thickening and wrinkling of the glomerular capillary basement membranes. Endothelial cells are swollen and the subendothelial space is widened by electron-lucent fluffy material. Platelet and fibrin thrombi may be present.

Main differential diagnosis
- Acute tubular necrosis (ATN) and cortical necrosis can be observed in malignant nephrosclerosis; however, the specific vascular changes of the latter are not seen in ischemic or toxic ATN.
- Primary glomerulonephritis can sometimes show vascular damages similar to malignant nephrosclerosis. The presence of glomerular hypercellularity is usually not seen in the latter. Glomeruli in malignant nephrosclerosis do not show any significant immune complex deposits by immunofluorescence or electron microscopy.
- Other causes of thrombotic microangiopathy include hemolytic uremic syndrome, thrombotic thrombocytopenic purpura, systemic sclerosis renal crisis, antiphospholipid antibody syndrome, and acute postpartum renal failure. Because histologic evaluation is usually not sufficient to differentiate the possibilities, clinical information is essential to make the correct diagnosis.

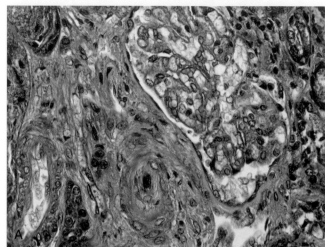
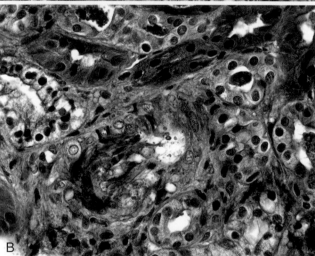

Fig 1. Malignant nephrosclerosis. The most characteristic lesion in malignant nephrosclerosis, which is also the prototypic histologic feature of all other thrombotic microangiopathies: intimal mucoid thickening with central fibrin occluding the lumen (**A,** Trichrome stain). Reactive endothelial cells, intimal mucoid thickening, and fragmented red blood cells in the intima are seen (**B,** Trichrome stain).

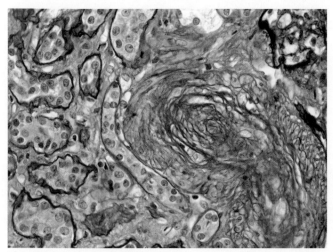

Fig 2. Malignant nephrosclerosis. An artery with occluded lumen by markedly thickened intima with concentric, ringlike layers (onion skin lesion; periodic acid–Schiff stain).

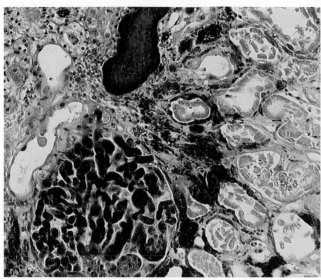

Fig 4. Malignant nephrosclerosis. In severe cases, infarcted cortical areas can be seen (periodic acid–Schiff stain).

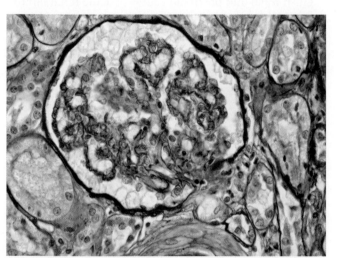

Fig 3. Malignant nephrosclerosis. Periodic acid–Schiff stain showing conspicuous thickening and wrinkling of the glomerular capillary walls (ischemic changes).

Definition
- A clinicopathologic entity with pathologic changes in the renal tubules when ischemic or toxic injuries affect the kidney

Clinical features
Epidemiology
- Acute tubular necrosis (ATN) is the most common cause of acute renal failure.
- Precipitating events include ischemic episodes and endogenous or exogenous nephrotoxins.
- Ischemia-induced ATN represents approximately 60% of the cases.

Presentation
- Rapid deterioration of the renal function with elevated blood urea nitrogen and serum creatinine
- Oliguria (urine output less than 400 mL/day) is present in 50% of patients.
- Urinalysis shows hyaline, granular, or pigmented casts.
- Complications include water and salt overload and metabolic acidosis.

Prognosis and treatment
- The morbidity and mortality rates depend on the clinical settings.
- Treatment is usually supportive.
- Recovery usually occurs during the first month after onset, but can be seen even after 1 year.

Pathology
Gross pathology
- Kidneys are usually enlarged with a pale cortex.
- The corticomedullary junction may be accentuated with deep red medullary regions.

Histology
- There is a spectrum of morphologic changes in the renal tubules:
  - Necrosis or severe vacuolation of tubular cells
  - Blebs formation or loss of the periodic acid–Schiff (PAS)-brush border of proximal tubular cells
  - Thinning of tubular epithelium with enlargement of the tubular lumens
  - Detachment of tubular cells to form tubular casts
  - Interstitial edema with scant peritubular inflammation
- Changes in ischemic cases are usually milder and more focal than toxic ATN.
- Nuclear atypia, mitotic figures, and basophilic cytoplasm are observed later in the regenerative stage.
- Pigmented casts often represent hemoglobin or myoglobin.

Immunopathology and electron microscopy
- Findings are nonspecific with no significant deposits of immunoglobulin or complement.
- Electron microscopic findings include simplification of tubular epithelium, various cytoplasmic vacuolization, loss or blunting of the brush border, and small gaps in the lining of the tubular epithelium.

Main differential diagnosis
- Acute interstitial nephritis and acute pyelonephritis will show tubular damages similar to ATN, but significant interstitial inflammation or leucocyte casts do not occur in ATN.
- Severe and acute primary glomerulonephritis is frequently associated with acute tubular damages, but glomeruli are abnormal. For example, glomeruli will show crescents, fibrinoid necrosis, and diffuse endocapillary proliferation. The interstitium will show significant inflammation.
- Thrombotic microangiopathy can show acute tubular damages similar to ATN, but intimal mucoid thickening in small arteries and glomerular thrombi are not seen in ATN.
- Bilateral urinary tract obstruction can cause tubular damages including dilatation and ruptured tubules. Clinical history and radiologic studies help to distinguish renal and postrenal causes of acute renal failure.
- Bilateral renal cortical necrosis will show fresh, infarcted parenchyma including tubules, glomeruli, and vessels.

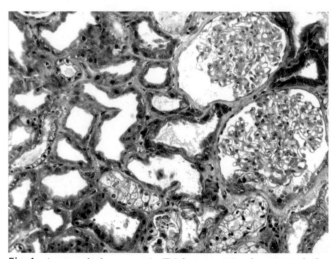

Fig 1. Acute tubular necrosis. Trichrome stain showing tubular dilatation and thinning of the tubular epithelium. Some tubules are also markedly vacuolated.

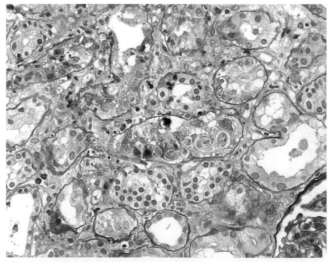

Fig 2. Acute tubular necrosis. Periodic acid–Schiff stain showing marked regenerative atypia in some tubules.

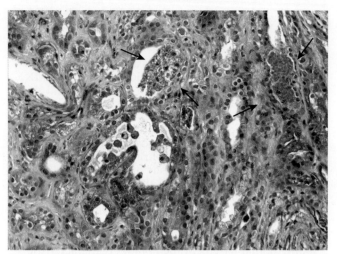

Fig 3. Acute tubular necrosis. Trichrome stain showing a dilated tubule with blebs formation and sloughing of tubular cells. Intratubular casts are seen *(arrows)*.

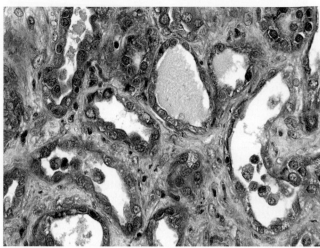

Fig 4. Acute tubular necrosis. Several tubules have thin epithelium with sloughing. Rare peritubular inflammatory cells are seen (trichrome stain).

Definition
- A clinicopathologic entity characterized by inflammation in the renal interstitium with various etiologies, often secondary to an allergic reaction to a drug

Clinical features
Epidemiology
- Acute interstitial nephritis (AIN) is the most common type of drug-induced renal injury.
- A large variety of drugs are implicated (e.g., nonsteroidal antiinflammatory drugs, antibiotics).
- It is most likely secondary to immune mechanisms (hypersensitivity reaction), with the drug acting as a hapten.

Presentation
- Classic triad includes fever, rash, and eosinophilia with acute renal failure approximately 2 weeks following exposure to the drug.
- Hematuria, mild proteinuria, and sterile leukocyturia are usually present.

Prognosis and treatment
- Cessation of the offending drug is usually followed by recovery with an excellent prognosis. Steroid therapy can hasten recovery.
- Irreversible progressive damage may occur (chronic interstitial nephritis).

Pathology
Histology
- The interstitium shows edema with various inflammatory cells, including lymphocytes, plasma cells, macrophages, eosinophils, and neutrophils.
- Eosinophils are frequently found in drug-induced allergic AIN, but represent a minor component of the inflammatory infiltrate.
- Tubulitis is common during the active phase.
- Some degree of tubular injury (tubular necrosis) can be found.
- Granulomatous inflammation is sometimes predominant.

Immunopathology and electron microscopy
- Immunofluorescence is generally negative or nonspecific.
- Rarely, intense linear staining for IgG along tubular basement membranes has been reported (in methicillin-induced AIN).
- Discrete granular staining for IgG along tubular basement membranes can be seen.
- Discrete electron-dense immune-type deposits can be found along the tubular basement membranes.

Main differential diagnosis
- ATN with secondary interstitial inflammation has been described; however, inflammation is sparse in ATN. Some drugs may induce both ATN and AIN for which the term *acute tubulointerstitial nephritis* can be used.
- Acute and severe primary glomerulonephritis is frequently associated with acute interstitial nephritis, but glomeruli are abnormal and may show crescents, fibrinoid necrosis, or diffuse endocapillary proliferation.

- Infectious interstitial nephritis and chronic pyelonephritis may show some histologic features of AIN. However, gross abnormalities of the calyces and the pelvis, scar, abscesses, and large necrotic areas are not observed in AIN. A clinical history suggestive of a drug-related disease and the absence of a specific infectious agent favor a diagnosis of AIN.
- Lupus-related interstitial nephritis and antitubular basement membrane antibody disease are specific types of interstitial nephritis that have to be distinguished from usual AIN. Strong granular deposits along tubular basement membranes and glomerular deposits with IgG, IgA, IgM, C3, and C1q are highly suggestive of lupus nephritis. Intense linear staining for IgG along tubular basement membranes is characteristic of antitubular basement membrane antibody disease. Serologic tests can help the differential diagnosis.
- Autoimmune diseases (e.g., sarcoidosis, Sjögren syndrome, Kawasaki disease) can cause AIN. Clinical history is essential to make the correct diagnosis.

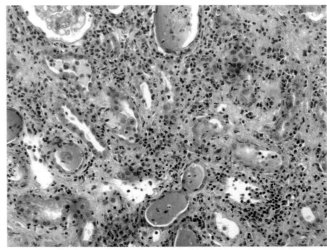

Fig 1. Acute interstitial nephritis. Marked interstitial inflammation with lymphocytes and plasma cells. Tubules show acute damages.

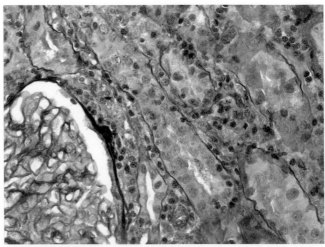

Fig 2. Tubulitis with intraepithelial lymphocytes found in the renal tubules (periodic acid–Schiff stain).

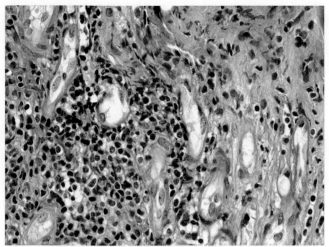

Fig 3. Acute interstitial nephritis. Many eosinophils were found in this case related to the use of nonsteroidal antiinflammatory drugs.

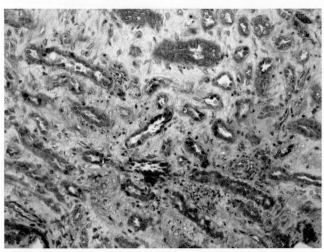

Fig 4. Acute interstitial nephritis. On Trichrome stain, interstitial edema appears pale blue. Edema is an important diagnostic criterion in acute interstitial nephritis. In more subtle cases, inflammation may only be present at the corticomedullary junction.

Definition
- Chronic infection of the renal parenchyma by a specific infectious agent

Clinical features

Epidemiology
- Uncommon, but more frequent in immunocompromised patients and transplant recipients
- Common bacteria and fungi are the most frequent causative agents during the early posttransplantation period. Viruses and tuberculosis are more common in the late period.
- Up to 20% of extrapulmonary tuberculosis cases involve the genitourinary system.

Presentation
- Decreased renal function, fever, flank pain, hematuria, tenderness at the costovertebral angle, and radiologic abnormalities
- Systemic (miliary tuberculosis, systemic fungemia, cytomegalovirus infection) or localized (cavitary tuberculosis of the kidney, BK viral nephropathy) infections

Prognosis and treatment
- Prognosis depends on many factors, including the nature of the infectious agent, the degree of immunosuppression, and the severity and chronicity of the renal lesions.
- Infections are usually treated medically.

Gross pathology
- Necrotic abscesses, hemorrhages, and destructive lesions (including papillary necrosis) are frequently observed.

Histology
- Tuberculous lesions are characterized by a granulomatous reaction surrounding caseous material. Fibrosis and interstitial inflammation with lymphocytes and plasma cells are also observed around foci of caseation necrosis.
- Aspergillosis and other fungal infections are usually characterized by interstitial inflammation with mononuclear cells and neutrophils, abscesses, and infarcts containing the fungus.
- BK virus nephropathy is characterized by nuclear inclusions in tubular epithelial cells, tubular necrosis, and interstitial inflammation composed of a heterogeneous mixture of lymphocytes, macrophages, plasma cells, and neutrophils. Tubulitis is usually inconspicuous but can be seen.
- Cytomegalovirus nephritis is characterized by the classic nuclear inclusions with a surrounding halo and the smaller cytoplasmic inclusions in endothelial cells as well as tubular epithelial cells.

Immunopathology
- Special stains or immunohistochemical studies are helpful to identify a specific infectious agent (PAS, Grocott methenamine silver stain, Ziehl-Nielsen, antibodies against common viruses).
- Microbial cultures and serum molecular analysis are also helpful.

Main differential diagnosis
- AIN can mimic infectious interstitial nephritis; however, abscesses and large necrotic areas are not observed in AIN. A clinical history suggestive of a drug-related disease and the absence of a specific infectious agent favor a diagnosis of AIN.
- Acute cellular rejection in a kidney allograft shows many histologic similarities with infectious nephritis (mostly virus-related infections). Severe tubulitis, mononuclear inflammation, and endarteritis favor rejection. The use of special stains and antibodies against viruses are essential.
- Chronic pyelonephritis, including obstructive or nonobstructive, can mimic infectious interstitial nephritis. However, a specific or causative infectious agent is usually not identified in chronic pyelonephritis.

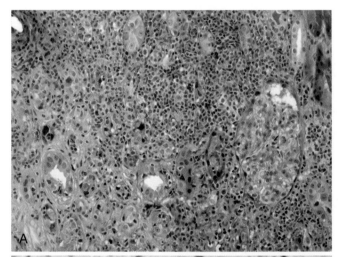

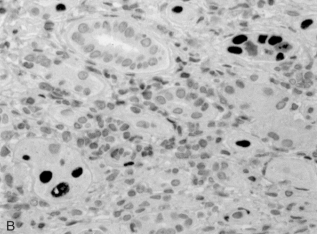

Fig 1. BK virus nephropathy. **A,** Nuclear viral inclusions are seen with interstitial inflammation. **B,** Immunostain for SV40 antigen confirms the diagnosis.

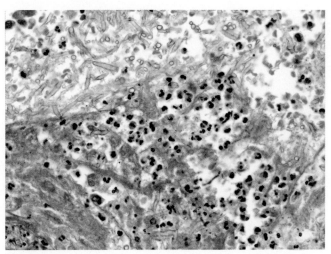

Fig 2. Renal aspergillosis with necrotic debris and branching septate hyphae (hematoxylin-phloxine-saffron [HPS] stain).

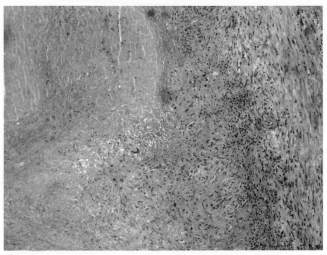

Fig 3. Renal tuberculosis. Caseating granulomas with epithelioid histiocytes and multinucleated giant cells are seen in the renal pelvis (HPS stain).

NEOPLASTIC DISEASE OF THE KIDNEY

Definition
- Epithelial tumor with tubulopapillary architecture, low nuclear grade, and a diameter of 5 mm or less

Clinical features
Epidemiology
- Increased incidence with age
- No gender predilection

Presentation
- Most are asymptomatic, detected in nephrectomy specimen or at autopsy

Prognosis and treatment
- Benign
- No therapy needed

Pathology
Gross pathology
- Well-circumscribed cortical nodules, 5 mm or less
- Yellow-tan to white-tan cut surface

Histology
- Tubulopapillary architecture
- Cells with scant amphophilic to basophilic cytoplasm
- Round to oval, small, uniform nuclei without prominent nucleoli
- Histiocytes and psammomatous calcification frequently present

Immunopathology (including immunohistochemistry)
- Positive for AE1/AE3, p504S/α-methylacyl-CoA racemase (AMACR), EMA, CK7, high-molecular-weight cytokeratin

Molecular diagnostics
- Gain of chromosome 7 and 17, and loss of Y chromosome in men

Main differential diagnosis
- Papillary renal cell carcinoma (RCC): larger than 5 mm, or has higher nuclear grade (≥3 Fuhrman grade 3)

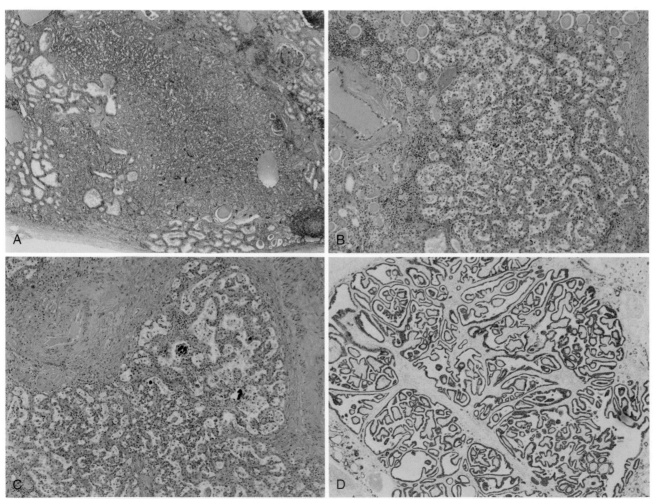

Fig 1. A 4-mm papillary adenoma **(A)** showing tubulopapillary architecture and low-grade nuclei **(B)**. Psammomatous calcifications are frequently seen **(C)**. Cytokeratin 7 is diffusely positive in papillary adenoma **(D)**.

Definition
- Benign renal epithelial neoplasm composed of round-to-polygonal cells with abundant mitochondria-rich eosinophilic cytoplasm, thought to arise from the intercalated cells in the kidney

Clinical features
Epidemiology
- Four percent to 8% of adult renal epithelial neoplasms in surgical cohorts
- Wide range of age distribution, with a peak incidence in the seventh decade of life
- Male-to-female ratio, 2:1
- Rare cases associated with Birt-Hogg-Dube syndrome

Presentation
- Asymptomatic presentation and incidental findings on imaging studies in most patients
- Classical triad associated with renal cancer (hematuria, flank pain, flank mass) seen in a small percentage of patients
- Appears as a solid homogenous mass in renal parenchyma on imaging studies and a central irregular area (scar), although not specific and not always present; suggestive of oncocytoma

Prognosis and treatment
- Benign with an excellent prognosis
- Often treated with partial or radical nephrectomy, the treatment option for any solid renal masses
- Active surveillance also considered for biopsy-proven cases
- Rare cases of "renal oncocytoma with metastasis" usually RCC mimicking oncocytoma

Pathology
Gross pathology
- A well-circumscribed but nonencapsulated solid mass is present.
- Color is dark brown or mahogany.
- A central stellate scar may be present in one third of cases.
- Hemorrhage and cystic changes are not common; necrosis is rare.
- Multiple oncocytomas in a kidney can be seen occasionally (oncocytosis).

Histology
- Tumor cells may form solid nests, acini, tubules or microcysts.
- Areas of edematous hypocellular stroma, particularly in the central scar, are frequently seen.
- Large, round-to-polygonal cells with abundant eosinophilic cytoplasm owing to cytoplasmic mitochondria are present and can be confirmed with electron microscopy.
- Uniformly round nuclei with inconspicuous nucleoli are present; scattered but not diffuse degenerative nuclear atypia can be seen.

- Oncoblasts are small tumor cells with minimal cytoplasm and dense hyperchromatic nuclei and are seen frequently.
- Although small papillae may be seen occasionally, the presence of extensive papillary architecture is not typical of oncocytoma and should raise the suggestion of an oncocytic papillary RCC.
- Extension to perinephric fat without stromal response can occur (20%).
- Extension into renal veins is reported in up to 5% of cases. Renal cell carcinoma should always be ruled out first.
- *Oncocytosis* refers to numerous oncocytic lesions involving the kidney.

Immunohistochemistry and special studies
- CD117 (C-Kit) diffusely positive
- CK7 negative or positive in single cells or small clusters of cells, which represent entrapped distal convoluted tubules.
- Vimentin negative in a majority of tumor cells, although focal positivity can be seen in tumor cells within septa
- Hale's colloidal iron showing luminal staining

Molecular diagnostics
- Unique molecular signature defined by gene expression microarrays and microRNA studies
- Minimal chromosomal alterations on cytogenetic studies, in contrast to multiple chromosomal losses seen in chromophobe RCC

Main differential diagnosis
- Renal cell carcinoma with oncocytic cytoplasm: the presence of the following features should raise the suggestion of an RCC:
  - Necrosis (more than focal)
  - Papillary architecture (more than focal)
  - Frequent mitosis (more than 1 per 20× field) or atypical mitosis
  - Clear cell or spindle cells
  - Presence of membrane-bound microvesicles on electron microscopy
  - Diffusely positive CK7, AMACR, or vimentin
- Chromophobe RCC: more prominent cell membranes and raisinlike or koilocytic nuclei, diffuse positive CK7, and Hale colloidal iron stain
- Clear cell RCC with eosinophilic cytoplasm: bright or golden yellow rather than dark brown in color on gross examination; distinctive "chicken wire" vascular pattern; generally has higher Fuhrman grade (grade 3 or 4)
- Oncocytic papillary RCC: more apparent papillary architecture
- Oncocytic tumor, not otherwise specified (or hybrid oncocytic tumor): cases with histologic and immunohistochemical features overlap between oncocytoma and chromophobe RCC. These cases can not be readily categorized into either diagnosis; however, this term should be reserved for the most difficult cases showing features of both tumors, because this term may cause confusion for clinical management.

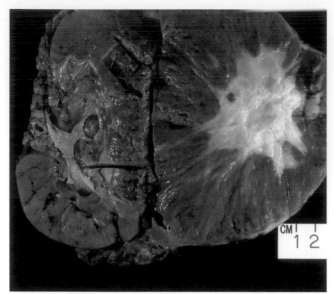

Fig 1. Grossly, oncocytoma forms a large, well-circumscribed renal mass with a distinct mahogany color and a central scar.

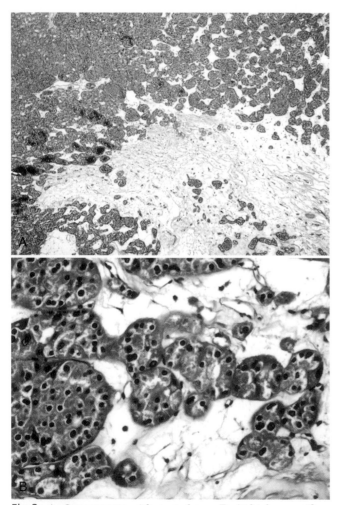

Fig 2. **A,** Oncocytoma with central scar. **B,** At high magnification, clusters of uniform oncocytic tumor cells are embedded in edematous stroma.

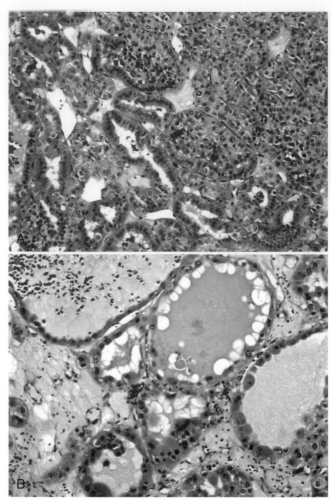

Fig 3. Oncocytoma with solid and tubular **(A)** and microcystic patterns **(B).**

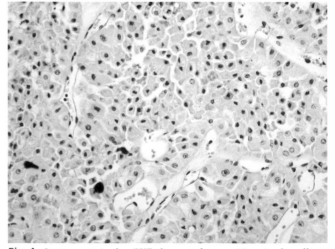

Fig 4. Immunostain for CK7 shows a few positive single cells or small clusters of cells that may represent entrapped tubular cells.

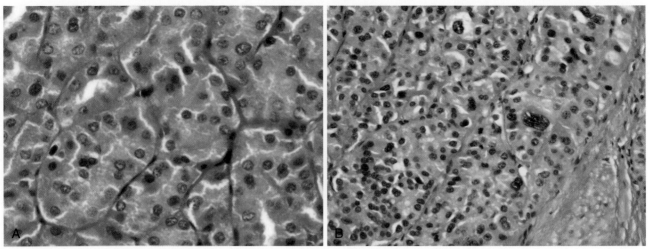

Fig 5. Oncocytoma with typical eosinophilic granular cytoplasm **(A)** and, infrequently, tumor cells may show focal nuclear atypia **(B).**

CLEAR CELL RENAL CELL CARCINOMA

Definition
- The most common histologic subtype of renal cell carcinoma (RCC), composed of cells with clear or eosinophilic cytoplasm and a prominent but delicate vascular network

Clinical features
Epidemiology
- Two percent of all malignancies and approximately 70% of RCCs
- Primarily in adults, sixth to seventh decades
- Male predominance (male-to-female ratio, 2:1 to 3:1)

Presentation
- Hematuria is the single most common presenting sign.
- An increasing number of cases are discovered incidentally.
- Less than 10% of patients exhibit the classic triad of flank mass, pain, and hematuria.

Prognosis and treatment
- Surgical excision offers the only hope for cure.
- Systemic chemotherapy is not effective against advanced disease.
- Fifteen percent to 20% advanced disease responds to immunotherapy.
- Tyrosine kinase inhibitors (e.g., sunitinib) are used for advanced stage disease.
- Approximately one third of patients with clinically localized disease develop local and distant recurrence after surgery.
- Approximately half of patients die of the disease.

Pathology
Gross pathology
- Solitary, well-circumscribed, lobulated renal cortical mass
- Characteristic golden-yellow color
- Necrosis, hemorrhage, and fibrosis common

Histology
- Nests and sheets of tumor cells are separated by delicate vascular network with dilated sinusoidal vascular spaces.
- Cystic changes with serosanguineous fluid or blood are often present.
- Other minor patterns include trabeculae, papillary, tubular, and microcystic.
- Tumor cells with optically clear cytoplasm contain abundant cytoplasmic lipid and glycogen.
- In high-grade tumor, cells can acquire eosinophilic and granular cytoplasm with a high nuclear grade (i.e., cytoplasm–nuclei synchrony).
- Rhabdoid or sarcomatoid differentiation with malignant spindle cells or heterologous elements may be present.

Immunohistochemistry
- Positive for CAM5.2, AE1/3, EMA, vimentin, CD10, RCC-Ag, CA9, PAX2, and PAX8
- Negative for K903; only rarely positive for S-100 and CEA

Molecular diagnostics
- Chromosome 3p alteration present in almost all the cases
- *VHL* gene alterations (mutation or promoter hypermethylation) in 50% to 70% of sporadic clear cell RCC

Main differential diagnosis
- Clear cell tubulopapillary RCC: small tumor arising in a cystic and fibrotic background; tumor cells of low nuclear grade form characteristic branching tubules and acini and clear cell ribbons; positive for CK7, but negative or only focally positive for CD10
- Chromophobe RCC: homogeneous, light-brown cut surface; prominent cell borders; translucent and reticulated cytoplasm; raisinoid nuclear atypia; diffuse CK7 positivity; positive Hale's colloidal iron stain; CA9 negative
- Papillary RCC, solid variant: characteristic papillary architecture with hemosiderin and histiocytes, positive CK7 and AMACR staining, negative CA9 staining
- RCC associated with Xp11.2/transcription factor E3 (*TFE3*) translocation: often affects children and young adults; papillae lined with abundant clear, granular cytoplasm; psammomatous calcification and hyalinized fibrovascular cores of papillae; epithelial markers frequently negative; TFE3 positive
- Adrenocortical carcinoma: negative for epithelial markers such as AE1/3 and EMA, although CAM5.2 frequently positive; positive for calretinin and inhibin
- Urothelial carcinoma: may be associated with pelvic urothelial carcinoma in situ or dysplasia; frequently positive for CK7, CK20, K903, and P63, but negative for PAX2 and PAX8
- Pure epithelioid angiomyolipoma: Multinucleated giant cells and cells with ganglion-like nuclei are often seen. Negative epithelial markers and positive melanocytic markers.

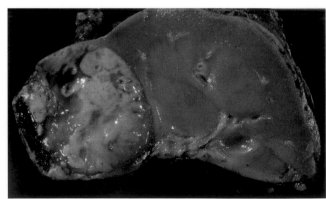

Fig 1. This partial nephrectomy specimen contains a well-circumscribed clear cell renal cell carcinoma with golden color and focal hemorrhage and fibrosis.

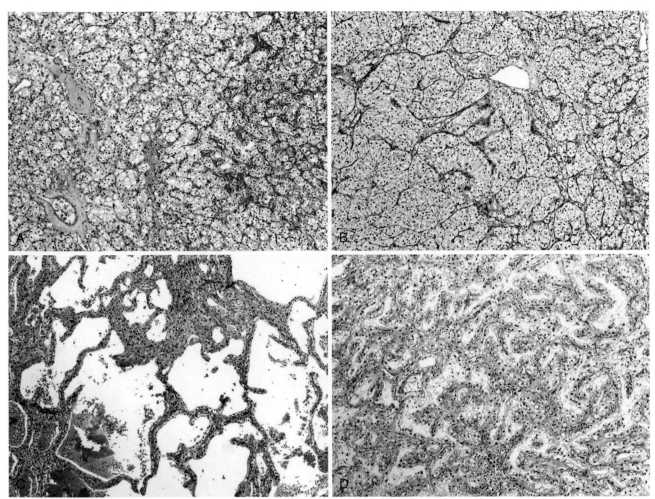

Fig 2. A typical clear cell renal cell carcinoma contains small nests of clear cells separated by a prominent delicate vascular network **(A).** Other architectural patterns include wide trabecular **(B),** cystic **(C),** and papillary **(D).**

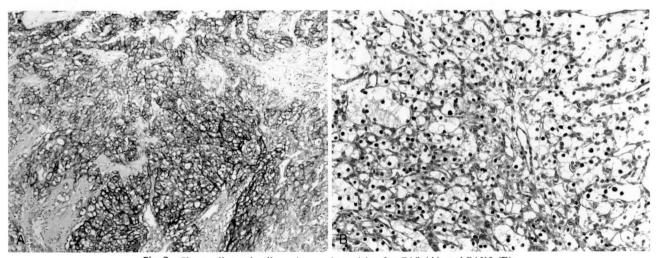

Fig 3. Clear cell renal cell carcinoma is positive for CA9 **(A)** and PAX2 **(B).**

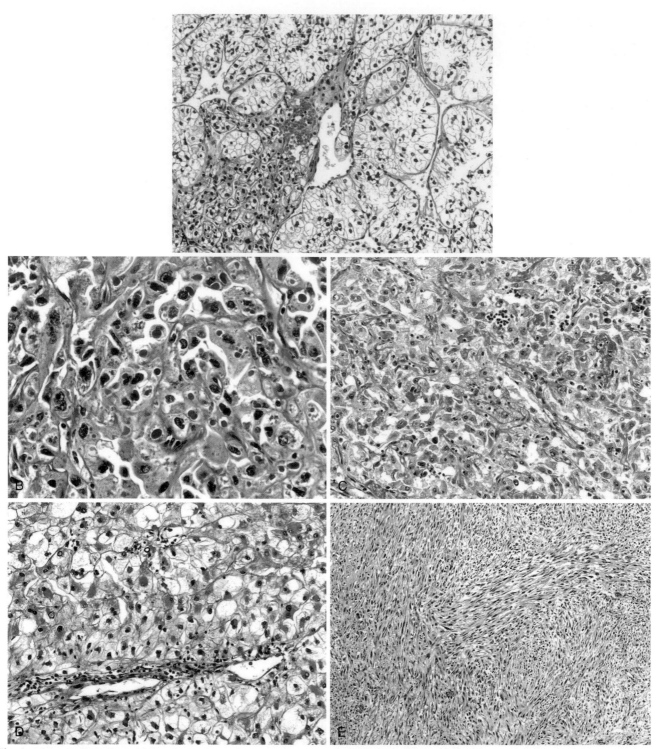

Fig 4. Tumor cells have optically clear cytoplasm and a distinct cell membrane **(A).** Cytoplasmic eosinophilic globules are typically seen in clear cell renal cell carcinoma **(B).** High-grade tumor tends to lose cytoplasmic clarity and acquire eosinophilic cytoplasm and a high nuclear grade **(C).** Rhabdoid cells **(D)** and malignant spindle cells **(E)** can be seen in high-grade tumors.

MULTILOCULAR CYSTIC RENAL CELL CARCINOMA

Definition
- A variant of clear cell RCC composed of multiple cysts lined with low-grade clear cells and no solid or expansile nodules

Clinical features
Epidemiology
- Four percent to 5% of all clear cell RCCs
- Age and gender distribution similar to clear cell RCC
- Usually lower stage (pT1N0M0) than other RCCs

Prognosis and treatment
- Partial or radical nephrectomy
- Excellent prognosis with no recurrence or metastasis reported after surgical resection

Pathology
Gross pathology
- Solitary, well-circumscribed entirely cystic mass
- No solid tumor mass or necrosis

Histology
- Cysts are lined by a single layer or focally stratified clear cells.
- Tumor nuclei are small, uniform, and round or oval without prominent nucleoli.
- Fibrous septa contain small nests of clear cells.
- No solid or expansile clear cell nodules are present.

Immunopathology (including immunohistochemistry)
- Positive: EMA, CD10, AE1/AE3

Molecular diagnostics
- Chromosome 3p deletion and *VHL* gene mutations

Main differential diagnosis
- Clear cell RCC with extensive cystic changes: cystic clear cell RCC with solid or expansile clear cell nodules, or high nuclear grade (Fuhrman grade 3 or greater) should not be diagnosed as multilocular cystic RCC.
- Cystic nephroma occurs almost exclusively in perimenopausal women; cystic walls are not lined with clear cells; ovarian-type stroma may be present.

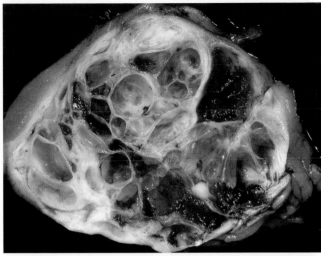

Fig 2. A partial nephrectomy specimen containing a multilocular cystic renal cell carcinoma with a thick, fibrous capsule and composed entirely of cysts of variable sizes. Some cysts are filled with serosanguineous fluid.

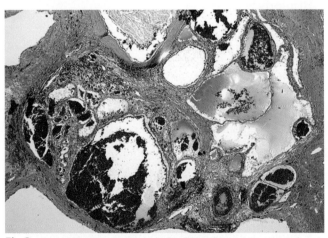

Fig 3. A multilocular cystic renal cell carcinoma consists of variably sized cysts.

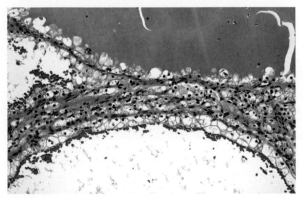

Fig 1. The clear cells have uniform, small, round or oval, and dense nuclei.

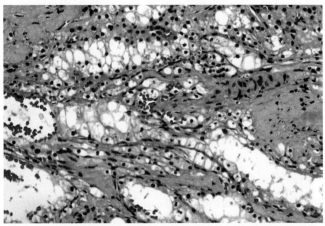

Fig 4. Small nests of clear cells are present within the fibrous septa.

Definition
- A histologic subtype of renal cell carcinoma (RCC) with predominant tubulopapillary architecture and characteristic genetic changes

Clinical features
Epidemiology
- Second most common RCC subtype
- Ten percent to 15% of all RCCs
- Age distribution similar to clear cell RCC
- Male predominance (male-to-female ratio, 2:1 to 4:1)

Presentation
- Most cases sporadic and unilateral
- More likely to be bilateral and multifocal than other RCC subtypes
- Rarely (2%) as part of hereditary papillary RCC syndrome or hereditary leiomyomatosis and RCC syndrome

Prognosis and treatment
- Prognosis generally more favorable than clear cell RCC but less favorable than chromophobe RCC
- Type 1 prognosis better than type 2
- Partial or total nephrectomy

Pathology
Gross pathology
- Fibrous pseudocapsule often present
- Extensive hemorrhage and necrosis often present

Histology
- Tumor cells form papillary fronds with central fibro-vascular cores and tubules.
- Papillae can coalescence to impart a solid growth patterns with glomeruloid structures.
- There is a variable amount of foamy histocytes, psammomatous calcification in papillary cores, hemosiderin deposition, and necrosis.
- Clear cell changes may be present, especially in areas adjacent to necrosis.
- They are further classified to type 1 and type 2 based on the following morphology:
  - Type 1: papillae lined with single layer of small cells with little, amphophilic cytoplasm and low grade (grade 1 or 2) tumor cells
  - Type 2: papillae lined with large cells with abundant eosinophilic cytoplasm, pseudostratified high-grade nuclei
- Rare sarcomatoid changes (5%)

Immunohistochemistry
- Diffusely positive for AMACR, CD10, RCC, Ber-EP4 and PAX2
- CK7 more frequently positive in type 1 (80%) than in type 2 (20%)
- Negative for high-molecular-weight cytokeratin, CA9

Molecular diagnostics
- Typically gain of chromosomes 7 and 17, and loss of chromosome Y in men
- Germline mutation of *MET* oncogene (7q31) in hereditary papillary renal carcinoma syndrome, or fumarate hydratase gene (1q42.3-43) in hereditary leiomyomatosis and RCC syndrome

Main differential diagnosis
- Papillary adenoma: less than 5 mm in size, low nuclear grade (Fuhrman nuclear grade 1 or 2)
- Xp11.2 translocation RCC: children and young adults; papillary structures lined with tumor cells with abundant clear and granular cytoplasm; epithelial markers frequently negative, positive for TFE3
- Clear cell tubulopapillary RCC: small tumors arising in a cystic and fibrotic stroma; clear cells forming branching acini and long clear cell ribbons; nuclei polarized away from basement membrane; positive for CK7, variably positive for CA9; very focally positive or negative for CD10, negative for AMACR
- Papillary urothelial carcinoma: arising in renal pelvis with urothelial dysplasia or carcinoma in situ, or both; solid nests of tumor cells with squamoid features; invasion with desmoplastic stroma; positive for CK7, CK20, K903, and P63; negative for PAX2
- Metanephric adenoma: well-circumscribed without capsule, tumor cells with little cytoplasm, uniform round or oval nuclei; cytokeratin negative, WT1 positive

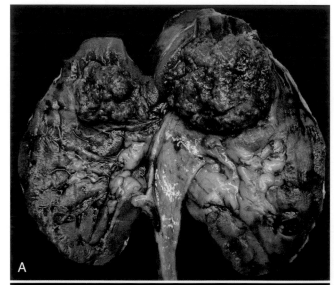
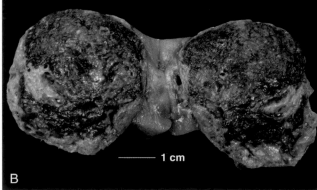

Fig 1. **A,** A well-defined papillary renal cell carcinoma showing variegated and hemorrhagic cut surface. **B,** Another tumor with extensive necrosis.

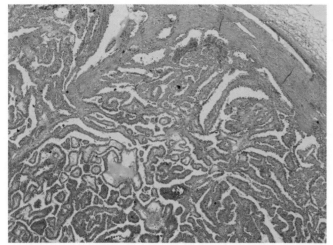

Fig 2. A papillary RCC invested by a fibrous pseudocapsule.

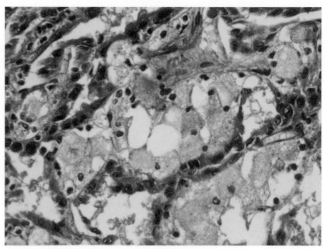

Fig 4. Aggregates of foamy histiocytes expanding the papillary fibrovascular cores.

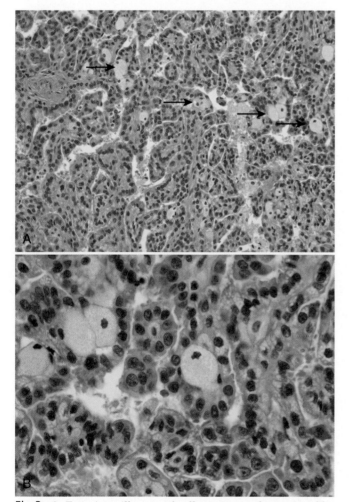

Fig 3. **A,** Type 1 papillary renal cell carcinoma characterized by a single layer of cuboidal cells. Foam cells are within the fibro-vascular cores *(arrows).* **B,** High magnification shows tumor cells containing scanty amphophilic cytoplasm.

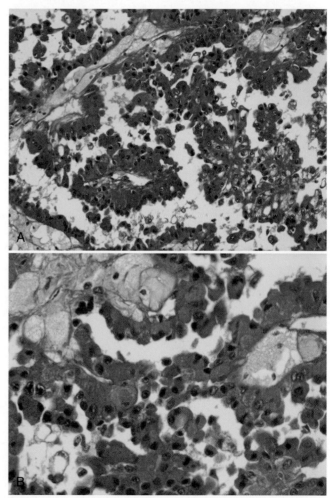

Fig 5. Type 2 papillary renal cell carcinoma composed of large eosinophilic tumor cells with pseudostratified nuclei **(A)** and abundant granular cytoplasm **(B).**

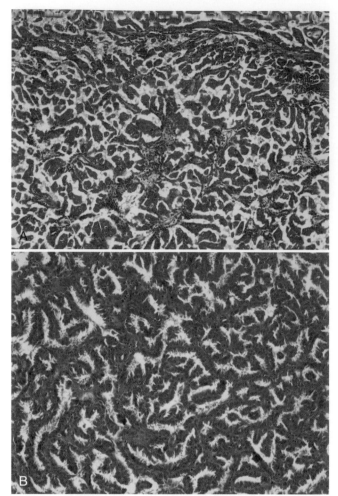

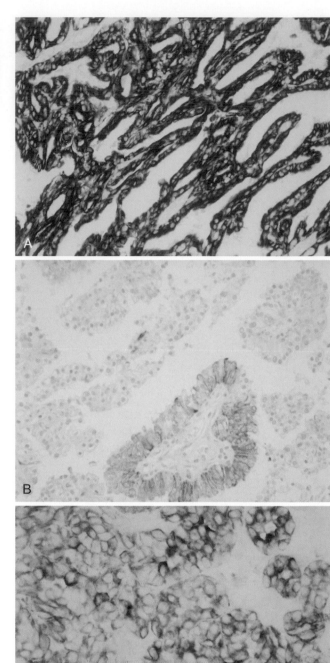

Fig 6. Papillary renal cell carcinoma composed chiefly of short papillae without conspicuous fibrovascular cores **(A)** and branching papillae **(B).**

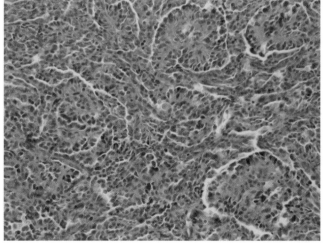

Fig 7. Solid variant of papillary renal cell carcinoma composed of closely packed tubules and acini. Vague glomeruloid structures are present.

Fig 8. **A,** Diffuse positivity for CK7 in type 1 papillary renal cell carcinoma (RCC). **B,** Focal CK7 positivity in type 2 papillary RCC. **C,** Diffuse immunoreactivity for CK7 in a solid variant of papillary RCC.

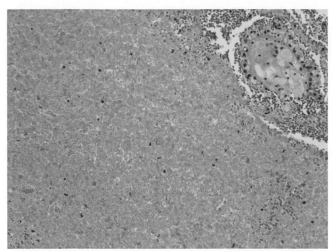

Fig 9. Tumor necrosis is common in papillary renal cell carcinoma. Residual tumor papillae are seen at upper right corner.

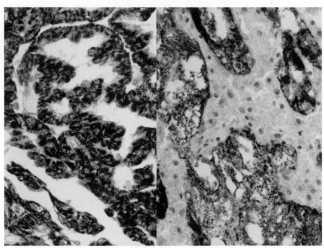

Fig 11. Strong cytoplasmic granular immunopositivity for AMACR in type 1 *(left)* and type 2 *(right)* papillary renal cell carcinoma.

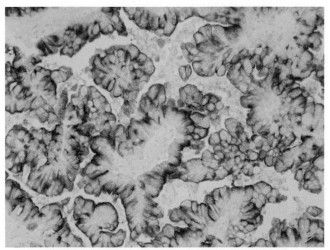

Fig 10. Luminal reactivity for renal cell carcinoma-Ag.

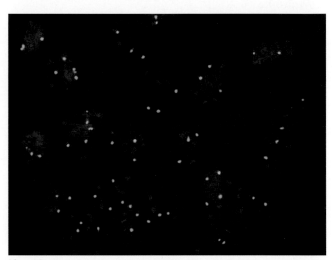

Fig 12. Fluorescence in situ hybridization with centromeric probes for chromosome 7 *(green)* and chromosome 17 *(red)* demonstrates frequent trisomy of chromosomes 7 and 17 in tumor nuclei.

CHROMOPHOBE RENAL CELL CARCINOMA

Definition
- A renal cell carcinoma (RCC) subtype comprising large pale and/or eosinophilic cells with prominent cell borders, irregular nuclei, and perineuclear halos

Clinical features
Epidemiology
- Five percent of RCCs
- Mean age, 50 to 60 years (range, 30 to 90 years)
- Male-to-female ratio, 1.5:1

Presentation
- Most tumors are asymptomatic and detected incidentally.
- Occasionally as a manifestation of Birt-Hogg-Dube syndrome

Prognosis and treatment
- Prognosis is much better than clear cell RCC, with mortality less than 10% and 5-year disease survival greater than 90%.
- Sarcomatoid features and perinephric extension are associated with worse outcomes.
- No prognostic difference exsists between classic and eosinophilic variants.
- An usual treatment is partial nephrectomy.

Pathology
Gross pathology
- Size range, 2 to 22 cm (mean, 8 cm)
- Solid and well circumscribed, but not encapsulated
- Homogeneous, light brown–tan cut surface
- Small areas of necrosis, hemorrhage, or scaring possibly be present, but not typical

Histology
- Classic type with large polygonal cells with pale and lightly reticulated cytoplasm
- Commonly mixed with smaller cells with granular eosinophilic cytoplasm
- Eosinophilic variant composed predominantly of intensely eosinophilic cells
- Prominent, plantlike, thick cell membranes imparting a cobblestone appearance
- Peripheral cytoplasm with variable degrees of eosinophilia and granularity, most prominent adjacent to the cytoplasm membrane
- Irregular, wrinkled, and angulated nuclei (raisinoid) with perinuclear clearing (halos)
- Medium-sized vessels with eccentrically hyalinized walls

Immunohistochemistry
- CK7 diffusely positive
- EMA, E-cadherin, paralbumin positive
- CD10 and RCC-Ag equivocal
- Vimentin negative
- Hale colloidal iron: diffuse and strong reticular cytoplasmic staining

Molecular studies
- Chromosomal losses involving chromosomes 1, 6, 10, 13, 17, 21, and Y

Main differential diagnosis
- Renal oncocytoma: round and uniform nuclei, without prominent cell borders; negative or focally positive C7 staining
- Clear cell RCC: cytoplasm optically clear compared with reticulated cytoplasm in chromophobe RCCs; CK7 negative, CA9 positive
- Epithelioid angiomyolipoma: significant nuclear pleomorphism with multinucleated cells; no perinuclear halos; adipose tissue and abnormal vessels may be found; positive for HMB-45 and melan A, but negative for CK7 and pankeratin

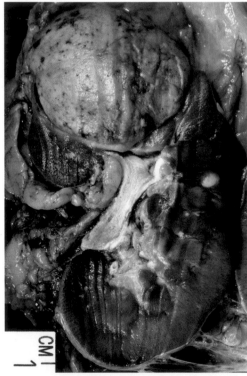

Fig 1. Grossly, chromophobe renal cell carcinoma forms a well-circumscribed mass with a light brown cut surface. Pin-point hemorrhage is present.

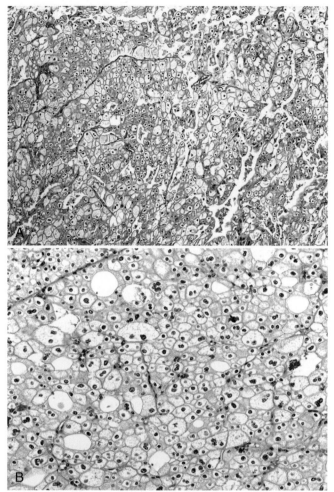

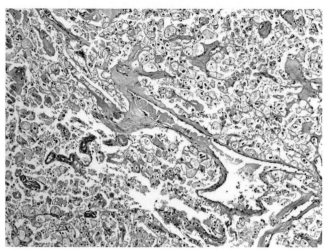

Fig 4. Eccentrically hyalinized blood vessels in a chromophobe renal cell carcinoma.

Fig 2. **A,** Tumor cells are of variable sizes, with thick and distinct cell borders imparting a cobblestone appearance. **B,** Higher magnification showing large polygonal pale or eosinophilic cells with flocculent cytoplasm, hyperchromatic and wrinkled nuclei, and perinuclear halos.

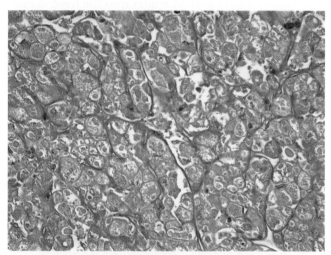

Fig 5. Hale colloidal iron stain showing diffuse cytoplasmic positivity.

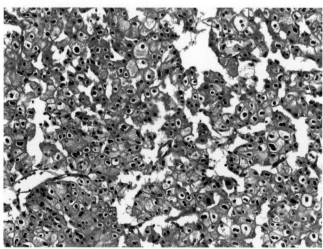

Fig 3. Eosinophilic variant of chromophobe renal cell carcinoma has smaller tumor cells with densely eosinophilic cytoplasm. Characteristic raisinoid nuclear atypia is present.

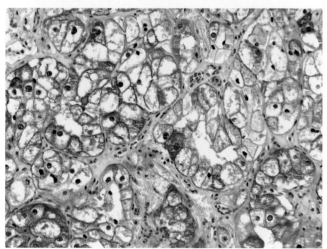

Fig 6. Strong positive staining for paralbumin in chromophobe renal cell carcinoma helps to distinguish from a renal cell carcinoma with granular cytoplasm.

Definition
- A highly aggressive type of renal carcinoma originating from collecting duct epithelium; also known as *carcinoma of the collecting ducts of Bellini*

Clinical features
Epidemiology
- Less than 1% of renal cancers
- Occurs mostly in adults; rare cases reported in children
- Age range, 13 to 83 years (mean, 55 years)
- Males more commonly affected

Presentation
- Hematuria, flank mass, or abdominal pain
- Some incidentally discovered on radiologic investigation
- On computed tomographic scans, normal outer contours usually maintained in affected kidneys; mass involves medulla and protrudes into the renal sinuses
- Positive urine cytology

Prognosis and treatment
- Very poor prognosis with most cases appearing at a high stage
- Approximately 45% with lymph node metastases, 30% distant metastases, commonly to liver, lungs, bone, and adrenal gland at presentation
- Two-year, disease-specific survival, 20%
- Standard therapy not well defined and of questionable efficacy
- Nephrectomy with adjuvant chemotherapy and immunotherapy

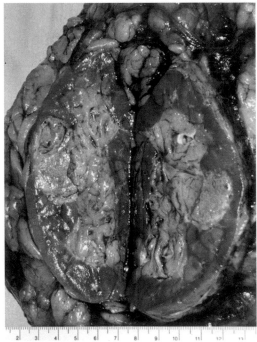

Fig 1. Collecting duct carcinoma is predominantly centrally located, with involvement of the medulla.

Acknowledgment: Brett Delahunt, Wellington School of Medicine and Health Sciences, Wellington, New Zealand

Pathology
Gross pathology
- Predominantly centrally located with involvement of medulla
- Irregular extensively infiltrating margins
- Necrosis and satellite nodules common
- Commonly involves renal sinus and perinephric fat and renal vein

Histology
- Irregular microcysts, tubulopapillae, and glands
- Cords and solid sheets of tumor cells; rarely signet ring cells
- Inflamed and desmoplastic stroma
- Intraluminal and intracytoplasmic mucin
- Eosinophilic cytoplasm
- High-grade nuclei and brisk mitosis
- Associated tubular dysplasia

Immunohistochemistry and special studies
- *Ulex europaeus* aglutinin-1, peanut agglutinin, CK19, high-molecular-weight cytokeratin, 34βE12, vimentin, PAX8 are usually positive.
- Variable staining for EMA and CD15
- α-Methylacyl–coenzyme A racemase, CD10, villin, aquaporin 1 and 2, and p63 negative

Molecular diagnostics
- Loss of heterozygosity on multiple chromosomal arms, including 1q, 6p, 8p, 13q, and 21q
- Loss of chromosome 3p rare
- Deletion located on 1q32.1-32.2
- HER2/neu amplification in 50% cases

Main differential diagnosis
- High-grade urothelial carcinoma with glandular differentiation: arising in the pelvocalyceal system; conventional invasive and in situ urothelial carcinoma component usually identified; PAX8⁻/p63⁺
- Papillary RCC: often showing a fibrous pseudocapsule and well-formed papillae that contain foamy histiocytes; CD10 and AMACR positive
- Metastatic adenocarcinoma: history; may be multifocal with location at corticomedullary junction; positive for lineage specific markers (e.g., TTF-1, CDX2)

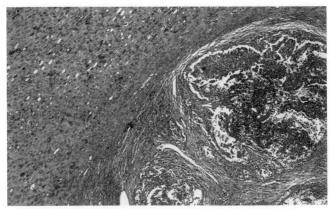

Fig 2. Collecting duct carcinoma involves a renal papilla.

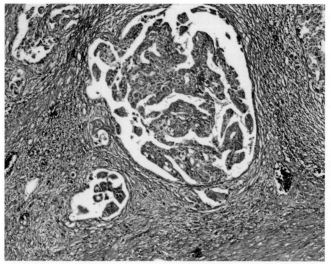

Fig 3. Collecting duct carcinoma with microcystic and papillary architecture. The margin is irregular and infiltrating.

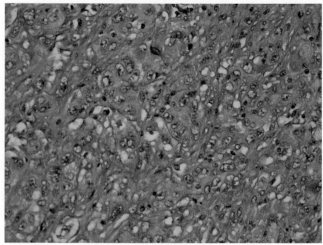

Fig 6. Solid nests of high-grade tumor cells in a collecting duct carcinoma.

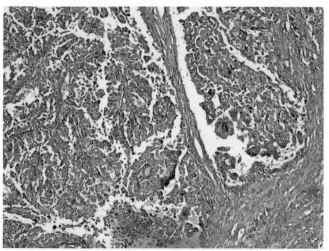

Fig 4. Collecting duct carcinoma with papillary architecture.

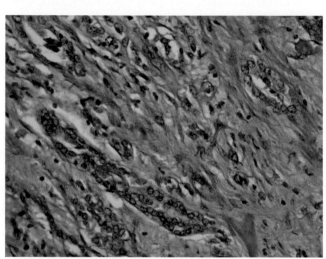

Fig 7. Associated tubular dysplasia.

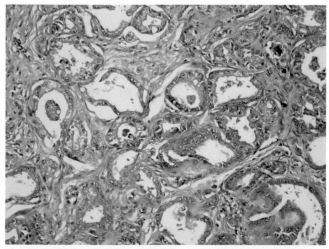

Fig 5. Collecting duct carcinoma with irregular tubules and glands embedded in desmoplastic stroma.

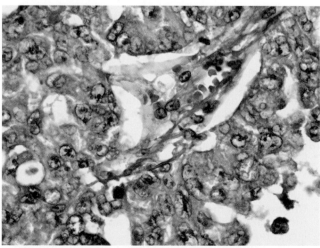

Fig 8. Tumor cells in collecting duct carcinoma have eosinophilic cytoplasm and highly pleomorphic nuclei.

Definition
- Rare, highly aggressive malignant renal tumor arising from the terminal collecting ducts, typically affecting individuals with sickle cell hemoglobinopathies

Clinical features
Epidemiology
- Affects young men with sickle cell hemoglobinopathies, mostly sickle cell trait
- Usually in blacks
- Male to female ratio, 1.9:1

Presentation
- Gross hematuria, flank or abdominal pain
- Symptoms associated with distant metastasis

Prognosis and treatment
- Prognosis is poor, with frequent metastasis at presentation.
- Common metastatic sites are lymph nodes, lung, liver, and adrenal gland.
- Rhabdoid features and absence of INI-1 expression are markers of aggressive behavior.

Pathology
Gross pathology
- Poorly circumscribed tumors arising from the renal medulla
- Hemorrhage and necrosis common

Histology
- The tumor assumes a reticular pattern reminiscent of testicular yolk sac tumor at low-power magnification.
- Microcystic, tubular, trabecular, solid, adenoid-cystic formations are present.
- Rhabdoid-like or plasmacytoid cells can be seen.
- Variable stromal desmoplasia is present.
- Suppurative necrosis resembles abscesses within tumor nests.
- Heavy inflammation is present at the interface between the tumor and the surrounding tissue.
- Sickled red cells can be seen.

Immunopathology and immunohistochemistry
- Tumor cells are positive for keratin, CEA, EMA, and CK19.

Molecular diagnostics
- Gene expression profiling shows renal medullary carcinoma to cluster with urothelial cancers.
- BRC/ABL translocation has been reported in some cases.

Main differential diagnosis
- Collecting duct carcinoma: a renal tumor with collecting duct carcinoma features affecting patients with sickle cell hemoglobinopathies is considered a medullary carcinoma.
- Urothelial carcinoma may contain pelvic mucosal urothelial carcinoma in situ and an exophytic papillary component.
- Acute pyelonephritis: florid tumor necrosis with neutrophils may be mistaken for acute pyelonephritis, but highly atypical tumor cells can usually be identified.

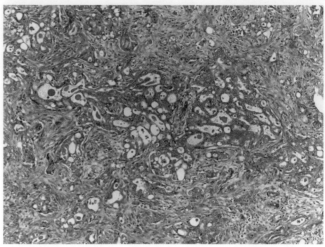

Fig 1. Fused tubular and adenoid cystic epithelial formations within a desmoplastic stroma in a renal medullary carcinoma. Eosinophilic globules are found within the glandular lumens.

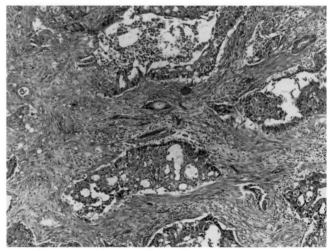

Fig 2. Necrosis is present within a glandular lumen.

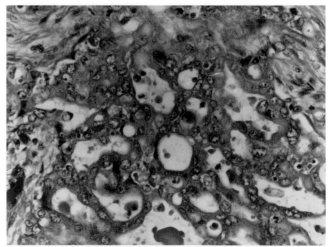

Fig 3. Higher magnification shows tumor cells with pleomorphic vesicular nuclei with prominent nucleoli.

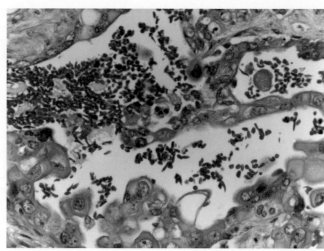

Fig 4. Sickled red blood cells within the lumens of malignant glands.

Definition
- Renal cell carcinoma occurring in long-term survivors of childhood neuroblastoma

Clinical features
Epidemiology
- Rare
- Male and female patients equally affected

Presentation
- Neuroblastoma diagnosed before 2 years of age
- RCC diagnosed at a median age of 13.5 years (range, 2 to 35 years)

Prognosis and treatment
- Prognosis correlated with tumor stage, similar to other RCC histologic subtypes
- Documented metastasis to liver, lymph nodes, adrenal glands, and bone
- Partial or radical nephrectomy

Pathology
Gross pathology
- Solitary tumors ranging from 3.5 to 8 cm
- One patient with multiple small tumors that measured from 1 to 2.4 cm; some cystic

Histology
- Morphologically heterogeneous
- Some tumors have solid and focally papillary architecture, monotonous population of cells with large eosinophilic cytoplasm that resemble oncocytomas
- Clusters of foamy histiocytes, as well as psammoma bodies, rarely present
- Translocation RCC also seen

Immunopathology
- Diffusely positive for epithelial membrane antigen, vimentin, cytokeratin 8, 18, 20
- Negative for cytokeratin 7, 14, S-100, and HMB-45

Main differential diagnosis
- Oncocytoma: postneuroblastoma RCC has higher-grade nuclei, distinct solid and papillary architecture, and the presence of foamy histiocytes. The loose myxoid background seen in oncocytomas is not present in postneuroblastoma RCC.
- Type 2 papillary RCC: foamy histiocytes, focal papillary architecture, and eosinophilic cytoplasm are commonly seen in both entities, but the age and clinical history will help distinguish the two.

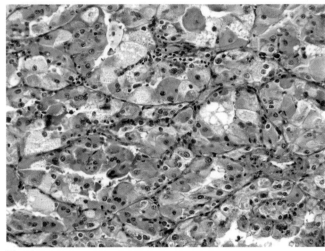

Fig 1. Carcinoma associated with neuroblastoma shows nests of cells with abundant eosinophilic and granular cytoplasm resembling renal oncocytoma. Some cells are vacuolated. Nuclei are of variable sizes and have moderately prominent nucleoli. (Courtesy Liang Cheng, Indianapolis, Ind.)

RENAL CELL CARCINOMA ASSOCIATED WITH XP11.2 TRANSLOCATION AND *TFE3* GENE FUSIONS

Definition
- Distinct subtype of RCC characterized by chromosomal translocation involving *TFE3* gene on chromosome Xp11.2

Clinical features
Epidemiology
- The majority of cases are reported in children and young adults.
- Incidence is rare in adults, but it is rising because of increased recognition.
- Some patients have a history of chemotherapy for other malignancies.

Presentation
- Similar to other RCCs

Prognosis and treatment
- Nephrectomy
- Indolent clinical behavior in lymph node positive and metastasis negative children; aggressive in metastasis positive children
- Aggressive clinical course in adult patients
- Anecdotal reports of response to sunitinib

Pathology
Gross pathology
- Not distinct from other RCCs

Histology
- RCC with different chromosomal translocations exhibiting somewhat different morphologic features
- ASPL-TFE3 RCC
  - Tumor cells with voluminous, partly clear, partly eosinophilic cytoplasm, discrete cell border, vesicular nuclei, and prominent nucleoli
  - Papillae or pseudopapillae lined with tumor cells with partly clear cytoplasm
  - Psammomatous calcification and hyalin nodules common
- PRCC-TFE3 RCC
  - There is a more compact nested and less papillary pattern.
  - Tumor cells have less abundant cytoplasm, fewer psammomatous calcification, and hyalinized fibrovascular cores.

Immunohistochemistry
- Confirmatory immunostain is nuclear protein TFE3.
- Approximately 50% of cases express epithelial markers such as cytokeratin and EMA, and the staining is often focal and weak
- RCC Ag and CD10 positive
- Melanocytic markers occasionally positive

Molecular diagnostics
- Characteristic chromosomal translocation involving *TFE3* gene on Xp11.2 and one of several partner genes
  - ASPL-TFE3, t(X; 17)(p11.2; q25)
  - PRCC-TFE3, t(X;1)(p11.2; q21)
  - PSF-TFE3, t(X ; 1)(p11.2; q34)
  - NonO-TFE3, inv(X)(p11; q12)
  - CLTC-TFE3, t(X ; 17)(p1.2 ; q23)
- Break-apart fluorescence in situ probes are available to detect *TFE3* gene fusion and aid the diagnosis of translocation RCC.

Main differential diagnosis
- Renal cell carcinoma, clear cell or papillary type: renal cell carcinoma is rare in children and young adults. Translocation RCC should always be considered and ruled out for any RCC in this age group.
- Epithelioid angiomyolipoma is uncommon in children and young adults unless in patients with tuberous sclerosis; fat and abnormal blood vessels are suggestive of angiomyolipoma; negative for epithelial markers and positive for at least one melanocytic marker.

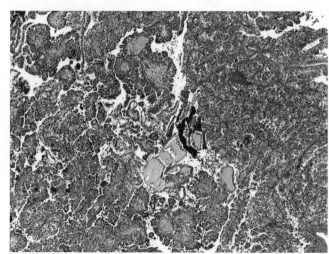

Fig 1. ASPL-TFE3 translocation renal cell carcinoma showing nested and papillary architecture.

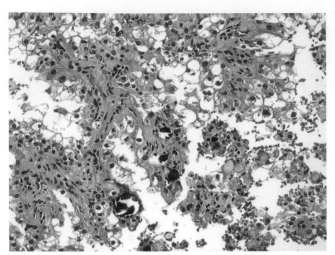

Fig 2. In ASPL-TFE3 translocation renal cell carcinoma, the papillae are lined with tumor cells with voluminous, partly clear, and partly eosinophilic cytoplasm. They have distinct cell borders, vesicular chromatin, and prominent nucleoli. Note the psammomatous calcifications.

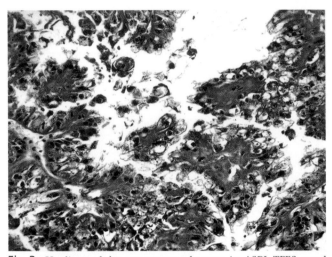

Fig 3. Hyalin nodules are commonly seen in ASPL-TFE3 renal cell carcinoma.

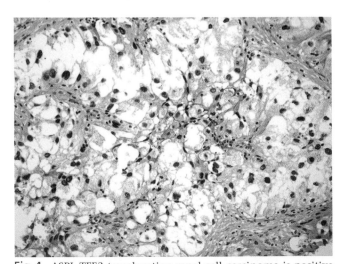

Fig 4. ASPL-TFE3 translocation renal cell carcinoma is positive for nuclear protein TFE3 by immunohistochemistry.

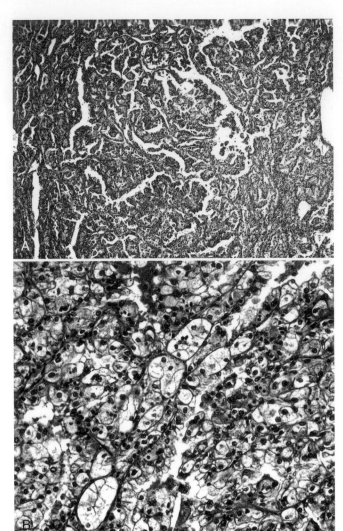

Fig 5. PRCC-TFE3 translocation renal cell carcinoma showing a more compact nested pattern **(A).** The tumor cells have distinct cell borders and have abundant, slightly eosinophilic cytoplasm **(B).**

MUCINOUS TUBULAR AND SPINDLE CELL CARCINOMA

Definition
- Low-grade renal epithelial neoplasm composed of tubules, spindle cells, and extracellular mucin

Clinical features
Epidemiology
- Usually occurs in adults, with a wide age range of 17 to 82 years (mean, 53 years)
- Occurs predominantly in female patients (male-to-female ratio, 1:4)

Presentation
- Usually asymptomatic and detected incidentally
- Can manifest with flank pain or hematuria

Prognosis and treatment
- Nephrectomy
- Excellent prognosis with only a few cases of metastasis reported

Pathology
Gross pathology
- Well-circumscribed mass with homogenous, gray to light tan cut surface

Histology
- Variable amounts of compressed and elongated tubules, spindle cells, extracellular mucin
- Bland, round or oval nuclei with inconspicuous nucleoli
- Stromal mucin variable, possibly scant
- Inflammatory cells and macrophages present in the stroma
- Sarcomatoid differentiation characterized by high-grade spindle cell proliferation with tumor necrosis occurring rarely

Immunohistochemistry
- Similar to papillary RCC, positive for CK7, AE1/AE3, CK19, EMA, AMACR, variably positive for high-molecular-weight keratin

Molecular diagnostics
- Losses of chromosome 1, 4, 6, 8, 9, 13, 14, 15, 18, 21, 22
- Gain of chromosome 7 and 17 and loss of Y chromosome usually not seen

Main differential diagnosis
- Papillary RCC: prominent papillary architecture, mucin absent or uncommon in the stroma, and gain of chromosome 7 and 17 and loss of Y chromosome
- Sarcomatoid RCC: other characteristic RCC component present and sarcomatoid component often present as malignant spindle cells
- Collecting duct carcinoma: high-grade tumor cells forming tubules and small cysts, prominent desmoplastic stromal reaction, and adjacent tubular dysplasia

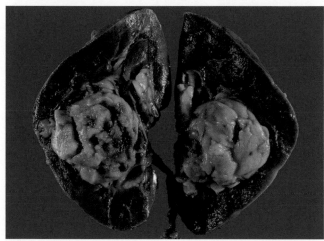

Fig 1. A well-circumscribed tumor with grayish, slightly glistering cut surface. (Courtesy Dr. Yosuke Iwata, Ohgaki, Japan)

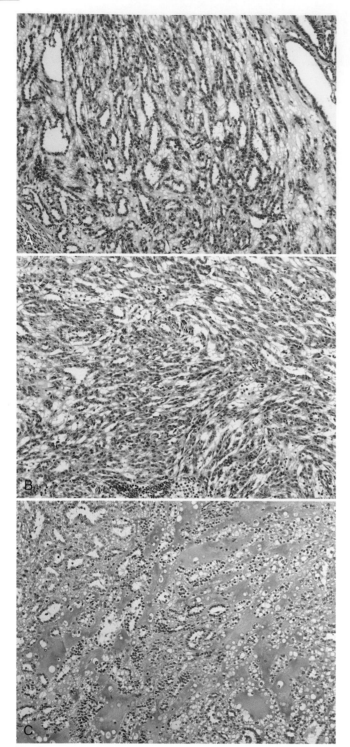

Fig 2. **A,** Round and closely packed elongated tubules embedded in extracellular mucin. **B,** Bland spindle cells are present. **C,** Stroma mucin is positive on Alcian blue stain.

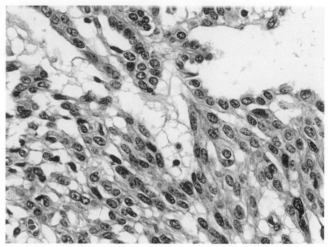

Fig 3. Tumor nuclei are round or oval with minimal atypia.

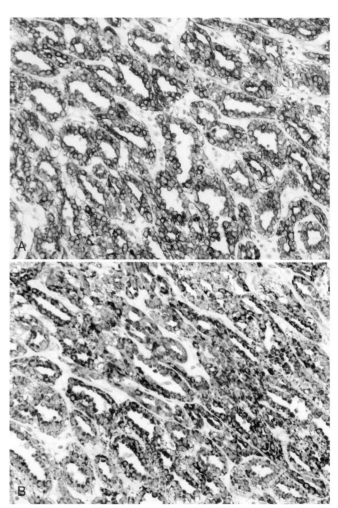

Fig 4. Tumor cells are positive for CK7 **(A)** and α-methylacyl–coenzyme A racemase **(B).**

Definition
- A group of RCCs whose morphology or growth pattern does not readily fit any of the RCC subtypes recognized by the current World Health Organization classification

Clinical features
Epidemiology
- Represents 3% to 5% of all RCCs

Presentation
- Similar to other renal cell carcinoma subtypes

Prognosis and treatment
- Prognosis and therapeutic responses are highly variable.
- Higher-grade tumor has a higher rate of metastatic disease and poorer clinical outcomes.
- Sarcomatoid differentiation may be an additional risk factor in some patients.
- Partial nephrectomy is the treatment of choice for the more indolent tumors.
- Radical nephrectomy or immunotherapy, or both, or chemotherapy for the higher-grade, more aggressive tumors.

Pathology
Histology
- Morphologic features do not fit in any one specific RCC subtype.
- A poorly differentiated or predominantly sarcomatoid component prevents classification using the current criteria.
- Occasionally several distinct patterns such as clear cell RCC and papillary RCC components are present in the same tumor.

Immunohistochemistry and special studies
- Immunostaining patterns are highly variable and in general do not conform to a specific RCC subtype.

Molecular diagnostics
- May be useful to subtype according to the genetic changes characteristic of known RCC subtypes, such as 3p deletions for clear cell RCC and trisomy of 7 and 17 for papillary RCC

Main differential diagnosis
- Collecting duct carcinoma: centrally located tumor; highly infiltrative growth pattern with high-grade cancer cells forming irregular glands, tubules and cysts embedded in a desmoplastic stroma; dysplastic changes in adjacent renal tubules
- Renal cell carcinoma with predominantly sarcomatoid differentiation: extensive sampling revealing an underlying epithelial element that can be used to subtype the tumor
- Metastatic carcinoma to the kidney: immunohistochemistry and clinical history important for a correct diagnosis

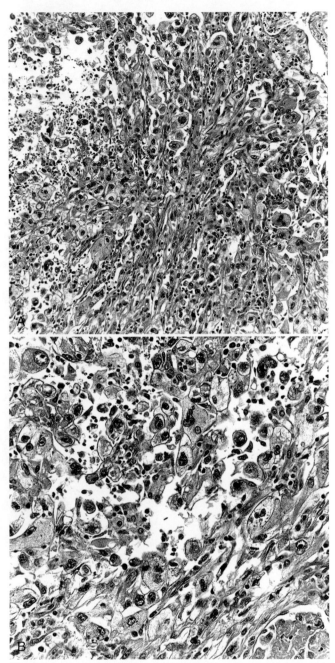

Fig 1. **A,** A poorly differentiated renal cell carcinoma with large pleomorphic cells with bizarre atypia. **B,** At higher magnification, some large pleomorphic cells have clear and others have eosinophilic cytoplasm. Note the atypical nuclear features, including macronucleoli in the pleomorphic cells. Although the tumor cells have somewhat clear cytoplasm, this neoplasm does not have the characteristic features of a clear cell renal cell carcinoma, nor does it have 3p deletion by molecular study; therefore it is classified as renal cell carcinoma, unclassified type.

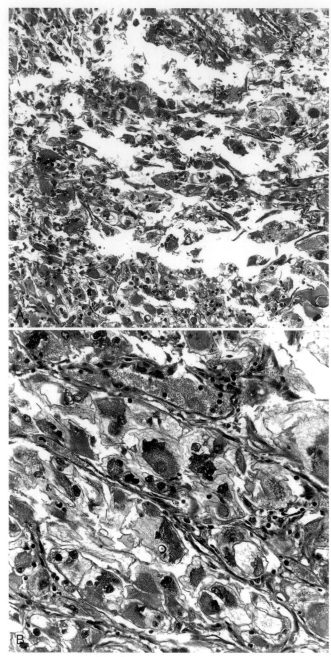

Fig 2. An unusual renal cell carcinoma characterized by prominent rhabdoid cells with eosinophilic cytoplasm. Note the eosinophilic cytoplasm with microvesicular appearance, leading to the unusual rhabdoid morphology of the tumor cells. These cells are cytokeratin positive and negative for muscle markers. This morphology is not readily classified into any one specific RCC subtype.

Definition
- A morphologic variant of renal carcinoma with predominantly tubular and cystic architecture

Clinical features
Epidemiology
- A rare variant of kidney epithelial neoplasm, with fewer than 100 cases reported in the literature
- Affects patients in fourth to ninth decades of life
- Average age, 57.2 years (range, 30 to 80 years)
- Striking male predominance, with a male-to-female ratio of 7:1

Presentation
- Most cases discovered incidentally
- Less commonly with nonspecific abdominal pain, distention, gross hematuria, or unintentional weight loss

Prognosis and treatment
- Surgical resection is the treatment of choice.
- Most cases are low grade with good to fair prognosis.
- Metastasis is seen in a small percentage of cases.
- There may be an association with papillary RCC.

Pathology
Gross pathology
- Mean tumor size, 4.3 cm (range 0.5 to 17.5 cm)
- Majority of tumors involve the renal cortex or the cortex and medulla
- Typically, the tumor arising as a single nodule; some cases associated with papillary renal cell neoplasms either adenomas or papillary RCC
- Well circumscribed but not encapsulated
- Composed of multilocular cystic spaces, some containing serosanguineous fluid, resembling sponge or Swiss cheese

Histology
- Carcinoma is composed of closely packed tubules and cysts separated by thin, fibrous septae that do not contain ovarian-type stroma or desmoplasia.
- Cysts are typically small, with variable sizes ranging from 0.05 to 2 mm, but can be as large as 1 cm.

- The tumor cells lining the cysts and tubules are large with eosinophilic cytoplasm and prominent nucleoli.
- Hobnail morphology is common.
- An association with papillary cell neoplasms is sometimes seen.
- Electron microscopy reveals features of both proximal convoluted tubules (abundant microvilli with brush border organization) and intercalated cells of the collecting duct (shorter, sparse microvilli with cytoplasmic interdigitation).

Immunohistochemistry and special studies
- Limited data on the immunohistoprofile
- AMACR positive
- CK7 positive, often heterogeneous and weak
- CD10 positive
- PAX2 positive

Molecular diagnostics
- Molecularly, this tumor is similar to papillary RCC by gene expression profiling.
- Comparative genomic microarray analysis and fluorescence in situ analysis have demonstrated gains of chromosome 17p and 17q (trisomy 17), typical for papillary RCC in a subset of cases.
- Trisomy 7, also characteristic of papillary RCC, was not identified in some cases, indicating the difference between the two tumors.

Main differential diagnosis
- Simple cortical renal cysts: single or several cysts with denuded, attenuated, or cuboidal lining cells that resemble normal renal tubules
- Cystic nephroma–mixed epithelial and stromal tumor: biphasic tumor with prominent epithelial and stromal components; cysts often lined by flattened or attenuated cells with inconspicuous nucleoli; prominent stroma that may contain dense collagen, smooth muscle, and ovarian-type stroma
- Multilocular cystic RCC: cysts lined by clear cells similar to clear cell RCC; nests of clear cells are also present in the walls of the cysts

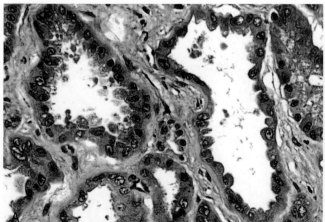
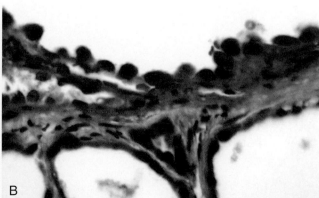

Fig 1. The tumor cells lining the cysts and tubules have abundant eosinophilic cytoplasm with prominent nucleoli **(A)** and a hobnail appearance **(B).**

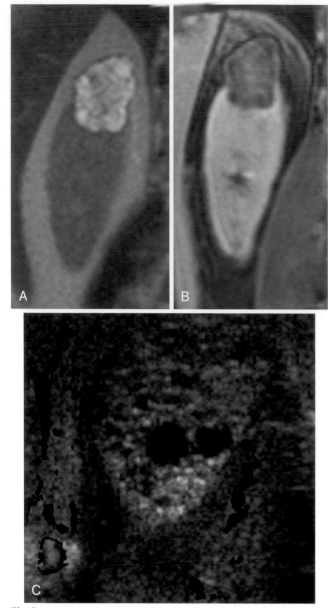

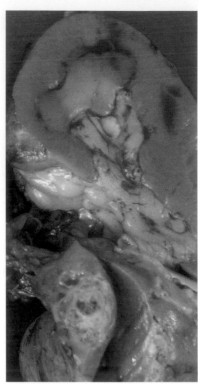

Fig 4. A tubulocystic carcinoma with multilocular cystic appearance in the lower pole of the left kidney.

Fig 2. A radiologic image of a tubulocystic carcinoma. **A,** Magnetic resonance imaging scan T2 image. **B,** T1 postcontrast image. **C,** Ultrasound image of another tubulocystic carcinoma. These images demonstrate a well-defined multilocular cystic lesion in the renal parenchyma.

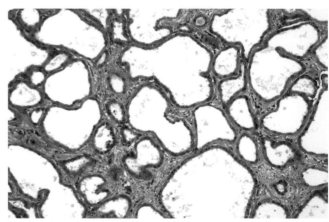

Fig 5. Renal tubulocystic carcinoma characteristically composed of tubules and cysts of variable sizes separated by fibrotic septa.

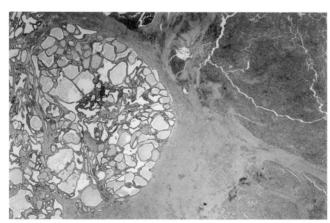

Fig 3. A tubulocystic carcinoma *(left)* coexists with a high-grade papillary renal cell carcinoma *(right)*.

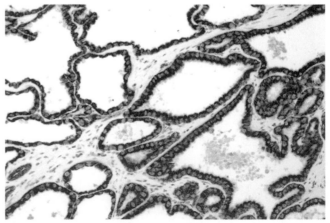

Fig 6. Strong and diffuse α-methylacyl–coenzyme A racemase immunoreactivity in tumor cells.

RENAL CELL CARCINOMA ASSOCIATED WITH ACQUIRED CYSTIC RENAL DISEASES

Definition
- Renal cell carcinoma developed in the acquired cystic kidney disease

Clinical features
Epidemiology
- Tumors develop in 3% to 7% of acquired cystic renal disease, and the risk is 100-fold that of the general population.
- Patients tend to be young and predominantly male.

Presentation
- Usually incidental findings during follow-up of the acquired cystic renal disease
- Occasionally flank pain and hematuria

Prognosis and treatment
- Surgical resection
- Prognosis considered more favorable than RCCs in non–end-stage kidneys

Pathology
Histology
- Approximately 40% of the tumors are classic clear cell, papillary, and chromophobe RCCs.
- The majority of the tumors are acquired cystic disease–associated RCC or clear cell papillary RCC.
- Acquired cystic disease–associated RCC is characterized by:
  - Various growth patterns including solid, papillary, acinar, cribriform, and tubulocystic
  - Tumor cells with abundant eosinophilic cytoplasm that may be markedly vacuolated and imparts a cribriform appearance
  - Large, round to oval nuclei with prominent nucleoli
  - Abundant intratumoral calcium oxalate crystals
- Clear cell papillary RCC is characterized by papillary architecture lined with clear cells with a low nuclear grade.

Immunohistochemistry
- Acquired cystic disease–associated RCC: positive for AE1/3, CD10, RCC-Ag, and AMACR
- Clear cell papillary RCC: positive for CK7, negative for CD10 and AMACR

Main differential diagnosis
- Papillary adenoma: common in end-stage kidney; diameter, 5 mm or less; low nuclear grade (equivalent to Fuhrman grade 1 and 2)
- Benign cysts: may have clear cell lining, which is a single layer, and lining cells have small dense nuclei; no clear cells within the stroma

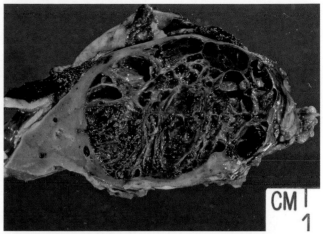

Fig 1. This end-stage kidney contains a multilocular cystic mass. The cysts are filled with blood. A hemorrhagic solid mass is found within several cysts.

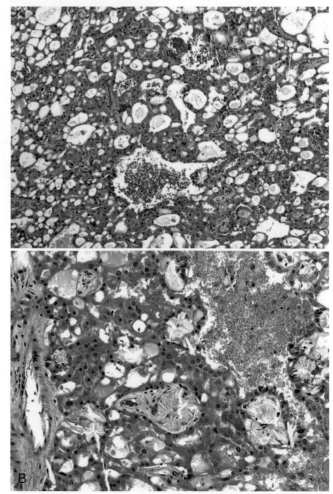

Fig 2. A, Acquired cystic disease–associated renal cell carcinoma showing tumor cells with abundant eosinophilic cytoplasm that is markedly vacuolated and imparts a cribriform appearance. **B,** Numerous intratumoral calcium oxalate crystals are present.

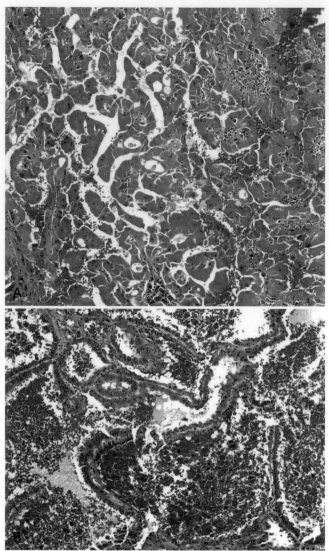

Fig 3. Acquired cystic disease–associated renal cell carcinoma showing papillary architecture lined with tumor cells with abundant eosinophilic cytoplasm **(A)** and tubulocystic pattern **(B).**

RENAL CELL CARCINOMA WITH SARCOMATOID DIFFERENTIATION

Definition
- Sarcomatoid component present in a RCC of any histologic subtype

Clinical features
Epidemiology
- Mean age, 60 years
- Patients, 60% men
- Usually stage 3 or 4
- Metastasis to the lung most common

Prognosis and treatment
- Prognosis is poor, even as a focal finding, and is an adverse prognostic factor independent of the pathologic stage or the grade of RCC.
- Five- and 10-year survival is 22% and 13% versus 79% and 76% for RCCs without sarcomatoid differentiation.

Pathology
Histology
- It is seen in any histologic subtype of RCC and represents a common pathway of transformation to a high-grade, poorly differentiated tumor.
- The most common pattern is focal or diffuse malignant spindle cells.
- It is less commonly composed of large polygonal pleomorphic or multinucleated giant cells.
- Sarcomas identical to the soft part counterparts, such as leiomyosarcoma, angiosarcoma, rhabdomyosarcoma, chondrosarcoma, osteosarcoma, and hemangiopericytoma, are rarely present.
- Renal cell carcinoma component is often present, but may be overrun by the sarcomatoid component.
- Diagnosis and classification are based on the identification of the RCC component and may require extensive tissue sampling.
- Immunostains demonstrate the epithelial differentiation in the sarcomatoid component if RCC component is not identified.

Immunohistochemistry
- Sarcomatoid component positive for PAX8 (the most sensitive marker, 80%), CD10 (70%), AE1/AE3 (60%), EMA (55%), PAX2 (50%), vimentin (50%), CAM 5.2 (40%), RCC-Ag (7%), desmin (rare), smooth muscle actin (rare)
- Negative for high-molecular-weight keratin 34βE12, p63

Main differential diagnosis
- Primary sarcoma of the retroperitoneum and kidney: no epithelial component; negative for PAX8, PAX2, RCC-Ag, and epithelial markers (focal positivity for keratin may be observed in leiomyosarcoma and synovial sarcoma); diagnosis made only after sarcomatoid RCC is ruled out
- Mucinous tubular and spindle cell carcinoma: low-grade tumor cells forming compressed tubules and spindle cells with mucinous stroma

- Renal cell carcinoma with reactive stromal cells: benign reactive fibroblasts lacking cytologic atypia
- Epithelioid angiomyolipoma: no RCC component; typical angiomyolipoma possibly present; positive for HMB45 or Melan-A, or both; negative for PAX8, PAX2, RCC-Ag, and epithelial markers

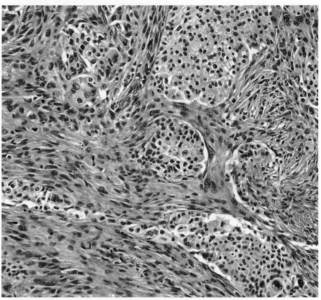

Fig 1. Chromophobe renal cell carcinoma with a sarcomatoid component.

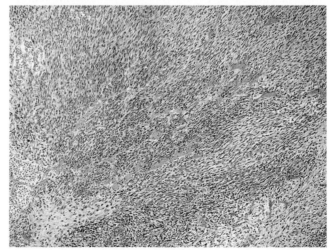

Fig 2. The most common pattern of sarcomatoid component is malignant spindle cells arranged either in sheets or interlacing fascicles. Chromophobe renal cell carcinoma is in the lower left.

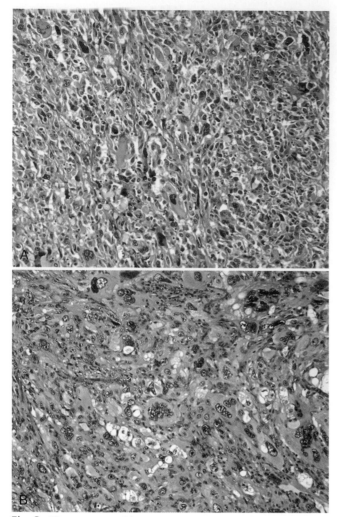

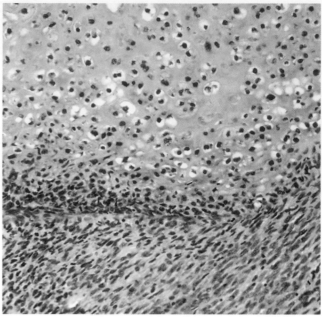

Fig 4. Sarcomatoid component showing malignant spindle cells and chondrosarcomatous differentiation.

Fig 3. The sarcomatoid component grows as large polygonal epithelioid pleomorphic cells **(A)** or large pleomorphic undifferentiated cells with frequent multinucleation **(B).**

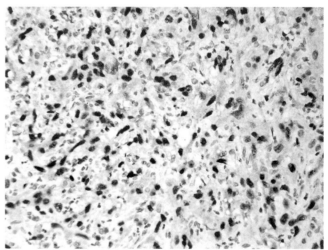

Fig 5. Sarcomatoid component stains positive for PAX8.

THYROID FOLLICULAR CARCINOMA–LIKE RENAL CELL CARCINOMA

Definition
- A newly described, rare morphologic variant of renal cell carcinoma (RCC) with a morphology that closely mimics well-differentiated thyroid follicular neoplasms

Clinical features
Epidemiology
- Rare with fewer than a dozen cases reported
- No gender or age preference in reported cases

Presentation
- Incidental findings in all reported cases

Prognosis and treatment
- Low malignant potential; aggressive behavior reported

Pathology
Gross pathology
- Solitary encapsulated mass, usually small (2 to 4 cm) but possibly as large as 12 cm
- Homogenous, tan to brown to dark brown cut surface
- Necrosis rare

Histology
- There is a prominent follicular architecture with microfollicles and macrofollicles containing a watery pink secretion or dense colloid-like material, with occasional calcifications.
- Tumor cells have a moderate amount of amphophilic to eosinophilic cytoplasm, round to oval nuclei, uniform chromatin, and inconspicuous nucleoli (mostly Fuhrman nuclear grade 2, rarely grade 3).
- Patchy lymphoid aggregates and foam cells may be seen in the background.

Immunopathology (including immunohistochemistry)
- Negative for thyroglobulin and TTF-1
- Typically negative for PAX2, WT1, CD56, vimentin, racemase, and RCC-Ag
- Occasionally positive for CK7 and CD10

Molecular diagnostics
- Gene expression profiles distinct from clear cell and chromophobe RCC

Main differential diagnosis
- Metastatic thyroid carcinoma: history of thyroid carcinoma; tumor cells positive for thyroid markers (TTF-1 and thyroglobulin)
- Oncocytoma: areas of classical oncocytoma with nests of oncocytic cells embedded in loose myxoid stroma
- Renal carcinoid: ribbons and trabeculae with hyalinized stroma; positive for neuroendocrine markers

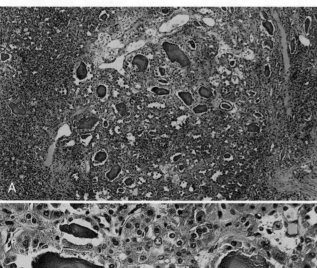

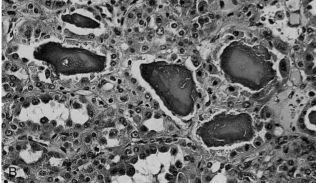

Fig 1. **A,** Thyroid follicular carcinoma–like renal cell carcinoma. The tumor displays prominent follicular architecture with some follicles containing dense colloid-like material in the lumen. **B,** Cells show hobnailing, densely eosinophilic cytoplasm, and round to ovoid nuclei with inconspicuous nucleoli.

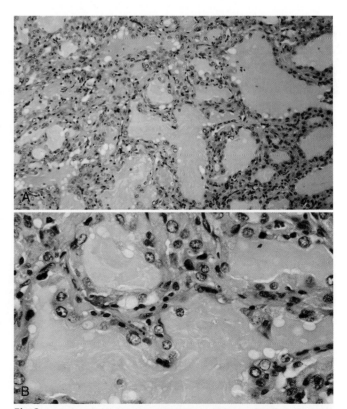

Fig 2. **A,** Thyroid follicular carcinoma–like renal cell carcinoma with watery secretion in the lumen. **B,** Cells show more prominent nuclear atypia with irregular nuclei, clumped chromatin, and conspicuous nucleoli.

Definition
- A recently described morphologic variant of RCC consisting of extensive tubulopapillary structures lined with clear cells

Clinical features
Epidemiology
- Mean age, 60.4 years (range, 26 to 88 years)
- Both genders equally affected

Presentation
- Most patients are asymptomatic and identified on imaging studies.
- Some patients have end-stage renal disease.

Prognosis and treatment
- Treatment is partial or radical nephrectomy.
- Limited follow-up shows no metastasis or recurrence after surgery.

Pathology
Gross pathology
- Small (mean size, 2.4 cm) mass in a cystic and fibrotic background

Histology
- Carcinoma is well-circumscribed with a fibrous capsule.
- Cystic and fibrotic stroma and smooth muscle bundles are infrequently present.
- Variable proportions of cysts, tubules, acini, papillae, and clear cell nests are present.
- Most characteristic patterns are branching tubules and anastomosing clear cell ribbons.
- There are closely packed tubules and acini, imparting a solid appearance.
- Cysts, tubules, and papillae are lined by cuboidal cells with a moderate amount of clear cytoplasm.
- The nuclei are round and uniform and polarized away from the basement membrane toward the luminal surface; nucleoli are not prominent (usually Fuhrman grade 1 or 2).
- There is no necrosis, perinephric, or vascular invasion.

Immunohistochemistry
- Positive for CK7 and variably positive for carbonic anhydrase IX, K903
- Negative for CD10, AMACR, and TFE3

Molecular diagnostics
- Lacks gains of chromosomes 7 and 17, and loss of chromosome Y (cytogenetic changes characteristic of PRCC)
- Lacks deletion of 3p (seen in clear cell RCC)

Main differential diagnosis
- Clear cell type RCC: no extensive papillary structures, positive for CD10, negative for CK7
- Papillary type RCC: no predominant clear tumor cells, positive for CD10 and AMACR
- Renal cell carcinoma associated with Xp11.2/TFE3 translocation: papillae lined with tumor cells with abundant clear and granular cytoplasm and high-grade nuclei; positive for TFE3

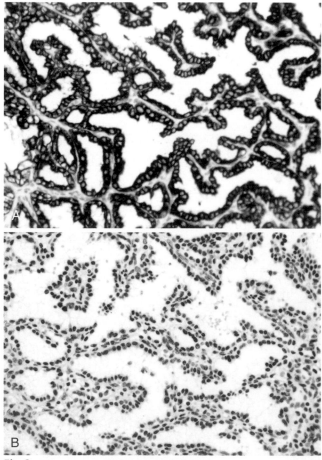

Fig 2. The tumor cells are positive for CK7 **(A)** but negative or only focally positive for CD10 **(B)**.

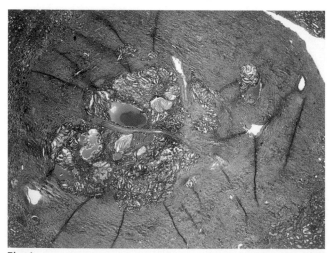

Fig 1. Low-power view of a clear cell tubulopapillary renal cell carcinoma shows prominent fibrotic stroma.

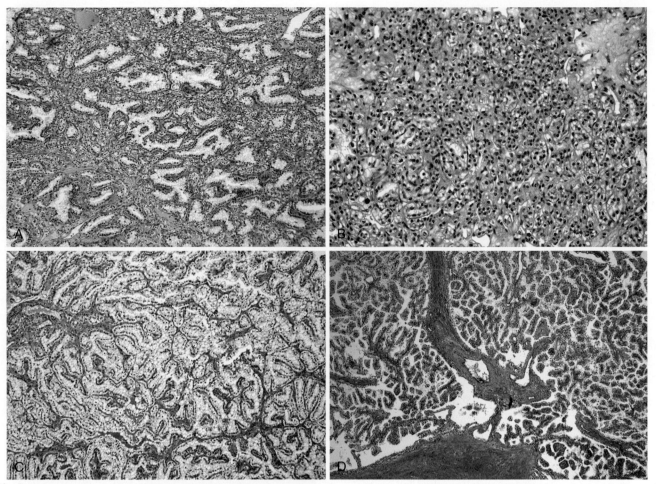

Fig 3. Several architectural patterns are observed in clear cell tubulopapillary renal cell carcinoma, including branching tubules and acini **(A)**, solid tubules and acini **(B)**, anastomosing clear cell ribbons **(C)**, and extensive papillae **(D)**.

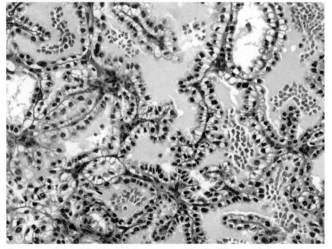

Fig 4. Tumor cells have small uniform nuclei with inconspicuous nucleoli. The nuclei are arranged away from the basement membrane and toward the luminal surface.

Definition
- A peculiar morphologic variant of renal cell carcinoma (RCC) with prominent smooth muscle–rich stroma that invests tumor cells

Clinical features
Epidemiology
- Rare, case reports in the literature
- Mean age, 54 years (range, 37 to 75 years)
- Male predominance

Presentation
- Incidental finding in the majority of cases
- Hematuria in 25% of patients

Prognosis and treatment
- Excellent prognosis in a limited study

Pathology
Gross pathology
- Small tumor (1.8 to 4 cm)
- Variegated appearance with mahogany brown, yellow, and semitranslucent white color
- Cystic changes, foci of necrosis, and calcification present

Histology
- Multinodular appearance at low power
- Tumor cells with optically clear cytoplasm
- Nests or trabeculae of tumor cells embedded in abundant fibrous stroma that contains smooth muscle bundles interspersed among tumor cells

Immunohistochemistry
- Epithelial component: positive for pancytokeratin, CK7, EMA, CD10, RCC-Ag, and CA9; negative for melanocytic markers
- Stromal component: positive for SMA, HHF35, and desmin; negative for ER and PR

Molecular diagnostics
- Inconsistent in a limited study
  - In some studies, molecular changes similar to clear cell RCC

Main differential diagnosis
- Conventional clear cell RCC: no conspicuous smooth muscle stroma, CK7 negative
- Clear cell tubulopapillary RCC: typical morphologic features, including branching tubules and clear cell ribbons; no conspicuous smooth muscle stroma; CD10 negative
- Epithelioid angiomyolipoma: melanocytic markers positive
- Mixed epithelial and stromal tumor: predominantly affecting perimenopausal female patients; clear cells not a predominant component; stroma may contain ovarian-type stroma that are positive for estrogen and progesterone receptors

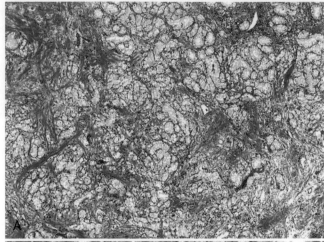

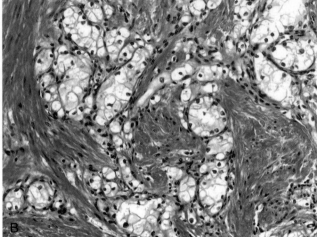

Fig 1. **A,** Renal cell carcinoma with leiomyomatous stroma showing nests and trabeculae of clear cells embedded in abundant fibrous stroma. **B,** Smooth muscle bundles are interspersed among tumor cells.

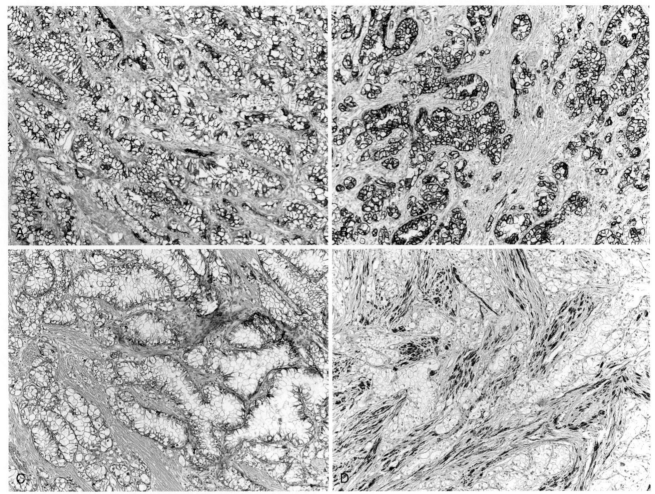

Fig 2. Immunophenotype of renal cell carcinoma with leiomyomatous stroma. The tumor cells are positive for CD10 **(A)** and CK7 **(B)** and weakly positive for CA9 **(C).** The desmin stain highlights the smooth muscle bundles between clear cell nests **(D).**

Definition
- A benign tumor recapitulating differentiation toward early embryonic metanephric tubules; also known as *embryonal adenoma* or *nephrogenic nephroma*

Clinical features
Epidemiology
- Female predominance
- Wide age range, from infants to elder individuals

Presentation
- Incidental finding of a unilateral, solitary, well-circumscribed renal mass
- Signs of a renal tumor (flank pain, hematuria, palpable mass) rare
- Polycythemia in 10% of cases

Prognosis and treatment
- Benign
- Surgical excision

Pathology
Gross pathology
- Well-circumscribed, nonencapsulated mass
- Gray to tan homogeneous cut surface

Histology
- Most tumors lack a tumor capsule and have a sharp interface between tumor and renal parenchyma.
- Tightly packed primitive tubules and acini are frequently intermixed with papillary or glomeruloid structures.
- Small, uniform tumor cells with scant cytoplasm are present.
- Nuclei are round or oval with smooth chromatin, inconspicuous nucleoli, and rare or absent mitosis.
- Stromal hyalinization, dystrophic calcification, psammomatous bodies, necrosis, and hemorrhage occur in some cases.

Immunopathology (including immunohistochemistry)
- Positive for WT1, PAX2, and CD57; negative for CK7, CD56, AMACR

Main differential diagnosis
- Papillary renal cell carcinoma often has a fibrous capsule; tumor cells may have abundant cytoplasm and prominent nucleoli and are positive for CK7 and AMACR, and negative for WT1.
- In epithelial-predominant Wilms tumor, a thick tumor capsule separates tumor from nonneoplastic renal parenchyma; tumor cells have columnar or elongated nuclei with frequent mitosis and are positive for CD56, but frequently negative for CD57.

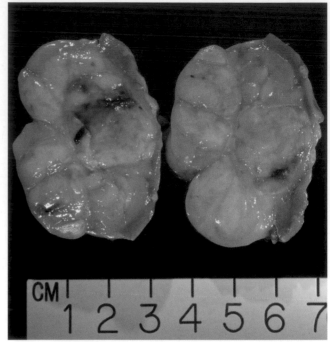

Fig 1. Metanephric adenoma forms a sharply circumscribed, unencapsulated, and lobulated mass with homogeneous tan cut surface.

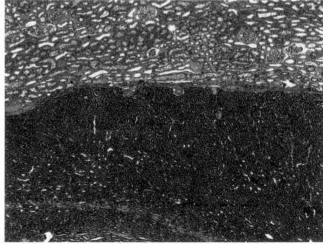

Fig 2. Metanephric adenoma forms a sharp interface with non-neoplastic kidney parenchyma without a tumor capsule.

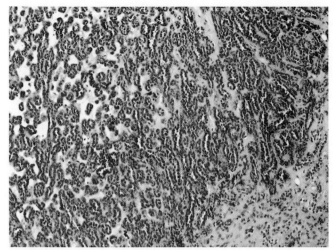

Fig 3. Metanephric adenoma with small tubules, papillae, and glomeruloid structures.

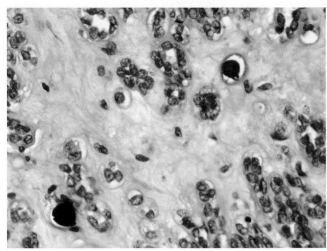

Fig 5. Metanephric adenoma often has dense hyalinized stroma. Psammomatous calcification is often seen.

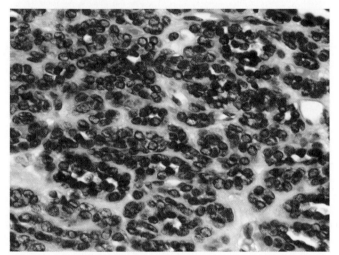

Fig 4. Tumor cells are uniform with scant cytoplasm and round nuclei with open chromatin and inconspicuous nucleoli.

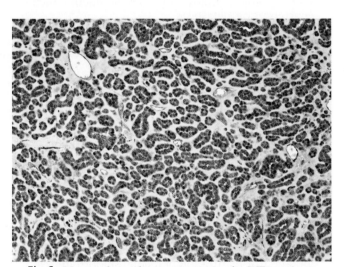

Fig 6. Metanephric adenoma is positive for WT1 antigen.

Definition
- Pediatric spindle cell renal tumor that is histologically identical to the stromal component of metanephric adenofibroma

Clinical features
Epidemiology
- Rare; fewer than 50 cases reported
- Mean age, 24 months (range, neonates to 15 years old)

Presentation
- Typically as abdominal mass
- Hypertension owing to juxtaglomerular cell hyperplasia in some patients

Prognosis and treatment
- Nephrectomy is curative; there are no documented recurrences or metastases.

Pathology
Gross pathology
- Three to 10 cm
- Typically well circumscribed
- May have cystic areas

Histology
- Low-power appearance is nodular because of alternating hypercellular and hypocellular regions.
- Cells are spindled or stellate with thin, tapered, hyperchromatic nuclei; some cases exhibit an epithelioid stroma.
- Cells surrounding entrapped renal tubules or blood vessels form concentric hypercellular or hypocellular onion-skin collarettes.
- Angiodysplasia of intratumoral arterioles with expansion and disorganization of medial smooth muscle is the most diagnostic feature, although it is not present in all cases.
- Entrapped tubules may become cystically dilated; entrapped glomeruli may show juxtaglomerular cell hyperplasia.
- Heterologous differentiation is common, including chondroid or primitive neuroectodermal-type cells.
- There is a scalloped, subtly infiltrative border with a normal kidney.

Immunopathology
- Spindle cells are positive for CD34, particularly in regions surrounding entrapped tubules.
- Desmin is negative.
- Keratins (CAM5.2, pan-cytokeratin) highlight entrapped tubules.
- S-100 may be positive in primitive neural elements.

Main differential diagnosis
- In cases of congenital mesoblastic nephroma (CMN), patients are typically somewhat younger, rarely older than 24 months; it is typically more deeply invasive and shows abrupt transitions in cellularity (linear versus nodular). Concentric collarettes around entrapped tubules are not seen in CMN; CMN is desmin positive.
- Clear cell sarcoma (CCS) is an important clinical distinction. CCS shows a branching capillary vascular pattern and lacks heterologous differentiation; CD34 is negative in CCS.
- Metanephric adenofibroma (MAF): metanephric stromal tumor (MST) and MAF form a spectrum. In MST, the normal tubular epithelial elements are entrapped and undergo embryonal hyperplasia and simulate the neoplastic epithelial element of an MAF. If the epithelial elements are present in a distinct nodule separated from normal renal parenchyma such that they are likely not entrapped, the lesion is best classified as an MAF.

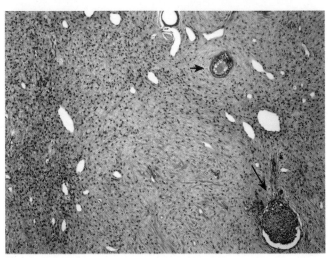

Fig 1. The appearance of alternating cellular and hypocellular areas is a characteristic low-power finding of metanephric stromal tumor. Entrapped tubules (*small arrow*) and juxtaglomerular hyperplasia (*arrow*) are also present.

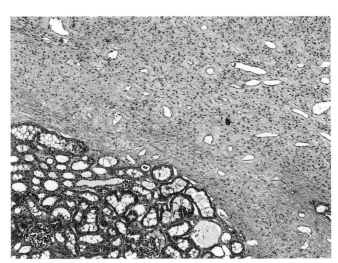

Fig 2. Scalloped border with normal kidney may be abrupt or subtly infiltrative.

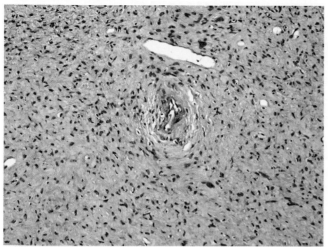

Fig 3. Cells surrounding blood vessels form hypocellular collarettes.

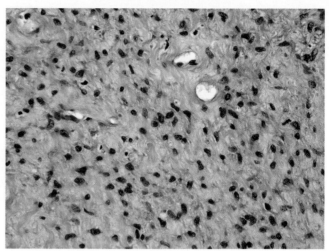

Fig 5. Cells are spindled or stellate with thin, tapered nuclei.

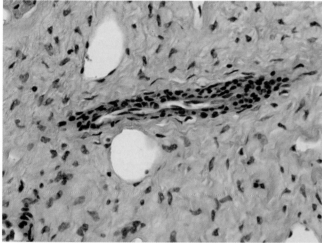

Fig 4. An intratumoral arteriole shows angiodysplasia, a diagnostic feature of metanephric stromal tumor.

Definition
- A renal tumor derived from the nephrogenic blastemal cells that recapitulate various stages of the developing kidney; also known as *nephroblastoma*

Clinical features
Epidemiology
- Affects 1/8000 to 1/10,000 children
- The most common renal tumor in children
- The most common genitourinary cancer in children
- Accounts for 8% of all pediatric cancers
- Ninety-eight percent of patients younger than 10 years
- Patient mean age: 37 months for males and 43 months for females

Presentation
- Most patients commonly have a palpable, nontender abdominal mass.
- Patients may have abdominal pain, hematuria, and acute abdomen secondary to rupture.
- Occasional paraneoplastic syndromes, including hypertension and polycythemia, are caused by renin and erythropoietin production.
- Ten percent of Wilms tumor cases are part of genetic syndromes.

Prognosis and treatment
- Treatment includes radical nephrectomy or chemotherapy, or both.
- Metastasis is most common in the regional lymph nodes, lungs, and liver.
- Most patients are at a low stage with a favorable histology, and the 4-year survival with a favorable histology approaches 90%.
- High-stage and nuclear anaplasia are unfavorable prognostic factors.

Pathology
Gross pathology
- Solitary or multinodular circumscribed mass
- Cut surface uniform, pale-pink or tan, and soft
- Cystic changes often present

Histology
- Most tumors show triphasic patterns: blastemal, epithelial, and stromal.
- In the blastemal component, there are small, closely packed, round or oval cells with scant cytoplasm forming anastomosing cords or trabeculae; the nuclei are overlapping and have evenly distributed chromatin and small nucleoli. There is frequent mitosis.
- The epithelial component recapitulates various stages of the normal nephrogenesis, ranging from primitive rosettelike structures to easily recognizable tubular or papillary elements; heterologous differentiation, such as mucinous and squamous differentiation, may be present.

- The stromal component commonly shows smooth muscle and fibroblastic differentiation; skeletal muscle, adipose tissue, cartilage, bone, ganglion cells, and neuroglial tissue may be seen.
- Anaplasia is seen in 5% of cases, is associated with a poor outcome, and is characterized by multipolar polyploid mitotic figures, marked enlarged nuclei (greater than threefold nonanaplastic nuclei), and hyperchromasia.
- Nephrogenic rests are seen in one third of kidneys.

Immunohistochemistry
- Positive for vimentin and CD56
- WT1 positive in primitive blastemal and epithelial components, but negative in differentiated epithelial and stromal components

Molecular diagnostics
- The *WT1* gene on chromosome 11p13
- *WT1* gene alterations more common in syndromic cases
  - Deletion of the *WT1* gene in WAGR syndrome (i.e., Wilms tumor, aniridia, genitourinary malformation, mental retardation)
  - Point mutation of the *WT1* gene in Denys-Drash syndrome (mesangial sclerosis, pseudohermaphroditism, and Wilms tumor)
- *WT1* gene alterations less common in sporadic Wilms tumor
  - Deletion of the *WT1* gene in one third of cases
  - Point mutation of the *WT1* gene in only 10% of cases

Main differential diagnosis
- Clear cell sarcoma: tumor cell nests demarcated by delicate, regularly spaced fibrovascular septa; tumor cells with clear cytoplasm and nuclei with finely dispersed chromatin
- Congenital mesoblastic nephroma: interlacing fascicles of fibroblastic cells with thin tapered nuclei and pink cytoplasm
- Rhabdoid tumor: vesicular chromatin, prominent cherry-red nuclei, and hyaline pink cytoplasmic inclusions
- Metanephric adenoma: no tumor capsule, uniform round or oval nuclei without nucleoli and mitosis
- Neuroblastoma: small round cells with Homer Wright rosettes; may have ganglionic differentiation and Schwannian stroma; neuroendocrine markers positive; WT1 negative
- Primitive neuroectodermal tumor (PNET)–Ewing sarcoma: sheets of monotonous polygonal cells with high nuclear-to-cytoplasmic ratio, uniform and hyperchromatic nuclei with fine chromatin and inconspicuous nucleoli; CD99 positive; WT1 negative

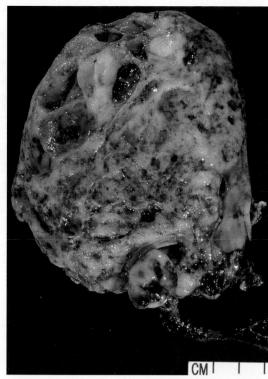

Fig 1. This Wilms tumor is well circumscribed with partially cystic and nodular cut surface. The tumor also invades into the renal vein.

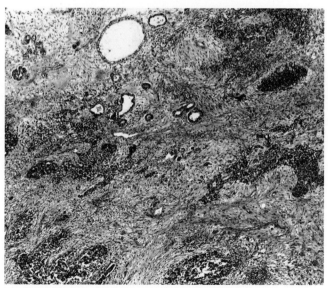

Fig 2. Wilms tumor shows typical triphasic patterns, with blastemal, tubular, and differentiated stomal components.

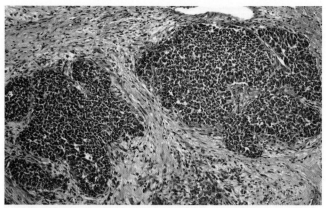

Fig 3. The blastemal component consists of small round cells with scant cytoplasm and overlapping nuclei. The blastemal cells are mitotically active.

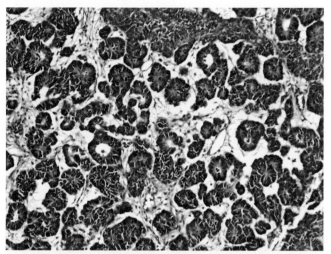

Fig 4. The epithelial cells form tubular structures.

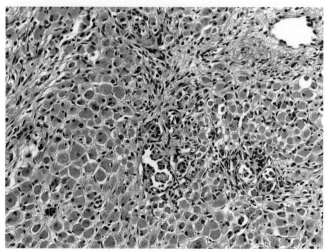

Fig 5. Skeletal muscle differentiation in the stroma.

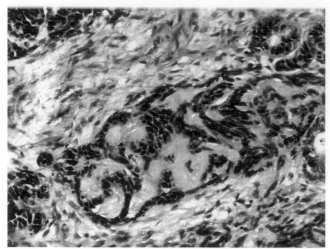

Fig 6. Wilms tumor shows mucinous differentiation in the epithelial component.

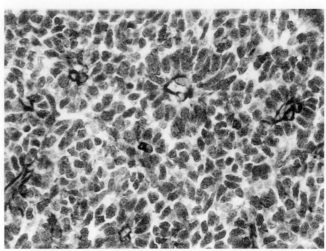

Fig 8. The tumor cells show nuclear immunoreactivity for WT1.

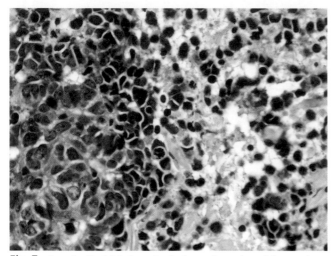

Fig 7. Anaplastic histology includes enlarged and hyperchromatic nuclei *(left)*.

NEPHROGENIC RESTS AND NEPHROBLASTOMATOSIS

Definition
- Nephrogenic rests are abnormally persistent embryonal cells that are associated with and capable of developing into nephroblastomas (Wilms tumor).
- *Nephroblastomatosis* is defined as the presence of diffuse and multifocal nephrogenic rests.

Clinical features
Epidemiology
- Encountered in 40% of patients with unilateral nephroblastoma and 90% of patients with bilateral nephroblastomas
- Observed in 1% of infant autopsies

Presentation
- Nephrogenic rests are found in nephrectomy specimens for Wilms tumor.
- Nephroblasmatosis can appear as diffusely enlarged kidneys or subtle subcapsular nodules on imaging

Prognosis and treatment
- Regression in most cases, but associated with an increased risk of synchronous or metachronous nephroblastoma
- Chemotherapy for diffuse hyperplastic nephroblastomatosis

Pathology
Histology
- Two distinct subtype: perilobar nephrogenic rests (PLNRs) and intralobar nephrogenic rests (ILNRs)
- PLNRs located in the periphery of renal lobules, sharply demarcated and usually multifocal, and composed of blastema, embryonal epithelial cells, and scant stroma
- ILPRs located randomly with the renal lobules, poorly circumscribed, usually unifocal, and composed of abundant stroma and fewer blastema cells
- PLNRs and ILNRs can pursue one or more of the following fates:
  - Incipient or dormant: microscopic lesions without proliferation
  - Sclerosing, regressing, or obsolete: mature tubular structures in a fibrotic stroma
  - Hyperplastic: enlarged foci with focal or diffuse proliferative overgrowth of blastemal and embryonal epithelial cells
  - Neoplastic: spherical clonal expansile lesion arising from nephrogenic rests
- Nephroblastomatosis applied for multifocal and diffuse nephrogenic rests

Immunohistochemistry and special studies
- Positive for WT1

Molecular diagnostics
- Cases associated with Wilms tumor have been found to share the same mutation of *WT1,* localized on chromosome 11p13.

Main differential diagnosis
- Wilms tumor: when clonal expansion develops within a PLNR, the resulting Wilms tumor is recognized by its spherical expansile growth and a peritumoral fibrous capsule that separates the tumor from the adjacent nephrogenic rests.
- Papillary adenoma is frequently encountered in adult kidney and lacks blastema; it is negative for WT1.

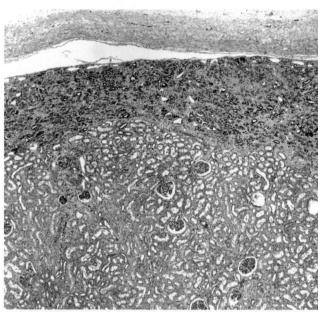

Fig 1. A perilobar nephrogenic rest is found at the periphery of the renal lobe and is composed of blastemal and primitive tubular structures.

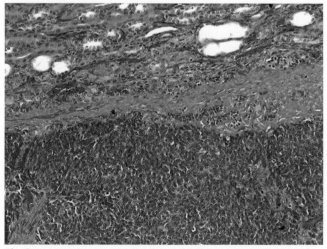

Fig 2. A hyperplastic perilobar nephrogenic rest is composed of oval collection of blastemal cells with increased mitosis.

Definition
Rare stromal neoplasm of infancy

Clinical features
Epidemiology
- Two percent to 4% of pediatric renal tumors
- Ninety percent occur in the first year of life
- Nearly all reported cases within less than 30 months of age
- Most common renal tumor diagnosed prenatally

Presentation
- Typically as a unilateral solitary abdominal mass
- Prenatal cases associated with hydramnios, hydrops fetalis, and premature delivery
- Hypertension, hypercalcemia, vomiting, and hyper-reninemia in the first days of life
- Prenatal cases sometimes diagnosed on ultrasound

Prognosis and treatment
- Excellent prognosis when completely excised
- Local recurrence and metastasis in 5% to 10% cases and confined to cases with cellular histology, stage III or greater, and involvement of intrarenal or sinus vessels

Pathology
Gross pathology
- Range, 1 to 14 cm in size (mean, 6 cm)
- Solitary, unilateral masses with soft or firm, bulging cut surface
- Cysts, hemorrhage, and necrosis common
- Most tumors centered near the renal hilus and involve the sinus

Histology
- Two major types: classic CMN and cellular CMN
- Classic CMN: 20% of CMN; morphologically similar to infantile fibromatosis
  - Intersecting fascicles of fibroblastic cells with thin tapered nuclei, eosinophilic cytoplasm, and low mitotic count
  - Abundant collagen
  - Highly irregular interface with kidney, with fascicles of tumor cells interdigitating with, but not distorting, renal parenchyma
  - Can infiltrate perinephric and renal sinus fat
- Cellular type: 60% of CMN cases; morphologically identical to infantile fibrosarcoma
  - More cellular than classic CMN
  - Closely packed cells with scanty cytoplasm, vesicular nuclei, and high mitotic count
  - Poorly formed fascicles and sheets
  - Necrosis and hemorrhage rarely seen
  - Circumscribed but unencapsulated border
- Mixed CMN; 20% of CMN cases
  - Multiple foci of cellular histology in the background of classic histology in majority of cases
  - Classic CMN at the periphery of a cellular CMN

Immunohistochemistry and special studies
- Markers of myofibroblasts, including vimentin and actin, are positive
- Desmin rarely positive
- WT1 rarely positive, but controversial
- CD34, cytokeratin, BCL2 negative

Molecular diagnostics
- Cellular CMN shares cytogenetic abnormalities with infantile fibrosarcoma, including translocation t(12;15)(p13;q25) and trisomy 11
- Classic CMN usually diploid

Main differential diagnosis
- Clear cell sarcoma: characteristic branching capillary network; tumor cells with moderate amounts of pale or clear cytoplasm and ovoid clear nuclei; actin and desmin stains are negative
- Metanephric stromal tumor: nodular appearance owing to alternating cellularity; onion-skin cuffing around entrapped renal tubules; heterologous differentiation and vascular alterations including angiodysplasia of entrapped arterioles; juxtaglomerular cell hyperplasia in entrapped glomeruli
- Wilms tumor, monophasic stromal type: blastemal and epithelial component usually present after extensive sampling; possible differentiation toward skeletal muscle or other stromal types; WT1 positive

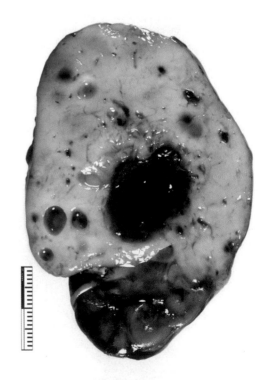

Fig 1. Congenital mesoblastic nephroma, cellular type, is well demarcated from the adjacent kidney. The tumor is fleshy with foci of cystic changes and hemorrhage.

Acknowledgments: Brett Delahunt, Wellington School of Medicine and Health Sciences, Wellington, New Zealand; and Joanna Perry-Keene and Diane Paton, Royal Brisbane Hospital, Brisbane, Australia.

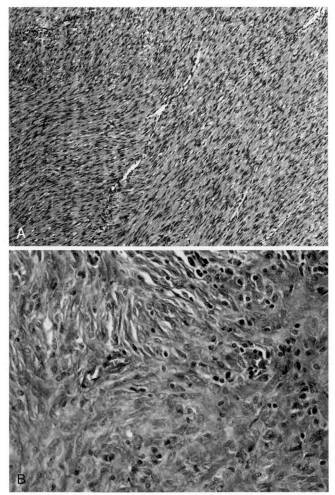

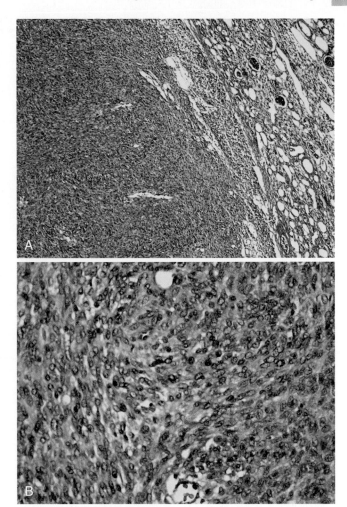

Fig 2. **A,** Congenital mesoblastic nephroma, classic type, composed of intersecting fascicles of spindle cells. **B,** The tumor cells have thin, tapered nuclei, eosinophilic cytoplasm, and low mitotic count. Abundant collagen is present.

Fig 4. **A,** Congenital mesoblastic nephroma, cellular type, displays a pushing border with the adjacent kidney. **B,** The tumor comprises sheets of closely packed plump cells with scant to moderate cytoplasm and vesicular nuclei.

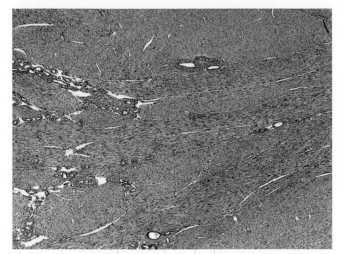

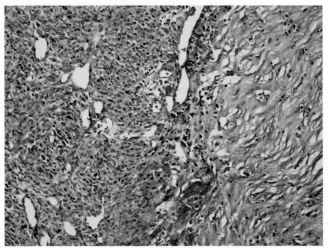

Fig 3. In congenital mesoblastic nephroma, classic type, the tumor interdigitates with renal parenchyma at the periphery.

Fig 5. Congenital mesoblastic nephroma, mixed type. The cellular type on left contrasts with the classic type on right.

RHABDOID TUMOR OF THE KIDNEY

Definition
- An aggressive childhood tumor composed of rhabdoid cells that resemble rhabdomyoblasts, although there is no true skeletal muscle differentiation

Clinical features
Epidemiology
- Two percent of pediatric renal tumors
- Virtually all patients younger than 5 years, with 80% being younger than 2 years

Presentation
- Hematuria, gross and microscopic
- Fever, hypercalcemia
- Abdominal and renal mass
- Acute abdomen from tumor rupture
- Brain tumors that resemble primitive neuroectodermal tumors in approximately 15% of patients

Prognosis and treatment
- Poor prognosis; 80% of patients dead of disease within 1 year of diagnosis
- Early metastases to distant sites
- Multimodality treatment, including surgery and chemotherapy, with no satisfactory results

Pathology
Gross pathology
- Large, hemorrhagic, and necrotic mass with invasive border

Histology
- Large polygonal tumor cells with vesicular nuclei, prominent nucleoli, and paranuclear cytoplasmic globular inclusions occur in monotonous sheets.
- The globular inclusions correspond ultrastructurally to whorled intermediate filaments.
- The tumor extensively infiltrates the adjacent renal parenchyma with many lymphovascular emboli.

Immunopathology (including immunohistochemistry)
- Tumor cells positive for vimentin and focally positive for EMA
- Negative for INI-1
- Inconsistent reactivity for cytokeratin, NSE, S100, CD99, desmin, and Leu7

Molecular diagnostics
- Biallelic inactivation of SMARCB1 (SNF5, INI-1) on chromosome 22q11, which is a component of the SWI/SNF chromatin remodeling complex via mutation, deletion, or whole chromosomal loss

Main differential diagnosis
- Wilms tumor characteristically has blastemal, epithelial, and mesenchymal components. Tumor cells are positive for WT1 antigens and CD56.
- Occasionally, rhabdoid tumor lacks the characteristic cytoplasmic inclusions and may resemble other small blue cell tumors of the childhood, including primitive neuroectodermal tumor/Ewing sarcoma and neuroblastoma. Immunostains including cytokeratin and other characteristic markers such as neuroendocrine markers and CD99 usually help to establish a correct diagnosis.

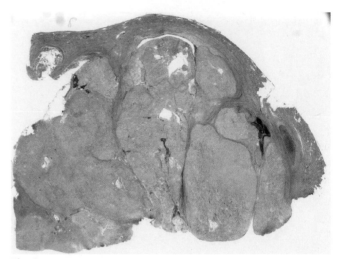

Fig 1. A 5-cm hemorrhagic and necrotic tumor in a 5-year-old boy shows a lobulated architecture and pushing border against the thinned renal cortex and capsule.

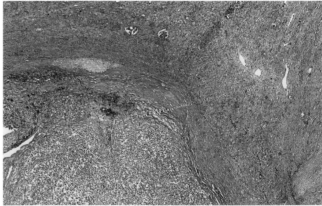

Fig 2. Sheets of loosely cohesive tumor cells. Several residual glomeruli are present within the fibrotic parenchyma.

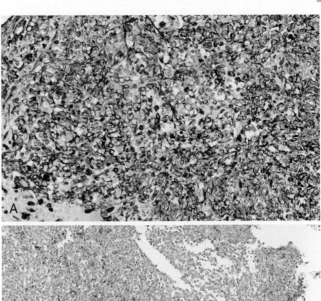

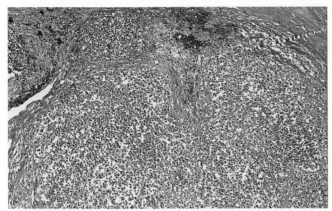

Fig 3. Alveolar nests of rhabdoid tumor cells with slender fibrous septa.

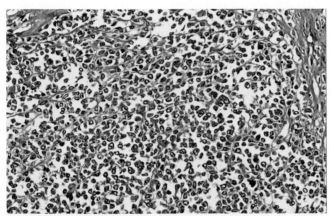

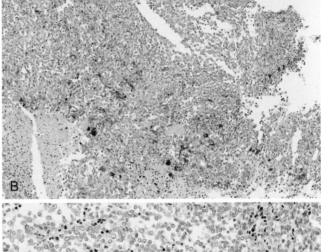

Fig 4. Tumor cells have pleomorphic vesicular nuclei with prominent nucleoli and eccentric pink cytoplasm. Some tumor cells appeared to have a cometlike appearance with cytoplasmic tails.

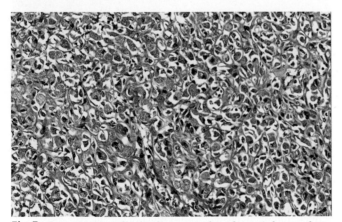

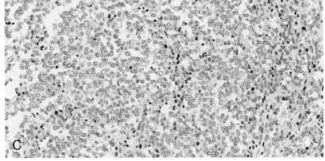

Fig 6. The tumor cells are diffusely positive for vimentin **(A)** and focally positive for epithelial membrane antigen. **(B).** INI-1 is negative in the tumor cells and positive in lymphocytes **(C).**

Fig 5. Some tumor cells display more abundant pink cytoplasm with compressed nuclei.

Definition
- Highly malignant mesenchymal tumor of pediatric kidney, also termed *bone-metastasizing renal tumor of childhood* because of its striking predilection to metastasize to bone

Clinical features
Epidemiology
- Accounts for 3% of the pediatric renal tumors, with approximately 20 new cases diagnosed annually in the United States
- Peak incidence between 12 and 36 months of age, with a sharp decline after that period
- Male-to-female ratio, 2:1 to 3:1

Presentation
- Abdominal mass, pain, hematuria, fever, and hypertension are frequent findings.
- Five percent have metastatic disease to bone, lung, abdomen, retroperitoneum, brain, and liver.

Prognosis and treatment
- Overall survival is worse than that for Wilms tumor and comparable to Wilms tumor with unfavorable histology.
- Bone metastasis is the most common form of relapse.
- Treatment is radical nephrectomy followed by radiotherapy and chemotherapy.

Pathology
Gross pathology
- Single, well-circumscribed mass
- Homogeneous light brown or tan, dense or firm, cut surface
- Multiple cysts common

Histology
- Plump, undifferentiated cells are arranged in cords or nests separated by a delicate chicken-wire vasculature
- Tumor cells are separated from each other by pale to clear mucopolysaccharide extracellular space that imparts a clear appearance.
- Tumor cells may contain dense, eosinophilic cytoplasm focally.
- Nuclei have smooth chromatin and often appear washed-out and do not have prominent nucleoli.
- Delicate vessels may be accompanied by proliferation of spindle cells or septal cells, which may be prominent.
- Tumor cells subtly infiltrate into the normal parenchyma at the periphery.

- Variant morphologic patterns have been described and include myxoid, sclerosing, cellular, epithelioid, storiform, and anaplastic.
- Anaplasia, defined by nuclear hyperchromasia, nuclear gigantism, and atypical mitoses, is usually mild and of uncertain significance.

Immunopathology
- Positive for vimentin
- Negativity for keratins and other markers
- Positivity for α1-antitrypsin and α1-antichymotrypsin

Main differential diagnosis
- Wilms tumor has a tendency to be multifocal and bilateral. Heterologous elements and nephrogenic rests rules out clear cell sarcoma of the kidney (CCSK). The borders of CCSK are usually subtly infiltrative, whereas Wilms tumor has a thick capsule. Wilms tumor is positive for WT1 and CD56.
- Conventional clear cell carcinoma of the kidney is rare in infancy. Tumor cells are positive for cytokeratin.

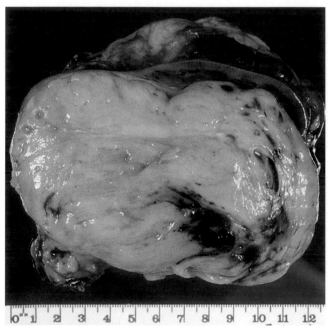

Fig 1. Clear cell sarcoma of the kidney forms a sharply circumscribed homogeneous mass with mucoid cut surface.

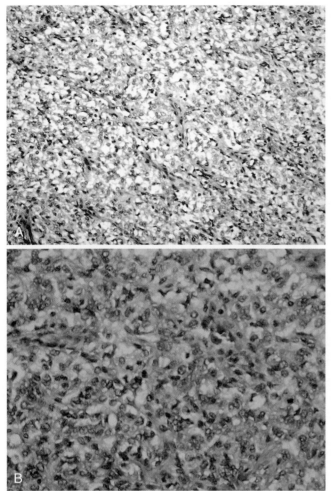

Fig 2. **A,** Clear cell sarcoma showing cords of spindled and epithelioid cells separated by thin fibrovascular septa at low magnification. The cells are separated by clear spaces. The nuclei have "washed-out" appearance with fine chromatin and inconspicuous nucleoli. **B,** There are some mitotic figures in this field.

Fig 3. Some clear cell sarcomas have more dense and eosinophilic cytoplasm. Note the "chicken-wire" vascular pattern.

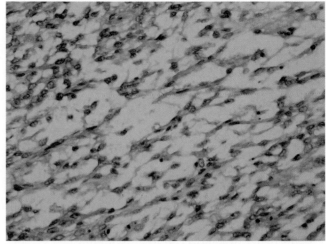

Fig 4. Clear cell sarcoma, myxoid pattern, with abundant mucoid material separating cords of tumor cells.

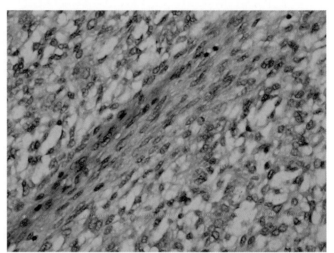

Fig 5. Clear cell sarcoma with focal spindle cell pattern.

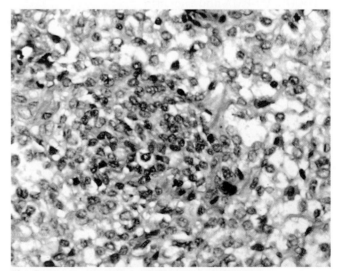

Fig 6. Clear cell sarcoma with circumscribed region of nuclear anaplasia.

OSSIFYING RENAL TUMOR OF INFANCY

Definition
- Intracaliceal mass composed of osteoid trabeculae, osteoblast-like cells, and a spindle cell component

Clinical features
Epidemiology
- Exclusively in infancy (age, 6 days to 17 months)
- Male predominant
- Left side predominant

Clinical features
- Gross hematuria most common symptom
- Palpable abdominal mass very rare
- Calcified mass by imaging studies

Prognosis and treatment
- Surgery
- Excellent; no recurrence or metastasis reported

Pathology
Gross pathology
- Well-circumscribed polypoid mass (range, 1 to 6 cm in diameter) attached to the renal pyramid
- Partially or entirely filled the pelvocalyceal system

Histology
- Three major components: osteoid trabeculae, osteoblast-like cells within and at the periphery of the trabeculae, and spindle cells
- Osteoblast-like cells with basophilic cytoplasm and a distinct border; large, eccentric nuclei
- Spindle cells ranging from elongated and fusiform to epithelioid

Immunohistochemistry
- Positive for EMA and vimentin
- Negative for cytokeratin

Main differential diagnosis
- Wilms tumor, stromal predominant type: older children; at least partially intraparenchymal location; blastemal and epithelial components present, even focally
- Extraskeletal osteosarcoma: neoplastic osteoid and bone, not infrequently together with neoplastic cartilage; tumor cells ranging from those that resemble fibrosarcoma to malignant fibrous histiocytoma

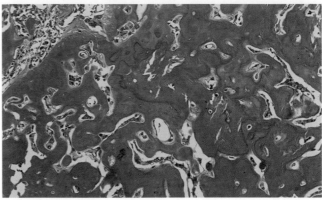

Fig 2. Osteoid trabeculae are focally lined with osteoblast-like cells.

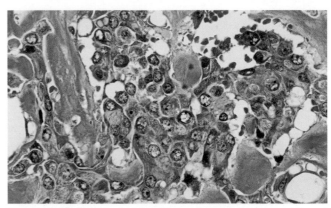

Fig 3. Epithelioid osteoblast-like cells with large nuclei and small nucleoli.

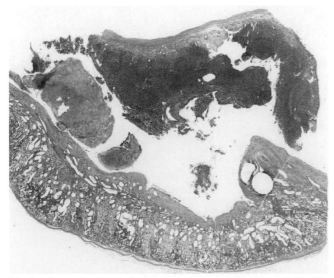

Fig 1. The tumor is attached to the renal medulla and partially fills the pelvocalyceal system. (Courtesy Dr. Yae Kanai, Tokyo, Japan.)

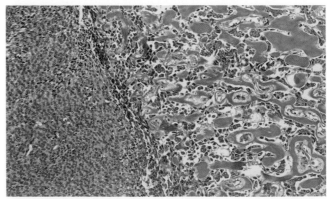

Fig 4. Transition between spindle cells and osteoid and osteoblast-like cells.

Definition

- Mesenchymal neoplasm comprising abnormal blood vessels, cells with smooth muscle features, and mature adipose tissue in variable proportions; believed to be derived from perivascular epithelioid cells, hence also named *PECOMA*

Clinical features

Epidemiology

- Accounts for 1% of all renal tumors in surgical cohorts
- Can be sporadic or associated with tuberous sclerosis (TS); sporadic angiomyolipomas (AMLs) fourfold to fivefold more common than TS-associated AMLs
- Patients with TS develop AML earlier (mean age at diagnosis is 25 to 35 years with TS versus 40 to 45 years without TS)
- More common in female patients (female to male ratio, 4:1 in patients without TS)

Presentation

- In patients with TS, AMLs are usually asymptomatic and detected by imaging studies.
- Patients without TS may have symptoms associated with a renal mass: flank pain, hematuria, or palpable mass.
- Intraabdominal bleeding owing to rupture could be an uncommon presentation initially or during follow-up.

Prognosis and treatment

- The vast majority of renal AMLs are benign and are cured by surgical resection.
- Large tumors may have the risk of hemorrhage.
- A small AML, if confirmed on needle biopsy, may be followed without immediate surgery.
- Epithelioid AML, an uncommon variant, demonstrates malignant behavior in 25% to 33% of cases.
- AML is occasionally associated with RCC.

Pathology

Gross pathology

- The majority are found in the renal parenchyma, but may be located on the capsule.
- They are typically well circumscribed with or without lobulation, sometimes with subtle infiltrative edges.
- Gross appearance depends on the relative amount of three components.
- Hemorrhage and cystic changes are common; necrosis is unusual.

Histology

- There are three components in various proportions: vessels, spindle cells, and adipose tissue.
- Vessels typically have an eccentrically thickened wall with spindle cells spun off the wall.

- Spindle tumor cells range from mature-appearing smooth muscle cells with blunt-end elongated nuclei and eosinophilic cytoplasm to immature spindle cells, epithelioid cells with or without clear cytoplasm, and bizarre cells with degenerative nuclear atypia.
- Mature adipocytes have cytologic atypia.
- Focal nuclear atypia or high cellularity is often present and is not associated with malignant behaviors.
- The presence of AML components in pelvic lymph nodes is not indicative of malignancy.
- Monomorphic (spindle cell) variant is composed predominantly of spindle cells with little or no vascular and adipose elements, typically small as incidental findings in the nephrectomy specimens.
- Cystic variant contains cystic spaces lined by benign cuboidal epithelial cells in addition to the typical components.
- Epithelioid variant contains significant amount of epithelioid cells, which are round, ovoid or pleomorphic in shape and have clear or granular cytoplasm; multinucleated or cells with a bizarre shape are common.
- Pathologic features seen in malignant AMLs are large size, tumor necrosis, atypical mitosis, and diffuse nuclear atypia.

Immunohistochemistry

- Positive for melanocytic markers, including HMB45, Melan-A, tyrosinase
- Use of a panel rather than single markers recommended; the stain with a single marker can be focal and weak
- Smooth muscle actin positive
- Keratins and other epithelial markers negative

Main differential diagnosis

- Renal cell carcinoma with eosinophilic cytoplasm: intratumoral fat exceedingly rare; epithelial markers positive; melanocytic markers negative
- Renal cell carcinoma associated with Xp11.2/TFE3 translocation: typically affecting children and young adults; characteristic features include papillae lined with clear or eosinophilic cells, psammomatous calcification and hyalinized fibrovascular cores; positive for TFE3
- Leiomyosarcoma: typically located on the renal capsule or extrarenal retroperitoneum rather than being in the renal parenchyma; high cellularity, frequent mitotic activity, and significant cytologic atypia; negative for melanocytic markers
- Myelolipoma: typically located in the adrenal gland or perirenal tissue; composed of adipose tissue and bone marrow elements; spindle cells not a component of the tumor

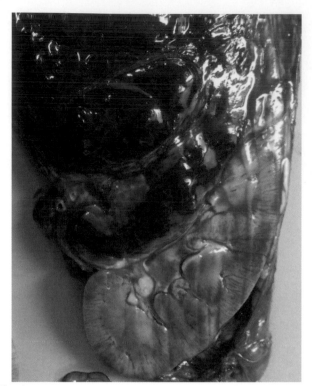

Fig 1. A large renal angiomyolipoma is 16 cm in the greatest dimension with a tan-yellow cut surface and extensive hemorrhage.

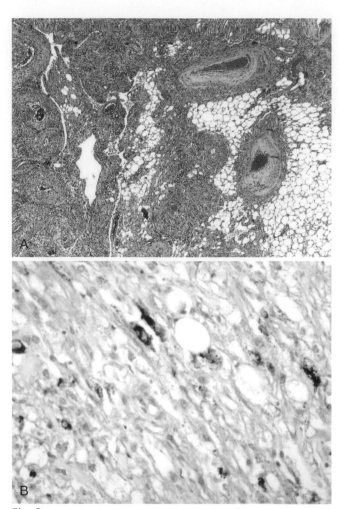

Fig 3. **A,** A typical angiomyolipoma has three components: spindle cells, adipose tissue, and blood vessels. The spindle cells appear to be spun off the abnormal thick-walled vessels. **B,** The spindle cells are positive for HMB45.

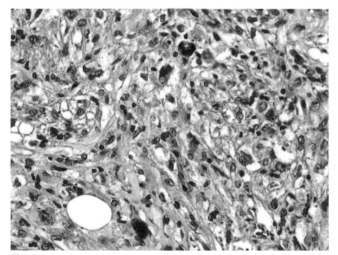

Fig 2. An angiomyolipoma showing nuclear atypia, which is degenerative with smudged chromatins.

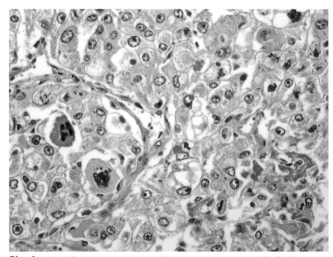

Fig 4. A malignant angiomyolipoma contains marked pleomorphic cells with bizarre nuclei and atypical mitotic figures.

Definition
- Angiomyolipoma composed predominantly of epithelioid cells, although there is no consensus on the percentage of epithelioid cells required for such a diagnosis

Clinical features
Epidemiology
- Eight percent of AMLs in surgical cohorts have epithelioid cells (10% or more of the tumor)
- Mean age, 38 years
- Both genders equally affected
- Greater than 50% of patients associated with tubular sclerosis (TS)

Presentation
- Symptoms associated with large renal mass (flank pain, palpable mass, hematuria)
- Some discovered through TS screening
- Little or no fat on radiologic study and may mimic RCC

Prognosis and treatment
- Treatment is surgical resection.
- Minor epithelioid component in an otherwise typical AML does not affect the outcome adversely.
- One fourth to one third of cases have malignant outcomes with retroperitoneal recurrence or distant metastasis.

Pathology
Gross pathology
- Usually large with an infiltrative border and invasion of extrarenal tissue and renal vessels
- Hemorrhage and necrosis possible

Histology
- Predominantly epithelioid cells forming nests and sheets; fat, smooth muscle, and thick vessels possibly present
- Epithelioid cells with cytoplasm ranging from scarce and pale to abundant, eosinophilic, and granular
- Nuclei ranging from small uniform to large and pleomorphic; multinucleated or ganglion-like cells often present but can be entirely absent
- Mitosis including atypical ones and necrosis possibly present
- Histologic features often seen in malignant tumors (three of these features predict malignant behavior): 70% or greater atypical epithelioid cells, two or more mitotic figures per 10× power fields, atypical mitosis, tumor necrosis

Immunohistochemistry
- Negative for epithelial markers (cytokeratins and EMA); rare cells positive for CAM5.2
- Positive for melanocytic markers; individual markers not always positive in 100% of cases; use a panel (e.g., HMB45, Melan-A)
- Positive for smooth muscle markers
- One third of cases positive for S100 (cytoplasmic staining, no nuclear staining)

Main differential diagnosis
- Renal cell carcinoma: extensive sampling may reveal areas characteristic of RCC; positive for epithelial markers; negative for melanocytic markers (with rare exception of translocation-associated RCC)
- Metastatic melanoma: history of malignant melanoma; multiple tumor nodules; S-100 usually diffusely positive with cytoplasmic and nuclear staining; smooth muscle markers negative

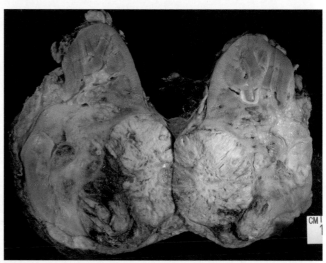

Fig 1. A large epithelioid angiomyolipoma replacing the middle and lower pole of the kidney. The tumor extensively infiltrates the perinephric fat and renal sinus. Large areas of necrosis and hemorrhage are evident.

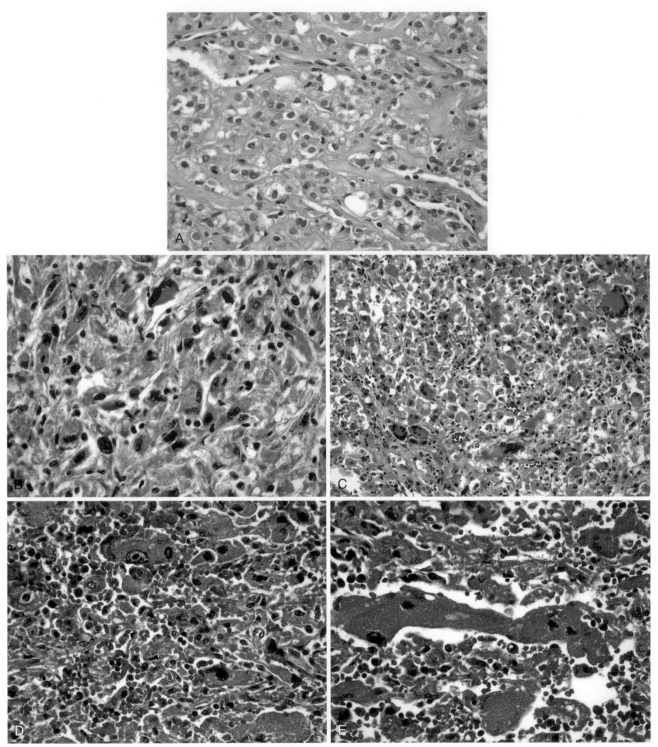

Fig 2. Cell types in epithelioid angiomyolipoma. **A,** In some cases, the epithelioid cells are relatively uniform in size and have a small amount of cytoplasm that is clear to wispy and eosinophilic and have uniform nuclei. **B,** Most cases contain large epithelioid cells that vary significantly in size and have abundant, densely eosinophilic cytoplasm. **C,** Multinucleation is present in some cases. **D,** Some tumor cells have prominent nucleoli and mimic ganglion cells. **E,** Occasionally, the tumor cells contain a large amount of cytoplasm and multiple nuclei scattered within the cytoplasm, resembling amoeboid cells.

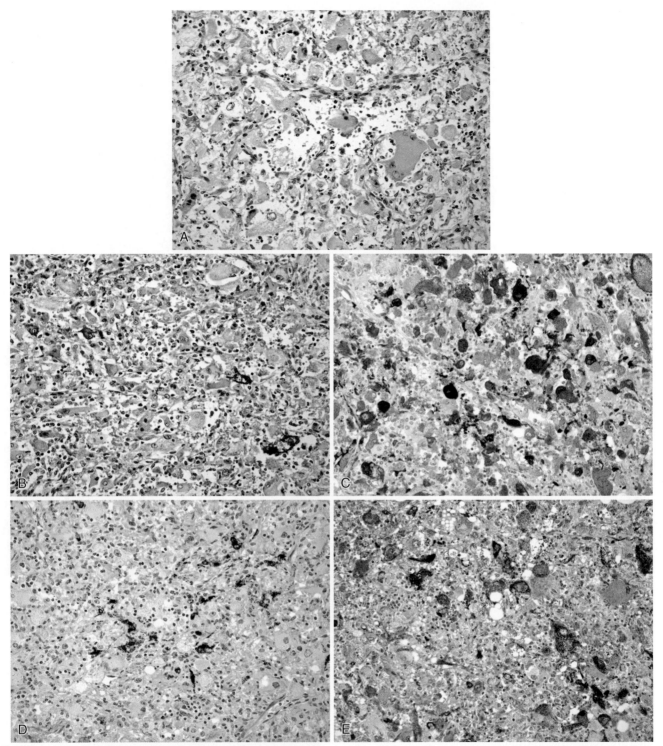

Fig 3. Immunohistochemical profile of an epithelioid AML. The tumor cells are negative for AE1/3 **(A)**, but rare cells are positive for CAM5.2 **(B)**. Melan-A is positive **(C)**, and HMB45 is focally positive **(D)**. S-100 is positive with staining in cytoplasm but not in nuclei **(E)**.

Definition
- A rare tumor differentiating toward specialized smoothmuscle cells found in the wall of the glomerular afferent arteriole; associated with excess renin production and hypertension

Clinical features
Epidemiology
- Rare tumor with less than 100 cases published
- Slight female predominance (female-to-male ratio, 2:1)
- Affects adolescents and young adults (mean age, 27 years)

Presentation
- Clinical presentation can be classified into three types:
  - Typical: hypertension, hypokalemia, hyperaldosteronism owing to high plasma renin
  - Atypical: hypertension but normokalemia
  - Nonfunctioning: normotensive and normokalemia

Prognosis and treatment
- These tumors were considered benign, but one metastatic case was recently reported.
- Treatment includes nephron-sparing surgery.

Pathology
Gross pathology
- Usually small (less than 3 cm), unilateral, cortical, and arises equally in both kidneys and either pole
- Well circumscribed, yellow-tan to gray-white, and may contain small cystic cavities

Histology
- Uniform population of round or polygonal or spindled tumor cells with granular and acidophilic cytoplasm
- Various growth patterns including trabecular, insular, solid, papillary, cystic, hemangiopericytic, and tubular
- Stroma frequently myxoid with prominent vasculature

Immunopathology and electron microscopy
- Tumor cells have cytoplasmic granules stained with modified Bowie stain, toluidine blue, and periodic acid–Schiff.
- Tumor cells are immunoreactive for renin, actin, vimentin, and CD34.
- Electron microscopy reveals characteristic rhomboid crystalline renin granules and round, electron-dense, mature, renin-like granules.

Main differential diagnosis
- The distinct clinicopathologic features this tumor are usually suggestive of the diagnosis.
- Renin secretion is not necessarily specific for this tumor because other tumors may secrete renin, and any tumor that compromises the renal artery blood flow may increase plasma renin levels.

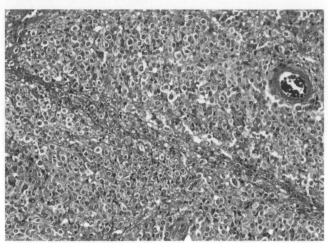

Fig 1. Juxtaglomerular cell tumor. Solid growth pattern with polygonal cells and perinuclear pale halos. (Courtesy Bernard Têtu.)

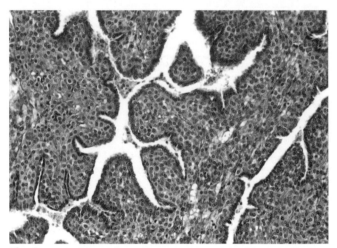

Fig 2. Juxtaglomerular cell tumor. Broad leaflike papillae are lined with uniform flat cells on the surface, and the cores are populated with polygonal cells with acidophilic cells. (Courtesy Bernard Têtu.)

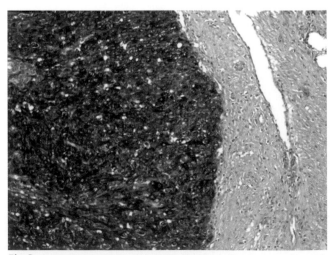

Fig 3. Juxtaglomerular cell tumor. Tumor cells are strongly positive for renin immunostain. (Courtesy Bernard Têtu.)

RENAL MEDULLARY FIBROMA (RENOMEDULLARY INTERSTITIAL CELL TUMOR)

Definition
- Mesenchymal tumor arising from the specialized interstitial cells of renal medulla

Clinical features
Epidemiology
- Found in up to 40% to 50% of autopsies
- No gender predilection
- Rare in the first two decades of life; increased incidence with age thereafter
- Multiple tumors in half of cases

Presentation
- Almost always asymptomatic lesions found incidentally in kidneys removed for other reasons or found at autopsy

Prognosis and treatment
- Benign lesions with no clinical significance

Pathology
Gross pathology
- Well-circumscribed, firm, gray-white round nodules in the medulla
- Usually less than 0.5 cm in diameter (range, less than 1 mm to 1 cm)
- Unencapsulated

Histology
- Composed of randomly arranged, benign-appearing, spindle or stellate-shaped cells
- Typically paucicellular with a loose collagenous or myxoid, faintly basophilic stroma
- Hyalinization or amyloid deposition in some lesions
- Entrapped medullary tubules at the periphery of the lesion
- No mitotic activity or features of malignancy

Immunohistochemistry and special studies
- Abundant acid mucopolysaccharides in stroma positive for periodic acid–Schiff or Alcian blue

Main differential diagnosis
- Leiomyoma: well-formed smooth muscle bundles positive for smooth muscle markers
- Metanephric stromal tumors: affects young pediatric patients; spindle tumor cell surrounding entrapped renal tubules or blood vessels form concentric onion-skin collarettes

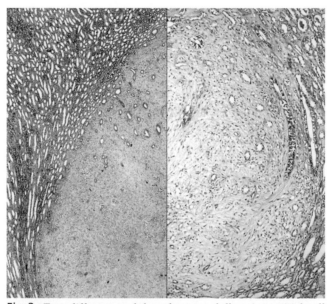

Fig 2. Two different nodules of renomedullary interstitial cell tumor. Unencapsulated hypocellular lesions composed of basophilic matrix and bland mesenchymal cells.

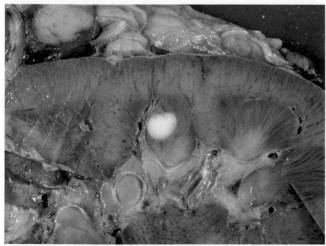

Fig 1. A renomedullary interstitial cell tumor appears as a well-circumscribed, gray-white, solid, firm nodule in the medulla.

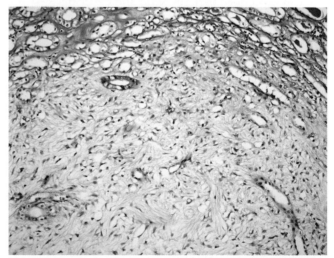

Fig 3. Medullary spindle or stellate-shaped interstitial cells, some with vacuolated cytoplasm, form a well-demarcated nodule. A few renal tubules are entrapped at the periphery.

CYSTIC NEPHROMA AND MIXED EPITHELIAL AND STROMAL TUMOR OF THE KIDNEY

Definition
- Cystic nephroma and mixed epithelial and stromal tumor (MEST) are benign neoplasms composed of epithelial and stromal components.
- They are categorized as different entities under an umbrella term *mixed mesenchymal and epithelial tumors* in the 2004 World Health Organization classification.
- Recent studies suggest that they represent different parts of the morphologic spectrum of the same lesion, based on their similar clinicopathologic and molecular features.

Clinical features
Epidemiology
- Adult patients
- Striking female predominance, with a female-to-male ratio of 7:1 to 8:1

Presentation
- Typically perimenopausal female patients
- A few case reports of male patients receiving estrogen therapy for prostate cancer or with liver disease
- Symptoms and signs associated with a kidney mass

Prognosis and treatment
- Nephrectomy
- Benign
- Sarcoma arising in MEST rarely reported, but MEST to sarcoma sequence questionable

Pathology
Gross pathology
- Cystic nephroma
  - Encapsulated and circumscribed, entirely cystic mass
  - No solid areas or necrosis
- MEST
  - Circumscribed partially solid and cystic mass
  - Often projects into the renal pelvis

Histology
- Cystic nephroma and MEST are composed of epithelial and stromal components in various proportions.
- Stroma ranges from hypocellular and hyalinized, hypocellular, hypercellular and ovarian stroma–like (only in female patients) to smooth muscle fascicles.
- Calcification, xanthomatous histiocytes, and thick-walled vessels can be seen in the stroma.
- Epithelial component ranges among tubules and cysts of variable sizes.
- Epithelial cells range among flat, cuboidal, hobnail, columnar, and urothelium-like; cytoplasmic clearing can be seen.
- Epithelial component tends to be more complex in MEST.

Immunohistochemistry
- Spindle stromal cells often positive for estrogen and progesterone receptors

Main differential diagnosis
- Cystic nephroma in pediatric patients: considered to be an entirely differentiated nephroblastoma; preferentially affecting boys (male to female ratio, 2:1) typically younger than 4 years
- Multilocular cystic RCC: multiple cysts lined with one or a few layers of clear cells; no significant amount of stroma
- Sarcomatoid RCC: both epithelial and stromal components exhibiting significant cytologic atypia
- Adult Wilms tumor: typically triphasic with blastemal, epithelial, and stromal components

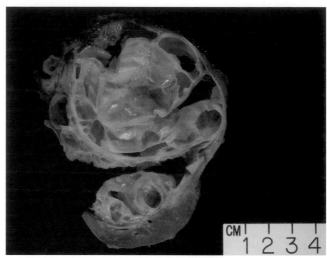

Fig 1. A partial nephrectomy specimen containing a cystic nephroma with a fibrous capsule and multiple cysts with thin septae. No solid areas are present.

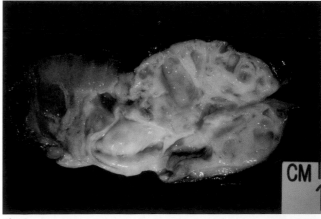

Fig 2. A partial nephrectomy specimen containing a mixed epithelial and stromal tumor. The tumor is well circumscribed and multicystic. Solid fibrotic areas are present.

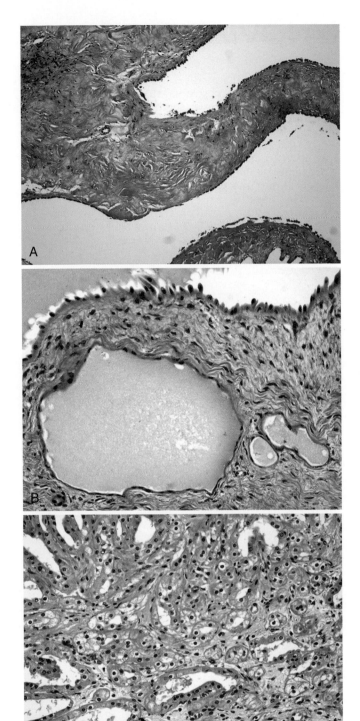

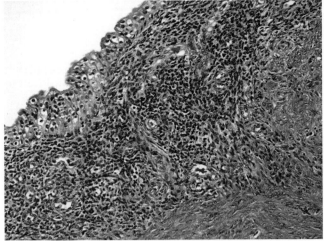

Fig 4. Hypercellular, ovarian-type stroma can be seen in both cystic nephroma and mixed epithelial and stromal tumor in female patients.

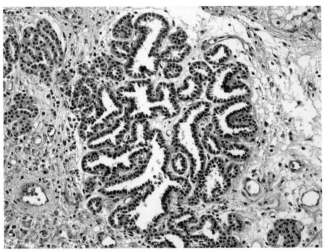

Fig 5. A mixed epithelial and stromal tumor containing glands with complex and branching contour.

Fig 3. **A,** A cystic nephroma showing paucicellular hyalinized stroma and cysts lined with cuboidal cells. **B,** In other areas, cysts are lined with hobnail cells. **C,** Cytoplasmic clearing is seen in a mixed epithelial and stromal tumor.

PRIMARY RENAL SYNOVIAL SARCOMA

Definition
- A extremely rare spindle cell tumor with rare epithelial differentiation and the characteristic translocation t(X;18)(p11.2;q11)

Clinical features
Epidemiology
- Wide age range (17 to 71 years), with a mean age of 39 years
- No sex predilection; male-to-female ratio, 1:1

Presentation
- Flank or abdominal pain; gross hematuria
- Rarely present as a palpable mass
- Some patients asymptomatic, with the mass as an incidental finding

Prognosis and treatment
- Highly aggressive tumor
- Metastatic disease common, with the lung being one of the most common sites
- No established treatment guidelines

Pathology
Gross pathology
- Large, necrotic, and grossly cystic
- Extension into the perirenal soft tissue or renal hilum, or both, present in many cases

Histology
- Most commonly monophasic, but poorly differentiated; biphasic pattern also possible
- Highly cellular with short intersecting fascicles
- Scant and ill-defined cytoplasm
- Oval to fusiform nuclei with coarse chromatin, variably sized nucleoli, and readily identifiable mitosis
- Prominent cystic component lined with hobnail cells with eosinophilic cytoplasm

Immunohistochemistry and special studies
- Tumor cells may be positive for EMA, calretinin, vimentin, CD99, and BCL2.
- Tumor cells are negative for cytokeratin, S100 protein, CD34, smooth muscle actin, and HMB45.

Molecular diagnostics
- Characterized by the translocation t(X;18)(p11.2;q11) that generates a fusion between the *SYT* gene on chromosome 18 and a member of the *SSX* family gene on chromosome X
- Monophasic primary renal synovial sarcoma (PRSS) more commonly associated with *SYT-SSX2*
- Biphasic PRSS more commonly associated with *SYT-SSX1*

Main differential diagnosis
- Mixed epithelial and stromal tumor: Lacks cytologic atypia and brisk mitosis seen in synovial sarcoma
- Primitive neuroectodermal tumor: small round blue cells growing in sheets and lobules; positive for CD99 and Fli-1; harbor t(11;22) or t(21; 22) translocations
- Adult Wilms tumors: blastemal component may predominate, but other epithelial and stromal components almost always present; WT1 positive but CD99 and Fli-1 negative
- Extrarenal synovial sarcoma: history of a primary synovial sarcoma or a large retroperitoneal synovial sarcoma with extension to the kidney

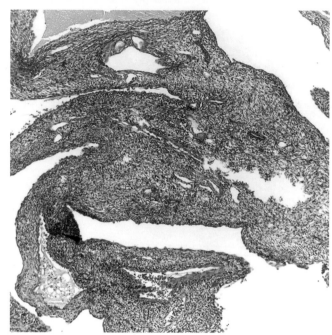

Fig 1. A primary renal synovial sarcoma with prominent cystic spaces that are surrounded by hypercellular spindle cells. The cysts are lined with hobnail cells with eosinophilic cytoplasm.

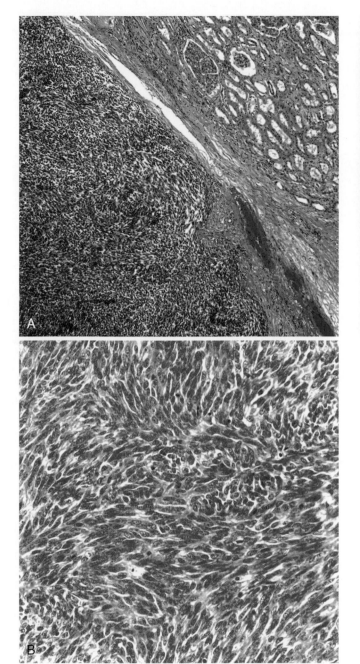

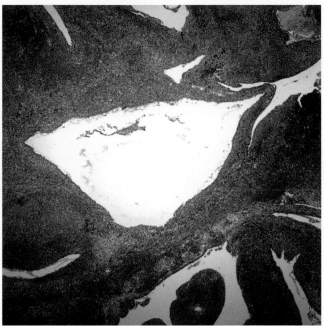

Fig 3. A primary renal synovial sarcoma with cystic spaces that are surrounded by solid sheets of blue spindle cells. The cysts are lined with bland eosinophilic cells.

Fig 2. A monophasic primary renal synovial sarcoma with adjacent benign renal parenchyma. **A,** The neoplasm consists of solid cellular sheets of plump spindle cells with a loosely fascicular growth pattern. **B,** At higher magnification, the tumor cells have scanty cytoplasm with plump nuclei. Some nuclei are round; others are more spindly. The chromatin is coarse. The mitosis brisk.

RENAL CARCINOID TUMOR

Definition
- Neuroendocrine neoplasm arising within the renal parenchyma

Clinical features
Epidemiology
- Rare tumor (fewer than 100 cases reported)
- Average age, 52 years (range, 27 to 78 years)
- No gender predilection
- May arise occasionally in a horseshoe kidney or renal teratoma

Presentation
- Flank pain
- Hematuria
- Abdominal mass
- Rarely present with symptoms of carcinoid syndrome

Prognosis and treatment
- Treatment involves surgical resection of the primary tumor.
- There is no standardized treatment for metastatic disease.
- Regional lymph node metastases are common at resection.
- Distant metastases to bone, liver, and lung can occur.

Pathology
Gross pathology
- Solid tan-brown homogenous appearance
- Average size, 6.4 cm (range, 2 to 17 cm)
- Majority unifocal, but possibly multifocal

Histology
- Tumor is well circumscribed with a distinct tumor-kidney interface.
- Tightly packed cords and trabeculae are present.
- Occasionally solid nests or glandlike lumina may be evident.
- Half of all cases demonstrate extracapsular extension through the renal capsule.
- Twenty-four percent of cases demonstrate calcification.
- Variable stroma may appear dense and sclerotic.
- Nuclei have finely granular chromatin with mild to moderate pleomorphism.
- Mitoses are usually limited to fewer than 2 per 10 high-power fields (HPF), although 3 to 4 per 10 HPF has been documented.

Immunopathology
- Approximately 90% of tumors show synaptophysin and Cam5.2 immunoreactivity.
- Chromogranin is positive in 65% of cases.
- Vimentin is positive in the majority of cases.

Main differential diagnosis
- Metastatic carcinoid tumor: history of a primary carcinoid tumor, possibly multifocal

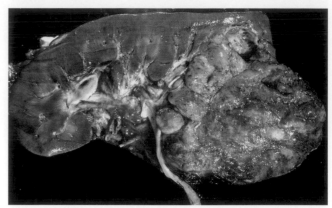
Fig 1. Grossly, renal carcinoid tumor is often tan-brown and homogenous.

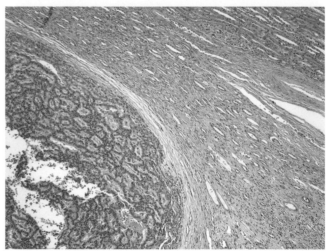
Fig 2. The junction between normal kidney and tumor is often sharply defined.

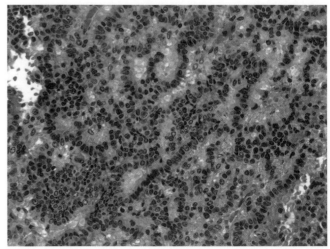
Fig 3. Compressed cords and trabeculae of cells are most commonly identified.

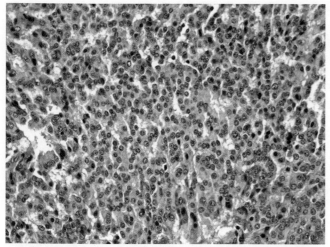

Fig 4. Rarely, tumors may demonstrate solid nests of cells.

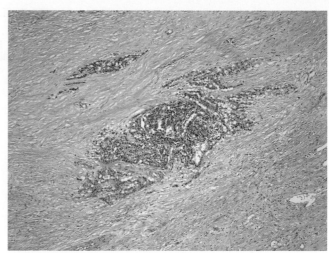

Fig 6. Stroma is variable, but may be dense and hyalinized in a subset of cases.

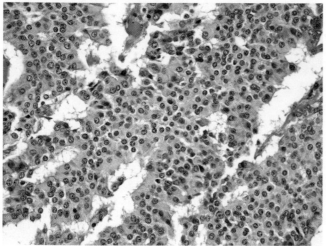

Fig 5. High magnification reveals relatively bland nuclei with finely stippled chromatin.

FUHRMAN GRADING SYSTEM FOR RENAL CELL CARCINOMA

Definition
- Histologic grading system based on nuclear size, shape, and nucleolar prominence

Comments
- Criteria of Fuhrman grading system:
  - Grade 1: nuclear size less than 10 μm, round nuclear shape, smooth nuclear contour, dense chromatin, inconspicuous nucleoli, no mitosis
  - Grade 2: nuclear size, 15 μm; round nuclear shape; slightly irregular nuclear contour; finely granular chromatin; nucleoli small but not visible at ×10 magnification; mitosis rare
  - Grade 3: nuclear size, 20 μm; round to oval nuclear shape; irregular nuclear contour; coarsely granular chromatin; nucleoli prominent and visible at ×10 magnification; occasional mitosis
  - Grade 4: nuclear size greater than 20 μm, pleomorphic and multilobate nuclear shape, irregular nuclear contour, clumped and hyperchromatic chromatin, macronucleoli, frequent mitosis
- How to assign Fuhrman grade
  - It is impractical to measure the diameter of nuclei.
  - Assessing nuclear feature (size, shape, chromatin pattern) and nucleoli at ×10 magnification is the key to Fuhrman grading.
  - Most RCCs are heterogeneous in nuclear grades, with two or more different grades in the same tumor.
  - Grading is based on the worst (highest) grade area of at least one 40× field, not counting scattered cells.
- Prognostic significance of Fuhrman grading system
  - Fuhrman grade is an independent prognostic predictor for clear cell RCC.

- Simplified two-tiered (G1-2 versus G3-4) or three-tiered (G1-2 versus G3 versus G4) Fuhrman systems have been proposed to improve interobserver agreement and still preserve its prognostic significance.
- The prognostic value of Fuhrman grading for non–clear cell RCC remains controversial.
- Fuhrman grading system is of little or no utility for chromophobe RCC.

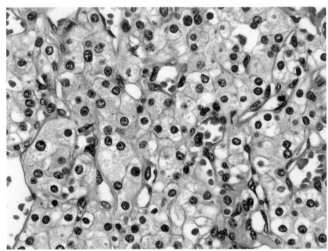

Fig 2. Fuhrman grade 2 in clear cell renal cell carcinoma. Nuclei are larger than those of grade 1 tumor cells and in general round. The chromatin is open. Nucleoli are only visible at ×20 magnification.

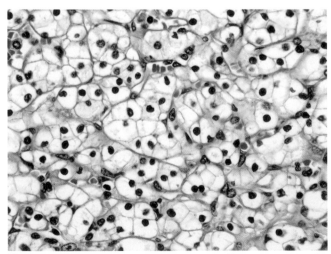

Fig 1. Fuhrman grade 1 in clear cell renal cell carcinoma. Nuclei are small and round with dense chromatin and inconspicuous nucleoli, like mature lymphocytes. Note the vascular endothelial cells have open chromatin and small nucleoli and could be mistaken for tumor nuclei.

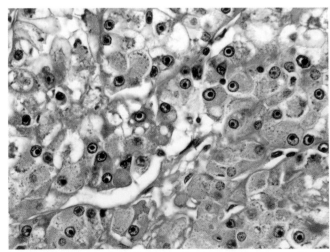

Fig 3. Fuhrman grade 3 in clear cell renal cell carcinoma. Nuclei are enlarged and irregular. Nucleoli are prominent and visible at ×10 magnification.

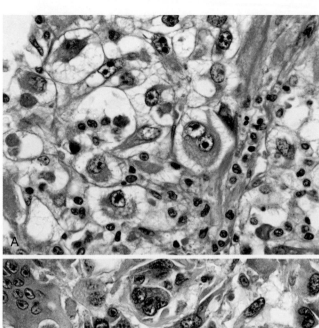

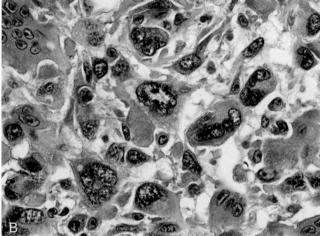

Fig 4. Fuhrman grade 4 in clear cell renal cell carcinoma. Nuclei are obviously irregular with one or more macronucleoli (A) or pleomorphic nuclei (B).

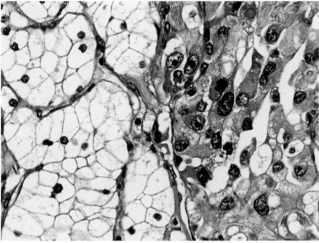

Fig 5. Fuhrman grade heterogeneity with grade 2 and grade 4 nuclei juxtaposed.

Definition
- Tumor–lymph node metastasis (TNM) staging for primary renal cell carcinoma (RCC)

Comments
- Careful gross examination of tumor extension in a nephrectomy specimen is important and should guide tissue sampling for histologic examination.
- Renal sinus fat involvement is often underrecognized. The renal sinus fat should be carefully examined and sampled.
- Direct and contiguous adrenal involvement by the renal tumor is classified as pT4. It is therefore important to distinguish from noncontiguous or metastatic involvement of adrenal gland by RCC (M1).
- Regional lymph node metastasis is staged as N1. Involvement of lymph nodes beyond the regional lymph nodes is staged as M1, not N1.
- TNM of RCC (2010)
  - Primary tumor (T)
    - TX: primary tumor cannot be assessed
    - T0: no evidence of primary tumor
    - T1: tumor 7 cm or less in greatest dimension, limited to the kidney
      - T1a: tumor 4 cm or less in greatest dimension, limited to the kidney
      - T1b: tumor more than 4 cm but not more than 7 cm in greatest dimension, limited to the kidney
    - T2: tumor greater than 7 cm in greatest dimension, limited to the kidney
      - T2a: tumor more than 7 cm but not more than 10 cm in greatest dimension, limited to the kidney
      - T2b: tumor more than 10 cm in greatest dimension, limited to the kidney
    - T3: tumor extends into major veins or perinephric tissue, but not into the ipsilateral adrenal gland and not beyond Gerota fascia
      - T3a: tumor grossly extends into the renal vein or its segmental (muscle containing) branches, or it invades perirenal or renal sinus fat, or both, but not beyond Gerota fascia
      - T3b: tumor grossly extends into vena cava below diaphragm
      - T3c: tumor grossly extends into vena cava above diaphragm or invades the wall of the vena cava
    - T4: tumor invades beyond Gerota fascia, including contiguous extension into the ipsilateral adrenal gland
  - Regional lymph nodes (N)
    - NX: regional nodes cannot be assessed
    - N0: no regional lymph node metastasis
    - N1: metastasis in regional lymph nodes
  - Distant metastasis (M)
    - M0: no distant metastasis
    - M1: distant metastasis

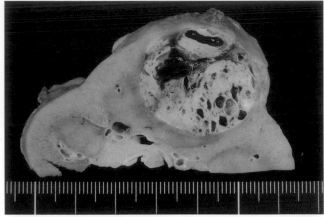

Fig 1. A 2.7-cm clear cell renal cell carcinoma grossly confined to the kidney, stage pT1a.

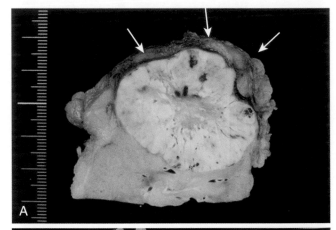

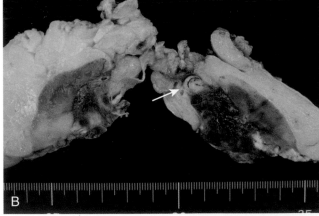

Fig 2. A, A clear cell renal cell carcinoma grossly invades into the perinephric fat. **B,** Another renal cell carcinoma grossly invades the renal sinus fat. The tumor-perinephric fat and sinus interface should be generously sampled to confirm the perinephric fat–renal sinus invasion and hence stage pT3a.

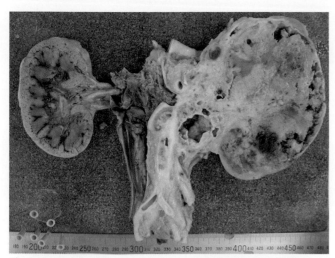

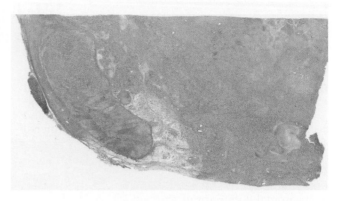

Fig 4. An RCC invaded the adrenal gland *(left)* contiguously from the tumor and was staged as pT4.

Fig 3. A postmortem examination of a patient with a large renal cell carcinoma that extended into subdiaphragmatic vena cava. This tumor would be staged as T3b in a surgical specimen.

Definition
- An autosomal dominant disease caused by germline mutations in the von Hippel-Lindau *(VHL)* gene and characterized by a constellation of neoplasms including renal cysts and clear cell RCC

Clinical features
Epidemiology
- Autosomal dominant disease
- Affects 1/36,000 to 1/45,000 births

Presentation
- Renal cysts and carcinoma affect 70% of patients.
- Renal tumors develop earlier in patients with VHL disease, with the mean age of onset of 37 years compared with 61 years for sporadic cases.
- Most renal tumors are asymptomatic and are detected in screening imaging studies.

Prognosis and treatment
- Metastatic RCC is the leading cause of death in patients with VHL disease.
- Early detection with nephron-sparing surgery is the key for treatment of RCC.
- Patients with renal involvement have a better prognosis than do their sporadic counterparts.

Pathology
Gross pathology
- Renal tumors tend to be bilateral and multifocal.
- In resected specimens, hundreds of microscopic tumor foci can be identified.
- Bright yellow, well-circumscribed, multiple masses are often associated with multiple renal cortical cysts containing clear fluid.

Histology
- Renal tumors in patients with VHL disease are clear cell RCC.
- Renal cysts are lined with clear cells.
- Small nodules of clear cells are present.

Immunohistochemistry and special studies
- IHC profile essentially the same as sporadic clear cell RCC

Molecular diagnostics
- The *VHL* gene is located on chromosome 3p25-26.
- VHL protein regulates hypoxia inducible factor and hypoxia-induced genes.
- Different mutations in the *VHL* gene are associated with variable phenotypes and distinct clinical manifestations.

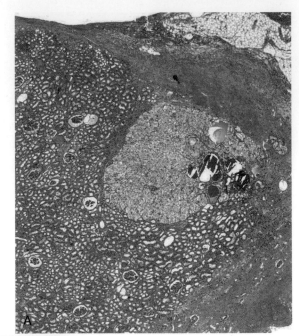

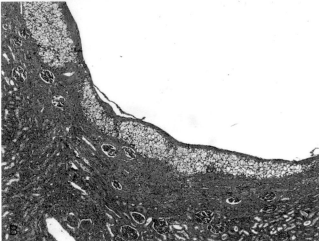

Fig 1. Clear cell renal cell carcinoma in von Hippel-Lindau disease. Characteristically, small clear cell renal cell carcinoma nodules are found within normal renal parenchyma **(A)** and the wall of a renal cyst **(B).**

Definition

- An autosomal dominant syndrome characterized by a constellation of benign skin follicle tumors, multiple renal cell neoplasms, and spontaneous pneumothorax

Clinical features

Epidemiology

- Rare autosomal dominant disease with an incidence of 1/36,000 to 1/45,000
- Mutations in *BHD* gene on chromosome 17
- *BHD* gene encoding folliculin protein

Presentation

- Patients exhibit cutaneous lesions (fibrofolliculomas), kidney masses, or spontaneous pneumothorax.
- In most cases, skins lesions are identified first.
- Renal tumors are found mostly by imaging studies; occasionally, patients exhibit symptoms and signs associated with RCC, including flank pain and palpable mass.
- Spontaneous pneumothorax can occur as the result of ruptured pulmonary cysts.

Prognosis and treatment

- The renal tumors can be malignant or benign. They are often multiple and bilateral. The treatment of the kidney tumors is the key to patient management.
- Close follow-up of the renal tumors, minimal surgery with local resection of tumors to conserve renal function, and multiple resections may be necessary.
- Skin lesions and pulmonary cysts are benign. Resection of skin or lung lesions is performed if necessary for confirmation of diagnosis and treatment.
- Surveillance of the first-degree relatives of a patient with Birt-Hogg-Dube (BHD) syndrome is important.

Pathology

Histology

- Diagnostic criteria of BHD syndrome include skin and kidney tumors and lung lesion (or pneumothorax)
- Skin tumors
  - Small lesions in the head, neck, and upper trunk are common.
  - Fibrofolliculoma is a circumscribed proliferation of collagen and fibroblasts that surround the distorted hair follicles from which blastoid cells protrude into fibromucinous stroma.
  - Other skins lesions such as acrochordon (fibroepithelial polyp) and trichodiscoma (fibrovascular tumor) are also reported as the defining lesions of BHD syndrome.
- Renal tumors
  - Lesions are typically multiple and well circumscribed (mean, 5.6 per kidney), with a tan to brown cut surface.
  - Histologically the tumors can be hybrid oncocytic tumors (50%). Morphologically they can resemble other renal tumors such as chromophobe RCC (34%), clear cell RCC (9%), oncocytoma (7%), or papillary RCC (2%).

- Hybrid oncocytic tumors have features between oncocytoma and chromophobe RCC and may contain clusters of tumor cells with clear cytoplasm.
- Lung lesions (pulmonary cysts)
  - Found in 24% of patients with BHD syndrome
  - Lined with a single layer of cuboidal or columnar epithelium, the rupture of which can lead to pneumothorax

Immunohistochemistry and special studies

- Hybrid oncocytic renal tumor cells positive for C-kit
- Patchy CK7 positivity in hybrid renal tumors

Molecular diagnostics

- Diagnosis of BHD syndrome can be established by identification of mutations in the *BHD* gene.
- Exon 11 of the *BHD* gene harbors hot spots for mutations in patients.

Main differential diagnosis

- Oncocytic papillary RCC: composed of tumor cells with eosinophilic cytoplasm and occasional papillary structures. This tumor is positive for CK7 and AMACR, but negative for C-kit.
- Metastatic oncocytic tumors to the kidney: malignant oncocytic tumors such as Hürthle cells carcinoma of the thyroid can metastasize to the kidney. However, oncocytic epithelial tumors develop in other organs in patients with BHD syndrome, especially in the thyroid, which should be distinguished from the metastatic oncocytic tumor of the kidney.
- Renal oncocytomas and chromophobe RCCs: when multiple oncocytic renal tumors are seen in young patients, the possibility of BHD syndrome should be considered. Clusters of clear cells are not found in a typical oncocytoma or chromophobe RCC. Genetic testing to confirm the diagnosis of BHD syndrome is important for the clinical management of the patients and for their families.

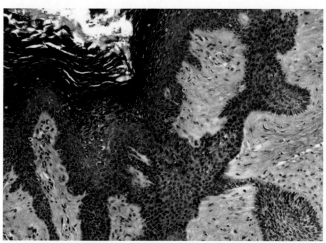

Fig 1. Skin fibrofolliculoma.

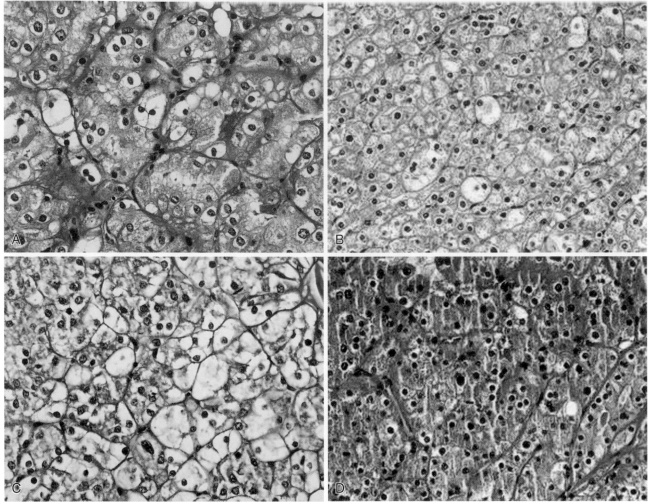

Fig 2. Renal tumors in patients with Birt-Hogg-Dube syndrome displaying morphology resembling several histologic variants of renal epithelial tumors including: hybrid oncocytic tumor with features of both oncocytoma and chromophobe renal cell carcinoma (RCC) and scattered clear cells **(A)**, chromophobe RCC **(B)**, clear cell RCC **(C)**, and oncocytoma **(D).**

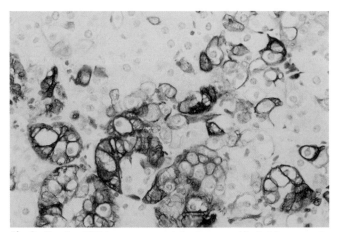

Fig 3. Patchy CK7 immunoreactivity in a renal hybrid oncocytic tumor.

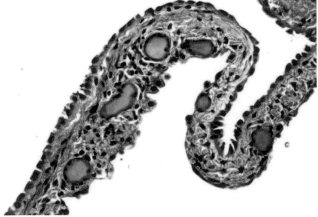

Fig 4. Lung cysts lined with a single layer of cuboidal cells.

HEREDITARY LEIOMYOMATOSIS AND RENAL CELL CARCINOMA SYNDROME

Definition
- Autosomal dominant hereditary cancer syndrome with stigmata of cutaneous leiomyomas, uterine fibroids, and papillary RCC of type II morphology

Clinical features
Epidemiology
- Rare; only a few more than 100 affected families reported around the world
- Cutaneous leiomyoma age of onset: mean, 25 years; range, 10 to 47 years
- Uterine fibroids age of onset: mean, 30 years; range, 18 to 52 years
- Renal tumors in 15% of patients, with a median age of 44 years

Prognosis and treatment
- Cutaneous leiomyoma rarely progresses to leiomyosarcoma.
- Uterine leiomyosarcoma occurs in a subset of female patients.
- Renal tumors are aggressive and have the propensity to grow quickly and metastasize early, and the distant metastasis is often detected at diagnosis.

Pathology
Gross pathology
- Cutaneous leiomyomas: firm, skin-colored to light-brown papules and nodules; the number increase with time; the number range from 10 to 1100, and the size range from 0.4 to 2.5 cm; disseminated or combination of disseminated and segmental distribution
- Uterine fibroids: numerous and large, ranging from 1 to 20 tumors and from 1.5 to 10 cm in diameter
- Renal tumors: solitary and unilateral

Histology
- Uterine lesions: majority benign fibroids; rare cases with atypia or leiomyosarcoma; very prominent nucleoli with perinucleolar clearing possible in tumor cells
- Renal tumors: majority are type II papillary RCC featuring papillae covered by large cells with abundant eosinophilic cytoplasm and very large nuclei with prominent, eosinophilic nucleoli with perinucleolar clearing, resembling cytomegalovirus nuclear inclusion; collecting duct RCC and oncocytic tumors rarely reported

Molecular diagnostics
- The gene is mapped to 1q42.3-43 and contains 10 exons that encode fumarate hydratase, which is involved in tricarboxylic acid cycle.
- The fumarate hydratase gene is a tumor suppressor, as biallelic inactivation is found in nearly all uterine leiomyomas and papillary RCC.

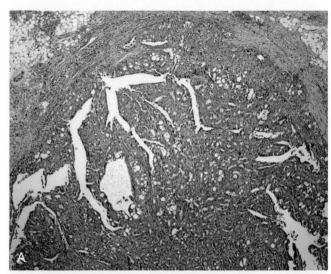
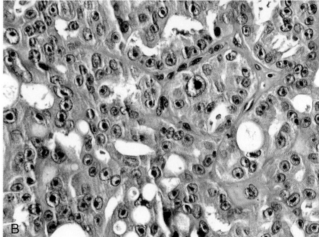

Fig 1. **A,** Low-power view of hereditary leiomyomatosis and renal cell carcinoma syndrome with cribriform architecture. **B,** At high power, the tumor cells have abundant granular cytoplasm and large eosinophilic nucleoli with perinucleolar halo reminiscent of cytomegaloviral inclusion bodies, a hallmark of these tumors.

Definition
- Renal tumors affecting patients with tuberous sclerosis complex (TSC)

Clinical features
Epidemiology
- TSC is the second most common genetic neurocutaneous disease, affecting 1 in 10,000 live births in the United States.
- It is transmitted in an autosomal dominant fashion.

Presentation
- Benign tumors involving multiple organ systems
  - Skin lesions: facial angiofibromas, periungual fibromas, shagreen patches, and hypopigmented macules
  - Central nervous system: subependymal nodules and giant cell astrocytomas
  - Cardiac rhabdomyomas, pulmonary lymphangioleiomyomatosis, and retinal hamartomas
  - Renal lesions: bilateral and multifocal angiomyolipomas of the kidneys, clear cell RCC, and oncocytomas
  - Renal angiomyolipoma in TSC
    - It is found in 80% of patients with TSC.
    - Renal masses are mostly incidental finding; occasionally, renal mass or hemorrhage can be the initial presentation in patients with TSC.
    - Patients with TSC develop angiomyolipomas earlier than sporadic patients do. The mean age at diagnosis is 25 to 35 years with TSC and 40 to 45 years without TSC.

Prognosis and treatment
- Angiomyolipomas are benign.
- Treatment is surgical resection.

Pathology
Histology
- Angiomyolipomas associated with TSC are histologically identical to the sporadic angiomyolipomas.
- Microscopic angiomyolipoma focus in grossly unremarkable renal parenchyma away from the main tumor in a majority of cases.
- Epithelioid angiomyolipoma is associated with TSC.
- An epithelial cyst is present within or at the periphery of an angiomyolipoma lined by flat to hobnail epithelial cells and is positive for pancytokeratin.

Immunohistochemistry and special studies
- Same as sporadic angiomyolipomas

Molecular diagnostics
- Two genes linked to TSC
- Tuberous sclerosis complex 1 (*TSC1*) gene, on chromosome 9q34, encodes hamartin
- Tuberous sclerosis complex 2 (*TSC2*) gene, on 16p13, encodes tuberin

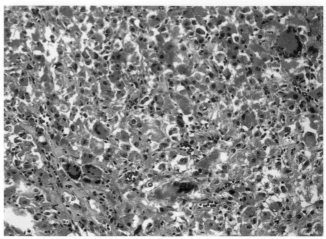

Fig 1. An epithelioid angiomyolipoma in a patient with tuberous sclerosis complex.

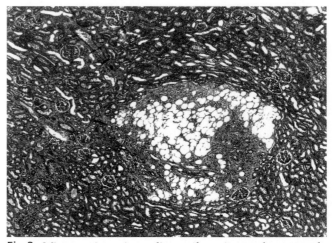

Fig 2. Microscopic angiomyolipoma focus in grossly unremarkable renal parenchyma away from the main angiomyolipoma in a patient with tuberous sclerosis complex.

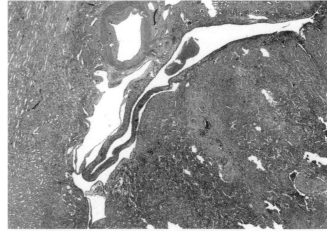

Fig 3. Epithelial cyst in angiomyolipoma associated with tuberous sclerosis complex.

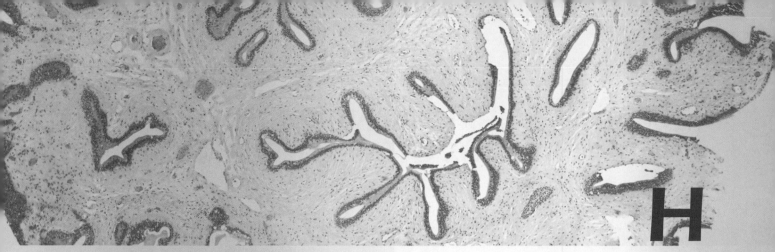

H

RENAL PELVIS AND URETER

PROLIFERATIVE URETERITIS, INCLUDING FLORID VON BRUNN NESTS AND URETEROPYELITIS CYSTICA ET GLANDULARIS

Definition
- Normal variation of urothelial histology, frequently associated with inflammation or other causes of reactive changes

Clinical features
Epidemiology
- Increased incidence with age, but less common than similar lesions of the urinary bladder (proliferation of von Brunn nests seen in 10% of normal ureters at autopsy versus 85% to 95% of bladders)
- No gender predilection

Presentation
- Associated with urinary tract infections, calculi, instrumentation, chemotherapy, and irradiation therapy
- Gross and microscopic hematuria
- May form a mass lesion mimicking a urothelial neoplasm

Prognosis and treatment
- Benign
- No treatment required

Pathology
Histology
- von Brunn nests
  - Invaginations of benign urothelial nests may show a connection with the surface urothelium.
  - Cells are cytologically bland but may be slightly larger than the overlying surface urothelial cells.
  - Nests are rounded and smooth and have an orderly spatial arrangement with a uniform maximal depth into the lamina propria (noninfiltrative base).
- Ureteropyelitis cystica
  - von Brunn nests have become cystically dilated with formation of a luminal space.
  - Cysts may contain eosinophilic fluid and occasionally inflammatory cells.
- Ureteropyelitis glandularis
  - Contains a cuboidal or columnar cell lining with mucin secretion
  - Possible presence of intestinal-type goblet cells
- These three patterns commonly present in the same biopsy specimen

Main differential diagnosis
- Nested variant of urothelial carcinoma: uneven and infiltrative base, cytologic atypia in the cells at the infiltrative base

- Inverted papilloma: interconnecting cords and trabeculae of urothelial cells with peripheral palisading and central streaming nuclei
- Adenocarcinoma: frank infiltrative growth with significant nuclear atypia

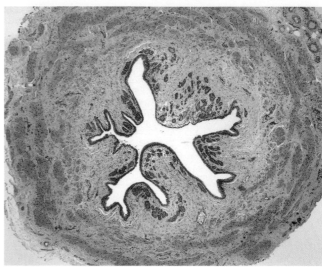

Fig 1. At low magnification, florid von Brunn nests maintain an association with the surface urothelium. The nests are rounded and smooth and have an orderly spatial arrangement with a uniform maximal depth into the lamina propria.

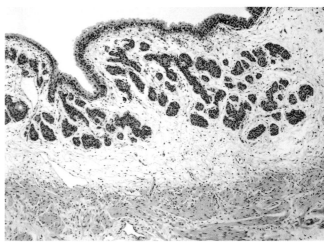

Fig 2. In florid ureteritis, urothelial nests are composed of relatively bland urothelial cells that extend to the same level in the lamina propria. The overlying urothelium is completely benign.

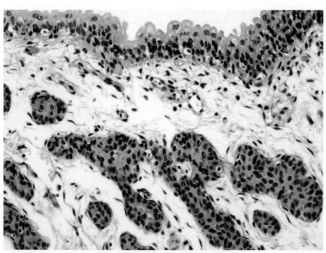

Fig 3. Cytologically the urothelial cells within von Brunn nests are similar to the basal and intermediate cells of the surface urothelium with only occasional atypia.

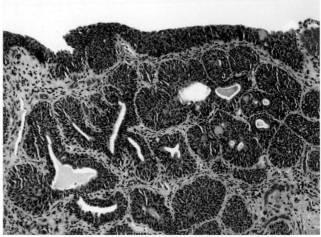

Fig 5. Ureteritis glandularis consists of cystically dilated von Brunn nests containing dense, pink secretions and a more secretory-appearing cuboidal or columnar surface epithelial layer.

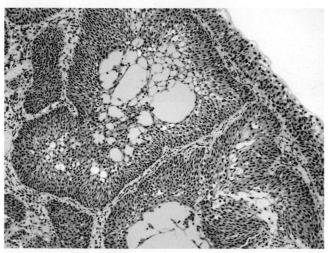

Fig 4. The term *ureteritis cystica* describes von Brunn nests with cystically dilated central spaces.

URETEROPELVIC JUNCTION OBSTRUCTION

Definition
- Obstruction of the urine flow from the renal pelvis to the proximal ureter owing to blockage at the ureteropelvic junction

Clinical features
Epidemiology
- Most cases sporadic
- Can appear at any age
- In children
  - Most common cause of pediatric hydronephrosis affecting 1 in 1000 to 2000 newborns
  - Twenty percent to 30% bilateral
  - Predominantly affecting boys (male-to-female ratio > 2:1 in neonates) and on the left side (67%)
  - Etiology
    - Defects in muscularis (75%)
    - Extrinsic compression by an aberrant renal vessel (6% to 24%)
    - Abnormally high insertion of ureter
- In adults
  - Most often unilateral
  - Predominantly in women
  - Etiology: kidney stones, upper tract inflammation, scarring from a past surgery or tumors

Presentation
- Periodic abdominal and flank pain
- Urinary tract infection
- Hematuria
- Rarely massive hydronephrosis filling the entire flank and abdomen
- Five percent to 20% associated with other urologic malformations in children

Prognosis and treatment
- Prophylactic antibiotic therapy in moderate-to-severe cases and close monitoring in patients with renal function better than 40%
- Surgical intervention (pyeloplasty) in patients with significant loss of renal function, recurrent urinary tract infection, and suspicion for tumor

Pathology
Gross pathology
- Funnel-shaped ureteropelvic junction
- May have valvelike intraluminal protrusion of edematous mucosa or muscularis
- Rarely stenotic obliteration

Histology
- Segmental smooth muscle attenuation, often with preponderance of longitudinal fibers
- Segmental absence of smooth muscle
- Stenotic lumen with normal smooth muscle

- Excess collagen deposition between muscle bundles on electron microscopic studies
- Diffuse lack of fascicular organization in pelvic muscles

Main differential diagnosis
- Retroperitoneal fibrosis: fibrosing process encasing the ureter; dense fibrosis with variable amount of chronic inflammation

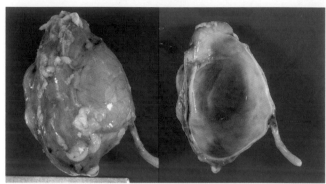

Fig 1. Nephrectomy specimen from a 1-year-old child with ureteropelvic obstruction leading to marked hydronephrosis and loss of renal parenchyma.

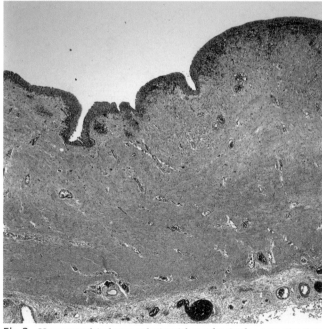

Fig 2. Hypertrophied muscularis without fascicular organization and excess collagen deposition in the renal pelvic wall proximal to the obstruction at the ureteropelvic junction.

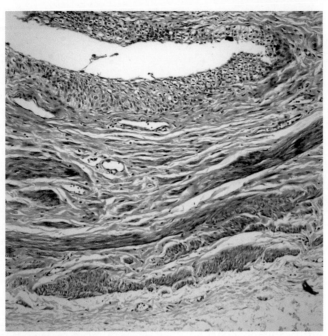

Fig 3. A section taken from a narrowed ureteropelvic junction. Preponderance of longitudinal smooth muscle fibers and increased collagen are noted on trichrome stain.

Definition
- Inflammatory and fibrosing process involving retroperitoneal structures with uncertain etiology

Clinical features
Epidemiology
- Wide age range with a peak in the fourth to sixth decades
- Men affected more frequently than women

Presentation
- Nonspecific complaints (flank, back, and abdominal pain)
- Abdominal mass on imaging
- Ureteral obstruction

Prognosis and treatment
- Most important issue is to identify any secondary cause of retroperitoneal fibrosis
- Surgical lysis of fibrosis encasing retroperitoneal structures
- Steroids and tamoxifen

Pathology
Histology
- Early stage: variably intense mixed inflammatory infiltrates with minimal fibrosis; plasma cells may predominate
- Late stage: dense collagen deposition with minimal inflammation; nerves and vessels often entrapped in the fibrosis and inflammation

Main differential diagnosis
- A variety of etiologies must be considered and ruled out clinically and pathologically.
  - Iatrogenic (drugs, surgery, radiation therapy)
  - Inflammatory (vasculitis, aneurysm, diverticulitis, inflammatory bowel disease)
  - Neoplastic processes (sclerosing lymphoma, metastatic carcinoma)

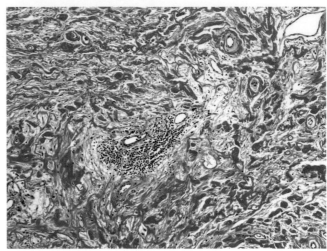

Fig 1. Retroperitoneal fibrosis. Dense fibrosis with minimal mixed lymphocytic infiltrates.

FIBROEPITHELIAL POLYP OF THE URETER AND RENAL PELVIS

Definition
- Benign urothelium-lined polypoid mesenchymal proliferation, etiology uncertain

Clinical features
Epidemiology
- Can occur at any age, the most common being benign polypoid lesion of the ureter in children
- Slightly male predominance (male-to-female ratio, 3:2)

Presentation
- Frequently involves the upper ureter, but can occur anywhere along the urothelium from renal pelvis to urethra
- Hematuria, urinary tract infection
- Flank pain or lower urinary tract symptoms, depending on the location
- Possibly associated with urogenital malformations

Prognosis and treatment
- Benign; no recurrence if completely excised
- Treated with endoscopic local resection

Pathology
Gross pathology
- Polypoid firm lesions ranging from 0.5 mm to 12 cm

Histology
- The polyp is composed of a loose fibrovascular stroma with overlying benign urothelium, in a fingerlike or polypoid architecture.
- The urothelium may show squamous metaplasia, glandular differentiation, and denudation.
- The stroma shows variable degree of fibrosis, smooth muscle, and vasculature proliferation.
- Degenerative atypia may be seen in both epithelium and stroma.

Main differential diagnosis
- Polypoid ureteritis, pyelitis, cystitis: associated with marked inflammation and edema
- Benign urothelial papilloma and inverted papilloma: florid urothelial proliferation forming papillae with thin and delicate fibrovascular cores; stroma not prominent

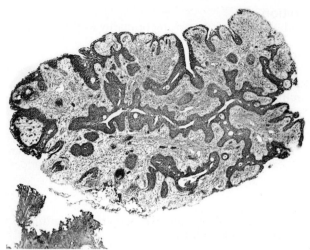

Fig 1. Fibroepithelial polyp, with prominent smooth muscle in the stroma.

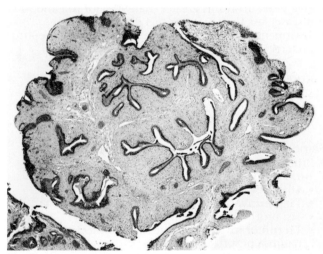

Fig 2. Fibroepithelial polyp, edematous fibrous stroma lined with benign urothelium and simple columnar epithelium.

Definition
• Urothelial carcinoma arising primarily in the ureter

Clinical features
Epidemiology
• Represents approximately 2% to 3% of all urothelial carcinomas
• More common in men than women (male-to-female ratio, 1.7:1 to 2:1)
• Tobacco use (strong risk factor)
• More than two thirds of patients with previous, concurrent, or subsequent urothelial carcinoma of the bladder

Presentation
• Hematuria
• Obstruction (hydroureter–hydronephrosis) leading to flank pain, pyelonephritis

Prognosis and treatment
• Stage is the only significant prognostic factor on multivariate analyses.
• Five-year survival is greater than 90% for pTa and pT1 disease; less than 50% for pT3 disease.
• Treatment includes partial ureterectomy, total nephro-ureterectomy, or chemotherapy.

Pathology
Histology
• Similar to urothelial carcinoma elsewhere in the urinary tract

Pathologic staging tumor node metastasis (TNM)
• Primary tumor (T)
  • Tx: cannot be assessed
  • T0: no evidence of primary tumor
  • Ta: noninvasive papillary urothelial carcinoma
  • Tis: urothelial carcinoma in situ
  • T1: tumor invades subepithelial connective tissue (lamina propria)
  • T2: tumor invades muscularis propria
  • T3: tumor invades beyond muscularis propria into periureteral soft tissue
  • T4: tumor invades adjacent organs or through the kidney into perinephric fat
• Regional lymph nodes (N)
  • Nx: cannot be assessed
  • N0: no regional lymph node metastasis
  • N1: metastasis in a single regional lymph node measuring 2 cm or less in greatest dimension
  • N2: metastasis in a single regional lymph node measuring greater than 2 cm but less than 5 cm in greatest dimension or metastases in multiple regional lymph nodes with none measuring greater than 5 cm in greatest dimension
  • N3: metastasis in a regional lymph node measuring greater than 5 cm in greatest dimension
  • Specify number of lymph nodes examined as well as number involved (any size)
• Distant metastasis (M)
  • Not applicable (do not include pM in pTNM staging unless status is pM1)
  • M1: distant metastasis pathologically documented (specify sites)

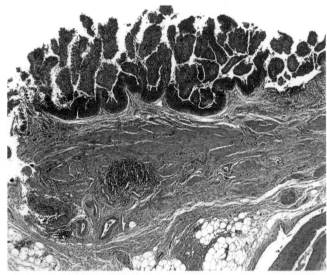

Fig 2. Noninvasive papillary urothelial carcinoma of the ureter (pTa).

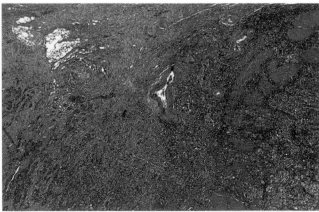

Fig 1. Urothelial carcinoma invading through the muscularis propria *(right)* to involve the periureteral soft tissue (pT3).

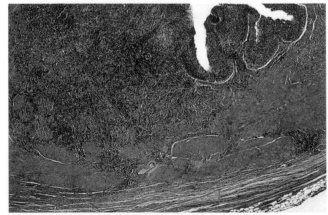

Fig 3. Urothelial carcinoma invading muscularis propria of the ureter (pT2).

Definition

- TNM staging for urothelial carcinoma arising from the renal pelvis, including the urothelium lining the renal papillae and minor and major calces
- Absent lamina propria (subepithelial connective tissue) beneath the urothelium lining the renal papillae in the pelvis and thin along the minor calyces
- For renal pelvic tumors, pagetoid spread of carcinoma into renal collecting ducts and renal tubules does not affect stage, while carcinoma invading into the renal parenchyma is pT3
- Primary tumor (T)
  - TX: primary tumor cannot be assessed
  - T0: no evidence of primary tumor
  - Ta: noninvasive papillary urothelial carcinoma
  - Tis: carcinoma in situ
  - T1: tumor invades subepithelial connective tissue
  - T2: tumor invades the muscularis propria
  - T3: tumor invades into the peripelvic fat or the renal parenchyma
  - T4: tumor invades adjacent organs or through the kidney into the perinephric fat
- Regional lymph nodes (N)
  - NX: regional lymph nodes cannot be assessed
  - N0: no regional lymph node metastasis
  - N1: metastasis in a single lymph node, 2 cm or less in greatest dimension
  - N2: metastasis in a single lymph node, more than 2 cm but not more than 5 cm in greatest dimension; or multiple lymph nodes, none more than 5 cm in greatest dimension
  - N3: metastasis in a lymph node, more than 5 cm in greatest dimension
  - Note: N classification not affected by laterality
- Distant metastasis (M)
  - M0: no distant metastasis
  - M1: distant metastasis

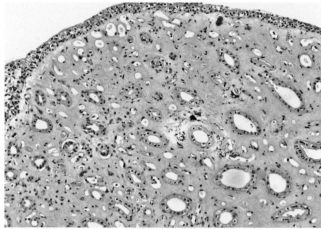

Fig 2. Urothelium juxtaposes on the renal parenchyma without a layer of lamina propria at the renal papillae.

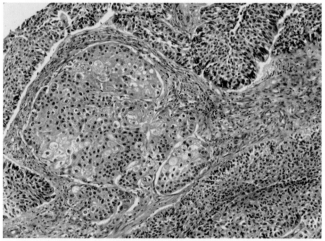

Fig 3. High-grade urothelial carcinoma invading into the subepithelial connective tissue, staged as T1. Flat urothelial carcinoma in situ is also present.

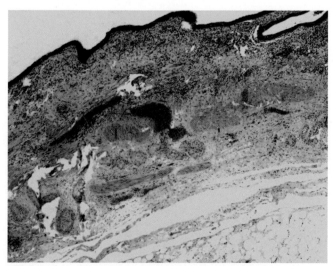

Fig 1. The renal pelvis is surrounded by a single layer of muscularis propria, which is not as well-formed as in the bladder proper.

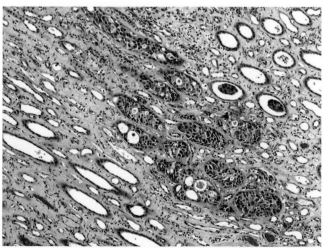

Fig 4. Urothelial carcinoma extending into the collecting ducts without invading the renal parenchyma. It is still staged as Tis.

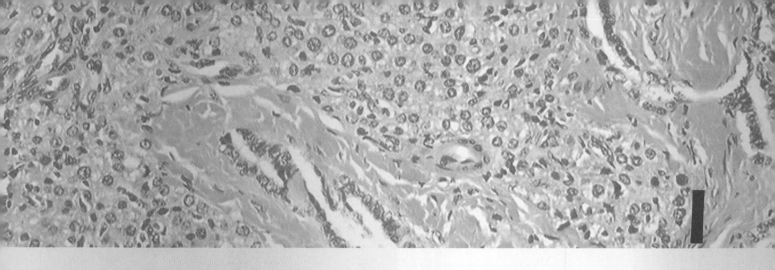

NONNEOPLASTIC DISEASE OF THE TESTIS

Definition

Anatomy

- Located within the scrotum, connected to the spermatic cord
- The scrotal wall consists of skin, dartos muscle, Colles fascia, and tunica vaginalis (parietal)
- Mean weight: 21.6 g for the right testis and 20.0 g for the left
- Mean volume: 20 mL
- Mean size: 4.5 × 3.0 × 2.5 cm

Pathology

Histology

- Includes testis, rete testis, epididymis, and spermatic cord
- Testis
  - Testis consists of seminiferous tubules (80%) and interstitium (20%). Seminiferous tubules are highly convoluted and tightly packed tubules, containing germ cells and Sertoli cells. The testicular interstitium contains Leydig cells in addition to macrophages, mast cells, blood vessels, and nerves.
  - Germ cells: spermatogonia (diploid) are the stem cells in spermatogenesis, replicate DNA, rest on the basal lamina, and are surrounded by the cytoplasm of Sertoli cells. Primary spermatocytes (diploid) lose contact with the basal lamina and produce two secondary spermatocytes through the first phase of meiotic division. Secondary spermatocytes (haploid) produce two spermatids through the second meiotic division. Spermatids (haploid) transform into spermatozoa (sperms) through spermatogenesis.
  - Sertoli cells are columnar cells extending from the basal membrane to the tubular lumen. The nucleus has pale chromatin and a prominent nucleolus. The number of Sertoli cells decreases with age. Sertoli cells are regulated by follicle-stimulating hormone (FSH) and androgen. Provide nutrition to germ cells and help proliferation and maturation of germ cells.
  - Leydig cells have a polyhedral shape, round nucleus with a large prominent nucleolus, and eosinophilic cytoplasm with numerous lipid-filled vesicles. They are adjacent to seminiferous tubules, produce testosterone, and are regulated by luteinizing hormone (LH).
- Rete testis
  - A network of channels that connect the seminiferous tubules with the efferent ducts
  - Lined by flat or cuboidal cells with focal areas of columnar cells with cilia and microvilli
  - Can be divided into three portions, septal, mediastinal, and extratesticular
- Epididymis
  - Highly coiled tubules with regular round lumens
  - Tubules lined mainly with principal cells (accounts for more than 90% of epithelial cells), which are tall columnar cells with stereocilia
  - Other lining cells: basal cells, clear cells, and apical cells
- Spermatic cord
  - It consists of vas deferens and blood vessels.
  - Vas deferens is lined with pseudostratified columnar cells with stereocilia, and basal cell vas deferens has a thick muscular wall, which includes inner and outer longitudinal layers and a middle circular layer.

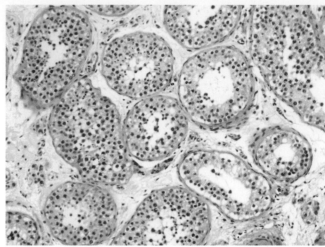

Fig 1. Testis showing tightly packed seminiferous tubules.

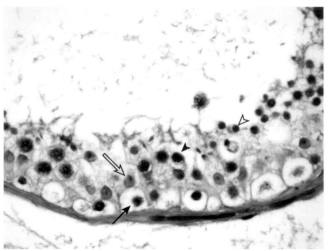

Fig 2. Seminiferous tubules contain spermatogonia *(black arrow)*, primary spermatocytes *(black arrowhead)*, spermatids *(white arrowhead)*, spermatozoa, and Sertoli cells *(white arrow)*.

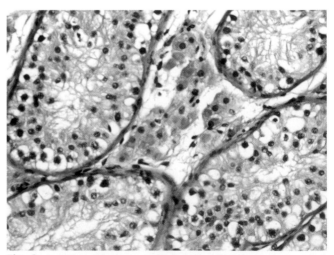

Fig 3. Leydig cells have eosinophilic cytoplasm and round nuclei with prominent nucleoli.

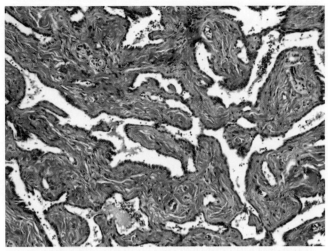

Fig 4. Rete testis shows irregular channels lined with flat or cuboidal cells.

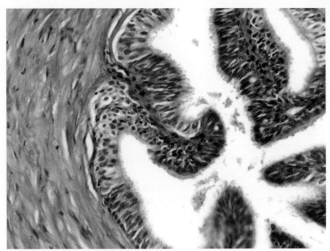

Fig 6. Vas deferens has an irregular lumen and is lined with pseudostratified, columnar cells with stereocilia.

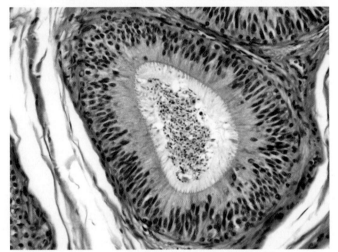

Fig 5. Epididymis tubules have a round lumen and are lined with columnar principal cells with stereocilia.

CRYPTORCHIDISM

Definition
- Failure of the testis to descend from an abdominal position through the inguinal canal into the scrotum during fetal development

Clinical features
Epidemiology
- It is the most frequent defect of the male urogenital tract at birth.
- Approximately 3% of full-term and 30% of premature infant boys are born with at least one undescended testis. Approximately 80% of cryptorchid testes descend by the first year of life (majority within 3 month).
- In the majority of affected children, the cause remains uncertain.
- Cryptorchidism is part of the testicular dysgenesis syndrome, which includes other male reproductive disorders such as hypospadias, increased risk of germ cell tumors, and infertility that shares a common pathogenic mechanism interfering with fetal testis development.
- There is a strong association between cryptorchidism and low birth weight caused by prematurity or intrauterine growth retardation.
- Risk factors include:
  - Exposure to polychlorinated pesticides, polybrominated flame retardants, and phthalates (most abundantly produced plasticizers that leach out from polyvinyl chloride plastics and disrupt androgen action)
  - Alcohol consumption, caffeine consumption (at least 3 drinks per day), or smoking during pregnancy
  - Gestational diabetes
  - Being a twin
- Acquired cryptorchidism can follow surgery in the region such as herniotomy, or it can be associated with severe hypospadias or mesothelial cysts of the spermatic cord.
- Primary cryptorchidism can be associated with Beckwith-Wiedemann syndrome, CHARGE syndrome (mutations most commonly in the CHD7 coding region inherited in an autosomal dominant manner), XY patients with gonadal dysgenesis, X-linked ichthyosis, Kallmann syndrome, Carpenter syndrome, Prader-Willi syndrome, Noonan syndrome, and cloacal exstrophy.
- A small percentage of isolated cryptorchidism is familial; it is reported in approximately about 4% of fathers and 6% to 10% of brothers of affected boys with cryptorchidism.
- Cryptorchidism occurs in 25% of boys with myelomeningocele.

Presentation
- Cryptorchidism is characterized by the absence of one or both testes from the scrotum.
- Approximately two thirds are unilateral. One third involves both testes.
- The undescended testis may be found in the abdomen retroperitoneally, in the inguinal canal, or in an ectopic location such as the thigh, perineum, opposite scrotum, or femoral canal.
- Pelvic ultrasound or magnetic resonance imaging is useful to find the location of the testis.
- The testis can be hypoplastic or absent (agenesis).
- The presence of a uterus on a pelvic ultrasound examination suggests persistent Müllerian duct syndrome (i.e., anti-Müllerian hormone deficiency or insensitivity)

Prognosis and treatment
- There is a high risk of infertility.
- Infertility is invariable in bilateral cases that are not treated at an early age.
- The rate of infertility is inversely proportional to the age at the time of orchidopexy.
- A major complication of undescended abdominal testis is the development of germ cell malignancy and is fivefold to tenfold more common than in a normally descended testis. The risk of malignancy does not completely normalize with orchidopexy, although it may decrease when orchiopexy is performed prepubertally.
- There is an increased risk of testicular torsion.
- Human chorionic gonadotropin or gonadotropin-releasing hormone treatments are not effective and may be harmful.
- Orchiopexy should be performed between 6 and 12 months of age, or soon after diagnosis if that occurs later.

Pathology
Histology
- Grossly normal undescended testes can appear histologically normal.
- In prepubertal cryptorchidism, a decreased tubular diameter is sometimes found. There are reduced numbers of germ cells, most marked between 2 and 4 years of age, and a 50% greater risk of germ cell depletion in nonpalpable relative to palpable undescended testis.
- In postpubertal cryptorchism, there are significant differences compared with normally descended testes, markedly reduced numbers of germ cells, increased thickness of peritubular connective tissue, failure of Sertoli cell maturation, Sertoli cell nodules (usually microscopic but rarely larger), or loss of Leydig cells in some cases.
- Atrophy can be associated with reactive hyperplasia of the rete testis.
- In longstanding cases, complete testicular atrophy can occur.

Molecular diagnostics
- Reverse transcriptase polymerase chain reaction shows elevation of p53 expression messenger RNA and decrease of Bax and BCL2 messenger RNA in cryptorchid testes.
- Expression of survivin 140 and 40 variants are strongly decreased.
- Mutations in the insulin-like factor 3 (INSL3) and RXFP2 genes cause cryptorchidism.
- Mutations of genes associated with androgen or anti-Müllerian hormone deficiency or insensitivity are present.

Main differential diagnosis
- Retractile testis
- Ectopic testis

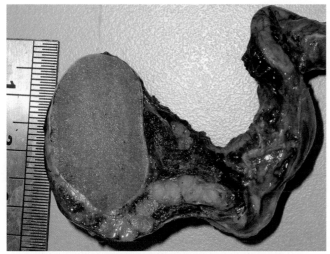

Fig 1. An atrophic testis in a case of cryptorchidism.

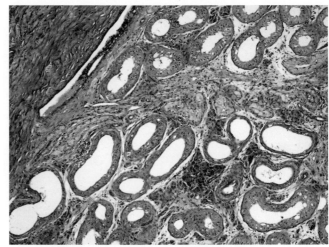

Fig 4. Marked atrophic cryptorchid postpubertal testis with seminiferous tubules reduced in size and containing only Sertoli cells.

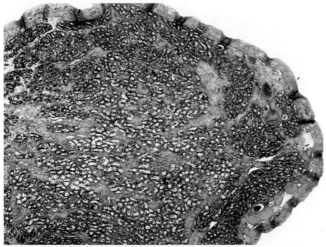

Fig 2. Cryptorchid prepubertal testis showing immature tubules.

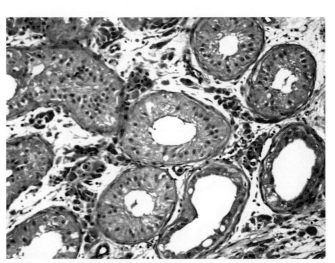

Fig 5. Cryptorchid postpubertal testis with seminiferous tubules reduced in size and containing only Sertoli cells.

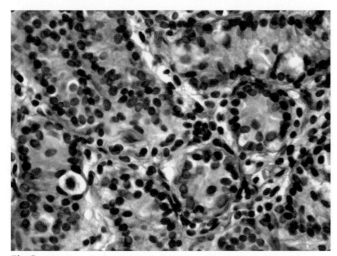

Fig 3. Cryptorchid prepubertal testis with immature tubules and reduced number of germ cells.

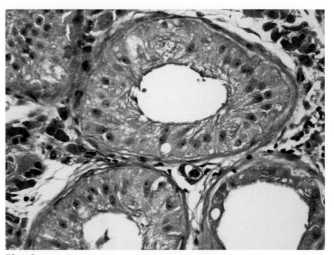

Fig 6. Cryptorchidism with seminiferous tubules containing only Sertoli cells.

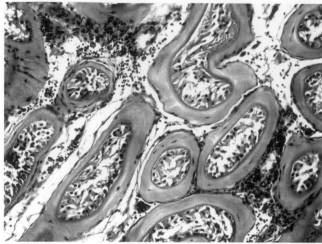

Fig 7. Seminiferous tubules contain only Sertoli cells. Thickening and hyalinization of peritubular connective tissue is observed.

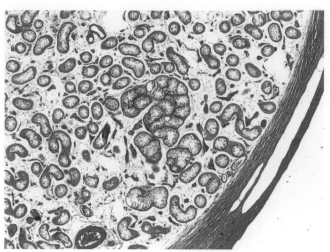

Fig 10. Sertoli cell nodule in a case of cryptorchidism.

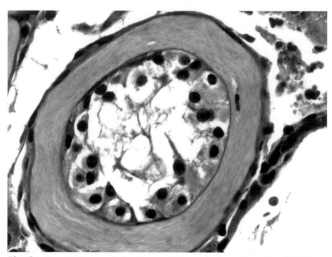

Fig 8. Seminiferous tubules contain only Sertoli cells. Thickening and hyalinization of peritubular connective tissue is seen.

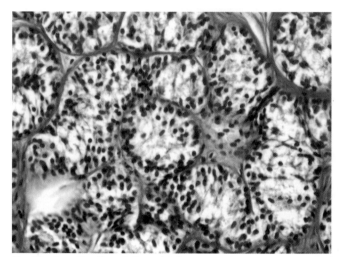

Fig 11. Sertoli cell nodule on higher magnification composed of closely packed nodules of seminiferous tubules containing only Sertoli cells.

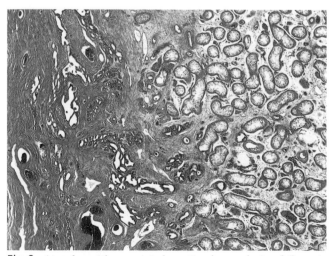

Fig 9. Atrophy with associated reactive hyperplasia of the rete testis.

Definition
- Rare congenital abnormality in which an ectopic spleen is connected to the testis owing to fusion of the developing splenic anlage with the gonadal mesoderm at approximately 5 weeks of intrauterine life

Clinical features
Epidemiology
- Affected individuals are younger than 20 years, with half being younger than 10 years.
- Gonadosplenic fusion can also occur in females, but the gender ratio is overwhelmingly in favor of males, with a male-to-female ratio of 20:1.

Presentation
- Cryptorchidism, usually left sided
- Testicular mass or swelling
- Testicular torsion
- Left indirect inguinal hernia
- Pain and enlargement of ectopic splenic tissue during strenuous exercise or systemic infections
- Acute intestinal obstruction from the cord of the continuous form of testiculosplenic fusion
- Congenital orofacial and limb abnormalities

Prognosis and treatment
- The condition is benign.
- Surgical removal of ectopic splenic tissue will prevent complications such as testicular infarction, torsion, and atrophy, allowing the preservation of fertility.
- Testiculosplenic fusion has been reported rarely with germ cell tumors arising from the testicular tissue, in which case the prognosis and treatment will depend on the characteristics of the malignant component.

Pathology
Histology
- There are continuous and discontinuous forms of testiculosplenic fusion—the former in which a band of splenic or fibrous tissue connects with the normal spleen, and the latter in which there is no such connection.
- Normal splenic tissue is present. Splenic tissue may show thrombosis, fibrosis, hemorrhage, hemosiderin deposits, and fatty degeneration.
- Testicular tissue can be normal or atrophic with fibrosis and Leydig cell hyperplasia.

Immunopathology (including immunohistochemistry)
- If present, the immunohistochemical profile of the germ cell component follows that described for the specific tumor subtypes.

Main differential diagnosis
- Lymphoproliferative disorder
- Teratoma

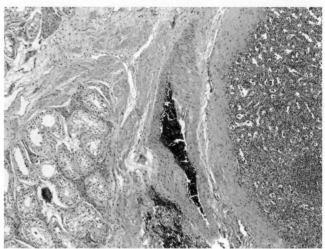

Fig 1. A case of testiculosplenic fusion showing testicular tissue *(left)* and spleen *(right)*.

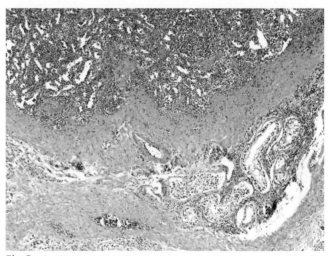

Fig 2. Testicular tissue *(lower right)* and spleen are connected by a dense band of fibrous tissue.

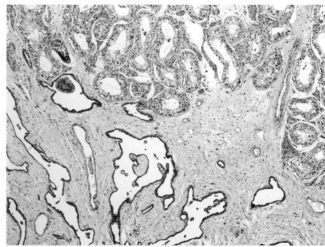

Fig 3. Seminiferous tubules showing hypospermatogenesis. Note also the rete testis *(lower field)*.

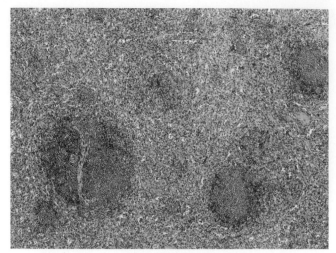

Fig 4. Splenic tissue is histologically unremarkable.

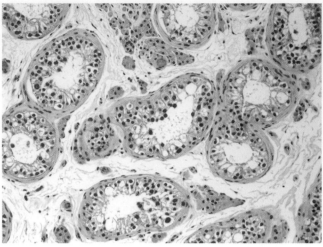

Fig 5. Seminiferous tubules showing hypospermatogenesis.

Definition

- Adrenal cortical rests, or heterotopia, are aggregates of ectopic adrenal tissue that may be present anywhere along the genitourinary tract.

Clinical features

Epidemiology

- Incidence is rare, but the true incidence is hard to establish because of their small size.
- They are usually an incidental finding.
- The prevalence seems to be higher in the pediatric population, suggesting that the lesions may regress in adulthood.

Presentation

- Typically an incidental diagnosis on herniorrhaphy or orchiectomy specimens
- Possibly present in hernia sacs, spermatic cord, epididymis, and rete testis; renal capsule also a common site

Prognosis and treatment

- No treatment is usually required.

Pathology

Histology

- Grossly they appear as small yellow nodules of approximately 1 to 5 mm in diameter, usually along the hernia sac or spermatic cord.
- Histologically, they are a well-circumscribed nodular collection of adrenal cortical cells that resemble the glomerulosa or fasciculate layers. The reticularis layer is usually seen only in older children. The nodules may have a thin capsule, and microscopic calcification may occur.
- Rarely, rests may have medullary adrenal tissue component.
- In Nelson syndrome or any condition of increased adrenocorticotropic hormone production, rests may be hyperplastic or harbor adenomas.
- Ectopic adrenal cortical carcinomas have been reported rarely.

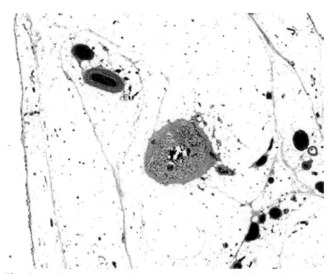

Fig 1. A low-magnification view of a spermatic cord section showing an island of epithelioid cells with clear cytoplasm vaguely arranged around a vessel.

Immunopathology (including immunohistochemistry)

- Adrenal cortical rests are positive for the same markers normally expressed in the topic gland—namely, calretinin, inhibin, and Melan-A.
- Cytokeratins are negative.

Main differential diagnosis

- Leydig cell nodules or tumors

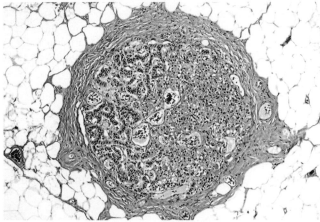

Fig 2. The architecture is of cords and nests, the vasculature is rich, and there is a rim of hyalinized tissue around the nodule.

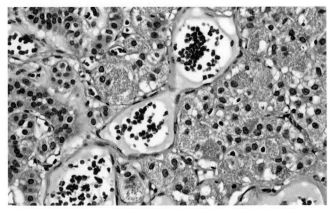

Fig 3. The cells of adrenal rests are similar to glomerulosa and fasciculate layers, with cells showing eosinophilic and granular cytoplasm, central nuclei, and conspicuous nucleoli.

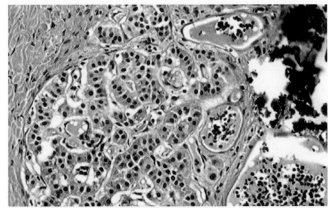

Fig 4. Calcification can sometimes be seen in association with adrenal cortical rests.

SPERMATIC CORD TORSION AND TESTICULAR INFARCTION

Definition
- Torsion is complete or incomplete twisting of the spermatic cord with or without associated ischemic necrosis of the testis as a consequence. Torsion may occur within the tunica vaginalis (intravaginal torsion) or outside to it (extravaginal torsion).

Clinical features
Epidemiology
- Intravaginal torsion generally occurs in adolescents and young adults, whereas extravaginal torsion is seen during infancy.

Presentation
- Acute onset of unilateral scrotal pain
- Scrotal swelling, nausea and vomiting, abdominal pain, fever, and urinary frequency
- Can occur related to physical activities or during sleep; antecedents of local trauma in some cases
- Related to the presence of a testicular tumor in rare instances

Prognosis and treatment
- Torsions lasting less than 6 hours probably will not cause testicular infarction.
- Torsions lasting more than 24 hours will certainly cause testicular infarction.
- Testicular atrophy, even if testicular infarction does not ensue as a consequence of torsion, appears in half of the patients if torsion lasts more than 10 hours.
- Treatment is orchiectomy if there is testicular infarction, but orchiopexy if testicular parenchyma is viable.

Pathology
Histology
- Venous congestion and interstitial hemorrhage, followed by infiltration by inflammatory cells, mainly polymorphonuclear leukocytes, between 2 and 6 hours after torsion
- Coagulative necrosis with extensive hemorrhage, between 6 and 12 hours after torsion
- Granulation tissue at 1 to 2 weeks and scaring at 1 to 2 months

Immunopathology (including immunohistochemistry)
- Not contributory

Main differential diagnosis
- Testicular torsion without infarction

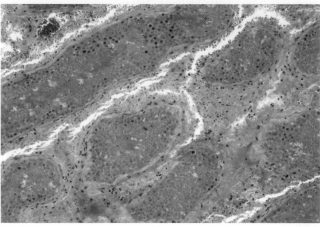

Fig 2. Testicular infarction showing coagulative necrosis of the seminiferous tubules and hemorrhage in the stroma.

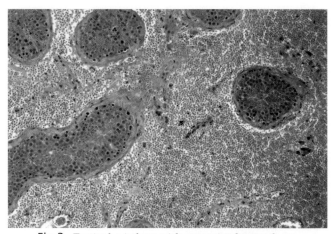

Fig 3. Testicular infarct with extensive hemorrhage.

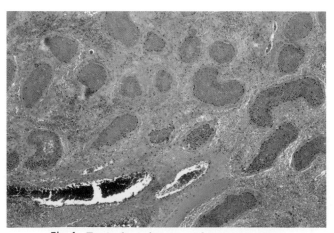

Fig 1. Testicular infarction at low-power view.

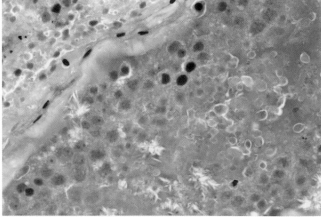

Fig 4. Necrotic seminiferous tubule in a case of testicular infarct.

Definition
- Presence of more than five foci of calcification less than 2 mm in diameter, randomly distributed in testicular parenchyma

Clinical features
Epidemiology
- Incidence of 0.6% in asymptomatic populations
- Can be seen both in children and adults
- Higher in whites than blacks
- Sixty-six percent bilateral
- Reported in cryptorchid (0.3%) and ex-cryptorchid (9.5%) testes, in infertility patients (4.6% to 20%), and in association with other benign conditions such as varicocele, scrotal trauma, mumps, epididymal cyst, testicular torsion, pulmonary alveolar microlithiasis, calcifications in parasympathetic nervous system, and neurofibromatosis
- Also reported in association with intratubular or invasive germ cell tumors (greater than 30%) in descended and undescended testes

Presentation
- Pain in patients without palpable testicular mass, owing to dilatation of seminiferous tubules secondary to obstruction by calcified concretions
- Multiple foci of calcification in asymptomatic patients detected by ultrasound

Prognosis and treatment
- Conflicting data in regard to microlithiasis being by itself a predisposing risk factor for testis malignancies
- Not an indication for monitoring in patients without other risk factors for germ cell tumors; yearly ultrasound examination, perhaps with testicular biopsy, suggested in microlithiasis patients with other risk factors (e.g., cryptorchidism, testicular atrophy, infertility, malignant intraepithelial germ cell neoplasia, gonadal dysgenesis, history of contralateral testicular germ cell tumor, exogenous estrogen administration to the mother when the patient was in utero)

Pathology
Histology
- Laminated intratubular calcifications are present in isolated or clustered seminiferous tubules, which arise as extratubular eosinophilic bodies that mineralize and pass into tubular lumina.
- There can be fibrosis in the adjacent testicular stroma.
- Mean tubular diameter and tubular fertility index are subnormal in tubules with microliths.
- Cystic dilatation is present in some tubules with microliths.
- If large, they can destroy seminiferous epithelium and be surrounded by peritubular cells.

Immunopathology (including immunohistochemistry)
- von Kossa stain to prove presence of calcium
- PLAP, CD117, or OCT3/4 to document intraepithelial germ cell neoplasia, if suspected

Main differential diagnosis
- Michaelis-Gutmann bodies
- Calcium deposits
- Hyaline globules
- Parasites, such as the giant kidney worm *Dioctophyme renale*

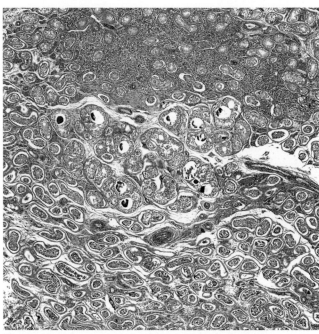

Fig 1. Numerous seminiferous tubules adjacent to seminoma containing small calcified intraluminal concretions (microliths).

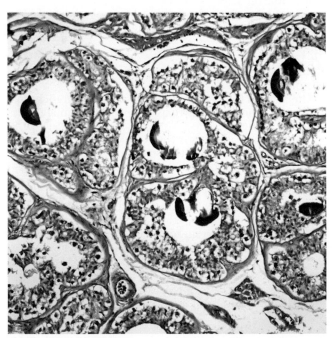

Fig 2. Intratubular germ cell neoplasia accompanied by calcifications within the lumina of seminiferous tubules.

Definition
- Testicular necrotizing vasculitis (inflammatory destruction of vessels with accumulation of fibrinoid material) that can be seen in various systemic disorders or as an isolated form

Clinical features
Epidemiology
- Testicular vasculitis is rarely the first manifestation of a systemic disease.
- Eighty percent of patients with polyarteritis nodosa have testicular or epididymal involvement found at autopsy (most frequent systemic vasculitis affecting the testis).
- Four percent of patients with Wegener granulomatosis have clinical testicular involvement.
- Vasculitis occurs as an isolated form in up to 33% of cases in small series.

Presentation
- Systemic disorders that can affect the testicular vessels include polyarteritis nodosa, Schönlein-Henoch purpura, antineutrophil cytoplasmic antibody vasculitis, Behçet disease, Cogan disease, rheumatoid arthritis, relapsing polychondritis, and dermatomyositis.
- Testicular pain, swelling, and tumorlike lesions are the most frequent presentation in isolated vasculitis.

Prognosis and treatment
- The prognosis is variable and depends on the etiology and the degree of systemic involvement.
- Prognosis is excellent in isolated forms.
- Strong immunosuppressive drugs are used to treat systemic diseases.
- Clinical, hematologic, and biochemical studies should always be performed after a diagnosis of necrotizing vasculitis.

Pathology
Histology
- The testis is frequently enlarged, and the parenchyma may show some hemorrhagic or necrotic remodeling and swelling.
- Necrotizing vasculitis is the key element.
- Fibrinoid necrosis and transmural inflammation with variable amount of neutrophils, lymphocytes, histiocytes, and plasma cells are observed.
- The composition of the inflammatory infiltrate depends on the etiology and the chronicity of the lesion.
- Thrombosis, aneurysm formation, fibrosis, and infarction can be seen admixed with more active lesions.

Main differential diagnosis
- Nonspecific orchitis or epididymitis
- Testicular torsion
- Testicular trauma

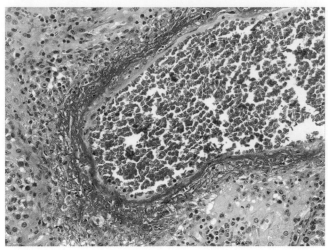

Fig 1. Intratesticular artery, severely injured, showing fibrinoid necrosis and transmural inflammation.

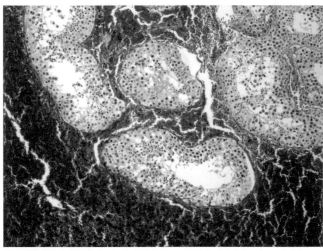

Fig 2. Interstitial hemorrhage is observed without significant inflammation. Vessels should always be carefully studied in cases without history of trauma to rule out vasculitis.

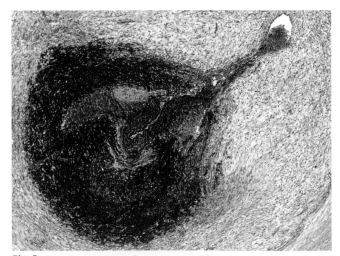

Fig 3. Trichrome stain showing intimal thickening, thrombosis, and fibrinoid necrosis in a large artery.

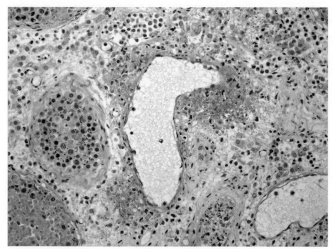

Fig 4. Fibrinoid necrosis and inflammatory cells are seen along this small intratesticular artery. Some tubules show necrotic changes.

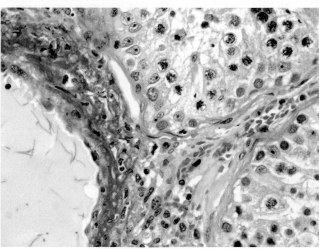

Fig 6. High-power view showing injured endothelial cells and fibrin in one artery. Tubules can be seen on the right side.

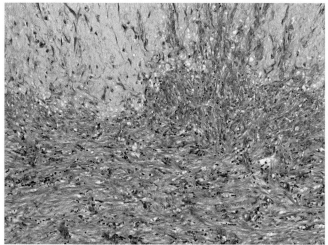

Fig 5. Periodic acid–Schiff stain showing cellular fibrosis with hemosiderin pigments at the border of a hemorrhagic infarct.

Definition
- Decreased production or delivery of spermatozoa or production of abnormal spermatozoa

Clinical features
Epidemiology
- Male infertility is common, affecting 5 million men in the United States.
- In infertile couples, male infertility is the primary and contributing cause in 40% and 20% of cases, respectively.

Presentation
- Infertility
- Possible history of cryptorchidism, orchitis, epididymitis, excurrent duct obstruction, varicocele, concurrent medical condition (diabetes), prior surgery (vasectomy, hernia repair, retroperitoneal dissection), chemotherapy or radiation therapy for malignancy, or substance abuse

Prognosis and treatment
- Testicular biopsy only performed in minority of cases, but can define the testicular alterations, distinguish obstructive versus nonobstructive etiology
- Testicular biopsy performed for sperm retrieval for assisted reproductive techniques

Pathology
Histology
- Hypospermatogenesis: all stages of spermatogenesis present but reduced to a variable degree; some tubules possibly showing Sertoli cell only or sclerosis
- Maturation arrest: complete arrest at a particular stage of spermatogenesis; no mature spermatids
- Germ cell aplasia: Sertoli cell only; no germ cells of any spermatogenesis stage
- Tubular and interstitial fibrosis: thickening peritubular basement membrane; lack of germ cells and Sertoli cells, interstitial fibrosis
- Prepubertal gonadotropin deficiency: small tubules, often aluminal, populated by prepubertal Sertoli cells, variable numbers of germ cells, interstitium loose with no recognizable Leydig cells
- Postpubertal gonadotropin deficiency: progressive change, from hypospermatogenesis, to maturation arrest, germ cell aplasia, and tubular sclerosis

Immunopathology (including immunohistochemistry)
- Not contributory

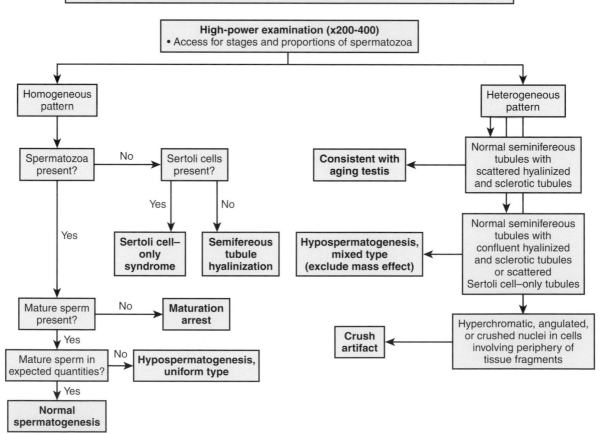

Fig 1. Diagnostic algorithm for testicular biopsy interpretation for infertility. (Modified from Cerilli LA, Kuang W, Rogers D: A practical approach to testicular biopsy interpretation for male infertility. *Arch Pathol Lab Med* 134:1197–1204, 2010.)

Definition
- Cessation of germ cell development beyond a specific (usually primary spermatocyte, rarely secondary spermatocyte or spermatid) stage in spermatogenesis

Clinical features
Epidemiology
- Can be idiopathic
- May have genetic etiologies including trisomy (XYY), balanced-autosomal anomalies (translocations, inversions) or deletions in the Y chromosome (Yq11)
- Can be secondary to postpubertal gonadotropin deficiency, varicocele, cryptorchidism, exogenous glucocorticoids, chemotherapy or radiotherapy, exposure to environmental toxins or heat, general diseases (liver or kidney insufficiency, sickle cell anemia)

Presentation
- Azoospermic infertility in complete arrest
- Oligospermic infertility in partial (incomplete) arrest

Prognosis and treatment
- Medical approach when needed
- Assisted reproductive techniques

Pathology
Histology
- Numerous spermatogonia, few spermatocytes, no maturation to elongate spermatids in seminiferous tubules in complete arrest, elongate spermatids focally present in partial (incomplete) arrest
- Prominent Sertoli cells owing to reduced germ cell number
- Frequent degenerating cells with irregular dense nuclei in tubules
- Intraluminal sloughing of arrested spermatocytes
- Reduced diameter of seminiferous tubules
- Usually normal findings in tunica propria, interstitium, Leydig cells

Immunopathology (including immunohistochemistry)
- Not contributory

Main differential diagnosis
- Hypospermatogenesis
- Normal spermatogenesis (in the cases of late-type maturation arrest)

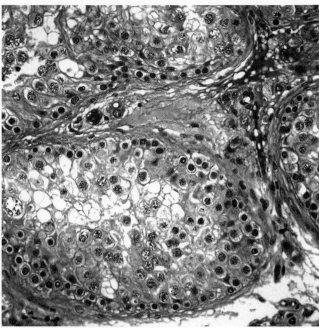

Fig 1. Maturation arrest at the level of primary spermatocyte. Spermatogonia and primary spermatocytes are the sole germ cell types existing.

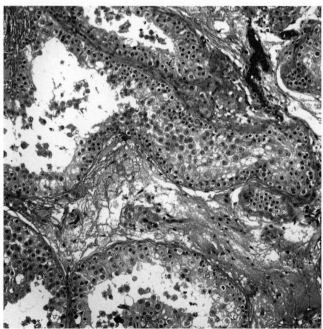

Fig 2. Maturation arrest. Normal morphology in tunica propria and interstitium.

Definition
- Reduced production of spermatozoa without a specific point of interruption

Clinical features

Epidemiology
- Common in infertile men who undergo testicular biopsy, which is usually performed only for patients with azoospermia without endocrine abnormalities
- Causes could include toxins, excess heat, varicocele, hypothyroidism, or hormonal dysfunction

Presentation
- Infertility

Prognosis and treatment
- Correct or remove the causes if possible. Testicular sperms can be collected for intracytoplasmic sperm injection.

Pathology

Histology
- There is a reduction in numbers of all types of germ cells with occasional elongated spermatids or spermatozoa.
- A thin epithelial layer with markedly decreased germ cell–to–Sertoli cell ratio is present (13:1 in normal young males).
- In mild forms occasional tubules are affected, and in severe forms there is a significant reduction in spermatogenesis in all seminiferous tubules. A report should include an estimate of percent of seminiferous tubules showing reduction.
- There is often thickening of tunica propria, focal interstitial fibrosis, and tubular sclerosis.
- Germ cell disorganization and sloughing into lumina are relatively nonspecific findings.
- Spermatogonia may show prominent nucleoli, mimicking intratubular germ cell neoplasia.

Immunopathology (including immunohistochemistry)
- Not contributory

Main differential diagnosis
- Maturation arrest
- Sertoli cell–only syndrome (germ cell aplasia)
- Intratubular germ cell neoplasia

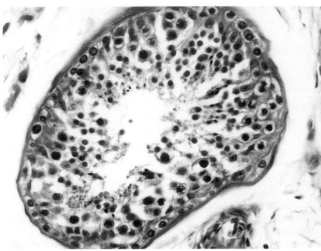

Fig 2. The numbers of all types of germ cells are decreased in this case of hypospermatogenesis.

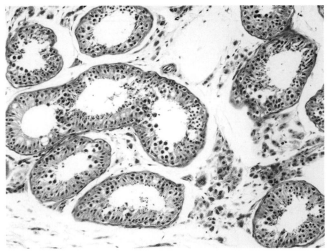

Fig 1. Marked hypospermatogenesis involving all seminiferous tubules of this 32-year-old man. Although there are some spermatids present, the ratio of germ cells to Sertoli cells is markedly decreased for the age. Leydig cell proliferation is seen in the interstitial.

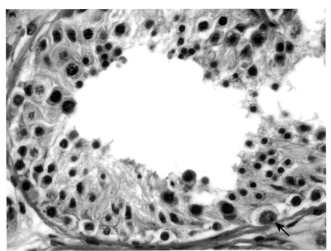

Fig 3. Spermatogonia at the periphery of tubules (arrow) occasionally show slightly enlarged nuclei and prominent nucleoli, mimicking intratubular germ cell neoplasia.

Definition
- Azoospermia with seminiferous tubules showing complete absence of germ cells and lined by Sertoli cells only

Clinical features
Epidemiology
- Occurs in 5% to 10% of male infertility cases
- Typically seen in men 20 to 40 years of age during infertility evaluation

Presentation
- Infertility, azoospermia, or hypogonadism
- Phenotypically normal males; some men may have small or atrophic testes
- Some cases possibly secondary to chemotherapy, especially regimens containing alkylating agents, or irradiation

Prognosis and treatment
- There is no known effective therapy.
- Hormone therapy may recover some spermatogenesis in the immature Sertoli cell type.
- Discontinuation of the offending agent in secondary germ cell aplasias sometimes restores spermatogenesis.

Pathology
Histology
- All seminiferous tubules show Sertoli cells only with complete absence of germ cells.
- The five variants are based on Sertoli cell morphology:
  - Dysgenetic Sertoli cells: varied Sertoli cell morphology between tubules; both mature and immature nuclear features present; overall increase in number of Sertoli cells; complete tubular hyalinization common; most often idiopathic, may be observed in cryptorchid testes
  - Adult Sertoli cells: mature Sertoli cells line each tubule; decreased tubular diameter; may be due to microdeletions in Y chromosome (i.e., azoospermia factor genes); Leydig cells are normal
  - Immature Sertoli cells: pseudostratified, prepubertal appearance of Sertoli cells that are markedly increased in number; decreased tubular diameter (lumina often absent); owing to childhood deficiency of LH and FSH
  - Involuting Sertoli cells: Sertoli cells show lobulated nuclei with irregular contours, coarse chromatin, and inconspicuous nuclei; basement membrane variably thickened; Leydig cells variably involuted; most common morphology seen with chemotherapy or irradiation
  - Dedifferentiated Sertoli cells: immature Sertoli cells in otherwise mature-appearing seminiferous tubules; tubular basement membrane thickened; markedly decreased tubular diameter; decreased number of Leydig cells; most commonly seen in patients undergoing androgen deprivation therapy or estrogen treatment

Immunopathology (including immunohistochemistry)
- Negative staining for germ cell markers (e.g., c-kit, Oct3/4, SALL4)

Main differential diagnosis
- Intratubular germ cell neoplasia
- Marked hypospermatogenesis or maturation arrest
- Tubular hyalinization

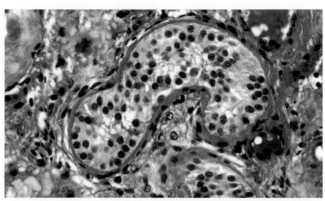

Fig 1. Seminiferous tubule with increased numbers of Sertoli cells, small tubular diameter, and virtually no lumen, suggestive of the immature variant. No germ cells are present.

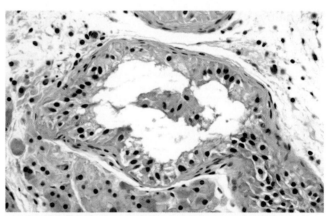

Fig 2. In this patient with germ cell aplasia, the tubules contain a mixture of mature and immature-appearing Sertoli cells with a relatively normal tubular diameter, most consistent with the dysgenetic variant of germ cell aplasia.

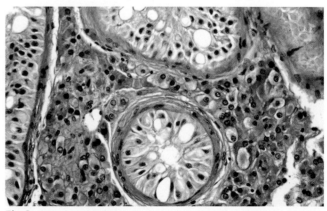

Fig 3. Decreased tubular diameter with mature-appearing Sertoli cells and unremarkable Leydig cells, suggestive of the adult variant of germ cell aplasia.

Definition
- Congenital or acquired obstruction of the epididymis or vas deferens, or both, leading to azoospermia or low sperm count

Clinical features
Epidemiology
- May be congenital or acquired
- Congenital: congenital bilateral absence of the vas deferens (seen with mutations of the cystic fibrosis transmembrane receptor gene), atrophy from secretions in cystic fibrosis
- Acquired: infection (usually epididymitis), sterilization, inadvertent surgical ligation of vas deferens

Presentation
- Azoospermia (if bilateral and complete obstruction) or low sperm count (if unilateral or incomplete obstruction)
- Normal size testes

Prognosis and treatment
- If a patient wishes to become fertile after vasectomy, the vasectomy site can be excised and a vasovasostomy or epididymovasostomy can be undertaken.

Pathology
Histology
- Active spermatogenesis is present with germ cell disorganization and sloughing and decreased number of Sertoli cells and spermatids.
- Variable interstitial fibrosis is a histologic feature most strongly associated with the rate of fertility after vasovasostomy.

- Sperm granulomas are present.
- There is no tubular basement membrane thickening.
- In biopsy specimens from men suspected of having excurrent duct obstruction, the number of elongate spermatids per tubule (counted in well-oriented cross-sections of 20 tubules) has been correlated with the sperm count in previous studies.

Immunopathology (including immunohistochemistry)
- Not contributory

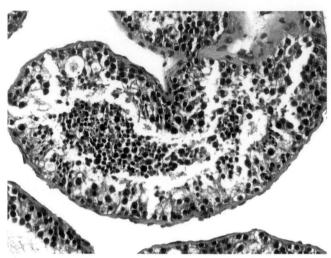

Fig 1. In excurrent duct obstruction, the seminiferous tubules show active spermatogenesis and sloughing of germ cells into the lumen of the tubules.

Definition
- Aspermatogenesis in adolescent or adult males who have never had normal secretion of gonadotropin hormones

Clinical features
Presentation
- Failure of pubertal development
- Other congenital anomalies when associated with a variety of syndromes
- May have deficiency of FSH or LH or both, with or without gonadotropin-releasing hormone deficiency, depending on the cause

Prognosis and treatment
- Treated with combinations of human gonadotropins
- Complete normal spermatogenesis and fertility possible after treatment

Pathology
Histology
- The morphology of testes is that of a prepubertal child and is abnormal only in that it is inappropriate for the patient's age.
- Small seminiferous tubules, generally without lumina, are composed of prepubertal Sertoli cells and scattered spermatogonia with no spermatogenesis.
- There is an absence of Leydig cells in the loose interstitium.

Immunopathology (including immunohistochemistry)
- Not contributory

Main differential diagnosis
- Postpubertal gonadotropin deficiency

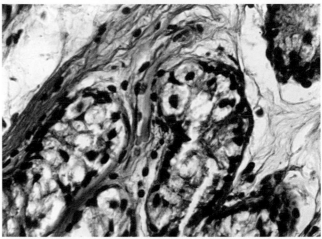

Fig 2. Higher magnification of the previous case. (Courtesy Howard Levin, Cleveland Clinic, Cleveland, Ohio.)

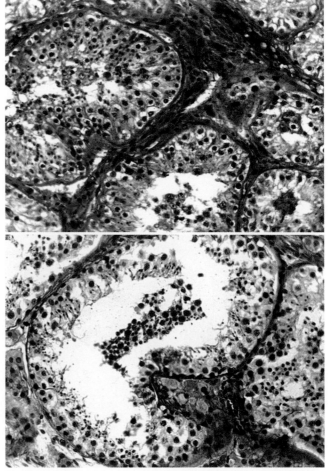

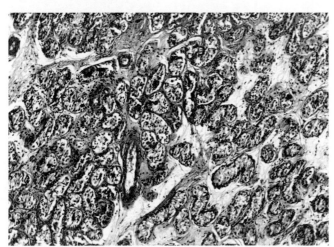

Fig 1. Testicular biopsy from a 19-year-old male with prepubertal gonadotropin deficiency showed morphology essentially of a prepubertal testis: small seminiferous tubules lined with prepubertal Sertoli cells and scattered spermatogonia with no spermatogenesis; loose interstitium with no Leydig cells identified. (Courtesy Howard Levin, Cleveland Clinic, Cleveland, Ohio.)

Fig 3. Testicular biopsy specimen after gonodotropin replacement. After treatment with hormones with predominantly luteinizing hormone activity, the biopsy specimen showed spermatogenesis in the tubules and Leydig cells in the interstitium. Sperm count was 1 million per milliliter. (Courtesy Howard Levin, Cleveland Clinic, Cleveland, Ohio.)

POSTPUBERTAL GONADOTROPIN DEFICIENCY

Definition
- Hypogonadism in postpubertal children or adults owing to LH and FSH deficiency

Clinical features
Epidemiology
- Hypothalamic and pituitary dysfunctions can be caused by trauma, surgery, neoplasm, irradiation, or estrogen therapy given to adult transsexual or prostate cancer patients

Presentation
- Often present with loss of libido, erectile dysfunction, depression, and lethargy
- May also have regression of secondary sexual characteristics, loss of muscle mass, and diminished intellectual capacity

Prognosis and treatment
- Treated by gonadotropin, gonadotropin-releasing hormone, or testosterone
- Possible to restore sexual function and fertility

Pathology
Histology
- Seminiferous tubules may have active spermatogenesis but usually show various deficiencies, including germ cell maturation arrest, hypoplasia, or aplasia.
- Seminiferous tubules can become sclerotic.
- Leydig cells are decreased or absent.

Immunopathology (including immunohistochemistry)
- Not contributory

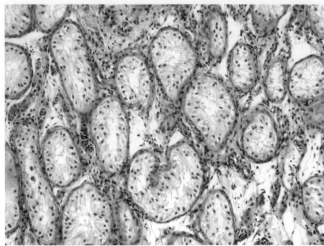

Fig 1. Germ cell aplasia in postpubertal gonadotropin deficiency.

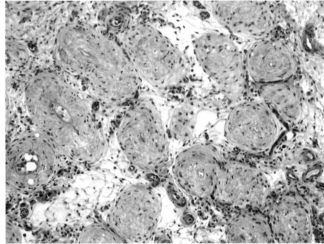

Fig 2. Tubular sclerosis in postpubertal gonadotropin deficiency.

Definition
- Inflammation of the testis due to viral infections, the most common agents being mumps and coxsackie B viruses

Clinical features
Epidemiology
- Postpubertal mumps in males is associated with a 40% likelihood of orchitis.
- Influenza, infectious mononucleosis, and other viruses can also be causative organisms for viral orchitis.
- Severe adult respiratory syndrome has also been reported to be associated with orchitis.
- With vaccination, the incidence of mumps orchitis has diminished.

Presentation
- Testicular pain, swelling, and fever are present.
- Bilateral symptoms occur in up to 25% of cases.
- Clinically and radiologically, the inflammation resembles a testicular neoplasm.
- When caused by the mumps virus, there can be preceding salivary gland enlargement, tenderness, and pain.
- Viral orchitis can lead to subfertility.
- Severe testicular damage can lead to hypergonadotropic hypogonadism, with low testosterone levels and regression of secondary sexual characteristics.

Prognosis and treatment
- Treatment is supportive, with the possibility of intravenous immunoglobulin infusion.
- Interferon-α administration has been used for viral epididymo-orchitis caused by mumps virus.
- Treatment includes mumps vaccination.

Pathology
Histology
- Testicular parenchyma is preserved.
- Edema and hemorrhage are present.
- Lymphohistiocytic infiltrates are present within seminiferous tubules and interstitium, with predominance of the intratubular inflammation.
- Testicular atrophy can occur with chronicity, tubular hyalinization, and hypospermatogenesis.

Immunopathology (including immunohistochemistry)
- CD68+ histiocytes, CD3+ T lymphocytes and fewer CD20+ B lymphocytes are present.

Main differential diagnosis
- Sertoli cell hyperplasia
- Intratubular germ cell neoplasia
- Seminoma
- Hematolymphoid neoplasia

Definition
- Granulomatous inflammatory condition affecting the testis and epididymis and caused mainly by *Mycobacterium tuberculosis*

Clinical features
Epidemiology
- High incidence in developing countries and immunosuppressed individuals
- Mainly in adults

Presentation
- Most cases are associated with involvement of other anatomic sites, such as the prostate (in adults) and lungs (especially in children).
- Most cases affect primarily the epididymis and from there spread to the testis.
- Mild testicular enlargement with tenderness is present.
- There is a possible association with systemic symptoms such as fever and weight loss.
- Bilateral involvement, hydrocele, or abscess formation is also possible.

Prognosis and treatment
- Excellent prognosis with current pharmacologic treatment
- Surgical resection of dead tissue if necessary

Pathology
Histology
- Caseating or noncaseating granulomatous inflammation composed of epithelioid histiocytes and multinucleated giant cells affecting the testicular parenchyma
- Chronic inflammatory infiltrate composed mainly of lymphocytes
- Fibrous tissue and scarring in chronic lesions

Immunopathology (including immunohistochemistry)
- Ziehl-Neelsen stains can show bacilli, but are not required for diagnosis.

Main differential diagnosis
- Granulomatous inflammation caused by fungi or other parasites
- Nonspecific granulomatous orchitis
- Seminoma with prominent granulomatous host reaction
- Malakoplakia
- Sperm granuloma

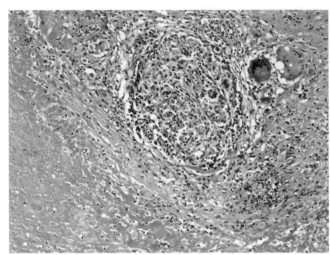

Fig 2. Tuberculous orchitis with caseous necrosis, granulomas, and giant cells.

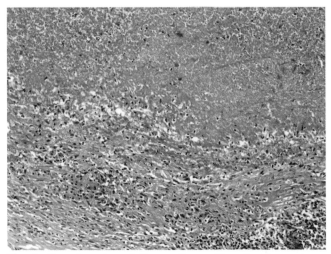

Fig 1. Granulomatous inflammation with extensive caseous necrosis *(upper field)*.

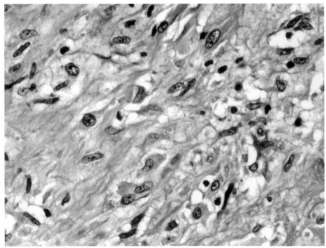

Fig 3. Granulomatous inflammation composed of epithelioid histiocytes.

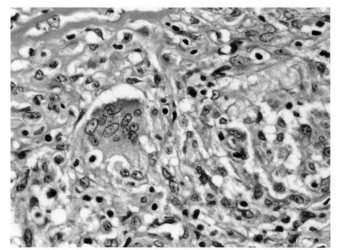

Fig 4. Epithelioid histiocytes and multinucleated giant cells.

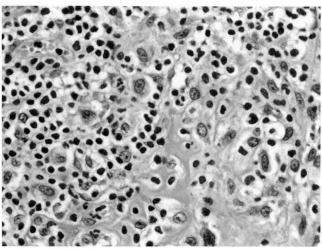

Fig 5. Granulomatous inflammation with epithelioid histiocytes and abundant lymphocytes intermixed with plasma cells and neutrophils.

Definition
- Nonspecific granulomatous orchitis is a rare and unusual disease with mixed chronic and granulomatous inflammation of an unknown etiology.

Clinical features
Epidemiology
- Unknown etiology; may be autoimmune, trauma, or infection
- Rare incidence
- More common in African Americans
- Age range, 25 to 80 years

Presentation
- Flulike symptoms
- Firm, enlarged, tender, or painless testicular mass, usually unilateral
- Scrotal discomfort varying in intensity from a dull ache to severe pain
- Associated urinary symptoms: increased frequency, dysuria, and nocturia, with associated urinary tract infection
- Epididymal enlargement and hydrocele; ultrasound examinations of affected testis showing diffusely hypoechoic testis or focal hypoechoic intratesticular areas

Prognosis and treatment
- Orchiectomy
- Antibiotics with variable or no response
- Steroid treatment

Pathology
Histology
- Grossly, solid nodular enlargement similar to lymphoma, leukemia, and malakoplakia
- Enlarged testis with a homogenous tan infiltrate obscures testicular architecture and may involve the epididymis and tunics.
- Chronic inflammation infiltrate within the interstitium, seminiferous tubules, tubular walls, and sometimes in the tubule lumens
- The inflammatory infiltrate consists predominantly of histiocytes, lymphocytes, and plasma cells.
- Although there are no true granulomas in nonspecific granulomatous orchitis, the tubular orientation of the inflammation, sometimes with histiocytes and occasional multinucleated giant cells, gives the lesion a somewhat granulomatous microscopic appearance.

Immunopathology (including immunohistochemistry)
- A CD68 stain will highlight the histiocytes.
- Gram stain, acid fast bacillus (AFB) stain, and Gomori methanamine silver (GMS) stain for microorganisms are used to exclude an infectious cause.
- Tissue should be cultured for bacterial, mycobacterial, and fungal organisms, and stained for spirochetes.

Main differential diagnosis
- Seminoma
- Testicular lymphoma
- Testicular malakoplakia
- Sarcoidosis

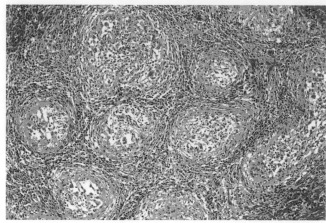

Fig 1. Nonspecific granulomatous orchitis with intratubular histiocytes and chronic inflammation infiltrating the interstitium, seminiferous tubules, and tubular walls.

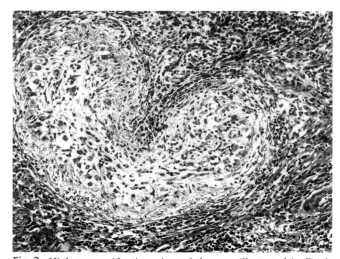

Fig 2. Higher-magnification view of the case illustrated in Fig 1. The inflammatory infiltrate consists predominantly of lymphocytes and plasma cells. The tubular orientation of the inflammation with histiocytes, lymphocytes, and occasional multinucleated giant cells gives the lesion a granulomatous microscopic appearance.

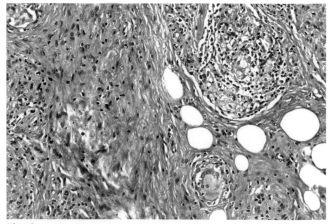

Fig 3. Late stage of nonspecific granulomatous orchitis with extensive fibrosis and tubular destruction.

CONGENITAL ADRENAL HYPERPLASIA

Definition
- Congenital adrenal hyperplasia, also known as *adrenogenital syndrome,* is a rare autosomal recessive condition caused by enzyme deficiency in the steroid synthesis pathway of the adrenal cortex, with the most commonly affected enzyme being 21-hydroxylase. Congenital adrenal hyperplasia is characterized by cortisol deficiency with or without aldosterone deficiency and androgen excess.

Clinical features
Epidemiology
- Classic, nonclassic, and cryptic forms are described. The classic form is characterized by severe enzyme deficiency presenting in childhood, whereas the nonclassic variety is associated with milder enzyme deficiency with signs and symptoms occurring in adolescence or adulthood. The cryptic form is asymptomatic.
- Incidence of the classic form is reported to range from 1/5000 to 1/15,000 live births in the white population.

Presentation
- Biochemical and clinical abnormalities depend on the specific enzyme that is affected and the severity of the enzyme deficiency.
- Salt wasting occurs when aldosterone production is affected, which can lead to death in the first few weeks of life.
- Ambiguous genitalia and virilization are seen in females with severe forms of congenital adrenal hyperplasia.
- In utero diagnosis can be achieved through molecular genetic analysis of fetal DNA obtained from amniocentesis or chorionic villus sampling.
- In moderate forms of 21-hydroxylase deficiency (nonclassic or late-onset variety), affected women have hyperandrogenism. Children may exhibit premature adrenarche and pubarche.
- Hyperandrogenic signs in women include acne, frontal hair loss, hirsutism, and irregular menstrual periods.
- Hypogonadism can also occur in men.
- Testicular tumors that develop in adolescence or young adulthood can be bilateral, painful, and tender.
- Iatrogenic Cushing syndrome
- Development of the metabolic syndrome predisposes patients to cardiovascular disease and diabetes.

Prognosis and treatment
- Prenatal treatment with dexamethasone of pregnant mothers with an affected fetus can reduce the likelihood of ambiguous genitalia.
- Oral glucocorticoid and mineralocorticoid administration is used to suppress adrenal androgens and compensate for adrenal steroid deficiency.
- Standard hormonal replacement might not lead to normal growth and development of affected children.

Pathology
Histology
- Grossly, the adrenal glands are enlarged with cortical gyriform folds and a light brown appearance.
- Adrenal cortical adenoma and carcinoma can occur in some patients with findings as described for these tumors.
- Testicular tumors are composed of Leydig cells with granular pink cytoplasm and round to oval nuclei and prominent nucleoli. No Reinke crystalloids are found.

Immunopathology (including immunohistochemistry)
- Not contributory

Molecular diagnostics
- 21-Hydroxylase deficiency is usually caused by mutations in the *CYP21A2* gene, located on the RCCX module. This chromosomal region is highly prone to genetic aberrations such as duplications, gross deletions, and gene conversions of variable extensions.
- Molecular genotyping of *CYP21A2* and the RCCX module has proved useful for a more accurate disease and prenatal diagnosis.
- HLA-Bw47, HLAB5, and HLA-B35 are the most common haplotypes usually found in the classical form, while the haplotype HLA-B14DR1 is most frequently seen in the nonclassical form of the disease.

Main differential diagnosis
- Leydig cell tumor

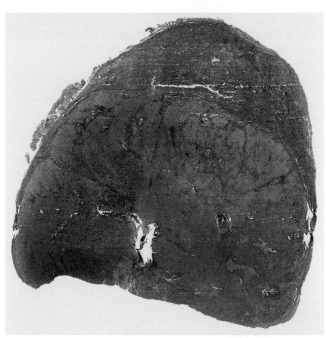

Fig 1. Section of a testicular lesion from a patient who was diagnosed with adrenogenital syndrome. Low magnification shows a circumscribed solid nodule. (Courtesy Fredrik Petersson, National University Hospital, Singapore.)

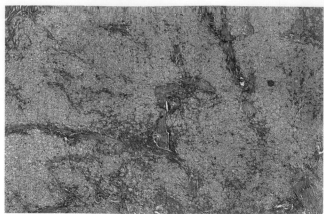

Fig 2. Medium magnification shows sheets of pink cells interspersed by fibrous strands.

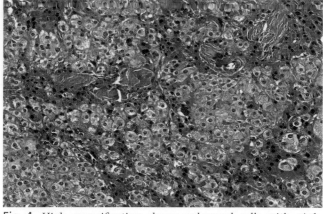

Fig 4. High magnification shows polygonal cells with pink, finely granular cytoplasm, and round vesicular nuclei with conspicuous nucleoli, typical of a Leydig cell tumor.

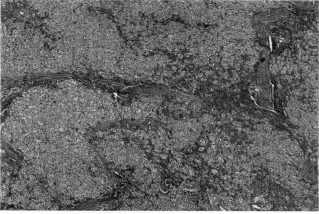

Fig 3. The pink cells show slight variability in nuclear size with ample, pink, microvesicular cytoplasm.

ANDROGEN INSENSITIVITY SYNDROME

Definition
- Resistance of target organs to androgen stimulation (owing to androgen receptor gene mutation on the X chromosome) leading to several syndromes with phenotypes varying from testicular feminization (severe form) to normal males with infertility (mild form)

Clinical features
Presentation
- Testicular feminization syndrome: most frequent cause of male pseudohermaphroditism (female phenotype with testis and absence of upper vagina, uterus, fallopian tubes, and ovaries); karyotype usually 46,XY and less commonly 47,XXY
- Bilateral cryptorchidism with testes present in the abdomen, inguinal canal, or labia majora
- Rarely diagnosed during childhood except in patients with hernia, inguinal tumor, or a family history of pseudohermaphroditism
- Primary amenorrhea principal presentation in adults

Prognosis and treatment
- Patients at increased risk of developing intratubular germ cell neoplasia, germ cell tumors, and sex cord tumors
- Gonadectomy recommended by puberty

Pathology
Histology
- Variably sized testis with small seminiferous tubules composed of Sertoli cells only, with sparse associated spermatogonia
- Leydig cell hyperplasia
- Ovarian-like stroma in the interstitium commonly seen
- Seventy percent of testes contain grossly visible white nodules consisting of Sertoli cell adenoma (nodular clusters of seminiferous tubules composed of Sertoli cells only)

Immunopathology (including immunohistochemistry)
- Not contributory

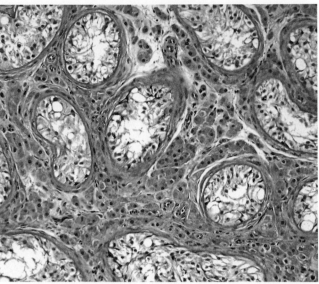

Fig 1. The two most common histologic findings in androgen insensitivity syndrome are seminiferous tubules composed of Sertoli cells only and Leydig cell hyperplasia in the intertubular areas.

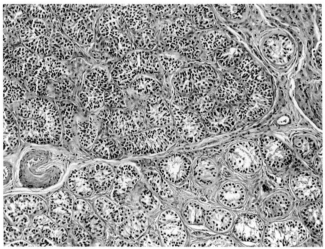

Fig 2. The testis commonly contains Sertoli cell adenomas that are nodular clusters of seminiferous tubules composed of Sertoli cells only.

Definition
- Klinefelter syndrome (or 47XXY or XXY syndrome) is a condition in which males have an extra X chromosome.

Clinical features
Epidemiology
- Klinefelter syndrome is the most common sex chromosome disorder in males and the second most common condition caused by the presence of extra chromosomes.
- Incidence is 1/1000 males.
- One in every 500 males has an extra X chromosome but does not have the syndrome.

Presentation
- Reduced body and pubic hair
- Gynecomastia in 40% to 80%
- High FSH
- Variable LH

Prognosis and treatment
- Increased risk of breast cancer

Pathology
Histology
- Firm and small testes
- Reduced number of intratubular germ cells
- Sertoli cell only in some tubules
- Leydig cell nodules, hyperplasia
- Tubular sclerosis
- Suboptimal spermatogenesis

Immunopathology (including immunohistochemistry)
- Not contributory

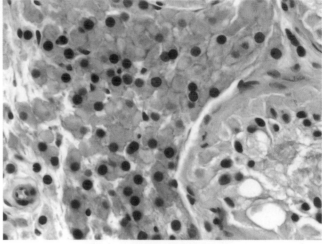

Fig 2. Leydig cell hyperplasia.

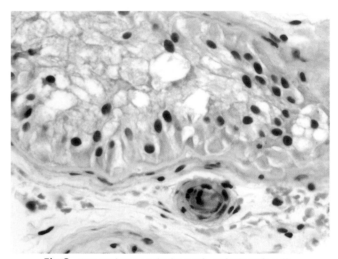

Fig 3. Seminiferous tubules with only Sertoli cells.

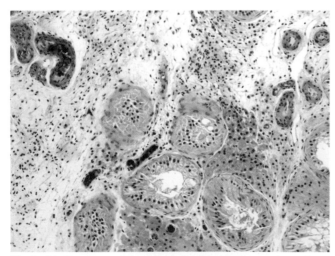

Fig 1. Medium-power view of a testicular biopsy specimen from a patient with Klinefelter syndrome.

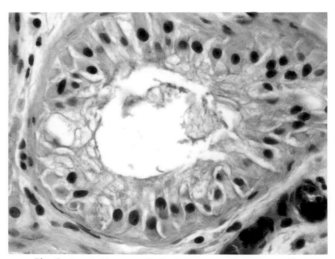

Fig 4. Seminiferous tubule showing only Sertoli cells.

TESTICULAR TUMOR OF THE ADRENOGENITAL SYNDROME

Definition
- Rare clinical entity found in young men with endocrine disorders

Clinical features
Epidemiology
- Rare; fewer than 100 cases reported in the English-language literature
- Predominantly affecting young adults (mean, approximately 20 years)
- Small proportion of the patients with androgenital syndromes develops these tumors

Presentation
- Most of the cases (80%) have a diagnosis of adrenogenital syndrome established before discovery of a testicular tumor.
- The presence of vomiting, diarrhea, dehydration, sudden collapse and death, enlargement of the genitalia, and sexual precocity call attention to adrenogenital syndrome.
- Tumors are often bilateral.
- Small tumors can be found as an incidental finding at autopsies in patients with adrenogenital syndrome.

Prognosis and treatment
- Prognosis is favorable. These tumors tend to decrease in size after therapy with corticosteroids.
- Treatment is usually followed conservatively, but partial resection and orchiectomy could be attempted.

Pathology
Histology
- Tumor size varies from less than 1 cm to 9 cm in diameter.
- Multifocality is common, with nodules in both the parenchyma and paratesticular soft tissue.
- Lesions are usually centered in the testicular hilum and associated with the rete testis.
- On light microscopy, tumor nodules are separated by fibrous bands.
- The tumor is composed of sheets, nests, and occasionally cords of cells.
- The cells are large and polygonal, with abundant eosinophilic cytoplasm, resembling Leydig cells. Cytoplasmic clearing is common.
- Lipofuscin pigment, inclusions, and scattered pleomorphism are common.
- The nuclear features also resemble those of Leydig cells, with mild atypia and central nucleoli.

Immunopathology (including immunohistochemistry)
- The few reported cases showed diffuse positivity with inhibin and Melan-A and focal positivity with calretinin.
- Synaptophysin can also be positive focally.
- Cytokeratins are uniformly negative in these tumors.

Main differential diagnosis
- Leydig cell tumor

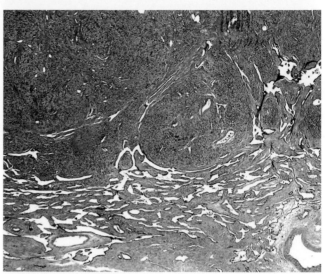

Fig 1. At low magnification, testicular tumors are located at the hilum in close association with the rete testis. The masses are multinodular with thin fibrous septa interspersed with the tumor.

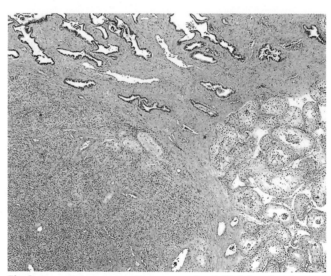

Fig 2. In a different case, the tumor edge is ill defined with some wrapping of seminiferous tubules *(center)*. The rete testis *(top)* is not involved by the tumor in this case.

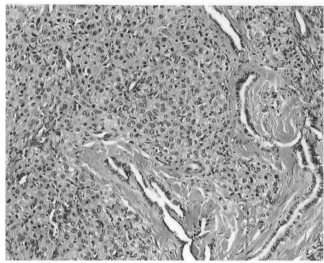

Fig 3. High magnification, same tumor as in Fig 1. The cytologic features are similar to those of Leydig cell tumors, with packed cells with abundant cytoplasm and a rich vasculature. The rete testis epithelium is entrapped.

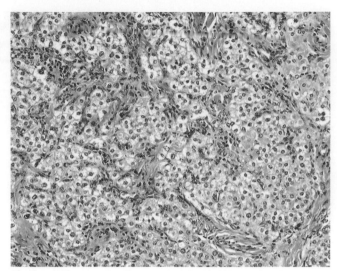

Fig 5. High magnification of testicular tumor of the adrenogenital syndrome showing cells with cleared cytoplasm in small nests and with a rich vasculature in the background. There is a mild lymphocytic infiltrate associated with the tumor.

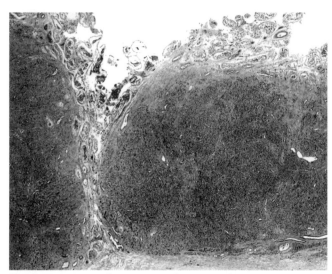

Fig 4. Low magnification, another case, showing two tumor nodules separated by an edematous testicular parenchyma. Note a few rete testis tubules on the top, surrounded by tumor cells.

Definition
- Also known as *bilateral vanishing testes syndrome*, embryonic testicular regression is an intersex condition in which testes vanish during embryogenesis in patients with an XY karyotype.

Clinical features
Epidemiology
- Usually sporadic with rare familial instances with recessive trait
- Unclear etiology, possibly regression of the testes in utero because of a genetic mutation, a teratogen, or bilateral torsion

Presentation
- Unilateral or bilateral anorchia
- Developmental defects of the Wolffian duct
- Variable Müllerian duct development
- Depending on chronology of gonadal injury, a spectrum of phenotypes ranging in severity from complete female to varying degrees of genital ambiguity to a normal male phenotype with microphallus and empty scrotum

Prognosis and treatment
- Dictated by the position of the patient in the clinical spectrum of the disease
- Estrogen supplement at the time of expected puberty in phenotypic females for the development of secondary sexual characteristics and vaginoplasty
- Long-term androgen replacement beginning at the time of expected puberty for the phenotypic males with placement of testicular prosthesis
- Individualized assessment to determine the optimal gender assignment
- No risk for development of germ cell tumor

Pathology
Histology
- Rudimentary cord structures; vas deferens or epididymis, or both, usually identified but no histologically recognizable testicular tissue at the biopsy from the ends of the ducts
- Tissue composed of fibrosis, hemosiderin deposition and dystrophic calcification at the site of former testis, sometimes with giant cell reaction, nerves resembling traumatic neuroma, and in some cases small groups of seminiferous tubules or Leydig cells near epididymis or proximal vas deferens
- Abnormally small spermatic vessels

Immunopathology (including immunohistochemistry)
- Inhibin stain to highlight Leydig cells, if present

Main differential diagnosis
- Cryptorchidism

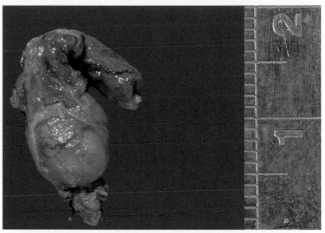

Fig 1. Testicular regression. Residual small nodular tissue (1-cm diameter) is seen at the end of spermatic cord.

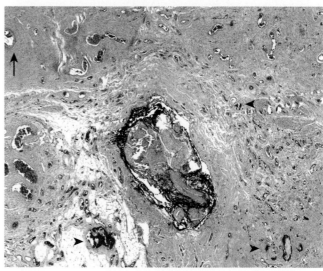

Fig 2. Same case as in Fig 1. No gonadal or testicular formation is noted. Instead, the nodule is composed of a fibrovascular tissue that contains calcified foci *(arrowheads)*. The *long arrow* indicates the rudimentary spermatic cord.

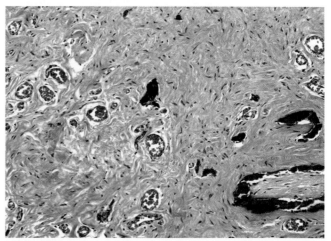

Fig 3. Regressed testis indicated by fibrosis, hemosiderin pigment, and calcifications.

Definition
- A spectrum of disorders with ambiguous genitalia, persistent Müllerian duct structures, Wolffian duct derivatives, and karyotypes having a Y chromosome

Clinical features
Epidemiology
- Second most frequent cause of ambiguous genitalia in newborns

Presentation
- Pure gonadal dysgenesis: bilateral streak gonads, internal Müllerian structures, 46XY karyotype, and female phenotype without signs of Turner syndrome
- Partial gonadal dysgenesis (dysgenetic male pseudohermaphroditism): bilateral dysgenetic testes, cryptorchidism, persistent Müllerian structures, XO/XY mosaicism, inadequate virilization, absent spermatogenesis
- Mixed gonadal dysgenesis (MGD): testis on one side and contralateral streak gonad, testis on one side and contralateral gonadal agenesis, hypoplastic gonads with rudimentary tubes in one, a streak gonad with contralateral tumor, or a germ cell tumor with contralateral gonadal agenesis; invariably present Müllerian structures, bilateral fallopian tubes bilaterally, poor development of ipsilateral Wolffian structures, and XO/XY mosaicism; normal male, ambiguous or normal female external genitalia (two thirds are raised as females), and signs of virilization in phenotypic females at puberty
- Rare patients have Denys-Drash syndrome (nephropathy, progressive renal failure, genital abnormalities, and Wilms tumor in infancy)
- Turner syndrome

Prognosis and treatment
- Gender determination
- Increased risk of gonadal neoplasms (9% to 30% in MGD), some of which occur in childhood
- Removal of gonads and Müllerian-derived organs at the time of diagnosis
- Screening for Wilms tumor in infancy
- Search for Denys-Drash syndrome in patients born with ambiguous genitalia and sex chromosome mosaicism

Pathology
Histology
- Streak gonads contain ovarian-type stroma with no primordial ovarian follicles. Rudimentary seminiferous tubules are present in some gonads.
- Dysgenetic gonads are composed of hypoplastic seminiferous tubules and ovarian-like stroma (sometimes it is not possible to describe the organ as *ovary* or *testis* because of a lack of differentiation).
- Morphology of seminiferous tubules ranges from totally sclerotic to having mild hypospermatogenesis. Sertoli cells may appear oxyphilic granular focally.
- Intratubular germ cell neoplasia in some cases. In half the cases, germ cells invade stroma as a seminoma.
- Gonadoblastoma is the most common tumor type developing in MGD (occurs in one third of MGD patients).

Immunopathology (including immunohistochemistry)
- CD117 and PLAP stains to show malignant germ cells in the case of gonadoblastoma or seminoma development
- Inhibin stain to identify gonadal stromal cells

Molecular diagnostics
- Cytogenetics and karyotyping: most common, 45 XO/46XY; second most common, 46XY; less frequently other mosaic karyotypes with Y chromosome

Main differential diagnosis
- Persistent Müllerian duct syndrome
- Complete androgen insensitivity syndrome
- Cryptorchidism

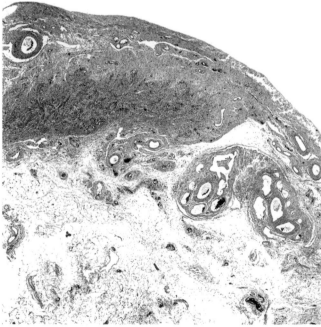

Fig 1. Gonadal dysgenesis. Elongated fibrotic tissue resembling ovarian stroma located adjacent to spermatic vessels.

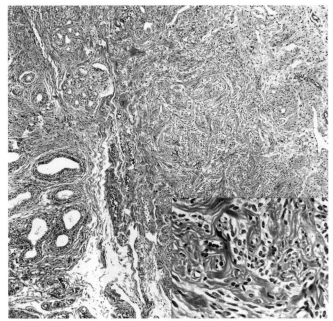

Fig 2. Streak gonad composed of ovarian-type stroma and atrophic sex cord–like structures. Rudimentary epididymal ducts are seen next to the gonadal formation.

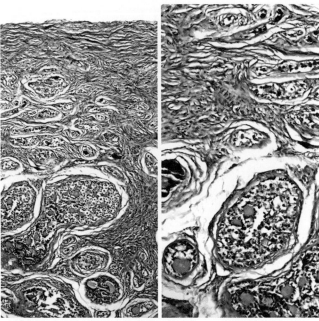

Fig 3. Gonadoblastoma developing in a dysgenetic gonad.

NEOPLASTIC DISEASE OF THE TESTIS

TESTICULAR INTRATUBULAR GERM CELL NEOPLASIA, UNCLASSIFIED

Definition
- Neoplastic germ cells develop within the seminiferous tubules, which are considered to be the precursor of the majority of malignant testicular germ cell tumors. Testicular intratubular germ cell neoplasia, unclassified (ITGCNU), is not an epithelial tumor or carcinoma. In addition, it should be distinguished from other types of invasive malignant germ cell tumors of the testis. Therefore the term *unclassified type of intratubular germ cell neoplasia* is used.

Clinical features
Epidemiology
- ITGCNU is derived from primordial (stem) germ cells.
- The true incidence in the general population is difficult to obtain without invasive procedures.
- The highest ITGCNU incidence was reported in a Danish population as 0.8%.
- One of the most important risk factors is cryptorchidism, in which 2% to 8% of patients will develop ITGCNU.
- The other major risk factor is the presence of a contralateral testicular germ cell tumor. In this group of patients, the risk of having contra lateral ITGCNU is 50-fold to 100-fold higher than general population, which is reported to be 4.9% to 5.7%.
- All other risk factors for developing testicular germ cell tumors are also risk factors for developing ITGCNU, such as infertility, androgen insensitivity syndromes, mixed gonadal dysgenesis, and a history of extragonadal germ cell tumors.

Presentation
- Patients are asymptomatic.
- There is no associated elevation of serum markers, unless coexisting with a malignant germ cell tumor. The elevated markers such as α-fetoprotein (AFP) or β-human chorionic gonadotrophin depends on the type of corresponding invasive tumor components.
- ITGCNU can be detected only in biopsy or surgically removed specimens.

Prognosis and treatment
- There are major differences in clinical management of patients with ITGCNU in different regions in the world. Because the latent period and risk of progression of ITGCNU to invasive GCTs is unknown, the approach is more conservative in the United States. Follow-up alone is recommended for a patient with ITGCNU without evidence of invasive malignant germ cell tumor.
- In some European countries, particularly Denmark, contralateral testicular biopsy is routinely offered in patients with germ cell tumor of the testis at the time of orchiectomy. Positivity for ITGCNU on a contralateral testicular biopsy specimen will be managed by offering sperm banking followed by low-dose radiotherapy to eradicate ITGCNU.

Pathology
Histology
- Testicular ITGCNU is characterized histologically by proliferation of neoplastic germ cells within tubules.
- Neoplastic cells have abundant vacuolated cytoplasm with enlarged hyperchromatic nuclei, often one or two prominent nucleoli (fried-egg appearance).
- Affected seminiferous tubules typically lack spermatogenesis and may have thickened peritubular basement membranes.

Immunopathology (including immunohistochemistry)
- Immunoprofile of ITGCNU similar to that of seminoma
- C-kit (CD117) positive (membrane staining)
- OCT3/4 positive (nuclear staining)
- Placental alkaline phosphatase (PLAP) positive (cytoplasmic staining), not specific
- Glypican 3 negative
- SALL4 positive (nuclear staining)

Molecular diagnostics
- Seminomas show relative overrepresentation of 12p chromosome sequences, but no consistent gain of 12p is detected in ITGCNU. These data indicate that overrepresentation of 12p is required for progression from preinvasive to invasive behavior.

Main differential diagnosis
- Nonneoplastic seminiferous tubules

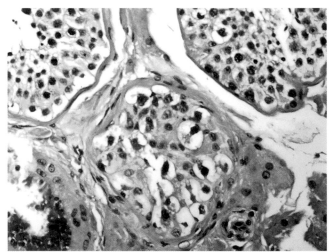

Fig 1. Intratubular germ cell neoplasia, unclassified, showing large neoplastic germ cells within a seminiferous tubule, with a fried-egg appearance.

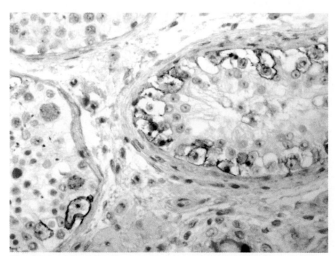

Fig 2. Immunostaining shows neoplastic germ cells of intratubular germ cell neoplasia, unclassified, are positive for C-kit (membranous staining).

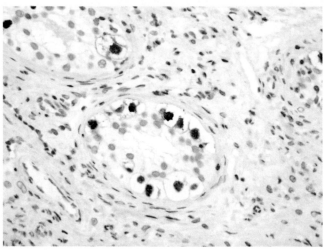

Fig 3. Immunostaining shows that neoplastic germ cells of intratubular germ cell neoplasia, unclassified, are positive for OCT3/4 (nuclear staining).

Definition
- GCT composed of uniform cells with clear cytoplasm and large round nuclei

Clinical features
Epidemiology
- Mean age, 40 years, 10 years older than patients with nonseminomatous GCT
- Rare in prepubertal children
- The most common histologic type of testicular GCT
- Pure seminoma accounting for 50% of all testicular GCT

Presentation
- There is usually painless enlargement of the testis.
- Two percent to 3% of patients may have gynecomastia or metastasis symptoms, such as low back pain, dyspnea, cough, hemoptysis, and headache.
- Serum human chorionic gonadotrophin (hCG) levels are slightly elevated in some patients because of scattered syncytiotrophoblast cells.
- Serum AFP level is normal.

Prognosis and treatment
- Thirty percent of patients develop metastasis at presentation.
- Patients are usually treated with radical orchiectomy.
- Radiation is usually used for stage I or nonbulky stage II disease.
- Chemotherapy is often used for bulky stage II or more advanced-stage disease: cisplatin-based multidrug regimens (cisplatin, bleomycin, etoposide, gemcitabine, vinblastine, ifosfamide).
- Overall survival rate is greater than 95%.

Pathology
Histology
- Usually a well-demarcated, tan-white multinodular mass with a creamy cut surface and various sizes, with an average of 4 cm.
- Most commonly shows diffuse solid sheets of tumor cells separated by fibrous septa; sometimes forms cords or tubular structures, more commonly in the periphery of the tumor
- Tumor cells uniform with distinctive cell borders and abundant clear to lightly eosinophilic cytoplasm; nuclei round to oval with granular chromatin and prominent nucleoli
- Often shows a robust mitotic activity (the use of "anaplastic" seminoma terminology in tumors with more than three mitoses per high-power field is not recommended given the lack of documented clinical significance)
- Septa usually containing abundant lymphocytes and chronic granulomatous reaction seen in up to 50% of cases
- Scattered syncytiotrophoblasts present in 10% to 20% of seminomas, causing slight elevations in serum hCG level
- Lymphovascular invasion common, but should be distinguished from carry-over artifact (floating loose cluster of tumor cells in vascular spaces, often associated with implants of similar cells on the tissue surface)

Immunopathology (including immunohistochemistry)
- Positive for PLAP, CD 117, OCT3/4 (nuclear staining), SALL4, and vimentin
- Negative for various cytokeratins, epithelial membrane antigen (EMA), CD30, AFP, and hCG

Molecular diagnostics
- Isochromosome (12p)
- Twenty percent with C-kit gene amplification and 12% have activating mutations of the C-kit gene (exon 17 or 11)

Main differential diagnosis
- Embryonal carcinoma
- Yolk sac tumor (solid pattern)
- Spermatocytic seminoma
- Testicular lymphoma

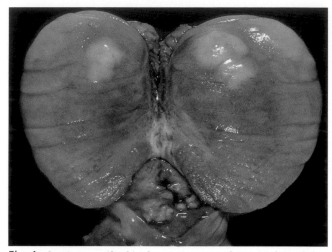

Fig 1. Seminoma (fresh) showing a tan-white, multinodular, and creamy cut surface.

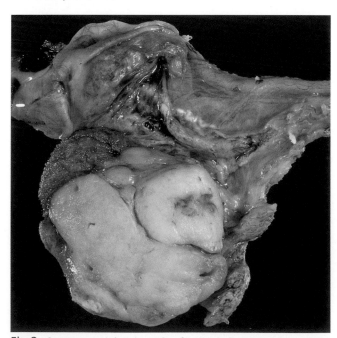

Fig 2. Seminoma (after formalin fixation) showing a tan-white, multinodular, sharply demarcated tumor in the testis.

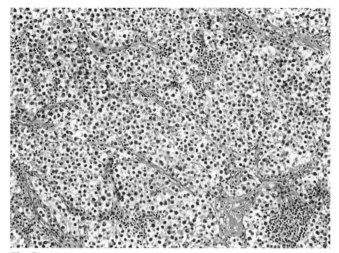

Fig 3. Seminoma showing a diffuse sheet growth pattern with fibrous septa.

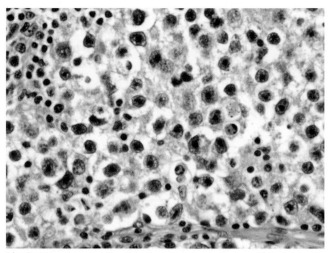

Fig 6. Seminoma cells showing abundant clear to slightly eosinophilic cytoplasm and round nuclei with prominent nucleoli.

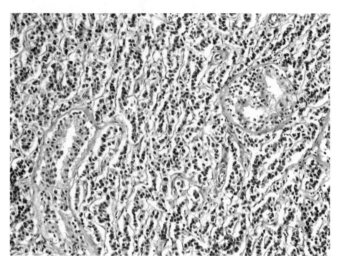

Fig 4. Seminoma cells forming cords infiltrating the interstitium between seminiferous tubules.

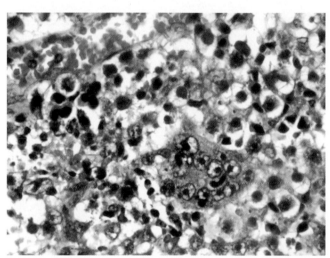

Fig 7. Syncytiotrophoblasts in seminoma containing mulberry-like multiple nuclei.

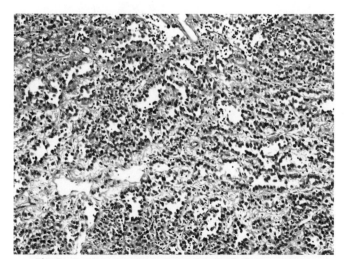

Fig 5. Seminoma cells forming focal tubular structures.

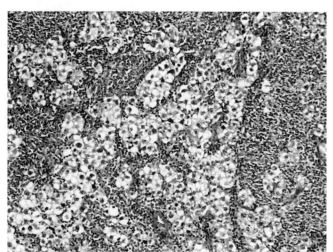

Fig 8. Seminoma showing abundant lymphocytes in the septa.

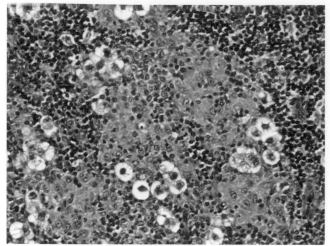

Fig 9. Seminoma showing prominent chronic granulomatous reaction.

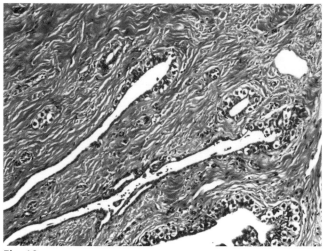

Fig 10. Seminoma cells involving the rete testis in a pagetoid pattern.

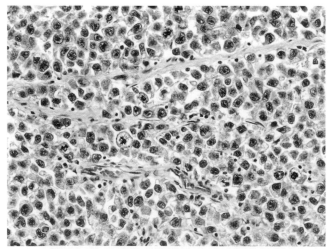

Fig 11. Seminoma showing abundant mitoses.

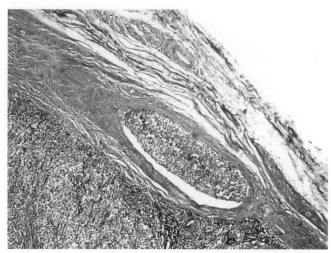

Fig 12. Seminoma invading a small vein in the tunica albuginea.

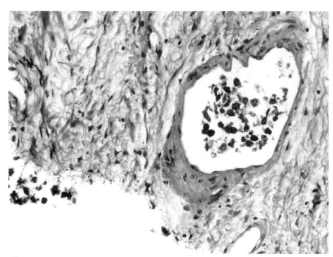

Fig 13. Seminoma showing a carryover artifact with floating loose cluster of tumor cells in vascular spaces and implants of similar cells on the tissue surface.

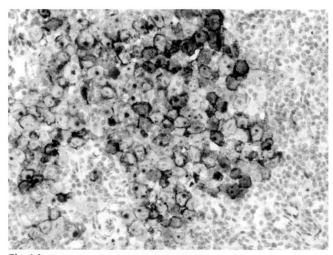

Fig 14. Seminoma cells show positive immunoreactivity for placental alkaline phosphatase in the membrane and cytoplasm.

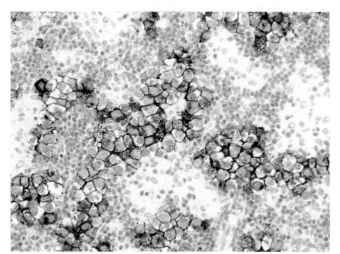

Fig 15. Seminoma cells show positive immunoreactivity for CD117 in the membrane and cytoplasm.

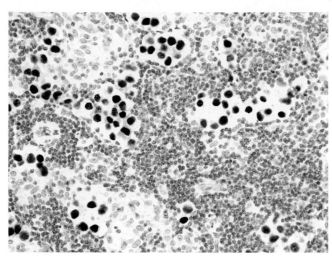

Fig 16. Seminoma cells show positive immunoreactivity for OCT3/4 in the nuclei.

Definition

- Spermatocytic seminoma is a rare germ cell tumor distinct from classical seminoma, both clinically and pathologically. Pathologically, it is characterized by three distinct cell types, lack of cytoplasmic glycogen, and scant to absent lymphocytic infiltrates.

Clinical features

Epidemiology

- Most cases in older white men, in the sixth decade of life
- Occurs exclusively in testis

Presentation

- Unilateral painless swelling of variable duration
- No associated history of cryptorchidism
- Patients typically have a negative tumor marker profile

Prognosis and treatment

- Spermatocytic seminomas rarely metastasize.
- Orchiectomy is the treatment of choice.

Pathology

Histology

- Grossly, a homogenous, solid, pale gray tumor, which may be well circumscribed, lobulated, or cystic, is observed, usually well circumscribed and encapsulated, and confined to the testis.
- Noncohesive tumor cells—with little or no intervening stroma and with no or scant lymphocytic infiltration and granulomatous inflammation—are present.
- Typically, there are three types of cells described. The predominant cell type is of medium size (15 to 20 μm), with a variable amount of dense eosinophilic cytoplasm and a round nucleus, often with a fine granular chromatin. The second type of cell is small (6 to 8 μm), with dark staining nuclei and scant eosinophilic cytoplasm resembling lymphocyte. The third cell type is large (80 to 100 μm) mononucleate, or rarely multinucleated giant cell with round, oval, or indented nuclei.
- Intratubular germ cell neoplasia is not present.

Immunopathology (including immunohistochemistry)

- Generally negative for germ cell markers such as OCT3/4, AE1/3, and CD30
- C-kit positive in approximately 50% of the spermatocytic seminomas

Molecular diagnostics

- The gain of chromosome 9 appears to be a consistent finding in all spermatocytic seminomas, but is not found in classic seminomas.
- Other genetic abnormalities include gain of X chromosome. Classic seminomas in contrast reveal a consistent structural chromosomal abnormality of isochromosome 12p.

Main differential diagnosis

- Seminoma
- Testicular lymphoma
- Embryonal carcinoma

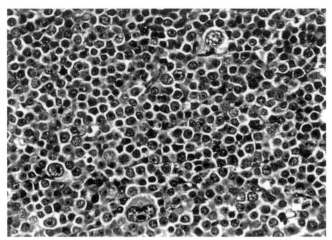

Fig 2. Low-magnification view of spermatocytic seminoma with a solid loose, sheetlike arrangement and distinctly lacking any fibrovascular septae. Note the absence of any lymphocytic or granulomatous inflammation.

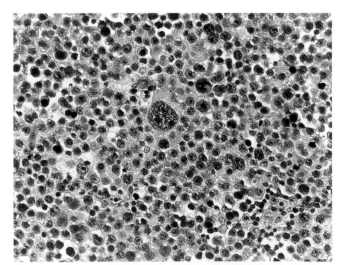

Fig 1. High-magnification view of a spermatocytic seminoma. Note the filamentous ("spireme") chromatin and prominent nucleoli in some of the larger cells. Mitosis and apoptosis is common.

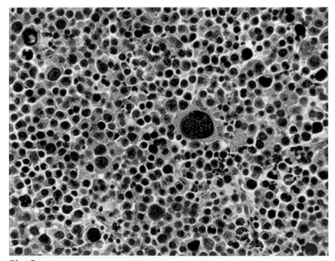

Fig 3. Spermatocytic seminoma with the presence of three cell populations with different cell sizes: small (6 to 8 μm), intermediate (15 to 18 μm), and occasional large cells (50 to 100 μm).

Definition
- GCT composed of primitive epithelial tumor cells recapitulating an early phase of embryonic development

Clinical features
Epidemiology
- Affects young men with a peak age of 30 years, 10 years younger than seminomas
- Rare in prepubertal children
- Common as a component of mixed GCTs, present in 40% of all mixed GCTs
- Rare in pure form; 2% to 10% of all GCTs

Presentation
- Usually painless swelling of the testis
- Occasional testicular pain
- Gynecomastia or metastasis symptoms, such as low back pain, dyspnea, cough, hemoptysis, and headache in 10% of patients
- Slightly elevated serum hCG level and normal AFP level

Prognosis and treatment
- Metastasis common at presentation, in more than 60% of cases
- Radical orchiectomy for all patients
- Retroperitoneal lymph node dissection for patients with regional metastatic disease, but controversial for patients without metastasis
- Possible use of cisplatin-based multidrug chemotherapy (cisplatin, bleomycin, etoposide, gemcitabine, vinblastine, or ifosfamide) as a neoadjuvant or salvage purpose
- Overall survival rate greater than 95%

Pathology
Histology
- Tumor is soft, tan-white, and poorly circumscribed with foci of hemorrhage and necrosis, often with bulges from the cut surface.
- Solid, glandular, and papillary growth patterns are present.
- Tumor cells are crowded with indistinct cell borders and overlapping nuclei. Nuclei have large and irregular with vesicular chromatin and prominent nucleoli. Some nuclei are degenerative with hyperchromatic and smudged chromatin, mimicking syncytiotrophoblasts.
- Mitotic figures are frequent and some are atypical.
- Scattered syncytiotrophoblasts may be present.
- Intratubular embryonal carcinoma may be present in adjacent testicular tissue.
- Lymphovascular invasion is common, but should be distinguished from carryover artifact (floating loose cluster of tumor cells in vascular spaces, often associated with implants of similar cells on the tissue surface).

Immunopathology (including immunohistochemistry)
- Positive for CD30, a highly sensitive and specific marker for EC
- Positive for OCT3/4, a distinct nuclear staining, but also positive in seminoma and intratubular germ cell neoplasia
- Positive for SALL4, nuclear pattern
- Positive for PLAP, but usually patchy and weaker than in seminoma
- Positive for various cytokeratins
- Focally positive for AFP in scattered tumor cells
- Negative for CD117, EMA, CEA, vimentin, and hCG

Molecular diagnostics
- Isochromosome (12p)
- Increased copy number of i(12p) associated with a more aggressive clinical course

Main differential diagnosis
- Seminoma
- Yolk sac tumor (solid type)
- Choriocarcinoma
- Large B cell lymphoma

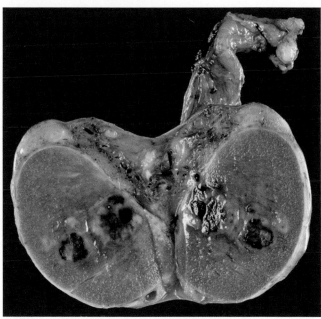

Fig 1. Embryonal carcinoma showing tan-white fleshy nodules with focal hemorrhage and necrosis.

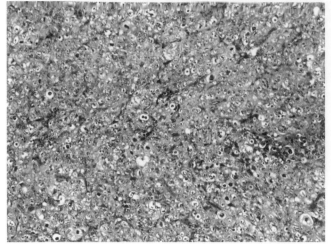

Fig 2. Embryonal carcinoma showing solid growth pattern.

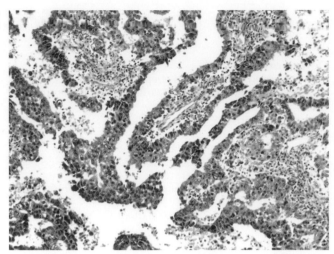

Fig 5. Embryonal carcinoma showing a papillary growth pattern.

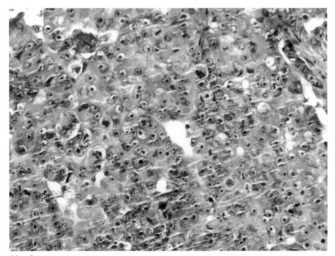

Fig 3. Embryonal carcinoma cells show overlapping nuclei with prominent nucleoli, indistinct cell borders, and active mitosis.

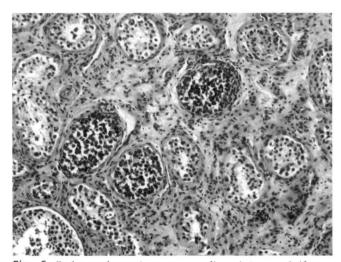

Fig 6. Embryonal carcinoma spreading into seminiferous tubules.

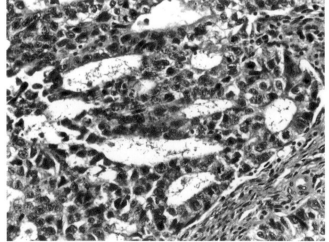

Fig 4. Embryonal carcinoma showing a glandular growth pattern.

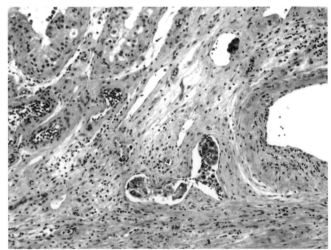

Fig 7. Embryonal carcinoma invading lymphovascular spaces.

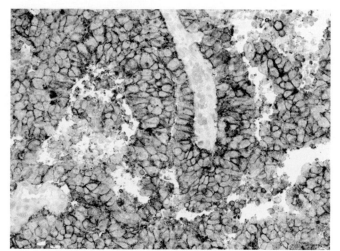

Fig 8. Embryonal carcinoma cells showing membranous staining for CD30.

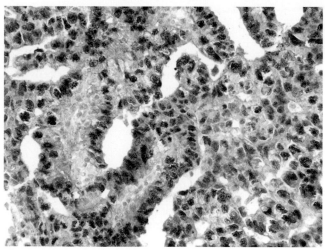

Fig 9. Embryonal carcinoma cells showing nuclear staining for OCT3/4.

Definition
- GCT composed of primitive epithelial tumor cells recapitulating the yolk sac, allantois, and extraembryonic mesenchyma; also called *endodermal sinus tumor*

Clinical features
Epidemiology
- Pure in prepubertal children
- The most common GCT in prepubertal children with a peak age of 16 to 17 months, accounting for 82% of all GCTs in prepubertal children
- Usually as a component of mixed GCT in postpubertal children and adults; present in 40% of nonseminomatous GCTs

Presentation
- Usually painless swelling of the testis
- Elevated AFP level in 90% of cases
- Metastasis at presentation in 10% to 20% of patients, most commonly to the retroperitoneal lymph nodes

Prognosis and treatment
- Radical orchiectomy for all patients
- Retroperitoneal lymph node dissection for patients with regional metastatic disease, but controversial for patients without metastasis
- Possible use of cisplatin-based multidrug chemotherapy (cisplatin, bleomycin, etoposide, gemcitabine, vinblastine, ifosfamide) as a neoadjuvant or salvage purpose, but possibly less effective
- Five-year survival rate greater than 90%

Pathology
Histology
- Well-demarcated, soft, gray to white tumor with gelatinous solid cut surface; cystic, hemorrhagic and necrotic changes possible
- Microcystic or reticular pattern: the most common pattern, characterized by tumor cells with intracellular vacuoles, producing a honeycomb or reticular appearance
- Macrocystic pattern: tumor cells forming large irregular cysts
- Solid pattern: sheets of polygonal cells with clear cytoplasm, distinct cell borders, and prominent nuclei; often associated with a peripheral microcystic pattern
- Glandular-alveolar pattern: tumor cells forming irregular alveoli, glandular or tubular structures
- Endodermal sinus pattern: characterized by Schiller-Duval bodies, composed of a thin-walled blood vessel surrounded by a layer of tumor cells
- Papillary pattern: tumor cells forming papillae projecting into cystic spaces
- Myxomatous pattern: tumor cells present in a myxomatous background

- Sarcomatoid: characterized of highly atypical spindle tumor cells
- Polyvesicular vitelline pattern: tumor cells forming irregular vesicle-like structures in an edematous background
- Hepatoid pattern: polygonal tumor cells with eosinophilic cytoplasm forming trabeculae, nests, or sheets; frequently produce intracellular hyaline globules of variable size (1 to 50 μm); positive for periodic acid–Schiff staining, resistant to diastase digestion
- Parietal pattern: tumor cells producing abundant extracellular basement membrane (parietal differentiation), irregularly shaped eosinophilic bands
- In most cases, several of these patterns present and mixed

Immunopathology (including immunohistochemistry)
- Positive for AFP in patchy pattern (50% to 100%), but negative staining does not exclude yolk sac tumor
- Positive for SALL4, α-1-antitrypsin and glypican-3, PLAP (usually patchy and weaker than in seminoma), and various cytokeratins
- Negative for CD117, OCT3/4, and hCG

Molecular diagnostics
- Loss of chromosomes 1p and 6q
- Gain of chromosomes 1q, 12q, 20q, 22

Main differential diagnosis
- Seminoma
- Embryonal carcinoma

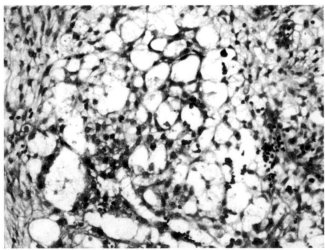

Fig 1. Microcystic or reticular pattern in yolk sac tumor.

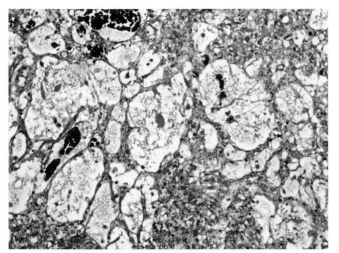

Fig 2. Macrocystic pattern in yolk sac tumor.

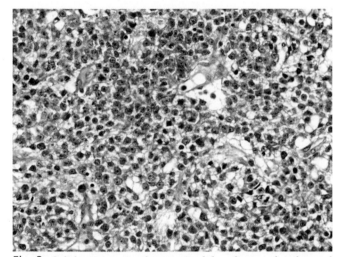

Fig 3. Solid pattern is characterized by sheets of polygonal tumor cells with clear cytoplasm, distinct cell borders, and prominent nuclei.

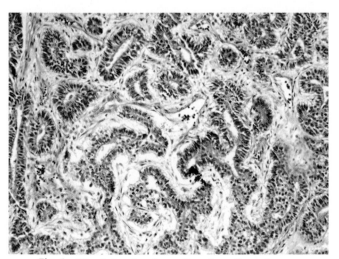

Fig 4. Glandular-alveolar pattern in yolk sac tumor.

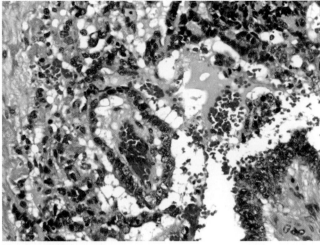

Fig 5. Endodermal sinus pattern is characterized by Schiller-Duval bodies with a thin-walled blood vessel surrounded by a layer of tumor cells.

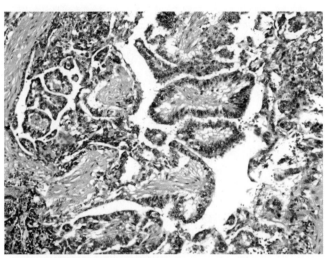

Fig 6. Papillary pattern in yolk sac tumor.

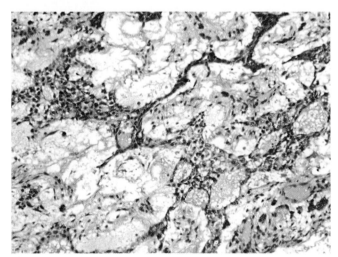

Fig 7. Myxomatous pattern is characterized by abundant myxoid stroma.

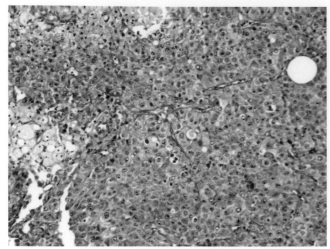

Fig 8. Hepatoid pattern is characterized by polygonal tumor cells with eosinophilic cytoplasm and intracellular hyaline globules.

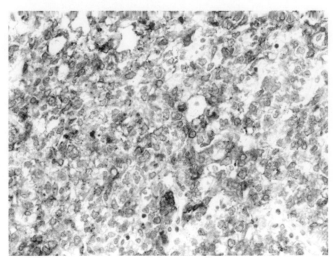

Fig 10. Yolk sac tumor cells are immunoreactive for α-fetoprotein.

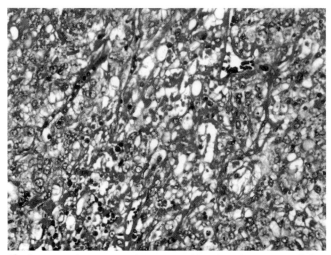

Fig 9. Parietal pattern is characterized by abundant extracellular, irregularly shaped eosinophilic bands.

Definition
- GCT composed of various types of somatic tissue originating from different germinal layers (endoderm, mesoderm, and ectoderm)

Clinical features
Epidemiology
- Occurs in two age groups: children and young adults
- In children, occurs in the first 2 years of life with a mean age of 20 months; the second most common tumor (after yolk sac tumor) and accounting for 24% to 36% of GCTs
- In young adults, rare pure form accounts for 2.7% to 7% of GCTs; commonly found mixed with other GCT components and seen in 47% to 50% of mixed GCTs

Presentation
- Usually painless swelling of the testis
- Normal or slightly evaluated serum hCG level and AFP level

Prognosis and treatment
- Teratomas are benign in prepubertal children and cured by orchiectomy.
- Teratoma is malignant in postpubertal patients. Metastases appear in 22% to 37% of cases, mostly synchronous but metachronous in 13% of cases, and may show different cellular composition from primary tumor. Treatment is the same as for nonseminomatous GCT.
- The presence of immature teratoma does not have any prognostic significance in primary testicular tumors. Designating immature or mature elements is required only in resected posttreatment metastatic lesions to determine response to treatment.
- The 5-year survival rate ranges from 70% to 100%.

Pathology
Histology
- There is a well-circumscribed nodular firm mass with a heterogeneous cut surface with solid cystic areas. Hair, cartilage, and bone may be seen grossly.
- Mature and immature elements are both malignant in postpubertal tumors.
- Mature teratoma elements consist of a variety of somatic-type tissue, including skin, cartilage, muscle, intestinal epithelium, nervous tissue, and others.

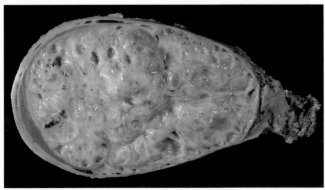

Fig 1. Teratoma showing a tan-white circumscribed lesion with mixed cystic and solid areas.

- Immature teratoma elements are common, but do not have any prognostic significance, and may include neuroepithelium, blastema, or embryonic tubules.
- Intratubular germ cell neoplasia is not present in prepubertal children.

Immunopathology (including immunohistochemistry)
- The differentiated elements express the immunophenotype expected for that specific cell type.
- AFP in 19% to 36% of cases with intestinal and hepatoid areas
- PLAP may also be focally positive in glandular structures.

Molecular diagnostics
- Normal diploid karyotype in prepubertal patents
- Isochromosome (12p) in postpubertal patients

Main differential diagnosis
- Dermoid cyst
- Epidermoid cyst

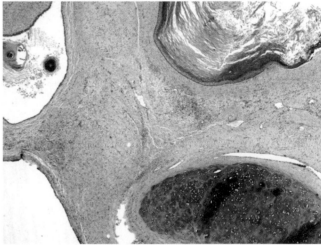

Fig 2. Teratoma showing cartilage, glandular and squamous components.

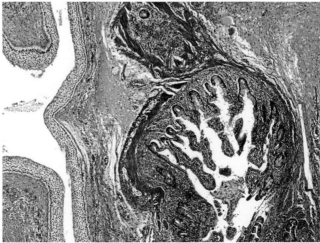

Fig 3. Teratoma showing intestinal and sebaceous glands.

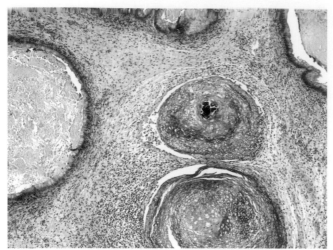

Fig 4. Teratoma showing intestinal glandular and squamous components.

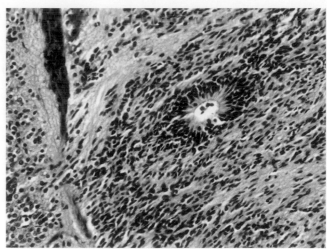

Fig 6. Teratoma showing an immature component characterized by neuroepithelial cells forming tubular structure.

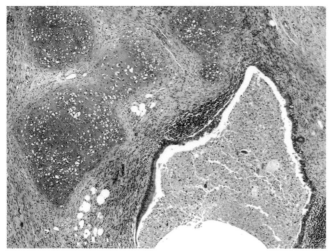

Fig 5. Teratoma showing cartilage and glands.

Definition
- Testicular germ cell tumor composed of more than one histologic type of germ cell tumor

Clinical features
Epidemiology
- Second most common germ cell tumor, representing 30% to 40% of all testicular germ cell tumors
- Most common in young adults (20 to 40 years old)

Presentation
- Testicular mass

Prognosis and treatment
- Prognosis depends on clinical stage, presence and proportion of embryonal carcinoma, and lymphovascular invasion.
- Treatment is similar to that for pure nonseminomatous germ cell tumor.

Pathology
Histology
- Embryonal carcinoma and teratoma represent the most common combination (25%), followed by embryonal carcinoma and seminoma (15%), and embryonal carcinoma, yolk sac tumor, and teratoma (10%); other combinations are less frequent.
- Histologic features are those corresponding to the pure forms of the tumors found in combination.

Immunopathology (including immunohistochemistry)
- Similar to the immunoprofile exhibit by the pure forms of the component tumors

Main differential diagnosis
- Pure germ cell tumor
- Metastatic carcinoma

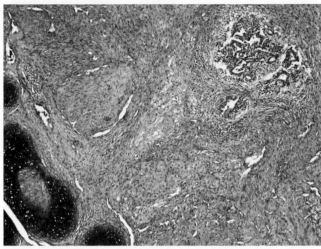

Fig 2. Mixed germ cell tumor with a predominant teratomatous component and foci of yolk sac tumor *(upper right field)*.

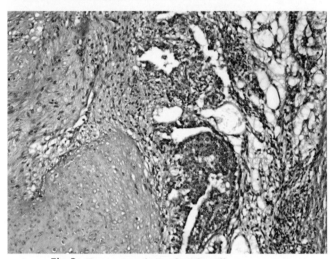

Fig 3. Teratoma admixed with yolk sac tumor.

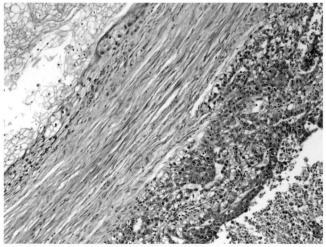

Fig 1. Mixed germ cell tumor composed of mature teratoma *(upper left field)* and embryonal carcinoma *(lower right field)*.

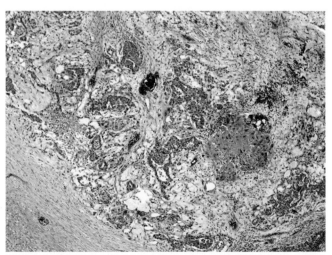

Fig 4. Embryonal carcinoma and choriocarcinoma in a mixed germ cell tumor.

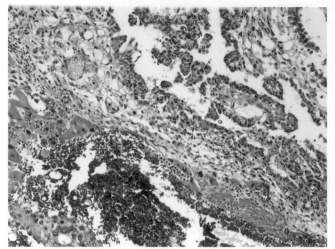

Fig 5. Embryonal carcinoma and choriocarcinoma.

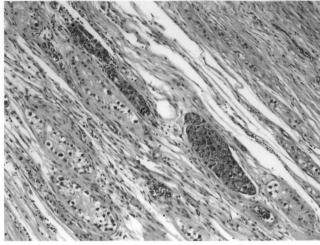

Fig 7. Lymphovascular invasion and intratubular germ cell neoplasia at the periphery of a mixed germ cell tumor.

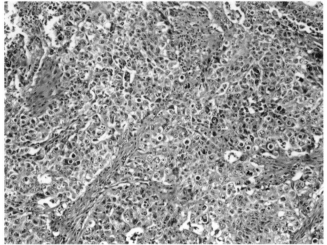

Fig 6. Solid embryonal carcinoma with areas of necrosis in a mixed germ cell tumor.

TERATOMA WITH SOMATIC-TYPE MALIGNANCIES

Definition
- A teratoma containing a secondary somatic (or non–germ cell) malignant component

Clinical features
Epidemiology
- Seen in 3% to 6% of GCTs containing a teratomatous component

Presentation
- Can be seen in primary or metastatic GCT
- Teratomatous component present in most cases, but absent in rare occasions

Prognosis and treatment
- Findings might not be clinically significant when limited to the primary tumor.
- Prognosis is poor if teratoma is present in metastasis.
- Patients are usually treated with surgical resection.
- Somatic malignancies do not respond to conventional GCT chemotherapy, but may respond to therapy designed for the specific type of somatic malignancy.

Pathology
Histology
- There is an expansive or infiltrative proliferation of cytologically atypical somatic cells overgrowing the surrounding teratoma or other GCT components. The atypical growth should be larger than a low-power (×4) field.
- Most common somatic components are sarcomas, including rhabdomyosarcoma, leiomyosarcoma, angiomyosarcoma, and primitive neuroectodermal tumor. Some are carcinomas, including adenocarcinoma, squamous carcinoma, and undifferentiated carcinoma. Hematopoietic malignancies have also been reported.

- This denomination can also be applied to an immature teratoma with similar overgrowth of the immature component.

Immunopathology (including immunohistochemistry)
- Immunoprofile characteristic of the somatic-type malignancy

Molecular diagnostics
- Most non-GCT malignancies also have isochromosome (12p).
- Some may show chromosomal rearrangement associated with the somatic tumor in a conventional location.

Main differential diagnosis
- Atypical stromal nodule
- Metastasis not associated with GCT components

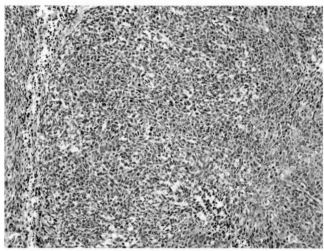

Fig 2. Poorly differentiated rhabdomyosarcoma in a teratoma.

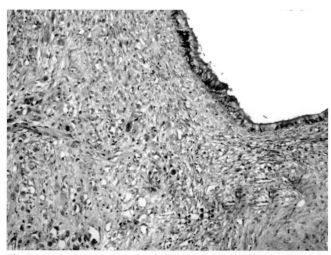

Fig 1. Teratoma with adenocarcinoma and primitive neuroectodermal tumor areas.

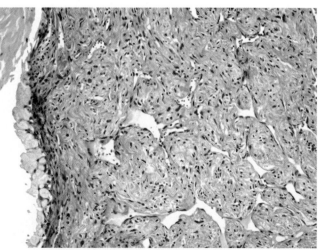

Fig 3. Well-differentiated angiosarcoma in a teratoma.

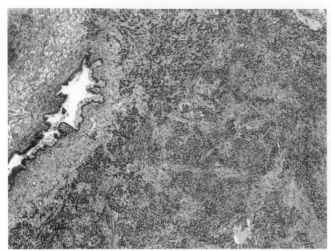

Fig 4. Primitive neuroectodermal tumor in a teratoma.

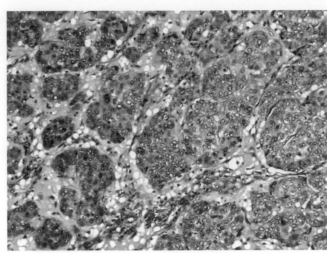

Fig 6. Poorly differentiated carcinoma in a teratoma.

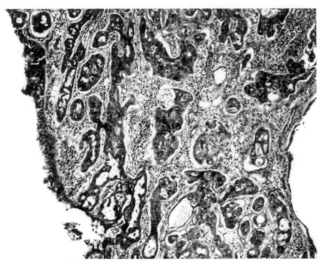

Fig 5. Adenocarcinoma in a teratoma.

Definition
- A monodermal teratoma composed of low-grade, well-differentiated neuroendocrine neoplasm

Clinical features
Epidemiology
- This tumor accounts for less than 0.5% of all testicular tumors.
- It occurs as a pure form in 75% of cases and is associated with a teratomatous component in the remainder of cases.
- Patient age ranges from 12 to 65 years, with a mean of 36 years.

Presentation
- The tumor is usually present with a testicular swelling that is sometimes be associated with pain.
- Twelve percent of patients can develop carcinoid syndrome, including diarrhea, hot flashes, palpitations, and others, and is more common in patients with metastasis.
- Serum AFP and HCG levels are normal, but serum serotonin is elevated.

Prognosis and treatment
- Most patients are cured by orchiectomy.
- Carcinoid syndrome and large size are associated with a poor prognosis.
- Metastatic carcinoid also has an indolent course.

Pathology
Histology
- Solid, tan-yellow, well-circumscribed tumor, with variable tumor size (0.8 to 8.0 cm; mean, 2.5 cm)
- Various patterns, the most common being an organoid pattern with solid nests and acini of cells in a fibrous or hyalinized stroma
- Uniform, polygonal tumor cells with eosinophilic granular cytoplasm and round nuclei with a punctuate or "salt and pepper" chromatin pattern
- Associated with focal epidermoid cyst or teratoma in 25% of cases
- Lacks intratubular germ cell neoplasia

Immunopathology (including immunohistochemistry)
- Positive for synaptophysin, chromogranin, neurospecific enolase, serotonin, substance P, gastrin, vasoactive intestinal polypeptide, and cytokeratin
- Also positive for argyrophil and argentaffin staining
- Pleomorphic neurosecretory granules on electromicroscopy

Main differential diagnosis
- Metastatic carcinoid tumor
- Sertoli cell tumor
- Granulosa cell tumor

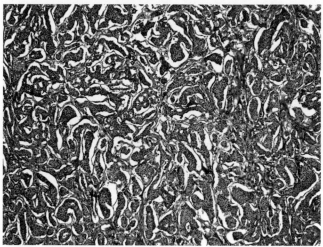

Fig 1. Testicular carcinoid tumor showing an organoid pattern with acini of tumor cells in a fibrous stroma. (Courtesy Wenle Wang.)

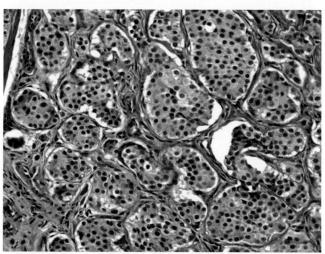

Fig 2. Testicular carcinoid tumor showing a nested growth pattern. (Courtesy Wenle Wang.)

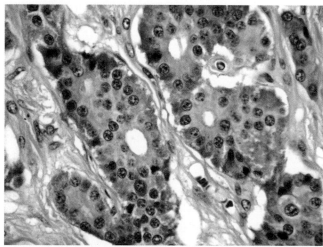

Fig 3. Testicular carcinoid tumor cells with abundant eosinophilic cytoplasm and small round nuclei with coarse chromatin.

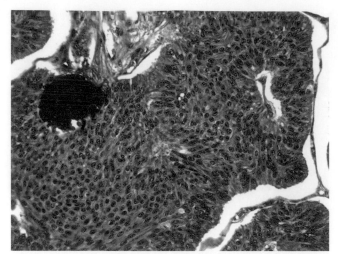

Fig 4. Testicular carcinoid tumor showing focal spindle cell features. (Courtesy Wenle Wang.)

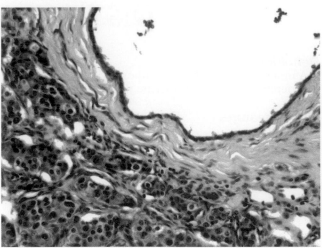

Fig 5. Testicular carcinoid tumor is associated with mature cystic teratoma. (Courtesy Wenle Wang.)

Definition
- Specialized benign, monodermal, and unicystic form of teratoma composed of keratinizing squamous epithelium and normal skin appendage structures

Clinical features
Epidemiology
- Extremely rare (less than 1% of all testis tumors)
- Typically seen in young adult males in the second to fourth decades of life; occasionally seen in prepubertal patients

Presentation
- Palpable, usually painless testicular mass

Prognosis and treatment
- Benign
- Surgical resection (either complete or partial orchiectomy)

Pathology
Histology
- Unilocular cystic structure composed of epidermis and dermis (normal-appearing skin)
- Epidermal layer composed of keratinizing squamous epithelium
- Dermal component contains skin adnexal structures (e.g., hair follicles, sebaceous glands, apocrine glands)
- Infrequently one can encounter other mature teratomatous elements as a minor component (e.g., ciliated epithelium, intestinal-type mucosa, thyroid, cartilage).
- Neither intratubular germ cell neoplasia nor any other germ cell tumor component should be present in the surrounding testis.
- Adjacent testis typically shows normal spermatogenesis; granulomatous reactions to cyst contents may be seen occasionally.

Immunopathology (including immunohistochemistry)
- Negative staining for germ cell markers (e.g., C-kit, OCT3/4, PLAP)

Molecular diagnostics
- Negative for isochromosome 12p

Main differential diagnosis
- Epidermoid cyst
- Mature cystic teratoma
- Malignant mixed germ cell tumor with teratomatous component

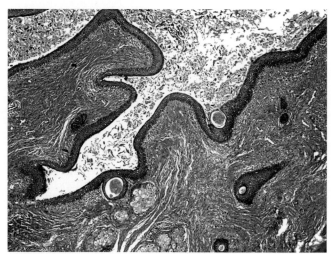

Fig 1. Testicular dermoid cyst lined by keratinizing squamous epithelium with hair follicles and sebaceous glands.

Definition
- Benign cyst lined by keratinizing squamous epithelium and lacking adnexal structures

Clinical features
Epidemiology
- Rare
- Male patients up to 40 to 50 years of age
- May arise from an epithelial inclusion from the overlying skin
- Entity suggested to represent a form of teratoma caused by identified chromosomal abnormalities in a subset of cases

Presentation
- Painless testicular mass that may slowly enlarge

Prognosis and treatment
- Surgical resection is the primary treatment.
- Course is benign.

Pathology
Histology
- Fibrous walled cyst, often intraparenchymal, lined by a keratinizing squamous epithelium with a granular cell layer; dense collections of keratin within the center of the cyst and lacking adnexal structures
- Not associated with intratubular germ cell neoplasia or teratomatous component
- Occasional rupture that can result in giant cell reaction

Immunopathology (including immunohistochemistry)
- Not contributory

Molecular diagnostics
- May demonstrate loss of heterozygosity on chromosomal analysis
- Lacks isochromosome 12p

Main differential diagnosis
- Malignant teratoma with pure mature cystic elements

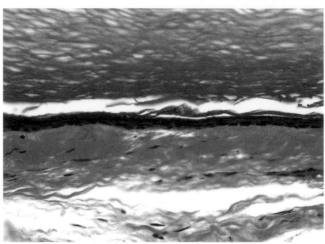

Fig 2. Epidermoid cysts lined by keratinizing squamous epithelium lacking adnexal structures.

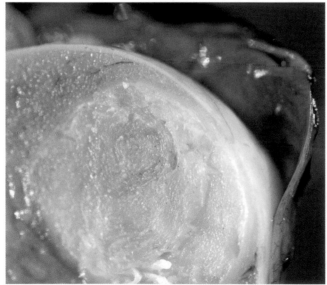

Fig 1. On gross examination, epidermoid cysts are well circumscribed and tan-white in appearance with a condensed center of keratin.

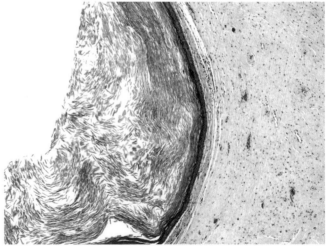

Fig 3. Testicular epidermoid cyst lined by keratinizing squamous epithelium without skin appendages.

Definition
- Malignant germ cell tumor composed of syncytiotrophoblast, cytotrophoblast, and intermediate trophoblast cells

Clinical features
Epidemiology
- Incidence of 0.8/100,000 overall
- Admixed in malignant mixed germ cell tumor in 8% of cases
- In pure form in less than 1% of cases
- Typically occurs in young men 25 to 30 years old

Presentation
- Most commonly appears with symptoms related to hematogenous metastases (hemoptysis, CNS symptoms, and hemorrhage in visceral sites)
- High hCG levels (greater than 100,000 mIU/mL)
- May result in gynecomastia or hyperthyroidism
- Testicular mass possibly present (primary site can regress)

Prognosis and treatment
- Typically appears with widely metastatic disease
- Stage-for-stage, may not behave much differently from other malignant germ cell tumors

Pathology
Histology
- Grossly, possible presence of a hemorrhagic nodule or scar
- Admixture of syncytiotrophoblast cells (large, multinucleated cells with large irregular nuclei), cytotrophoblast cells (pale cytoplasm with single large nucleus and prominent nucleolus), and intermediate trophoblast cells (clear cytoplasm, larger than cytotrophoblasts with single nuclei)
- Background of extensive hemorrhage and necrosis
- Vascular invasion possibly prominent

Immunopathology (including immunohistochemistry)
- All cell types stain for cytokeratin.
- Syncytiotrophoblasts are positive for hCG, inhibin, and EMA.
- Intermediate trophoblasts are positive for human placental lactogen (hPL).

Main differential diagnosis
- Seminoma with syncytiotrophoblasts
- Embryonal carcinoma
- Other trophoblastic neoplasms

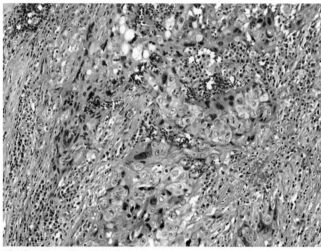

Fig 2. Two cell types are noted. Syncytiotrophoblasts are larger multinucleated cells with abundant eosinophilic cytoplasm, whereas admixed cytotrophoblasts have pale cytoplasm and a single nucleus.

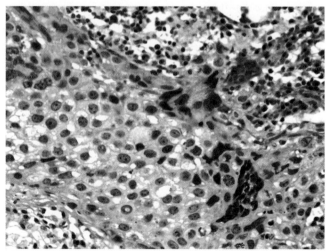

Fig 3. Cytotrophoblasts with single nucleus and prominent nucleolus, juxtaposed with syncytiotrophoblasts, which have larger nuclei and more prominent cytologic atypia.

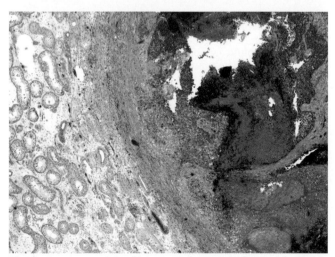

Fig 1. Extensive central hemorrhage and necrosis are characteristic of choriocarcinoma.

Definition
- Neoplasm of the Leydig cells, which are normally located in the interstitium of the testis

Clinical features
Epidemiology
- Leydig cell tumors (LCTs) are most common in prepubertal boys (5 to 10 years old) and in young adults (30 to 60 years old).
- LCTs are more common in whites than in African Americans and Asians. Similar to germ cell tumors, patients with cryptorchidism, atrophy, and infertility are at a slightly increased risk.
- Benign LCTs are not uncommon, representing approximately 1% to 3% of testicular neoplasms, and are the most common sex cord–stromal tumors in all ages.
- It is estimated that 10% of LCTs are malignant, but fewer than 200 cases appear in the English-language literature. The only established criterion for defining malignant disease is the presence of metastasis.

Presentation
- Diagnosis is typically incidental on imaging.
- Patients may have a palpable, painless mass.
- Prepubertal boys with androgen-secreting tumors may exhibit precocious puberty.
- Adults with androgen-secreting tumors are generally asymptomatic.

Prognosis and treatment
- The prognosis is good, with cure in the vast majority of cases. LCTs are primarily managed with surgical resection using radical inguinal orchiectomy. Testis-sparing surgery with enucleation of the mass has been tried, especially in children and young adults.
- For malignant cases, chemotherapy with the bleomycin-etoposide-platinum regimen used for germ cell malignancies has been used, but with limited efficacy.
- The tyrosine kinase inhibitor imatinib has shown some chemotherapeutic activity in animal models, and it may be a promising alternative regimen in aggressive cases.

Pathology
Histology
- Usually well-circumscribed, yellow or tan, solid intratesticular masses, measuring up to 5 cm in diameter. Necrosis or hemorrhage is uncommon and may be a feature of aggressive disease. Extension to paratesticular tissue can be seen grossly or microscopically in approximately 10% of cases and does not indicate malignant behavior.
- Leydig cells are characteristically polygonal with abundant eosinophilic cytoplasm, round nuclei with variation in size, and central nucleoli.
- LCTs are composed of a well-circumscribed collection of Leydig cells. Association with Leydig cell hyperplasia is seen in selected cases. Reinke crystals, cytoplasm inclusions that are only seen in Leydig cells, are reportedly found in approximately 40% of LCTs. Lipofuscin deposition is a common feature, and fibrous bands separating tumor nodules are also seen in some cases. Scattered larger cells are common and can be seen in most cases. These cells should not be interpreted as malignant transformation.

- Several histologic variants exist, including solid (most common), cordlike, pseudoglandular, adipose-like, and microcystic. Focal spindle cell morphology can occur in some cases and is not diagnostic of sarcomatoid transformation.
- Diagnostic criteria for malignant LCTs have not been established, and metastatic disease is the only pathognomonic finding. However, features that are suggestive of aggressive behavior and should be mentioned in the report are large tumor size (greater than 5 cm), increased mitotic figures, overt cytologic atypia, vascular or capsular invasion, infiltrative pattern, and tumor necrosis.

Immunopathology (including immunohistochemistry)
- Diffusely positive for vimentin, calretinin and inhibin A
- Negative for keratins (CAM5.2, pancytokeratin)
- May be positive for Melan-A, p53, and BCL2

Main differential diagnosis
- Leydig cell hyperplasia
- Adrenogenital syndrome–associated tumors
- Metastatic carcinoma, especially high-grade prostatic carcinoma
- Adrenal rests

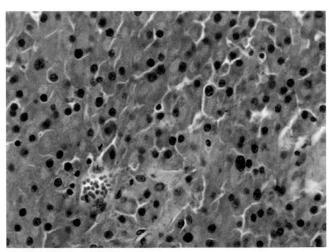

Fig 1. Classic Leydig cell cytologic features with abundant, densely eosinophilic cytoplasm and central nuclei. Some variation in nuclear size is common.

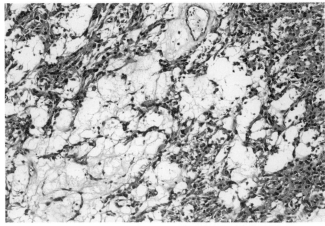

Fig 2. Leydig cell tumor with mucinous stroma.

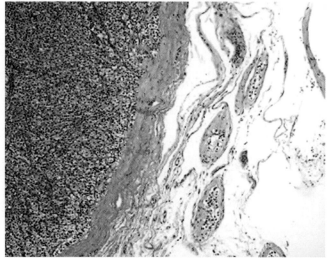

Fig 3. Most Leydig cell tumors are well circumscribed with a thin pseudocapsule separating the tumor from the adjacent parenchyma. In this case, the testis is atrophic.

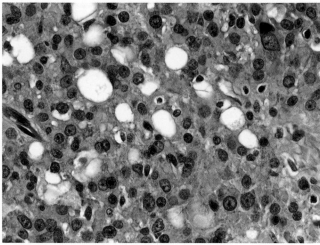

Fig 6. Focal vacuolization in tumor cells of Leydig cell tumors is a common finding.

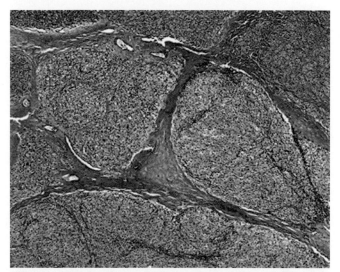

Fig 4. Intralesional fibrous bands are commonly found in Leydig cell tumors.

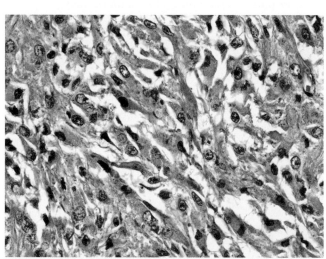

Fig 7. Spindle cells are sometimes seen. In this case, there is also mild cytologic atypia.

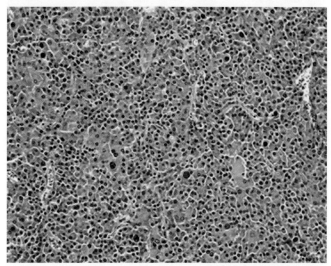

Fig 5. Scattered, large, more atypical cells can be seen in most cases.

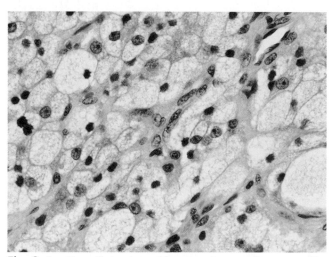

Fig 8. Leydig cell tumor with extensive xanthomatous-like changes.

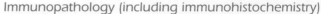

Definition
- Sex cord–stromal tumor of the testis composed of cells showing features of Sertoli cells

Clinical features
Epidemiology
- Less than 1% of testicular neoplasms
- Mostly in adults; 15% in children

Presentation
- Painless testicular mass
- Occasional gynecomastia
- Some associated with androgen insensitivity syndrome, Carney syndrome, and Peutz-Jeghers syndrome

Prognosis and treatment
- Mostly benign (90%)
- Surgical excision
- No response to radiation and chemotherapy

Pathology
Histology
- Generally small and well circumscribed, yellow-gray, and lobulated on cut surface
- Solid, tubular, cordlike growth patterns observed
- Ovoid or spindle-shaped nuclei without prominent nucleoli, without overt atypia, low mitotic count, eosinophilic or clear cytoplasm, and variably scanty, edematous, hyalinized, or sclerotic connective stroma
- Size larger than 5 cm, cellular atypia, increased mitotic activity, necrosis, infiltrative pattern, extratesticular extension, and vascular invasion associated with aggressive behavior

Immunopathology (including immunohistochemistry)
- Positive for vimentin, cytokeratin, EMA, and inhibin (less frequently than in LCTs)
- Negative or very focally positive for PLAP, OCT3/4, CD30

Main differential diagnosis
- Seminoma with tubular pattern
- LCT
- Adenomatoid tumor

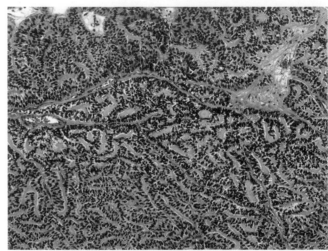

Fig 2. Cord-like disposition of tumor cells in a Sertoli cell tumor.

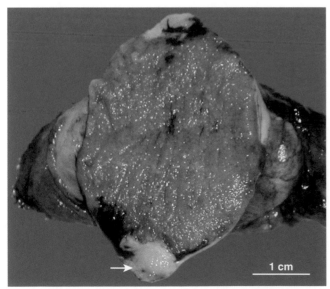

Fig 1. Bisection of the testis showing a well-demarcated gray-white Sertoli cell tumor *(arrow)*.

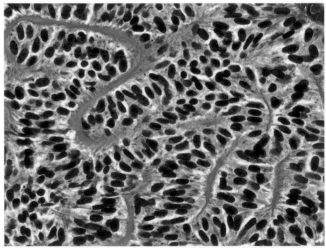

Fig 3. Closely packed cords of tumor cells surrounded by scanty paucicellular stroma.

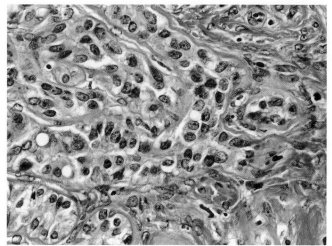

Fig 4. The tumor cells have clear to pale cytoplasm and ovoid nuclei.

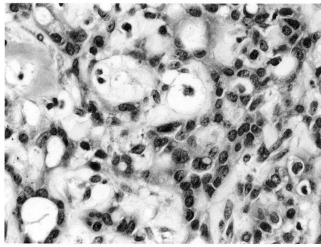

Fig 7. Sertoli cell tumor with mucinous stroma.

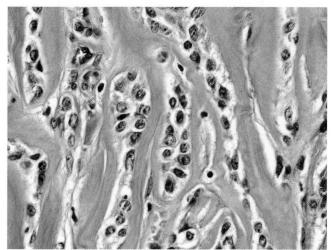

Fig 5. Sertoli cell tumor with discrete small cords and nests among a hyalinized stroma.

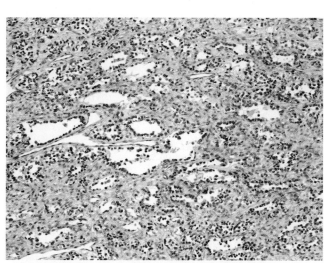

Fig 8. Sertoli cell tumor with retiform pattern.

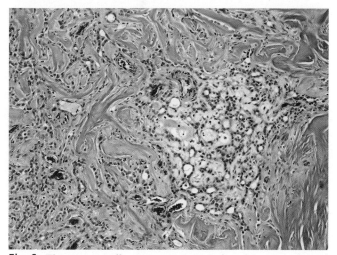

Fig 6. The tumor cells aggregate into trabeculae or cords and hyalinized stroma.

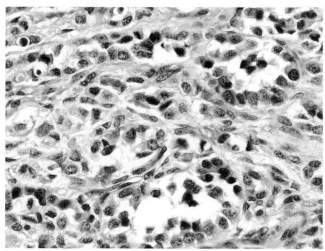

Fig 9. Malignant Sertoli cell tumor with atypia and mitotic figures.

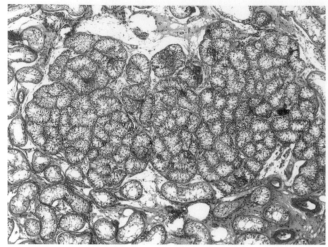

Fig 10. A Sertoli cell adenoma in a patient with androgen insensitivity syndrome. The nodule is composed of well-circumscribed proliferation of closely packed tubules.

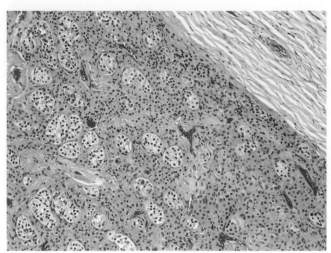

Fig 12. Sertoli cell adenoma with associated Leydig cell hyperplasia.

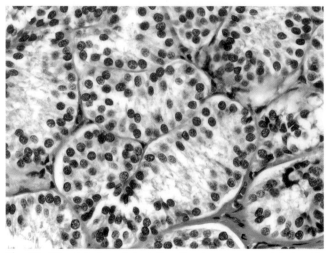

Fig 11. The tubules of Sertoli cell adenoma associated with androgen insensitivity syndrome are lined with immature Sertoli cells.

SCLEROSING SERTOLI CELL TUMOR

Definition
• Rare variant of Sertoli cell tumor with prominent sclerosis

Clinical features
Epidemiology
• Mean age, 35 years (range, 18 to 80 years)

Presentation
• Testicular mass or nodule
• Incidental finding

Prognosis and treatment
• Good; benign outcome in most cases
• Orchiectomy

Pathology
• Usually unilateral, well-circumscribed, but unencapsulated tumors smaller than classic Sertoli cell tumors (mean diameter, 1.5 cm), showing a solid white to yellow-tan cut surface
• Histologically cords, solid or tubular nests of Sertoli cells intimately admixed with a densely sclerotic stroma, variably sized nuclei with pale and vacuolated cytoplasm, and low mitotic activity

Immunopathology (including immunohistochemistry)
• Neoplastic cells positive to vimentin, inhibin, and S-100

Main differential diagnosis
• Trabecular carcinoid tumor

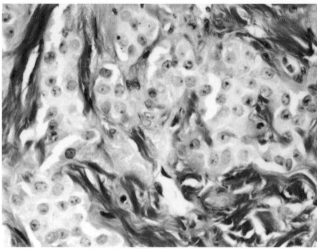

Fig 2. Tumor cells are polygonal, with clear cytoplasm, indistinctive cellular borders, and round nuclei with evident nucleoli.

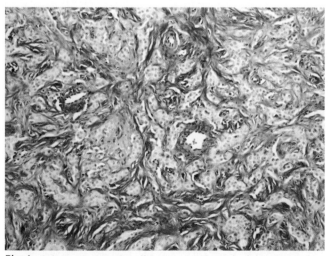

Fig 1. Sclerosing Sertoli cell tumor composed of dense interlacing bands of fibrous tissue.

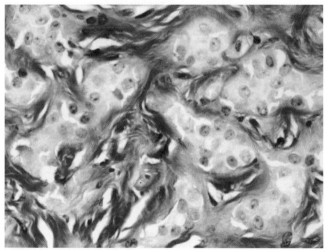

Fig 3. Dense bands of fibrotic tissue are observed interspersed between the Sertoli tumor cells.

LARGE CELL CALCIFYING SERTOLI CELL TUMOR

Definition
- Variant of Sertoli cell tumor composed of large polygonal Sertoli cells with calcification

Clinical features
Epidemiology
- Extremely rare

Presentation
- Painless testicular mass
- Bilateral in 40%
- Sporadic (60%) or associated with Carney or Peutz-Jeghers syndromes
- Endocrine syndromes, precocious puberty, or gynecomastia present in some patients

Prognosis and treatment
- Mostly benign (80%)
- Surgical excision

Pathology
Histology
- Tumors are generally small and well circumscribed with a yellow-gray and lobulated cut surface.
- Solid, tubular, and cordlike growth patterns can be observed.
- Tumor cells are large polygonal with abundant eosinophilic, finely granular cytoplasm, vesicular nuclei with prominent nucleoli, within a myxohyaline stroma. Distinct calcifications characterized by large, laminated calcified nodule, psammoma bodies and focal ossification, and neutrophilic infiltration can be also found.

- Size larger than 5 cm, cellular atypia, increased mitotic activity, necrosis, extratesticular extension, and vascular invasion are associated with aggressive behavior.

Immunopathology (including immunohistochemistry)
- Positive for vimentin, EMA, melan-A, and inhibin

Main differential diagnosis
- Sertoli cell tumor
- LCT

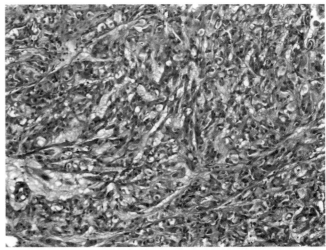

Fig 2. Tumor cells with a solid pattern of growth.

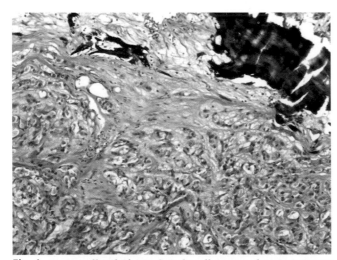

Fig 1. Large cell calcifying Sertoli cell tumor showing tumor cells within a hyalinized stroma and prominent foci of irregular tissue calcification.

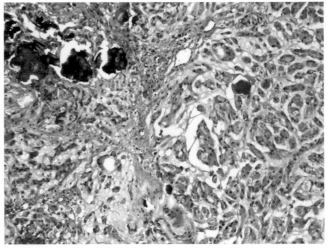

Fig 3. Tumors cells forming cords and nests within a hyalinized and fibromyxoid stroma and foci of distrophic calcification.

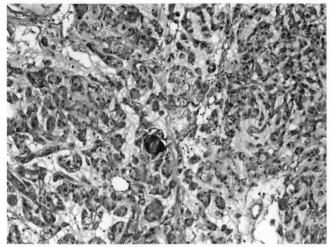

Fig 4. A psammomatous body (*center of the field*) surrounded by cords and nests of Sertoli cells. Note the fibromyxoid stroma.

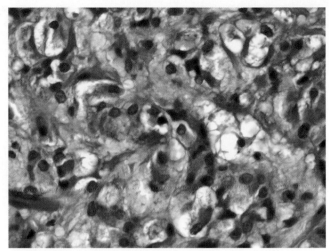

Fig 6. Tumor cells are polygonal, with ample eosinophilic cytoplasm, round nuclei, and evident nucleoli. Note the absence of nuclear atypias or mitotic activity.

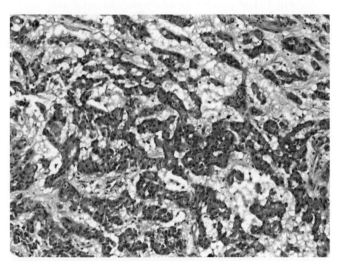

Fig 5. Large cell calcifying Sertoli cell tumor with a predominant cordlike pattern of growth.

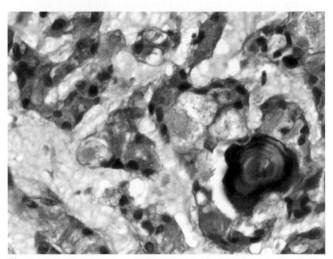

Fig 7. A laminated psammomatous body in a large cell calcifying Sertoli cell tumor.

Definition
- Testicular sex cord–stromal tumor resembling ovarian granulosa cell tumor

Clinical features

Epidemiology
- Extremely rare
- No specific age predominance for adult cases (average, 44 years)
- Juvenile granulosa cell tumor occurs in the first year (in more than 90% of cases before 4 months old)

Presentation
- Painless testicular mass, well circumscribed, sometimes encapsulated
- Occasionally associated with gynecomastia (approximately 25%)
- Ambiguous genitalia and gonadal dysgenesis in 20% of patients with juvenile granulosa cell tumor, all showing abnormal karyotypes, including 45X/46XY mosaicism or structural anomalies of Y chromosome

Prognosis and treatment
- Mostly indolent course, but with malignant potential (metastasis in 20% of cases)
- Surgical excision
- Long-term follow-up

Pathology

Histology
- Microfollicular (most common), solid, trabecular, insular, macrofollicular, or cystic growth patterns are described.
- Tumors are round to ovoid with little cytoplasm, nuclear grooves, occasional cytologic atypia, and Call-Exner bodies.
- Malignant features include large size (greater than 7 cm), high mitotic count (greater than four of ten high-power fields [HPFs]), hemorrhage, necrosis, and lymphovascular invasion.
- Juvenile granulosa cell tumor is characterized by cystic structures lined by inner granulosa cells and outer theca cells.

Immunopathology (including immunohistochemistry)
- Positive for vimentin, inhibin, Melan-A, calretinin, smooth muscle actin, CD99
- Occasionally positive for cytokeratins
- Nonreactive for EMA, PLAP, OCT3/4, AFP, CD30, hCG

Main differential diagnosis
- Other sex cord–stromal tumors
- Yolk sac tumor for juvenile granulomas cell tumor

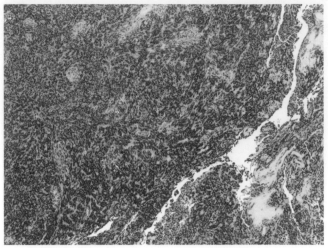

Fig 1. Low-power view of a granulosa cell tumor.

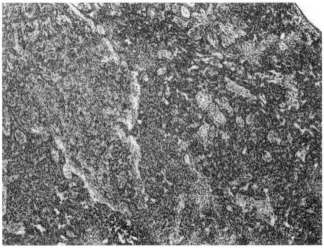

Fig 2. Granulosa cell tumor with a predominant solid pattern of growth.

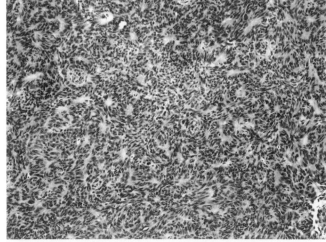

Fig 3. Granulosa cell tumor with a solid pattern of growth.

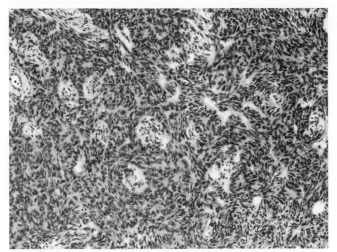

Fig 4. Granulosa cell tumor at medium-power view.

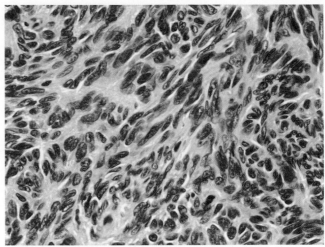

Fig 6. Granulosa cell tumor composed of tumor cells with irregular nuclear membranes and occasional nuclear grooves, ample amphophilic cytoplasm, and indistinctive borders.

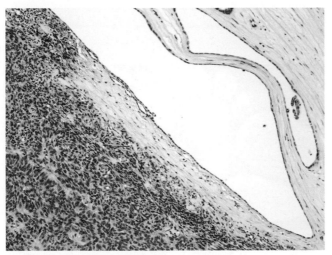

Fig 5. Granulosa cell tumor extending to the rete testis.

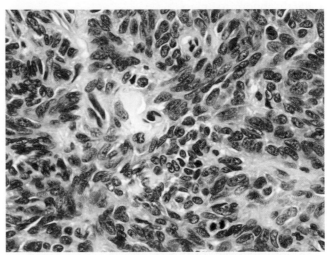

Fig 7. Granulosa cell tumor with a single mitotic figure *(lower right field)*.

JUVENILE GRANULOSA CELL TUMOR

Definition
- Rare benign testicular gonadal stromal tumor

Clinical features
Epidemiology
- Typically occurs in children 4 years old or younger, with most cases occurring before 1 year of age
- Accounts for 1% to 5% of all prepubertal testis tumors
- Most common congenital testicular neoplasm and the most common cause of testicular enlargement in newborns younger than 6 months
- Rare cases reported in adults
- Approximately 30% reported in patients with cryptorchidism
- Usually unilateral; rare bilateral cases reported

Presentation
- Testicular or inguinal swelling or mass
- Rarely abdominal mass
- On ultrasound, complex, hypoechoic mass with multiple septae
- Association with ambiguous genitalia, mixed gonadal dysgenesis, and hypospadias
- No associated gynecomastia or endocrine disorders with normal testosterone, β-hCG, and inhibin levels

Prognosis and treatment
- Excellent prognosis
- Inguinal orchiectomy is main form of treatment
- Testis-sparing enucleation also found to be successful
- Recurrences or metastases never reported

Pathology
Histology
- Grossly, multicystic tumors have solid foci within fibrotic and loose myxoid stroma that are partially encapsulated and 0.8 to 5 cm in size.
- Cysts are lined by multilayered cells, with inner cells resembling granulosa cells and the outer cells resembling theca cells. Granulosa-like cells have round nuclei, even chromatin, inconspicuous nucleoli, and scanty vacuolated cytoplasm. Theca-like cells are elongated and have scanty cytoplasm. Occasional Call-Exner bodies can be found.
- Cyst contents are amorphous proteinaceous but can be mucinous.

Immunopathology (including immunohistochemistry)
- Granulosa-like cells diffusely positive for vimentin, cytokeratins, and S100 protein and focally positive for anti-Müllerian hormone
- Theca cells diffusely positive for vimentin, smooth muscle actin, and focally to desmin
- α-Fetoprotein negative
- Cytoplasmic expression or nuclear under expression of SOX9
- Nuclear expression of FOXL2

Molecular genetics
- Constitutional chromosome 4 abnormality is present.
- All cases with ambiguous genitalia have karyotypic abnormalities, 45X/46 XY mosaicism, or structural anomalies of Y chromosome.

Main differential diagnosis
- Yolk sac tumor

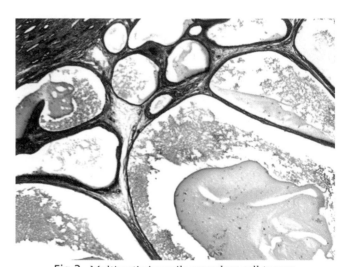

Fig 2. Multicystic juvenile granulosa cell tumor.

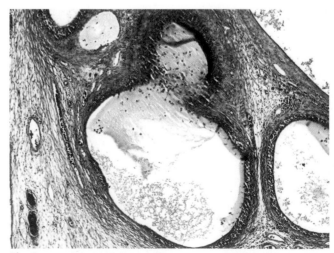

Fig 3. Juvenile granulosa cell tumor. Cysts are present within fibrotic and loose myxoid stroma and contain an amorphous and proteinaceous secretion.

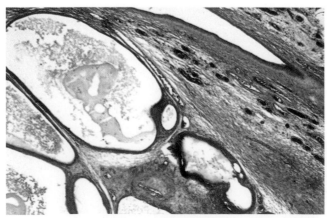

Fig 1. Multicystic juvenile granulosa cell tumor in an infantile testis.

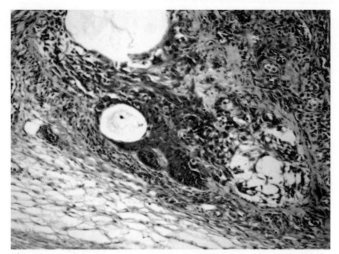

Fig 4. Juvenile granulosa cell tumor. Solid nests and microcysts are present within a loose myxoid stroma.

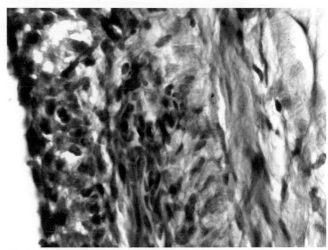

Fig 7. Juvenile granulosa cell tumor. Granulosa-like cells have round nuclei, even chromatin, inconspicuous nucleoli, and scanty vacuolated cytoplasm. Theca-like cells are elongated and have scanty cytoplasm.

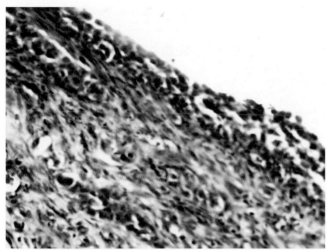

Fig 5. Juvenile granulosa cell tumor. Cysts are lined by multilayered cells. Inner cells resemble granulosa cells and the outer cells resemble theca cells.

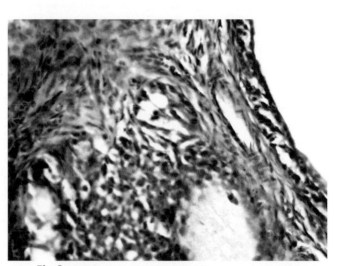

Fig 8. Solid nests of cells resembling granulosa cells.

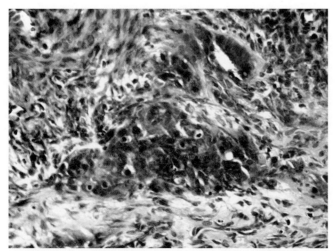

Fig 6. Juvenile granulosa cell tumor displaying solid nests of cells.

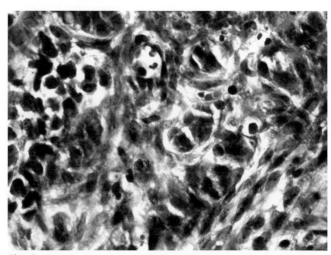

Fig 9. Nests of cells resembling granulosa cells in a juvenile granulosa cell tumor.

Definition
- Testicular stromal tumor resembling its ovarian counterpart of fibrothecoma

Clinical features
Epidemiology
- Extremely rare

Presentation
- Unilateral testicular mass
- Not associated with hormonal alterations
- Well-circumscribed, solid, yellow-white mass without necrosis and hemorrhage

Prognosis and treatment
- Prognosis is good.
- Surgical excision is the preferred treatment.

Pathology
Histology
- Fusiform spindle cells resembling ovarian stromal cells, with a fascicular or storiform pattern of growth
- Slightly collagenous stroma with numerous small blood vessels
- Usually scant mitotic figures, but mitotic counts up to four per HPF reported

Immunopathology (including immunohistochemistry)
- Positive for vimentin and smooth muscle actin
- Occasionally positive for cytokeratins, desmin, and S100 protein
- Nonreactive for inhibin and CD99

Main differential diagnosis
- Leiomyoma
- Solitary fibrous tumor
- Primary testicular sarcomas

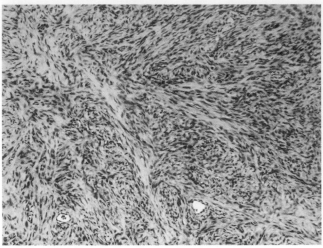

Fig 1. Fibrothecoma composed of interlacing fascicles of tumor cells.

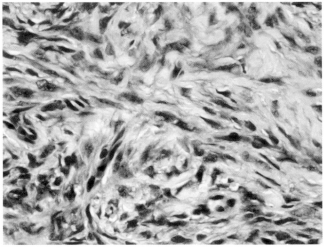

Fig 2. Fibrothecoma showing fusiform cells and abundant small blood vessels.

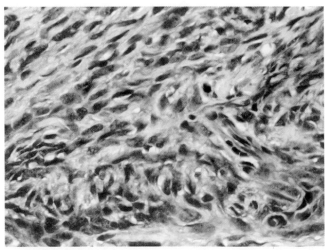

Fig 3. Fibrothecoma tumor cells within a fibrous stroma.

STROMAL TUMOR OF THE TESTIS, UNCLASSIFIED TYPE

Definition
- Sex cord–stromal tumors not showing a specific histologic differentiation, such as LCTs, granulosa cell tumors, or Sertoli cell tumors, are considered *unclassified type*.

Clinical features
Epidemiology
- Incidence is low and variable in the literature.
- Unclassified tumors seem to be more common in children.

Presentation
- Similar other sex cord–stromal tumors
- Usually asymptomatic, unilateral testicular mass
- Rare hormonal manifestations, such as gynecomastia

Prognosis and treatment
- Unclassified sex cord–stromal tumors of the testis that are other than very small and cytologically innocuous are considered potentially malignant although a malignant course seems to be less common in children than in adults.
- Radial orchiectomy is the mainline treatment.

Pathology
Histology
- Unclassified testicular tumors usually show epithelial and stromal components in variable proportions.
- Cords and tubules are usually present, but most tumors are predominantly solid. The tubules are lined by cells that resemble Sertoli cells.
- Focally, islands and masses of cells resembling granulosa cells and containing Call-Exner–like cells may also be present, but the tumor should not be solely composed of granulosa cell tumor by definition.
- Stromal cells with abundant cytoplasm may resemble Leydig cells, but Reinke crystals are absent.
- The stromal component may be cellular or hyalinized.
- Poorly differentiated tumors exhibit varying degrees of nuclear pleomorphism and mitotic activity.

Immunopathology (including immunohistochemistry)
- Unclassified stromal tumors variably express antigens that are expressed by Leydig cell, granulosa, and Sertoli cell tumors.
- Positivity for calretinin and inhibin is usually present.
- Variable, focal keratin expression has been reported in less differentiated tumors.
- S-100 and smooth muscle actin with a pattern also seen in both adult and juvenile granulosa cell tumors have been observed.

Main differential diagnosis
- LCTs
- Sertoli cell tumors
- Metastatic tumors, such as metastatic melanoma or carcinoma
- Sex cord–stromal tumors of the testis with entrapped germ cells

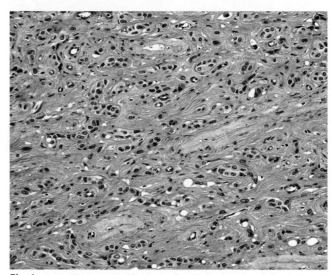

Fig 1. A medium magnification showing an area of short chords and small tubules in a fibrotic background. The cells have an eosinophilic cytoplasm that resembles Leydig cells, but in other areas the tumor showed well-formed tubules and spindled cells (not shown).

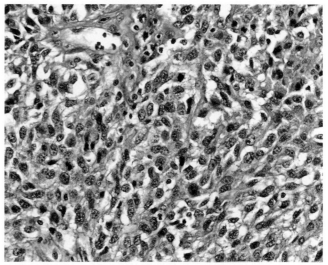

Fig 2. Epithelioid and vaguely spindled cell area with atypia and mitotic activity. The tumor is poorly differentiated. On immunohistochemical studies (not shown), the tumor cells were positive for smooth muscle actin and focally for calretinin.

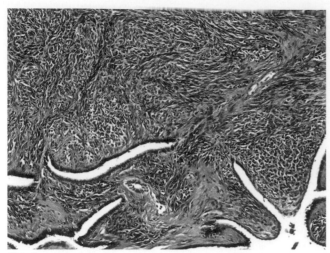

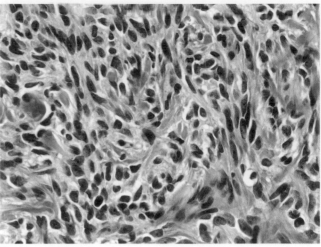

Fig 3. Unclassified sex cord–stromal tumor with prominent spindle cell features.

Fig 4. Unclassified sex cord–stromal tumor with a fusiform pattern of growth.

Definition
- A tumor composed of a mixture of seminoma-like large germ cells and small cells with sex cord features

Clinical features
Epidemiology
- Related to mixed dysgenetic gonad Y-chromosomal material, such as 45X, 46XY
- Left side predominant
- Usually arise in dysgenetic patients with an intersex syndrome
- Eighty percent phenotypically female, 20% male
- Some cases related to Turner syndrome
- Rarely, gonadoblastoma in genotypical and phenotypical male patients

Prognosis and treatment
- Treatment is surgery (usually bilateral gonadectomy).
- Prognosis is excellent prognosis, even when malignant components are present.
- The most common malignant germ cell arising from gonadoblastoma is seminoma, but nonseminomatous germ cell tumors also occur.

Pathology
Histology
- Rounded or irregularly shaped tumor nodules are composed of two cell types: a seminoma-like cell with large, pale cytoplasm, and a sex cord–like cell with small, dark, angular cytoplasm surrounded by hyaline material.
- Calcification may be present in tumor nodules and is usually associated with hyaline material.
- Mitotic figures are sometimes seen in the seminoma-like cells.

Immunopathology (including immunohistochemistry)
- Seminoma-like cells are positive for PLAP, C-kit, and OCT3/4.
- Sex cord–like cells are positive for inhibin, WT1, and calretinin.

Molecular diagnosis
- Most cases are aneuploid.
- 45X/46XY mosaicism is identified by fluorescence in situ hybridization.

Main differential diagnosis
- Seminoma
- Nonseminomatous germ cell tumor
- Sex cord tumor with annular tubules
- Sex cord–stromal tumor, unclassified

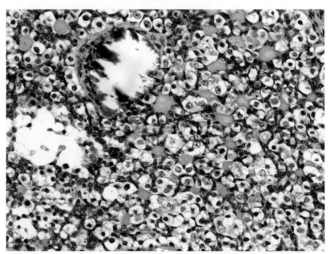

Fig 2. Gonadoblastoma composed of seminoma-like and sex cord–like cells, with hyaline material deposition and calcification.

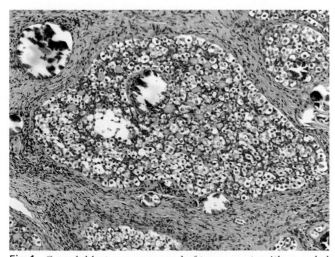

Fig 1. Gonadoblastoma composed of tumor nests with rounded contours.

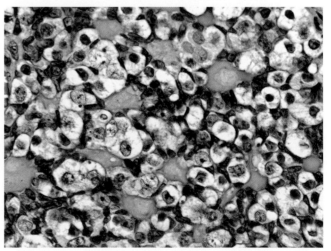

Fig 3. Gonadoblastoma composed of seminoma-like cells.

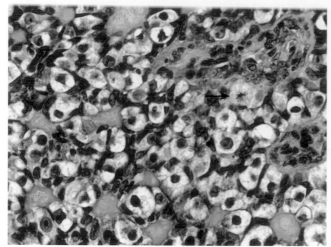

Fig 4. Seminoma-like cell with mitosis *(arrow)*.

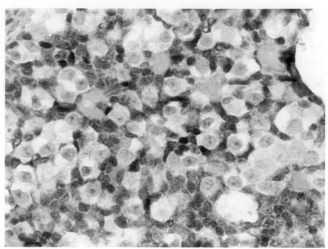

Fig 6. Sex cord stroma–like cells are positive for calretinin.

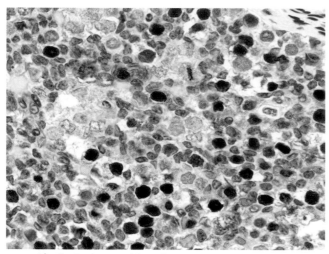

Fig 5. Seminoma-like cells are positive for OCT3/4.

Definition
- Malignant neoplasm of lymphocytes arising from or involving the testis

Clinical features
Epidemiology
- Testicular lymphomas can be seen in men ranging from 16 to 90 years old, but they typically occur in older patients with a mean age of 60 years, which is different from that of patients developing testicular germ cell tumors such as seminoma (mean age, 40 years) and nonseminomatous germ cell tumors (mean age, 30 years).
- Lymphoma of the testis usually represents as a secondary involvement of the testis from extratesticular lymph node primary. Rarely, primary lymphoma can develop in the testis initially without nodal involvement.
- Testicular lymphomas account for 5% of testicular tumors; however, in men older than 60 years, 50% of the testicular malignancies are lymphoma.

Presentation
- The majority of patients have a painless testicular mass.
- Some patients may have systemic symptoms such as fever, sweats, and weight loss.
- Most patients with testicular lymphomas will be found to have nodal or other organ involvement during the clinical work-up.
- Twenty percent of cases are bilateral.

Prognosis and treatment
- The stage of the testicular lymphoma will be the determining factor for the prognosis. Patients with early-stage lymphoma will have a better prognosis. The 5-year tumor-free survival is 60% for early-stage patients, and less than 20% for the advanced-stage patients.
- The prognosis of testicular lymphoma is typically worse than nodal lymphoma. One of the reasons is probably that most cases of testicular lymphomas are not primary tumors. The other possibility is the presence of a possible blood-testicular barrier, which could limit the chemotherapy drugs' access to tumor cells in the testis.
- The reported recurrence rate is high, up to 80% in some retrospective studies of testicular lymphoma.
- Orchiectomy is not the treatment of choice for testicular lymphomas. However, the majority of the testicular lymphomas encountered in surgical pathology are found in orchiectomy specimens, without prior clinical suspicion.

Pathology
Histology
- Grossly, lymphoma either can diffusely replace the testicular parenchyma without a discrete mass or form a single or multinodular tumor. The cut surface is fleshy and white to tan.
- The most common type of lymphoma of the testis in adults is diffuse large B cell lymphoma, which accounts for up to 75% of all testicular lymphomas.
- Lymphoma cells exhibit a typical interstitial growth pattern, with tumor cells surrounding but not replacing the seminiferous tubules. Although some of the seminiferous tubules may be eventually replaced and destroyed, tubule sparing is often observed in most cases.
- Large B cell lymphoma typically is composed of large tumor cells with diffuse growth patterns. The tumor cells are large with vesicular nuclei and prominent nucleoli and brisk mitotic activity.
- Granulomas and abundant, small, mature lymphocytes are usually not found, although common in seminomas.

Immunopathology (including immunohistochemistry)
- Large diffuse B cell lymphomas are positive for CD45 and CD20 and negative for CD3
- Negative for germ cell markers such as AFP, hCG, C-kit or OCT3/4, SALL4, and epithelial markers such as AE1/AE3 or Cam5.2

Main differential diagnosis
- Germ cell tumors, especially seminoma
- Reactive lesions such as lymphoid hyperplasia and chronic orchitis

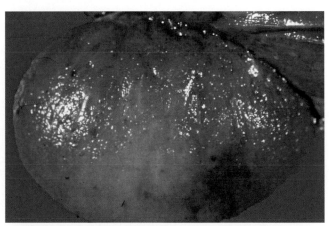

Fig 1. Testicular lymphoma entirely replacing the testis.

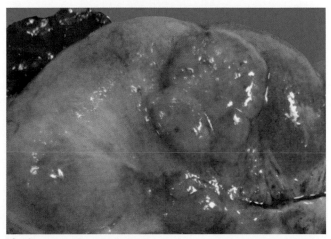

Fig 2. Testicular lymphoma forming multiple nodules without capsule.

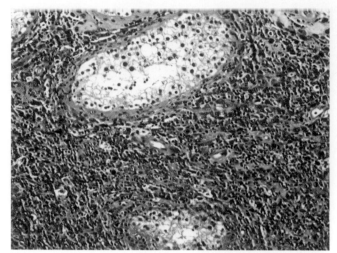

Fig 3. Lymphoma cells showing an interstitial-pattern growth, sparing seminiferous tubules.

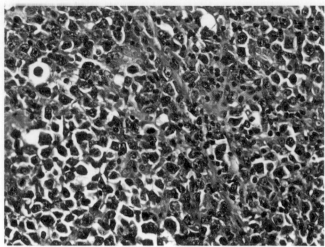

Fig 4. Large B cell lymphoma of the testis showing large neoplastic cells with cytologic atypias and frequent mitoses.

Definition
• Tumors of the testis resembling surface epithelial tumors of the ovary

Clinical features
Epidemiology
• Very rare
• Wide age range (14 to 68 years old)

Presentation
• Majority of the patients have a painless testicular mass, swelling, or associated hydrocele.
• Ovarian epithelial–type testicular tumors can also be located in the tunica or paratesticular area.

Prognosis and treatment
• Surgical resection of the testicular tumor is the treatment of choice.
• Good prognosis in cystadenomas and borderline tumors. Cystadenocarcinoma can lead to intraabdominal spread.

Pathology
Histology
• Cystic lesions usually correspond to serous borderline tumors or mucinous cystadenoma, whereas solid areas tend to be malignant.
• The microscopic morphology is identical to their ovarian counterparts. Most cases correspond to serous carcinomas, but endometrioid carcinomas, mucinous cystadenomas, and borderlines have also been encoutered. In addition, cystadenocarcinomas, clear cell carcinomas, and Brenner tumors have been reported.

Immunopathology (including immunohistochemistry)
• Findings are similar to the immunoprofile seen in ovarian tumors.
• Immunohistochemistry may be necessary in some cases to distinguish these tumors from mesothelioma. Mesothelioma is positive for AE1/AE3, EMA, vimentin, and calretinin, and negative for CEA, B72.3, Leu M1, and Ber-Ep4.

Main differential diagnosis
• Carcinoma of the rete testis
• Papillary mesothelioma
• Metastatic adenocarcinoma

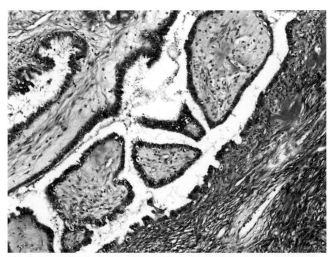

Fig 2. Detached papillae are a common finding in serous borderline tumors. No stromal invasion is seen.

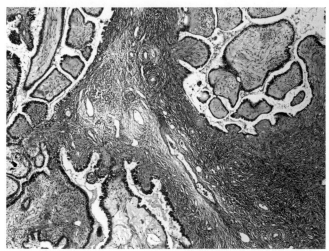

Fig 1. Serous borderline tumor with ovarian-type stroma.

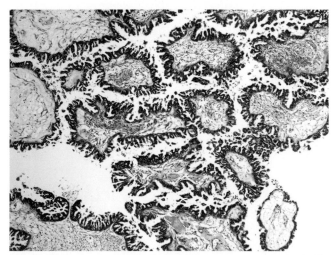

Fig 3. Testicular serous borderline tumors are morphologically identical to their ovarian counterparts.

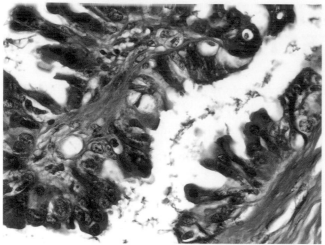

Fig 4. Papillae are lined by atypical columnar cells.

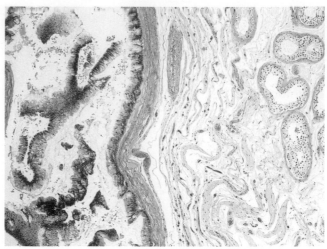

Fig 7. Mucinous borderline tumor of the testis.

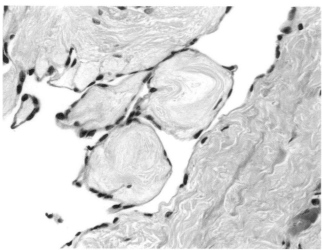

Fig 5. Papillary mesothelioma should be distinguished from ovarian epithelial–type tumors. Clues are in the features of the lining cells.

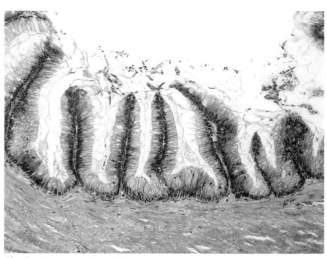

Fig 8. Mucinous borderline tumor showing prominent papillae.

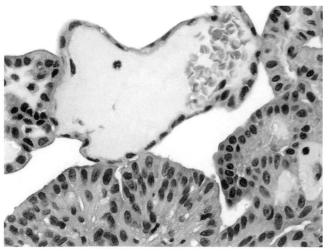

Fig 6. Papillary mesothelioma of the tunica vaginalis.

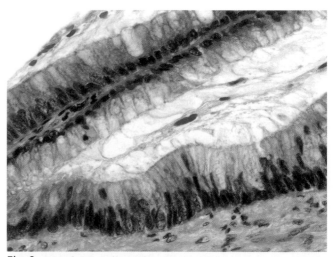

Fig 9. Neoplastic cells with intestinal-type features and slight atypia.

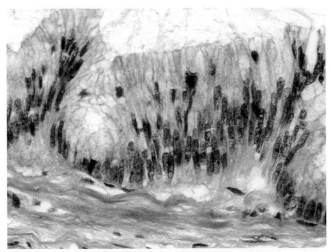

Fig 10. Mucinous borderline tumor showing endocervical-like features with mild atypia, nuclear crowding, and loss of polarity.

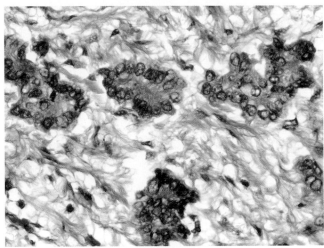

Fig 13. Serous adenocarcinoma infiltrating the testicular stroma.

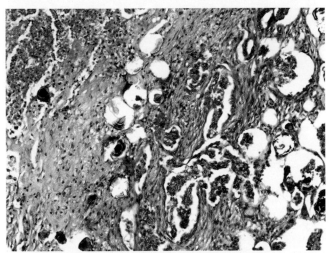

Fig 11. Serous cystadenocarcinoma with infiltrating malignant glands *(right field)*, psammomatous bodies, and tumor necrosis *(left field)*.

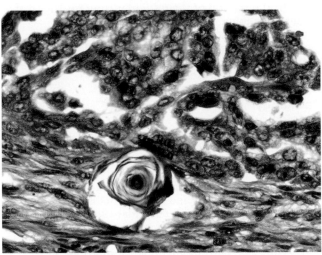

Fig 14. Calcified concentric bodies are a common feature of serous cystadenocarcinomas of the testis.

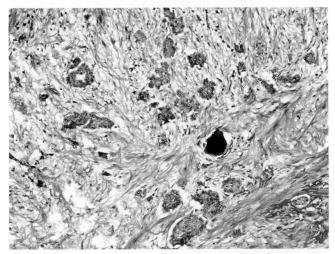

Fig 12. Infiltrating malignant glands eliciting an intense stromal reaction. Note also the psammomatous body.

Definition
- Benign or malignant tumors of rete epithelial origin

Clinical features
Epidemiology
- Unusual tumors
- Malignant tumors predominantly in the fourth to eighth decades of life

Presentation
- Majority of the patients have a painless hilar mass (range, 1 to 10 cm) with ill-defined borders.
- Tenderness or lumbar pain is present.
- It may be masked by an inguinal hernia, hydrocele, fistula, sinus, or epididymitis.

Prognosis and treatment
- Surgical resection of the testicular tumor is the treatment of choice.
- Rete testis adenocarcinoma can disseminate to regional and systemic lymph nodes and to viscera and bone. Approximately half of the patients die of disseminated disease.

Pathology
Histology
- Benign tumors (adenomas) show a tubular pattern resembling Sertoli cell tumor (sertoliform cystadenoma).
- Malignant tumors (adenocarcinomas) require the presence of a solid pattern of growth, histologic transition from unaffected rete testis, tumor centered on the testicular hilum, and no identifiable conventional (germ or non–germ cell) testicular tumor or similar extratesticular primary.
- Rete testis adenocarcinoma shows large tumor nodules intermingled with smaller ones, sometimes with necrotic foci. These nodules protrude in the dilated channels of the rete testis. Papillary excrescences may be observed but should be focal and not prominent.

Immunopathology (including immunohistochemistry)
- Similar to the immunoprofile seen in ovarian tumors

Main differential diagnosis
- Mesothelioma
- Ovarian-type serous cystadenocarcinoma

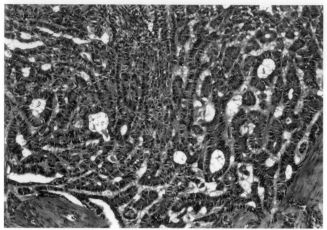

Fig 2. Sertoliform adenoma of the rete testis with a cordlike pattern of growth.

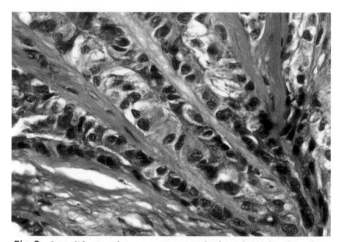

Fig 3. Sertoliform adenoma composed of cords and trabeculae.

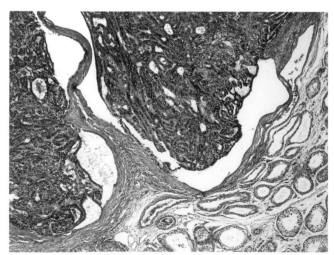

Fig 1. Sertoliform adenoma of the rete testis at low-power view. Note the testicular parenchyma *(lower right field)*.

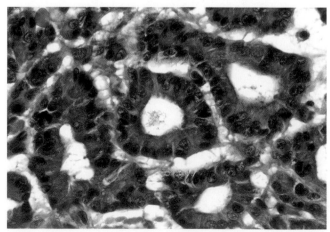

Fig 4. Glandular configuration in a sertoliform adenoma of the rete testis. Note the absence of overt atypia.

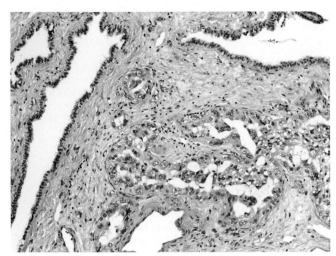

Fig 5. Adenocarcinoma infiltrating the rete testis.

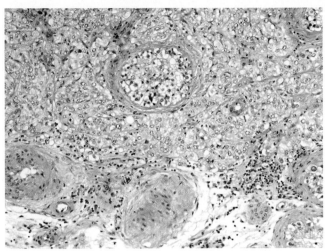

Fig 8. High-grade carcinoma of the rete testis infiltrating the testicular parenchyma between the seminiferous tubules.

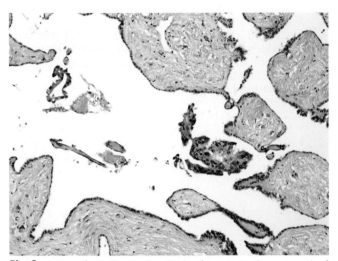

Fig 6. Areas of carcinoma in situ in the rete testis are required for the proper diagnosis of adenocarcinoma of the rete testis.

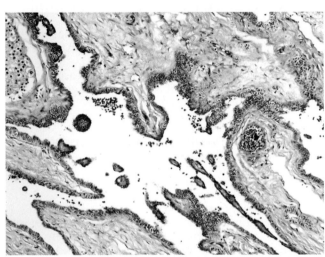

Fig 9. Papillary hyperplasia of the rete testis can simulate a borderline serous tumor, but its location and absence of atypia provide clues for the correct diagnosis. In addition, papillary hyperplasia of the rete testis is usually an incidental finding.

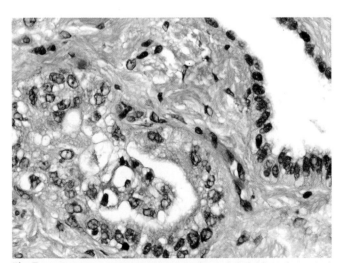

Fig 7. Infiltrating malignant glands *(lower left field)* and atypical changes in the intervening rete testis *(upper right field)*.

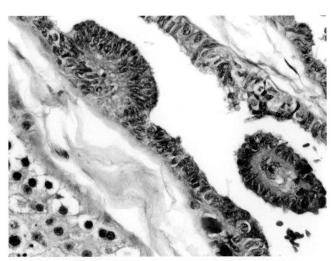

Fig 10. Papillae in papillary hyperplasia of the rete testis are lined by nonatypical columnar cells. Note a seminiferous tubule in the lower left field.

- American Joint Committee on Cancer (AJCC) system
  - The Classification of Malignant Tumors (TNM) staging system proposed by the American Joint Committee on Cancer (most common)
  - Primary tumor (T)*
    - pTX: primary tumor cannot be assessed
    - pT0: no evidence of primary tumor
    - pTis: intratubular germ cell neoplasia
    - pT1: tumor confined to the testis and epididymis without lymphovascular invasion; tumor invading into the tunica albuginea but not the tunica vaginalis
    - pT2: tumor confined to the testis and epididymis with lymphovascular invasion; tumor invading through the tunica albuginea into the tunica vaginalis
    - pT3: tumor invading the spermatic cord
    - pT4: tumor invading the scrotum
  - Regional lymph nodes (N)
    - NX: regional lymph nodes cannot be assessed
    - N0: no regional lymph node metastasis
    - N1: metastasis with a lymph node measuring 2 cm or less in greatest dimension and five or fewer positive nodes
    - N2: metastasis with a lymph node measuring greater than 2 cm but 5 cm or less in greatest dimension; or more than five positive nodes, each 5 or less cm in greatest dimension; or extranodal extension of tumor
    - N3: metastasis with a lymph node mass greater than 5 cm in greatest dimension
  - Distant metastasis (M)
    - MX: distant metastasis cannot be assessed
    - M0: no distant metastasis
    - M1: distant metastasis
    - M1a: nonregional nodal or pulmonary metastasis
    - M1b: distant metastasis other than to nonregional nodal or pulmonary metastasis
  - Serum markers (S)†
    - SX: marker studies not available or not performed
    - S0: marker levels within normal limits
    - S1: lactate dehydrogenase (LDH) < 1.5 N, hCG (mIU/mL) < 5000, and AFP (ng/mL) < 1000
    - S2: LDH 1.5 to 10 N, hCG (mIU/mL) 5000 to 50,000, or AFP (ng/mL) 1000 to 10,000
    - S3: LDH > 10 N, hCG (mIU/mL) > 50,000, or AFP (ng/mL) > 10,000
- Children's Oncology Group (COG) system
  - The clinical staging system proposed by the COG is another system commonly used.
  - Stage I: tumor confined to the testis; no evidence of disease beyond the testis by clinical, histologic, or radiographic examination; an appropriate decline in serum markers has occurred after radical orchiectomy (AFP half-life of 5 days or hCG half-life of 16 hours)
  - Stage II: microscopic disease located in the scrotum or high in the spermatic cord (less than 5 cm from the proximal end); retroperitoneal lymph node involvement present (less than 2 cm); serum AFP persistently elevated
  - Stage III: retroperitoneal lymph node involvement (greater than 2 cm) present; no visible evidence of visceral or extra abdominal involvement
  - Stage IV: distant metastasis
- Correlation between the AJCC and the COG systems
  - Stage 0: T, pTis; N, N0; M, M0; S, S0
  - Stage I: T, pT1-4; N, N0; M, M0; S, S0
  - Stage II: T, any pT/Tx; N, N1-3; M, M0; S, S0 or S1
  - Stage III: T, any pT/Tx; N, N1-3; M, M0; S, S2 or S3
  - Stage IV: T, any pT/Tx; N, any N; M, M1; S, any S

---

*The primary tumor should be assessed on a radical orchiectomy specimen. For mixed GCT, all histologic types and their percentage should be provided in the pathology report.
†The serum tumor marker levels should be measured before orchiectomy. N indicates the upper limit of normal for an LDH assay.

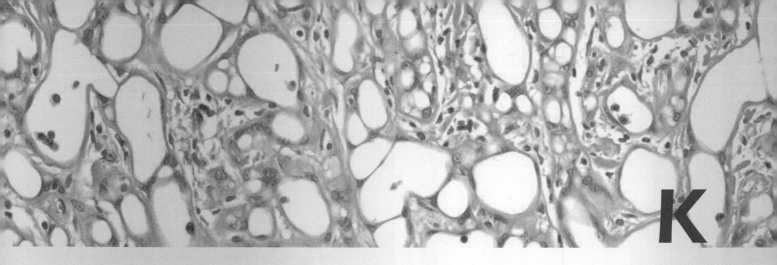

K

SPERMATIC CORD AND TESTICULAR ADNEXA

Definition
- A vestigial remnant of the Müllerian duct present on the upper pole of the testis and attached to the tunica vaginalis; also called *hydatid of Morgagni*

Clinical features
Epidemiology
- Present in more than 90% of testes at autopsy

Presentation
- One third of patients have a palpable blue-dot discoloration on the scrotum, diagnostic of this condition
- May cause acute testis if torsed

Prognosis and treatment
- Surgical resection if torsed

Pathology
Gross pathology
- Frequently found in the groove between the testis and the epididymal head or on the superior surface of the testis
- Polypoid or nodular excrescence attached to the visceral tunica vaginalis

Histology
- Surface epithelium is cuboidal or low columnar Müllerian-type and continuous with the tunica vaginalis at the base.
- Delicate loose connective tissue stroma is present; invagination of the surface epithelium is common.

Main differential diagnosis
- Appendix epididymis: located on the superior surface of the epididymal head; flat mesothelial cells line the surface

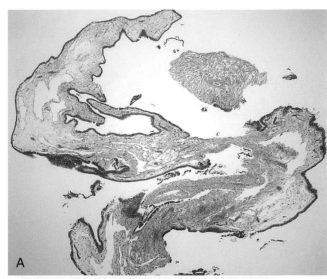

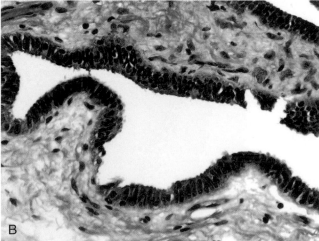

Fig 2. Appendix testis **(A)** with columnar Müllerian-type surface epithelium and delicate loose connective tissue stroma **(B)**. Invagination of the surface epithelium into the stroma is often present.

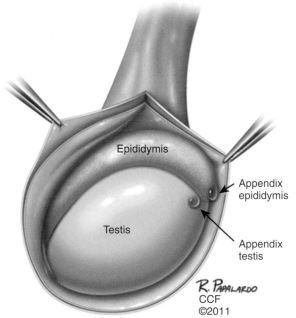

Fig 1. The location of appendix testis and appendix epididymis. (Copyright Cleveland Clinic Foundation, 2011.)

Definition
- A remnant of the most cranial portion of the meso-nephric duct (Wolffian duct) attached to the head of the epididymis

Clinical features
Epidemiology
- Present in approximately 23% to 25% of testes

Presentation
- Incidental finding at the time of surgery
- Testicular swelling and pain if torsed, which is common in children

Prognosis and treatment
- Benign
- May require surgical excision for persistent pain from torsion

Pathology
Gross pathology
- A pedunculated spheric cystic structure filled with amorphous secretion attached to the head of the epididymis

Histology
- Cuboidal or low columnar and often ciliated epithe-lium lines the cystic space, which is attached to the epididymis by a fibrovascular stalk.
- The external surface is covered by mesothelial cells.

Main differential diagnosis
- Appendix testis, found in the groove between the testis and the epididymal head or on the superior surface of the testis

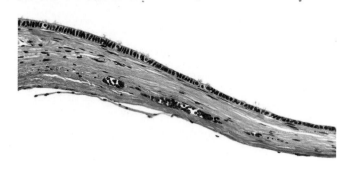

Fig 1. Appendix epididymis lined with cuboidal epithelium. Some cells are ciliated.

GLANDULAR INCLUSIONS IN INGUINAL HERNIORRHAPHY SPECIMENS

Definition
- Glandular and ductal structures found in inguinal hernia sac specimens, as the remnants of Wolffian and Müllerian ducts and infolding of coelomic epithelium

Clinical features
Epidemiology
- Uncommon, less than 0.5% of pediatric herniorrhaphy specimens

Presentation
- Incidental findings in herniorrhaphy specimens

Pathology
Histology
- Vas deferens–like inclusions: a single or a few separate ducts of similar sizes, lined with pseudostratified ciliated columnar epithelium, and encircled with a distinct cellular stromal cuff, but lacking well-formed muscular coating

- Epididymis-like inclusions: aggregates of numerous tubules of similar sizes, evenly distributed, lined with simple to pseudostratified ciliated cuboidal to columnar epithelium with occasional peg cell–like clear ovoid cells, with or without a distinct cellular stromal cuff, but lacking well-formed muscular coating
- Müllerian duct–like inclusions: a few tubules or glands of variable sizes and shapes, unevenly distributed in the fibrovascular tissue, lined with simple ciliated cuboidal to columnar epithelium, no distinct stromal cuff; may show a close association with dilated capillaries

Immunopathology (including immunohistochemistry)
- Epithelial cells are negative for CD10 in vas deferens and Müllerian duct–like inclusions but may be positive in epididymis-like inclusions.

Main differential diagnosis
- Vas deferens and epididymis: well-formed concentric smooth muscle coating; epithelial cells positive for CD10

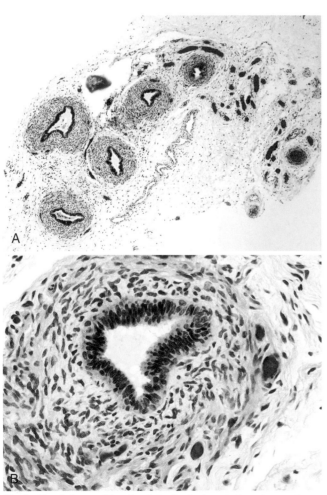

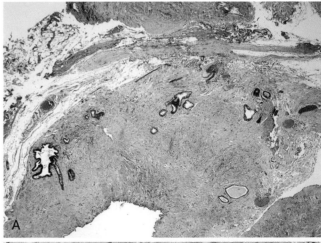

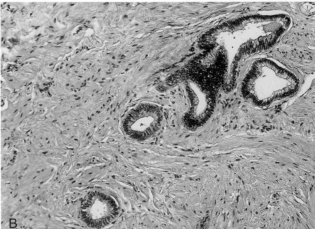

Fig 1. Vas deferens–like glandular inclusions in hernia sac, showing a few ducts **(A)** lined with pseudostratified ciliated columnar epithelium and encircled with a distinct stromal cuff **(B).**

Fig 2. Müllerian duct–like glandular inclusions in a hernia sac, showing a few unevenly distributed glands of different sizes and shapes **(A),** lined with simple columnar epithelium and lack of a distinct stromal cuff **(B).**

Definition
- Accumulation of serous fluid between the parietal and visceral layers of tunica vaginalis surrounding the testicle or along spermatic cord

Clinical features
Epidemiology
- Up to 10% of male infants have a hydrocele at birth, but most disappear without treatment within the first year of life.
- Adult men can develop a hydrocele as the result of an imbalance between fluid production and absorption owing to inflammation, injury, or tumor.
- Rarely involves canal of Nuck in women (pouch of peritoneum extending into labia majora), a structure analogous to the processus vaginalis in men

Presentation
- Painless scrotum swelling

Prognosis and treatment
- Benign; many spontaneously regress
- Enlarging or symptomatic hydroceles can be surgically removed or managed by needle aspiration in nonsurgical candidates

Pathology
Histology
- Mesothelium-lined cystic fibrous connective tissue, often with chronic inflammatory infiltrate, fibrosis and squamous metaplasia
- Reactive mesothelial proliferation ranges from mild to very prominent, but usually associated with inflammation and no infiltrative growth

Immunohistochemistry
- Positive for mesothelial markers (pancytokeratin, calretinin, CK5/6, WT1, D2-40)

Main differential diagnosis
- Mesothelioma: extensive and more infiltrative growth in tunica and underlying connective tissue; frank cytologic atypia
- Spermatocele: retention cyst developed from tubules of rete testis or epididymis containing spermatozoa; lined by flattened epithelium; negative for mesothelial markers

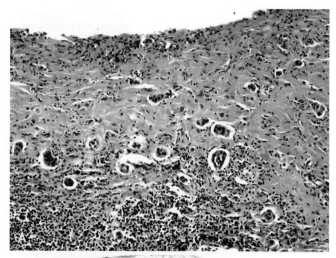

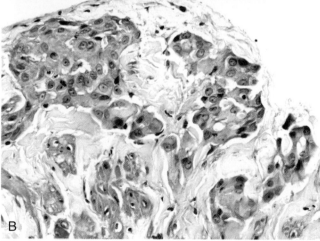

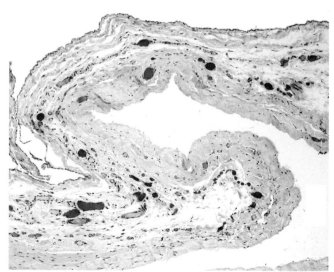

Fig 1. Hydrocele sac is characterized by mesothelium-lined loose fibrous connective tissue.

Fig 2. **A,** Reactive mesothelial proliferation in hydrocele, which is associated with inflammation and has a noninfiltrative growth front. **B,** Prominent mesothelial proliferation mimics mesothelioma.

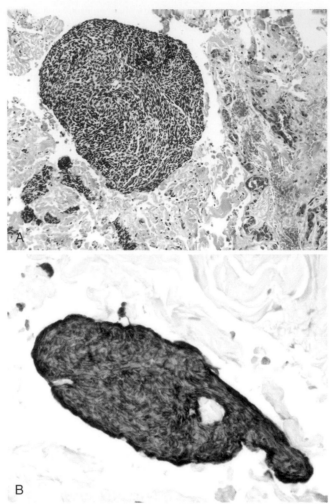

Fig 3. Sloughed rete testis epithelial cells are occasionally found in hydrocele specimens and can mimic small cell carcinoma **(A).** They appear to have a high nuclear-to-cytoplasmic ratio, and the nuclei are closely related to each other with the appearance of molding. However, the cells lack mitotic figures or apoptotic bodies. These cells are positive for CD56 **(B),** but negative for synaptophysin and chromogranin.

Definition
- Cystic dilatation of an efferent ductule, proximal rete testis, or head of the epididymis

Clinical features
Epidemiology
- Typically younger men (20 to 50 years old) but can occur at any age postpuberty

Presentation
- Mass, pain, or both are most common complaints.
- Acute testis due to torsion is rarely encountered.

Prognosis and treatment
- Benign lesion treated surgically
- Recurrence infrequent

Pathology
Gross pathology
- Unilocular or multilocular thin-walled cystic lesion filled with clear to slightly yellow serous fluid

Histology
- Cyst lined by columnar, cuboidal, or flattened ciliated epithelial cells

- Cyst wall composed predominantly of fibrous connective tissue with an occasional smooth muscle component and chronic inflammation
- Spermatozoa within the cyst contents required for the diagnosis

Main differential diagnosis
- Hydrocele: lined with mesothelial cells; sperms not found in the cystic content

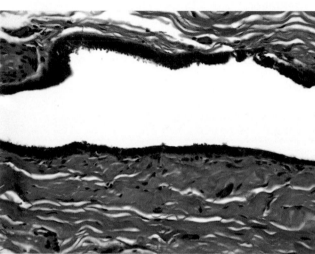

Fig 2. The cystic wall is lined with cytologically bland columnar, cuboidal, or, in the case of marked distention, flattened ciliated epithelial cells.

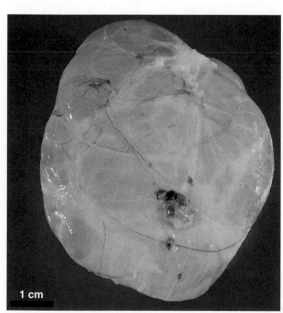

Fig 1. Grossly, spermatoceles appear as cystic masses containing clear fluid.

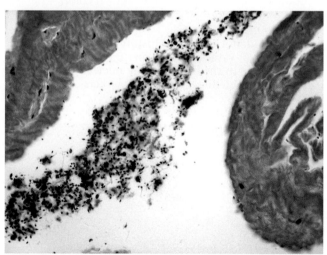

Fig 3. Sperms and histiocytes are frequently seen within the cystic spaces.

Definition
- Benign ductular proliferation in reaction to obstruction of the vas deferens

Clinical features
Epidemiology
- Typically young men with a mean age of 36 years
- Lesion results from damage to the vas deferens ducts, typically post-vasectomy

Presentation
- Produces either a fusiform enlargement of the vas deferens or solitary or multiple indurated nodules
- Usually an asymptomatic lesion caused by vasectomy and encountered at the time of vasovasostomy or herniorrhaphy
- Rarely idiopathic

Prognosis and treatment
- Benign

Pathology
Histology
- Diffuse or nodular ductular proliferation
- Spermatozoa often present in the ductular lumina in the early phase
- Ductules lined with a single layer of cuboidal cells with pale cytoplasm and prominent single nucleoli
- Perineural or vascular invasion by proliferating ductules occasionally encountered
- Variable chronic inflammation and sperm granulomas with ceroid pigment deposition (lipid degradation product of sperm with a yellow-brown color)

Main differential diagnosis
- Prostatic adenocarcinoma: history of prostatic cancer; no history of vasectomy; no sperm granulomas and spermatozoa in the lumen; frank nuclear atypia; positive for prostate lineage–specific markers

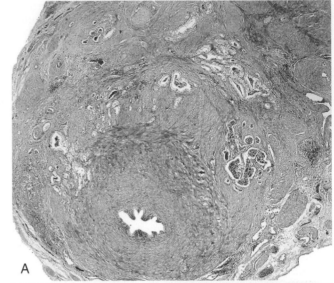

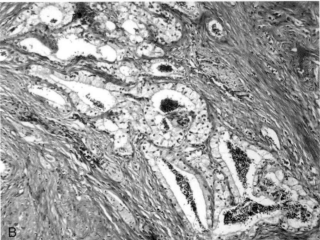

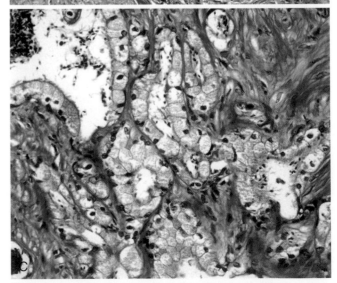

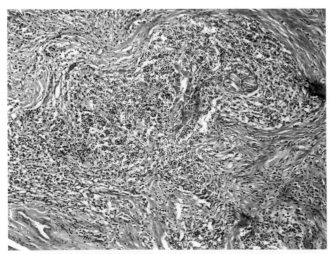

Fig 1. Chronic inflammation and nonnecrotizing granulomatous reaction to the extravasated sperms are often present.

Fig 2. Low-power view of vasitis nodosa showing proliferation ductules in the hypertrophic muscular wall of the vas deferens. The ductules have an infiltrative growth pattern. Sperms are found within the lumens **(A).** The ductules are lined with a single layer of cuboidal cells with pale cytoplasm **(B)** and conspicuous nucleoli **(C).**

Definition
- Granulomatous inflammation surrounding extravasated spermatozoa resulting from injury or inflammation of vas deferens or epididymis

Clinical features
Epidemiology
- A wide age range (18 to 75 years), more common in young adults

Presentation
- A small painful nodule (up to 4 cm) involving the epididymis or vas deferens
- Often with a history of vasectomy (in approximately 90% of cases), trauma, or epididymitis

Pathology
Gross pathology
- A small, firm, well-circumscribed nodule that may contain soft, yellow-white foci

Histology
- In early stage, there is extensive acute inflammation mixed with histiocytic reaction surrounding pools of spermatozoa, adjacent to injured ducts or tubules; central necrosis may be seen.
- In late stage, chronic granulomatous inflammation and fibrosis, affected tubules, or ducts may show squamous metaplasia.
- It is associated with vasitis nodosa or epididymitis nodosa in 30% of cases.

Main differential diagnosis
- Infectious etiology (i.e., *Histoplasma capsulatum*): necrotizing inflammation and abscesses; 2- to 4-m fungal spores visualized on Grocott's methenamine silver (GMS) stain

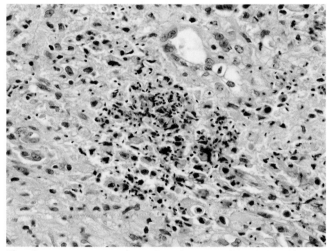

Fig 2. Sperm granuloma, showing granuloma reaction to numerous extravasated spermatozoa.

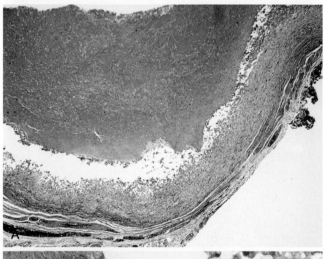

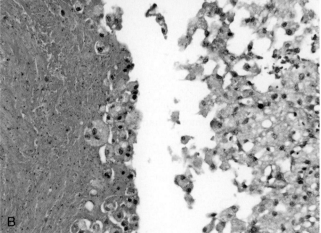

Fig 1. Sperm granuloma, showing a nodule with necrotic debris in the center **(A)**, surrounded by histiocytic reaction and fibrosis **(B).**

Definition
- A benign tumor of mesothelial origin in the testicular adnexa

Clinical features
Epidemiology
- The most common tumor in the testicular adnexa, including the epididymis, tunica albuginea, and spermatic cord
- Accounts for 32% of all tumors at this site
- Occurs in the late teens up to 79 years of age, with a mean age of 36 years

Presentation
- Usually asymptomatic or as a small, slow-growing intrascrotal tumor
- Imaging studies show an extratesticular tumor most commonly in the epididymis and occasionally in the spermatic cord and tunica albuginea
- Normal serum markers

Prognosis and treatment
- Benign tumor with no metastatic potential
- Usually treated with orchiectomy, but intraoperative frozen section may allow a local resection of the extratesticular tumor with preservation of the testis

Pathology
Gross pathology
- Usually less than 2.0 cm (range, 0.4 to 5.0 cm)
- Well-circumscribed, round tumor with a tan-white homogenous cut surface

Histology
- Tumor cells form solid cords, nests, irregular tubules, or glandular-like spaces.
- Tumor cells are cuboidal or flat with small vesicular nuclei and eosinophilic cytoplasm.
- Intracytoplasmic vacuoles can be prominent and impart a signet ring cell or microcystic appearance.

Immunohistochemistry
- Positive for cytokeratin AE1/3, calretinin, WT1, and EMA
- Negative for MOC-31, Ber-Ep4, CEA, B72.3, LEA 135, Leu M1, and CD34

Electromicroscopy
- Show mesothelial features, including slender microvilli, intermediate filaments, intracellular canaliculi, and desmosomes

Main differential diagnosis
- Yolk sac tumor: occurs within the testicular parenchyma; several patterns usually present, including microcystic, Schiller-Duval bodies, and glandular-alveolar; positive for AFP; negative for calretinin and WT1
- Leydig cell tumor: intratesticular location; tumor cells grow in sheets and aggregates; positive for inhibin, but negative for WT1
- Metastatic prostatic carcinoma: history of prostatic carcinoma; uniform nuclei with prominent nucleoli; positive for prostate specific markers; negative for calretinin and WT1
- Malignant mesothelioma: large size with invasion into adjacent organs; malignant cytologic features

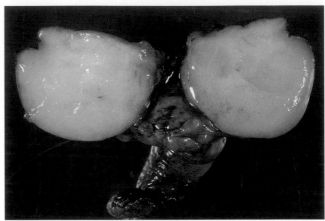

Fig 1. A tan-white firm adenomatoid tumor involving the epididymis.

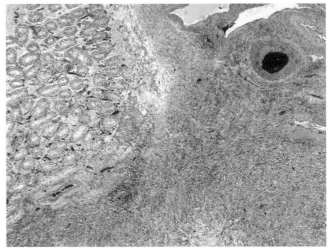

Fig 2. Adenomatoid tumor is sharply demarcated from the testicular parenchyma.

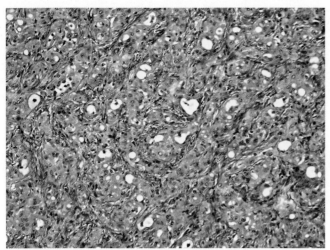

Fig 3. Adenomatoid tumor cells form solid cords or tubules.

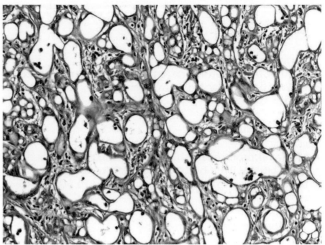

Fig 5. Adenomatoid tumor cells with markedly vacuolated cytoplasm, creating a microcystic pattern.

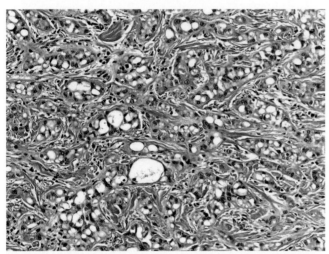

Fig 4. Adenomatoid tumor cells show prominent cytoplasmic vacuoles, imparting a signet ring cell appearance.

Definition
- Nonneoplastic proliferation of fibrous tissue admixed with inflammatory cells frequently involving the tunica vaginalis

Clinical features
Epidemiology
- Most common in the third through sixth decades of life
- Associated with a hydrocele in 50% of cases
- Prior trauma or inflammation reported in 30% of cases

Presentation
- Palpable scrotal mass
- May be painful

Prognosis and treatment
- Benign reactive
- Often treated by radical orchiectomy because of its mimicry of a primary testicular neoplasm

Pathology
Gross pathology
- Appears nodular, with an occasional cystic component
- Single or multiple
- Involves the tunica vaginalis in 75% of cases; can involve the epididymis, spermatic cord, or tunica albuginea

Histology
- Dense hyalinized fibrous tissue with scattered fibroblasts present in varying amount
- Variable inflammatory infiltrates
- Calcification and ossification may frequently occur
- May have mild cellular atypia

Immunopathology
- Reactivity to cytokeratin and vimentin is often present.
- Mesothelial markers such as calretinin are typically negative.

Main differential diagnosis
- Solitary fibrous tumor: spindle cells with variable amount of collagenous stroma arranged in "patternless" pattern; hemangiopericytoma-like vessels

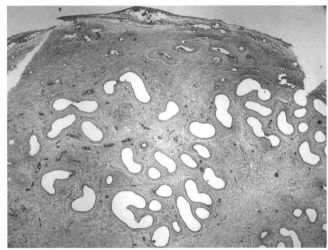

Fig 2. Low magnification reveals involvement of the epididymis.

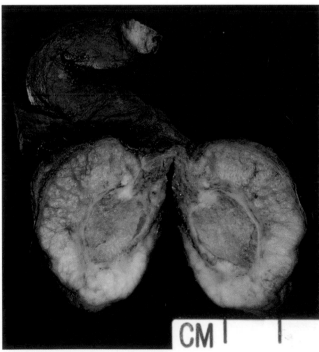

Fig 1. This fibrous pseudotumor involves the epididymis and tunica vaginalis and clinically mimics a primary testicular tumor.

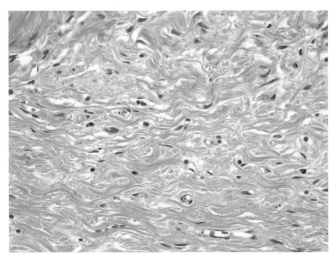

Fig 3. Dense hyalinized fibrous tissue with bland nuclear features and scattered inflammatory cells characterize this lesion.

PARATESTICULAR IDIOPATHIC SMOOTH MUSCLE HYPERPLASIA

Definition
- Haphazard overgrowth of the native smooth muscle between or around vessels or efferent ducts in the paratesticular region or the spermatic cord

Clinical features
Epidemiology
- Mean age, 63 years (range, 46 to 81 years)
- Etiology not clear; may represent hamartomatous proliferation
- Epididymal or vas deferens ductal ectasia in some cases suggestive of an obstruction as a cause

Presentation
- Asymptomatic or mimicking an intrascrotal mass

Prognosis and treatment
- Orchiectomy
- No recurrences after surgical excision

Pathology
Gross pathology
- Most commonly in the spermatic cord or the epididymis
- Present as discrete or ill-defined nodules, or thickened or enlarged paratesticular structures
- Firm and white to tan cut surface

Histology
- Hyperplastic smooth muscle fascicles with periductal, perivascular, interstitial pattern, or mixed growth pattern are present.
- Concentric proliferation around ducts of the vas or epididymis is most characteristic.

Immunohistochemistry and special studies
- Positive for smooth muscle markers

Main differential diagnosis
- Leiomyoma: cohesive, well-circumscribed proliferation of interlacing smooth muscle fascicles.

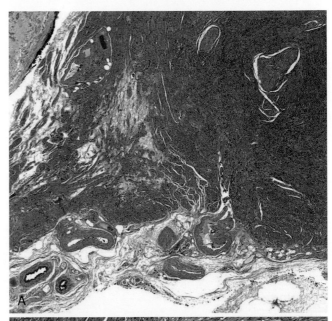
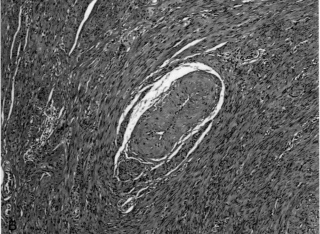

Fig 1. Idiopathic smooth muscle hyperplasia manifests as a hyperplastic smooth muscle nodule in a paratesticular region (**A**) surrounding vessels (**B**). Efferent ductules are seen in the left lower part of **A**.

PAPILLARY CYSTADENOMA OF THE EPIDIDYMIS

Definition
- A benign papillary epithelial tumor of the epididymis

Clinical features
Epidemiology
- Rare, but accounts for one third of primary epididymal tumors
- Seen in 40% of patients with von Hippel-Lindau disease
- Mean age, 35 years (range, 16 to 76 years)

Presentation
- Mass or swelling
- Incidental finding
- Some cases discovered during infertility work-up
- Bilateral disease in 40% and more common in von Hippel-Lindau disease

Prognosis and treatment
- Benign

Pathology
Gross pathology
- Size range, 1.6 to 6 cm
- Solid or cystic cut surface

Histology
- Cysts with intracystic papillary proliferation
- Colloid-like secretion within the lumens
- Cysts and papillae lined with cuboidal or low columnar cells with glycogen-rich clear or vacuolated cytoplasm
- Fibrous connective tissue in the fibrovascular cores and ductal walls

Immunohistochemistry
- Positive for pancytokeratin AE1/3, Cam5.2, CK7, EMA
- Negative for CD10, renal cell carcinoma antigen (RCC-Ag)

Main differential diagnosis
- Metastatic clear cell renal cell carcinoma: negative for CK7 and positive for CD10 and RCC Ag; opposite staining pattern for papillary cystadenoma of the epididymis (positive for CK7 and negative for CD10 and RCC Ag)
- Papillary mesothelioma: tumor cells with eosinophilic rather than clear cytoplasm; positive for calretinin
- Serous borderline tumor of the paratestis: broad papillary structures lined with stratified cells; no clear cells; occasional psammoma bodies

Molecular diagnostics
- Mutations of *VHL* gene (3p25-26) have been detected in sporadic and von Hippel-Lindau–associated cases.

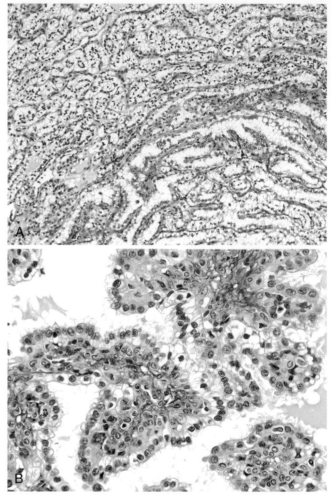

Fig 1. Papillary cystadenoma of the epididymis showing florid papillary and tubular proliferation **(A).** The papillae are lined with a single layer of cuboidal cells with clear cytoplasm and small uniform nuclei **(B).** (Courtesy Hakan Aydin, Cleveland, Ohio.)

Definition
- Benign tumor comprising mature adipocytes of the paratesticular region

Clinical features
Epidemiology
- The most common tumor of the paratesticular region
- Most frequent in the fourth and fifth decades of life

Presentation
- Painless mass of the scrotum
- Enlarged scrotum

Prognosis and treatment
- Benign
- Surgical resection

Pathology
Histology
- Resembles normal mature fat
- Variant histology including angiolipoma, fibrolipoma, myxolipoma, myolipoma
- Possible secondary changes, such as fat necrosis

Main differential diagnosis
- Atypical lipomatous tumor (well-differentiated liposarcoma): characterized by variation in the size of adipocytes, with occasional atypical, hyperchromatic nuclei; pleomorphic, multinucleated stromal cells often found in fibrous septa; ring chromosome 12

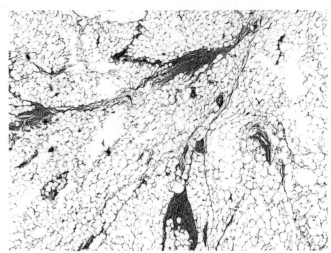

Fig 1. A lipoma of the spermatic cord resembles normal fat with no irregular fibrous bands. The adipocytes show no pleomorphism.

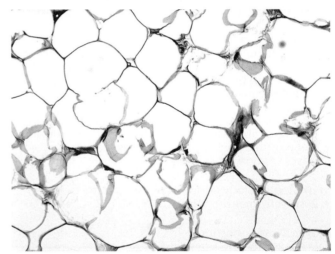

Fig 2. Higher magnification of a lipoma shows minimal variation in size and shape of the adipocytes with uniform nuclei.

Definition
- Malignant tumor of adipocytic origin, arising from the spermatic cord or paratesticular region

Clinical features
Epidemiology
- Most common sarcoma of the spermatic cord or paratesticular region in adults
- Mean age, 56 years (range, 16 to 90 years)

Presentation
- Paratesticular or testicular mass

Prognosis and treatment
- Good outcomes in patients with completely resected, well-differentiated liposarcoma
- Relatively high rate of local recurrence and may recur as dedifferentiated liposarcoma

Pathology
Gross pathology
- Lobulated mass with yellow cut surface
- Average size, 12 cm (range, 3 to 30 cm)

Histology
- Well-differentiated liposarcoma, including lipoma-like and sclerosing liposarcoma, most common and with scattered atypical cells and occasional lipoblasts
- Myxoliposarcoma with prominent chicken-wire vasculature
- Dedifferentiated liposarcoma with component reminiscent of fibrosarcoma or malignant fibrohistocytoma
- Pleomorphic liposarcoma and round cell liposarcoma least common

Immunopathology (including immunohistochemistry)
- Positive: vimentin, S-100, CD36, MDN2, CDK4

Molecular diagnostics
- MDM2$^+$, CDK4$^+$
- Well-differentiated liposarcoma: 12q14-q15 amplification
- Myxoid and round cell liposarcoma: t(12;16)(q13:p11)

Main differential diagnosis
- Large lipoma: uniform size and shape of adipocytes, lacks atypical lipoblasts
- Sclerosing lipogranuloma: associated with histiocytic and granulomatous inflammation, including giant cells; no atypical lipoblasts

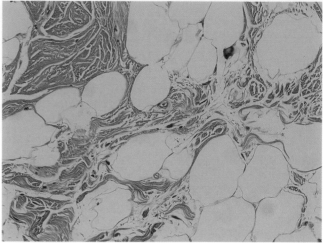

Fig 1. A well-differentiated liposarcoma containing several atypical lipoblasts in paratesticular region.

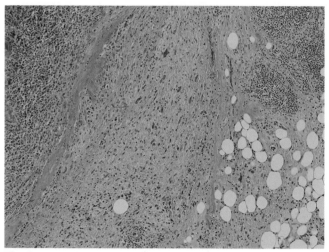

Fig 2. A paratesticular, well-differentiated liposarcoma *(right)* with transformation to a dedifferentiated liposarcoma *(left)*.

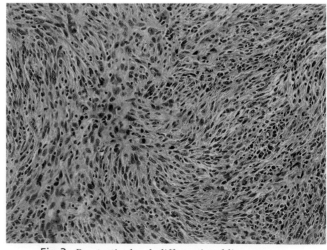

Fig 3. Paratesticular dedifferentiated liposarcoma.

PARATESTICULAR RHABDOMYOSARCOMA

Definition
- Malignant tumor of skeletal muscle (rhabdoid) differentiation, arising from the spermatic cord or paratesticular region

Clinical features
Epidemiology
- Most common sarcoma of the spermatic cord or paratesticular region in children
- Mean age, 9 years (range, 5 to 40 years)
- Paratesticular tumors accounts for 4% of all rhabdomyosarcomas

Presentation
- Paratesticular or testicular mass
- Possible distant metastasis (lung, retroperitoneal lymph nodes, and bone)

Prognosis and treatment
- Multimodality regimen including chemotherapy, surgery, or radiation
- Better prognosis for spindle cell and embryonal variants than for alveolar or pleomorphic variants

Pathology
Gross pathology
- Lobulated mass with gray-tan gelatinous cut surface
- Focal hemorrhage and cystic changes
- Average size, 5 cm (range, 1 to 20 cm)

Histology
- Most commonly embryonal variant with small round cells with variable number of myoblasts and myxoid stroma
- Spindle cell variant with elongated fusiform cells arranged in fascicles
- Alveolar variant, 6%
- Pleomorphic variant rarely seen

Immunopathology (including immunohistochemistry)
- Positive: MYOD1, myogenin, desmin, myoglobin, actin HHF35, vimentin

Molecular diagnostics
- PAX3/FKHR fusion
- PAX7/FKHR fusion (better prognosis in alveolar rhabdomyosarcoma)

Main differential diagnosis
- Myxoid liposarcoma can be mistaken for embryonal rhabdomyosarcoma, but has prominent plexiform vascular network.
- Leukemia or lymphoma: they are positive for lymphoid markers and negative for desmin; the presence of occasional myoblasts suggests rhabdomyosarcoma.
- Leiomyosarcoma can be mistaken for the spindle cell variant of rhabdomyosarcoma, but has more consistent fascicular arrangement and is positive for smooth muscle actin.

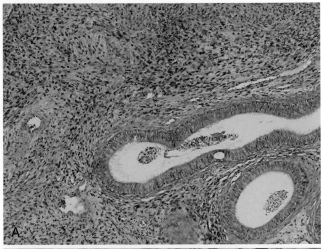
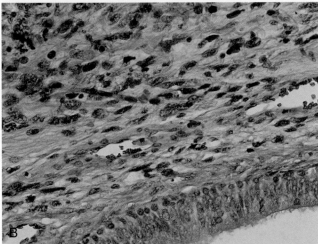
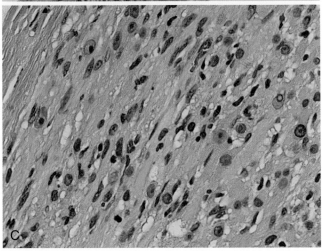

Fig 1. A rhabdomyosarcoma involving the epididymis **(A)**. Note the strap-shaped rhabdomyoblast **(B)** and cross-striations in several cells **(C)**.

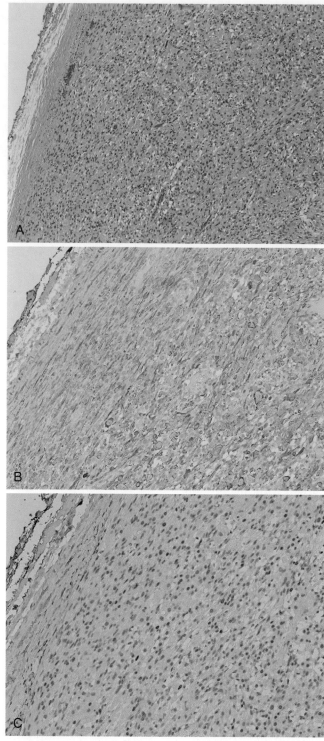

Fig 2. A rhabdomyosarcoma composed of malignant cellular spindle cells with abundant eosinophilic cytoplasm **(A)**, which are positive for desmin **(B)** and focally positive for MyoD1 **(C).**

LEIOMYOMA OF THE SPERMATIC CORD AND TESTICULAR ADNEXA

Definition
- Benign smooth muscle tumor arising in the spermatic cord and testicular adnexa

Clinical features
Epidemiology
- Rare
- Most patients in fifth to seventh decades of life
- Occasionally bilateral, especially epididymal leiomyomas

Presentation
- Painless mass

Prognosis and treatment
- Benign
- Excision

Pathology
Histology
- Morphology identical to its counterpart in other body sites
- Good circumscription without infiltrative growth
- Interlacing fascicles of spindle smooth muscle cell
- Rare or no mitotic figures
- Minimal cellular atypia
- Absence of necrosis

Immunohistochemistry
- Positive for vimentin, actin, and desmin

Main differential diagnosis
- Leiomyosarcoma: infiltrative border, necrosis, cellular atypia, mitosis
- Solitary fibrous tumor: spindle cells arranged in "patternless" pattern with deposition of intercellular collagen; positive for CD34 and BCL2; negative for desmin
- Idiopathic smooth muscle hyperplasia: haphazard arrangement of smooth muscle bundles, often around vessels or epididymal ducts

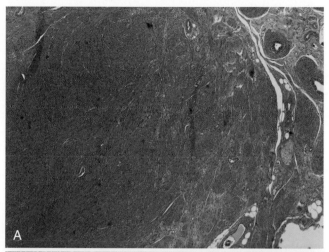

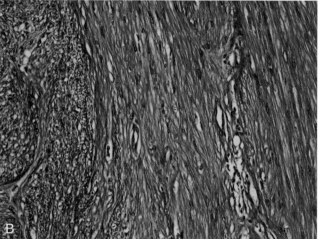

Fig 1. **A,** A well-circumscribed leiomyoma in the spermatic cord. **B,** The tumor is composed of bland, spindle-shaped smooth muscle cells with low cellularity and without nuclear atypia.

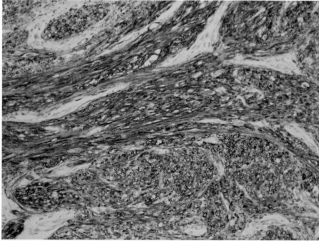

Fig 2. The tumor cells are diffusely positive for smooth muscle actin.

Definition
- A rare malignant mesenchymal tumor of smooth muscle differentiation

Clinical features
Epidemiology
- Most commonly arising from the spermatic cord, but may also arise from the epididymis
- Wide age range, but most commonly in men older than 40 years

Presentation
- Paratesticular mass

Prognosis and treatment
- Local recurrence or metastatic disease is dependent on tumor grade and stage.
- Radical orchiectomy is often the treatment.
- Surgery, radiation, or chemotherapy, or a combination, may be offered to the patient.

Pathology
Gross pathology
- Solid, grayish white with whirled cut surface
- Hemorrhage and necrosis in high-grade tumor

Histology
- Spindle cells are arranged in fascicles or occasionally in a herringbone pattern.
- Cigar-shaped hyperchromatic nuclei with inconspicuous nucleoli are present.
- Paranuclear vacuoles may be present.
- Cytologic atypia may be prominent with an occasional pleomorphic component.
- A high number of mitotic figures are usually present.
- Epithelioid cells may be present.

Immunohistochemistry and special studies
- Positive for smooth muscle actin, desmin, and vimentin
- Negative for S-100 or C-kit

Main differential diagnosis
- Embryonal rhabdomyosarcoma with prominent spindle cell morphology: positive for MYOD1, myogenin, and desmin
- Leiomyoma: usually small in size, well circumscribed, with bland appearance and low mitotic activity; may be difficult to differentiate from low-grade leiomyosarcoma; use low diagnostic threshold for leiomyosarcoma at the paratesticular site
- Metastatic sarcomatoid carcinoma with prominent spindle cells: positive cytokeratin expression

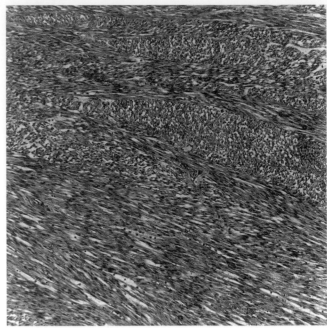

Fig 1. Leiomyosarcoma with interweaving spindle cells arranged in interlacing fascicles.

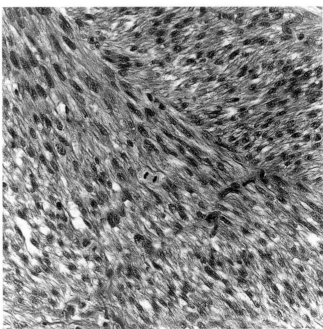

Fig 2. Higher magnification of a leiomyosarcoma shows an increased number of mitosis with occasional atypical mitotic figures. Neoplastic cells have cigar-shaped hyperchromatic nuclei and inconspicuous nucleoli.

AGGRESSIVE ANGIOMYXOMA OF THE MALE GENITAL REGION

Definition
- Distinctive, locally aggressive fibromyxoid tumor of the pelvic and genital region

Clinical features
Epidemiology
- Rare; approximately 150 cases reported to date
- Predominantly affecting females with males rarely affected (female-to-male ratio, 7.5:1)
- Mean age, 46 years (range, 1 to 82 years); most commonly in the third and fourth decades of life

Presentation
- Mass or swelling in the scrotum, inguinal region, or lower abdomen
- Typically a slow-growing lesion
- Presenting symptoms possibly related to compression by the expanding tumor
- Not associated with urethral or rectal obstruction

Prognosis and treatment
- Locally infiltrative; recurrence in 9% of cases
- No metastasis reported
- Wide local resection is treatment of choice

Pathology
Gross pathology
- Tumors not encapsulated, with lobulated contours, and infiltrating the surrounding soft tissues
- Semitransparent and gelatinous in appearance, sometimes showing a cystic and glistening cut surface

Histology
- Poorly circumscribed infiltrative tumor with myxoid stroma
- Sparse population of cytologically bland, spindled, and stellate cells with delicate cytoplasmic processes that surround small and medium-sized blood vessels
- Cells showing fibroblastic or myofibroblastic features
- Tumor cells displaying no atypia or mitotic figures
- Numerous randomly distributed arteries, veins, venules, arterioles, and capillaries in the stroma

Immunohistochemistry and special studies
- Positive for vimentin, variably positive for muscle-specific actin, CD34
- Negative for α-smooth muscle actin, and S-100 protein
- Focal nuclear and cytoplasmic staining for factor XIIIa
- Androgen, estrogen, and progesterone receptors can be positive

Molecular diagnostics
- Rare clonal chromosomal translocation –t(8;12) detected

Main differential diagnosis
- Superficial angiomyxoma: in contrast to the deeply infiltrative aggressive angiomyxoma, superficial angiomyxoma is a benign myxoid tumor involving subcutaneous tissues; these are composed of moderately to sparsely cellular angiomyxoid lobules containing scattered spindle cells and stellate cells in abundant myxoid stroma.
- Cellular angiofibroma (male angiomyofibroblastoma-like tumor) is a circumscribed, lobulated tumor composed of a cellular spindle cell component and numerous small to medium-sized thick-wall blood vessels, some of which are hyalinized.
- Myxoid or spindle cell lipoma typically occurs in the neck, shoulder, and back of adult men and rarely in other locations; this is a circumscribed tumor with bland spindle cells and fat.
- Myxoid neurofibroma can superficially resemble aggressive angiomyxoma; however, features of a nerve sheath tumor are typically evident.

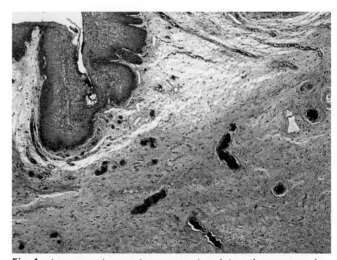

Fig 1. An aggressive angiomyxoma involving the scrotum has numerous vessels.

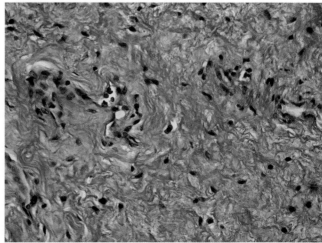

Fig 2. Sparsely cellular and bland, spindled, and stellate cells with delicate cytoplasmic processes that surround small and medium-sized blood vessels.

Definition

- Benign, highly cellular, and richly vascular mesenchymal tumor that usually arises in the superficial soft tissue of the inguinoscrotal region of men and vulva in women
- Synonym: angiofibroblastoma-like tumor in men

Clinical features

Epidemiology
- Rare

Presentation
- Painless intrascrotal or inguinal mass
- May be associated with hernia or hydrocele

Prognosis and treatment
- Benign
- Excision

Pathology

Histology
- Well circumscribed
- Numerous small to medium-sized vessels
- Variable cellularity of bland spindle cells with an oval to fusiform nucleus and a scanty amount of lightly eosinophilic cytoplasm
- Rare or no mitoses
- Focal perivascular fibrosis, epithelioid cells, and a intralesional fatty component
- Occasional intravascular thrombi and extravasation
- Scattered mast cells

Immunohistochemistry
- Variably positive for CD34, estrogen, and progesterone receptors, smooth muscle actin, desmin

Main differential diagnosis
- Aggressive angiomyxoma; poorly circumscribed with infiltrative border

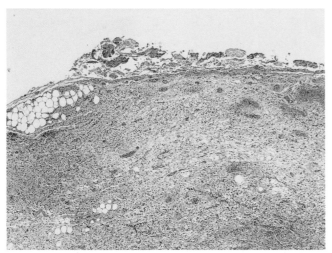

Fig 1. Cellular angiofibroma has a well-circumscribed border. (Courtesy Dr. Pal Chih-Hsueh Chen, Taipei, Taiwan.)

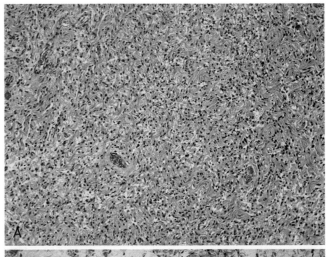

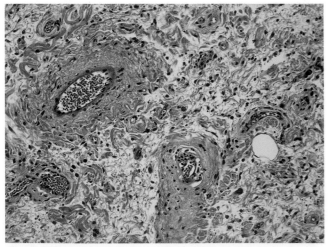

Fig 2. Numerous small to medium-sized vessels with hyaline wall. Bland spindle cells are present in the stroma.

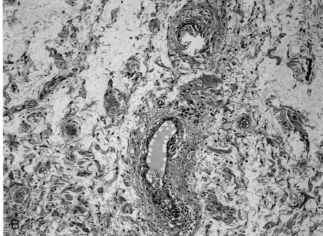

Fig 3. Cellular spindle cells (A) and hypocellular stromal cells (B) are present in a cellular angiofibroma.

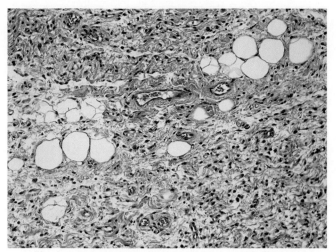

Fig 4. Intralesional aggregates of adipocytes are seen.

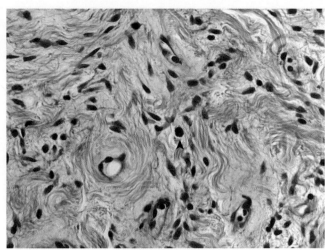

Fig 6. The stromal mast cells *(arrowhead)* are always present.

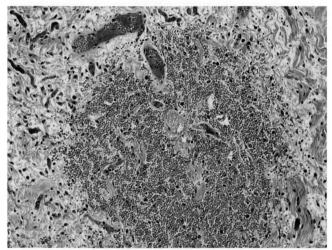

Fig 5. Red cell extravasation and thrombi in the vessels are occasionally seen.

Definition
- Highly aggressive tumor arising from the mesothelial lining of the tunica vaginalis, and less commonly from the spermatic cord or epididymis

Clinical features
Epidemiology
- Rare, accounts for less than 1% of all malignant mesotheliomas
- Usually affecting old patients (mean age, 65 years); some pediatric cases reported
- Association with asbestos exposure weaker than pleural and peritoneal mesotheliomas in approximately one fourth of cases

Presentation
- Hydrocele of unknown origin
- Intrascrotal mass

Prognosis and treatment
- Aggressive tumor is capable of widespread local invasion and distant metastasis.
- Recurrence occurs in 60% within 2 years.
- Median survival is 24 months.
- Treatment generally requires radical orchiectomy.

Pathology
Gross pathology
- Multiple friable nodules involving thickened tunica vaginalis
- Mass can infiltrate into testis and hilar structures

Histology
- Similar to pleural mesotheliomas
- Seventy-five percent of cases: epithelial type with papillary and tubulopapillary architecture
- Twenty-five percent of cases: biphasic with epithelial and sarcomatoid components
- Tumor cells with varying amount of eosinophilic cytoplasm, moderate nuclear atypia with vesicular nuclei, and prominent nucleoli

Immunopathology
- Positive for wide-spectrum cytokeratins, EMA, calretinin, D2-40, WT1, thrombomodulin, and CK5/6
- Negative for CEA, CK20, BerP4, MOC31, and CD15

Differential diagnosis
- Well-differentiated papillary mesothelioma is an unusual variant of mesothelioma with borderline behavior, more common in the peritoneum of women, and rarely seen in the tunica vaginalis of men. It is a papillary neoplasm covered with a single layer of relatively uniform flat or cuboidal mesothelial cells with minimal atypia. Small nests of tumor cells may be found along the fibrovascular cores, but solid and complex architecture and stromal invasion are not seen.
- Florid mesothelial hyperplasia is almost always a microscopic finding, and the presence of a mass lesion and studding of hydrocele sac is inconsistent with such a diagnosis; it exhibits predominantly tubular pattern, does not exhibit the complex growth pattern seen in mesothelioma, and is often associated with intense inflammation.
- Adenomatoid tumor is also a tumor of mesothelial origin, also termed *benign nonpapillary mesothelioma* because it lacks the papillary fronds. Cytoplasmic vacuoles are characteristic. Atypia is minimal to absent.
- Metastatic adenocarcinoma, especially prostatic carcinomas, may line the mesothelium of the tunica and mimic mesotheliomas. History and immunohistochemical stains are essential in this circumstance.

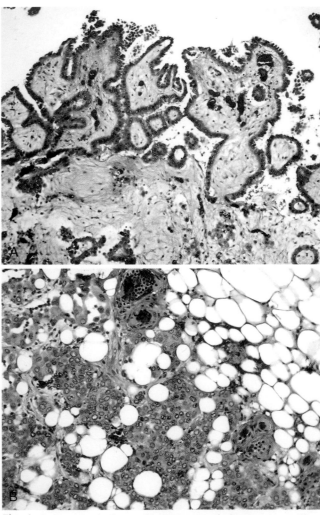

Fig 1. In paratesticular malignant mesothelioma, a papillary component is virtually always present, at least focally **(A)**. In another area, solid nests of mesothelioma cells invade the fatty tissue **(B)**.

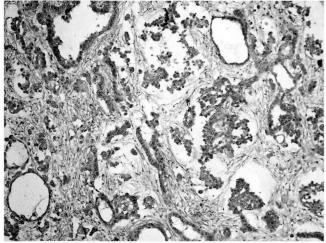

Fig 2. The architecture is varied microcysts, cords, nests, and vague papillary formation.

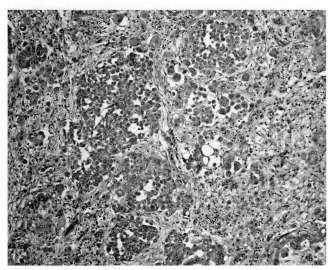

Fig 4. A solid area in a malignant mesothelioma.

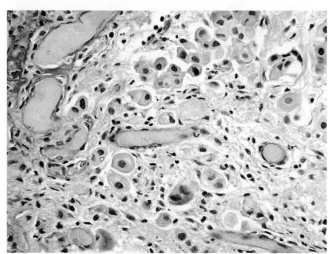

Fig 3. Malignant mesothelioma grows in single cells with abundant cytoplasm and more pronounced nuclear atypia.

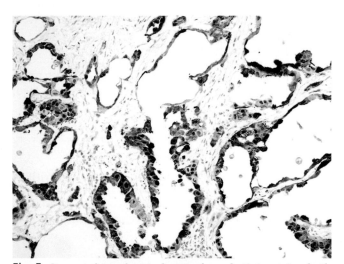

Fig 5. Immunohistochemical stain for calretinin stains both nuclei and cytoplasm in a malignant mesothelioma.

Definition
- Paratesticular tumors equivalent to the ovarian-type epithelial tumors

Clinical features
Epidemiology
- Extremely rare
- Wide age range of 14 to 77 years

Presentation
- Mass in the testicular or paratesticular region
- Hydrocele in some patients

Prognosis and treatment
- Radical orchiectomy
- Good prognosis for borderline tumors, worse prognosis for invasive carcinoma

Pathology
Histology
- Histology is identical to their ovarian counterparts.
- Serous borderline tumor is the most common.
- Other types, including mucinous, endometrioid, Brenner, and clear cell carcinoma, have been reported.

Immunohistochemistry
- Positive for CK7, WT1, CA125, CEA

Main differential diagnosis
- Carcinoma of rete testis is located in the hilus, with microscopic evidence of occurrence in the rete testis; immunostains are of little value because it is positive for WT1, PAX2, and PAX8.

- Malignant mesothelioma can be mistaken for a serous borderline tumor of the tunica vaginalis, but the papillae of a well-differentiated mesothelioma are not as broad and do not exhibit the same degree of cellular budding and stratification; tumor cells positive for calretinin.
- Mucinous and endometrioid carcinoma of the paratesticular regions should be differentiated from a metastatic adenocarcinoma. Clinical history is critical.

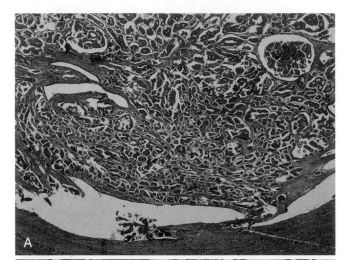

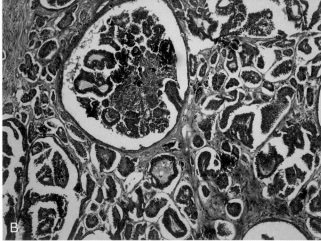

Fig 2. **A,** Borderline serous carcinoma composed predominantly of micropapillae, which are lined with hobnail cuboidal cells with eosinophilic cytoplasm. **B,** Note the frequent psammoma bodies.

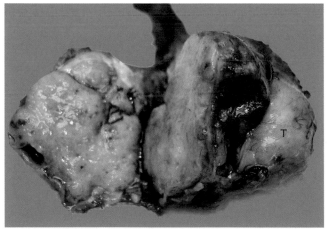

Fig 1. A solid mass of serous borderline carcinoma arising in the paratestis. The testis *(T)* is intact.

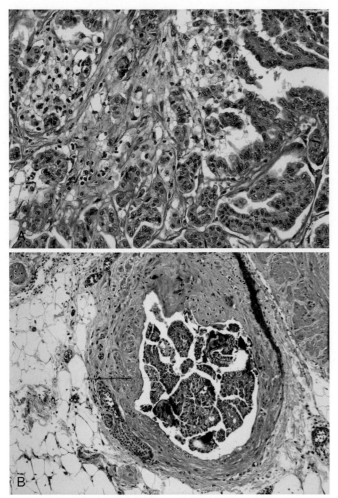

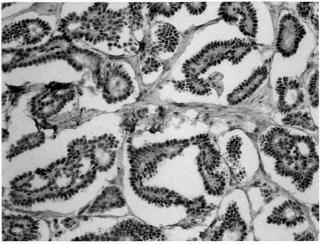

Fig 4. The tumor cells reveal nuclear reactivity for estrogen receptor.

Fig 3. Stromal invasion **(A)** and vascular invasion **(B)** in a serous carcinoma.

EPITHELIAL TUMORS OF THE RETE TESTIS

Definition
- Neoplasms arising from the epithelial lining of the rete testis

Adenoma of the rete testis
Clinical features
- Exceedingly rare
- Age range, 21 to 79 years
- Some patients have von Hippel-Lindau disease
- Appears as a slow-growing palpable mass
- Benign and treated with local resection

Pathology
- A tan-white heterogenous tumor with cystic and solid areas, centered in the rete testis
- Cysts, tubules, or papillae are lined with flat, cuboid, or columnar cells with minimal cytologic atypia
- Adenoma, cystadenoma, adenofibroma, and Sertoliform cystadenoma

Adenocarcinoma of the rete testis
Clinical features
- Most patients older than 60 years (range, 8 to 91 years)
- Present with an enlarging mass and scrotal pain
- Often associated with hydroceles
- Often develop lymphatic and hematogenous metastasis

Prognosis and treatment
- Treatment is radical orchiectomy.
- Survival is dismal, with a mean of 8 months.

Pathology
- Diagnostic criteria
  - Tumor centers in the testicular hilum
  - Morphology incompatible with any other type of testicular or paratesticular tumor
  - Absence of an extrascrotal tumor with similar histology
  - Presence of a transition between the unaffected rete testis and the tumor
- Size ranges from 1 to 10 cm
- A tan-white heterogenous tumor with solid and cystic areas
- Often involve spermatic cord
- Tumor shows glandular, tubular, papillary, and solid patterns
- Tumor cells usually cuboidal with eosinophilic cytoplasm and moderate to severe nuclear atypia
- Tumor necrosis and inflammatory and desmoplastic changes response common
- Residual rete possibly dilated and containing intraluminal tumor nests

Immunohistochemistry
- Positive for PAX2 and PAX8

Main differential diagnosis
- Metastatic adenocarcinoma: usually multifocal and bilateral, frequent lymphovascular invasion, and clinical history of a primary carcinoma
- Mesothelioma: ill-defined tumor involving the tunica vaginalis, tubulopapillary pattern, positive immunostaining for calretinin and WT1
- Malignant Sertoli cell tumor: located in the testicular parenchyma, positive for inhibin, negative for PAX2 and PAX8

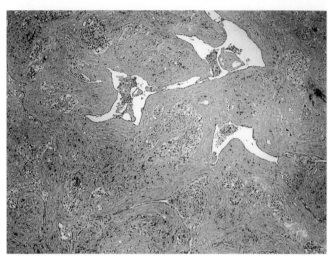

Fig 1. Adenocarcinoma of the rete testis involves the rete channels and stroma.

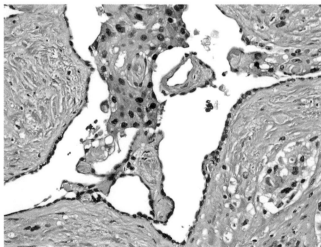

Fig 2. Adenocarcinoma of the rete testis involves the rete channels and forms intraluminal papillary structures.

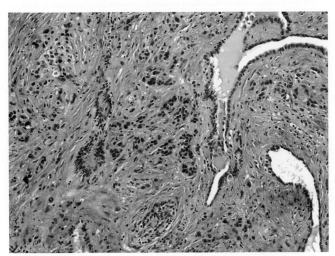

Fig 3. Adenocarcinoma of the rete testis invades the stroma and induces desmoplastic changes and displays marked nuclear atypia.

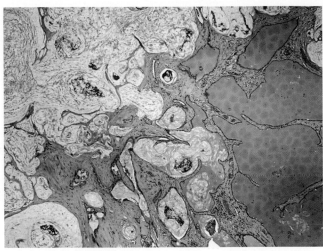

Fig 4. Metastatic mucinous adenocarcinoma of the colon involves the rete testis.

L

DISEASE OF THE PENIS, URETHRA, AND SCROTUM

FIBROEPITHELIAL POLYP OF THE URETHRA

Definition
- Polyp composed of fibrovascular stroma covered by urothelium

Clinical features
- Symptoms of urinary obstruction
- Asymptomatic in some adults
- Polypoid lesions in the posterior urethra on urethroscopy

Epidemiology
- Marked male predominance
- Majority of cases reported in infants and children; some cases related to urogenital malformations
- Rarely seen in adults

Prognosis and treatment
- Conservative transurethral resection
- Benign

Pathology
Gross pathology
- Polypoid mass on narrow stalk protruding into the urethra
- Sometimes shows "Medusa head" features

Histology
- Several low-power growth patterns: tall fingerlike, clublike, or cloverleaf-like

- Papillary structures composed of central fibrovascular stromal cores
- Surface of the polyp lined by normal urothelium
- Urothelium may show florid cystitis cystica et glandularis or squamous metaplasia
- Stromal cells may show degenerative atypia
- Nerves and smooth muscle bundles in one third of cases

Main differential diagnosis
- Urothelial papilloma: proliferation of urothelium forming simple papillary structures with thin and delicate fibrovascular cores
- Polypoid urethritis: thick, edematous papillary structures with marked inflammation; may overlap with fibroepithelial polyp morphologically in some cases
- Prostatic type urethral polyp: papillary structures and glands are lined with prostatic glandular epithelium
- Urothelial carcinoma: proliferation of urothelial cells with cytologic atypia
- Rhabdomyosarcoma: polypoid tumor with a central hypocellular and myxoid stroma with condensation of tumor cells beneath the surface urothelium (cambium layer)

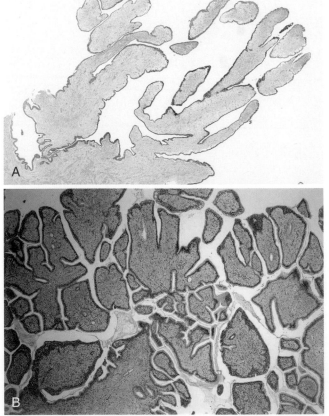

Fig 1. Cystoscopic appearance of a fibroepithelial polyp. The narrow stalk is characteristic.

Fig 2. The architectural patterns observed in fibroepithelial polyps include tall fingerlike (A) and clublike or cloverleaf-like (B).

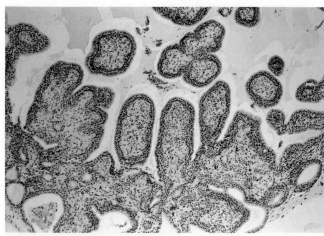

Fig 3. Papillary structures are lined with normal-appearing urothelium and contain fibrovascular stromal cores.

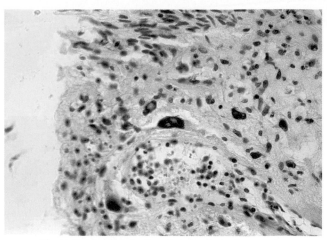

Fig 5. Stromal cells showing degenerative atypia.

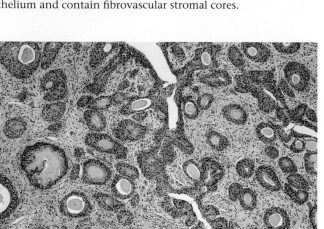

Fig 4. Squamous cell metaplasia and glandular metaplasia in a fibroepithelial polyp.

Definition
- A polypoid inflammatory lesion involving the distal urethra, particularly the posterior urethral orifice

Clinical features
Epidemiology
- Most cases seen in postmenopausal women; rarely reported in young girls
- Believed to result from focal prolapse of the posterior urethral wall

Presentation
- Most are asymptomatic
- Occurs occasionally with irritative symptoms such as frequency, urgency, pain, and dyspareunia, particularly when the lesion is inflamed
- Bloody spotting typically seen when there is trauma to the lining epithelium

Prognosis and treatment
- Benign reactive lesion
- Conservative treatment such as warm sitz baths, topical creams, and antiinflammatory drugs
- Surgical treatment occasionally performed for symptomatic cases or cases with suspicion for neoplastic lesions or special infections

Pathology
Gross pathology
- Reddish or fleshy polypoid lesion protruding from the posterior lip of urethral orifice
- Usually small, up to 1 to 2 cm in diameter

Histology
- Proliferative surface epithelium, either urothelial or squamous
- Prominent vessels in the lamina propria; thrombosis or hemorrhage can be seen
- Acute or chronic inflammation

Main differential diagnosis
- Urothelial carcinoma: urothelial cells are cytologically atypical.
- Inflammatory pseudotumors (inflammatory myofibroblastic tumor) are typically larger and may display infiltrative growth. Atypical mesenchymal cells are present, and stromal cells are positive for myoepithelial markers.

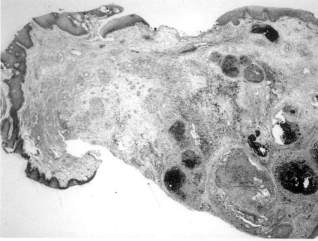

Fig 1. A urethral caruncle forms an elongated polypoid lesion with dilated vessels in the stroma and is covered by benign squamous epithelium.

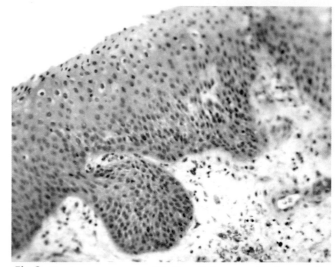

Fig 2. Benign squamous epithelium lining a urethral caruncle.

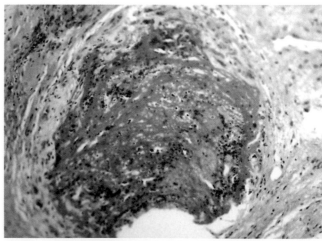

Fig 3. A dilated blood vessel with thrombosis and hemorrhage in the stroma of a urethral caruncle.

Definition
- Diverticulum arising from the urethra

Clinical features
Epidemiology
- Affecting predominantly women
- Mostly in adults (third to sixth decades) and acquired after infection, trauma, or obstruction
- Rarely congenital

Presentation
- Most commonly at the dorsolateral wall of the midurethra
- Bulging mass usually palpated in the anterior vaginal wall
- May be asymptomatic but can present with irritative symptoms
- Often complicated with infection, calculi, and obstruction

Prognosis and treatment
- Treatment is surgical repair.
- Malignancy (adenocarcinoma or squamous cell carcinoma [SCC]) is the most ominous complication.

Pathology
Histology
- Urothelial lining with frequent squamous or glandular metaplasia
- Frequent mucosal denudation, ulceration, exudation, and inflammatory changes
- Edematous, inflamed, or fibrotic wall containing attenuated smooth muscle

Main differential diagnosis
- Urethral cyst: affecting boys; parameatal location; resulting from obstruction of paraurethral ducts or faulty preputial separation from the glans along the sulcus; cyst wall lined with urothelial or squamous as well as columnar epithelium

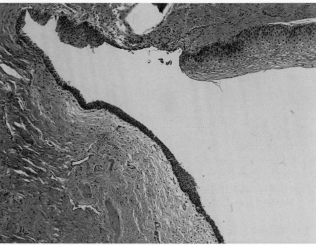

Fig 2. The diverticular wall is lined by urothelium and metaplastic squamous epithelium.

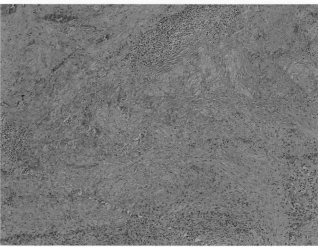

Fig 3. The diverticular wall is markedly fibrotic and inflamed, and contains a discontinuous muscular layer.

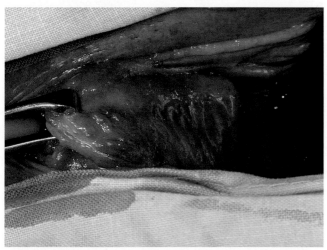

Fig 1. Urethral diverticulum presenting as a bulging mass protruding from the anterior vagianl wall. (Courtesy Alex T. L. Lin, Taipei Veterans General Hospital, Taiwan.)

Definition
- Narrowing of the urethra caused by various etiologies including congenital anomalies, trauma, infection, and neoplasia

Clinical features
Epidemiology
- Risk factors include history of sexually transmitted disease, instrumentation, radiotherapy of the urinary tract, trauma to the pelvic area, and repeated episodes of urethritis.
- Incidence is more common in men, involving membranous portion of the urethra.
- Congenital strictures are rare.
- Stricture is a risk factor for carcinoma of the urethra.

Presentation
- Obstructive voiding symptoms
- Signs or symptoms related to a specific etiology (e.g., infection, calculus, radiotherapy)

Prognosis and treatment
- Early detection and treatment usually result in an excellent outcome.
- Repeated urethral dilation or urethroplasty may be needed.

Pathology
Histology
- Dense hyalinized fibrosis with or without chronic inflammation is seen most commonly.
- A keratinizing squamous epithelium frequently covers the scarred stroma.
- Nephrogenic adenoma, polypoid urethritis, urethral diverticula, and pseudosarcomatous fibromyxoid changes in the stroma can also be noted in some cases.

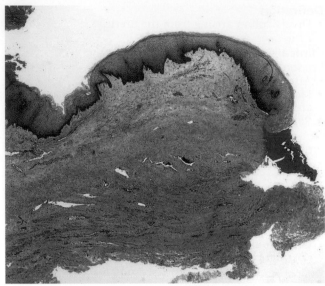

Fig 1. Urethral stricture showing a thick keratinizing squamous epithelium overlying fibrotic subepithelial connective tissue.

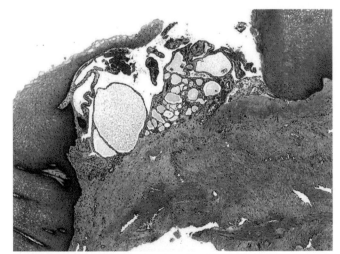

Fig 2. Urethral stricture showing focally eroded mucosa with a focus of nephrogenic adenoma.

Definition
- Polypoid or papillary exaggeration of the urethral mucosa in response to inflammation or irritation

Clinical features
Epidemiology
- Frequency unknown
- Invariably associated with urinary tract infection or mechanical irritation

Presentation
- Single or multiple polypoid or papillary growth
- Commonly found in prostatic urethra near verumontanum

Prognosis and treatment
- Nonneoplastic lesion
- Usually resolves spontaneously after removal of the inflammatory stimulus
- Does not recur or rarely recurs after resection

Pathology
Gross pathology
- Polypoid protrusions of the urothelial mucosa with wide base or thinner papillae

Histology
- Normal surface urothelium, sometimes hyperplastic or with squamous metaplasia or ulceration
- Edematous lamina propria with variably dilated thin-walled vessels and chronic inflammatory infiltrate
- von Brunn nests or urethritis cystica in lamina propria

Main differential diagnosis
- Urothelial neoplasms: papillae with thin fibrovascular cores without significant inflammation or edema; may have significant cytologic atypia
- Squamous papilloma: papillae with thin fibrovascular cores without significant inflammation or edema
- Prostatic-type urethral polyp: composed of benign prostatic glands
- Caruncle: granulation tissue, often denuded without overlying mucosa
- Condyloma acuminatum: papillae lined with squamous epithelium with changes related to human papilloma virus (HPV)

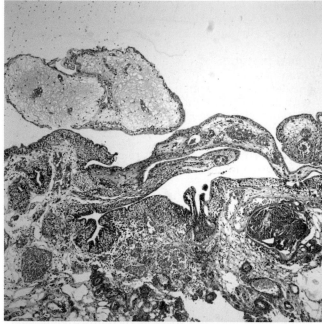

Fig 1. Polypoid urethritis. Polypoid or papillary fronds are broad with edematous and inflamed lamina propria.

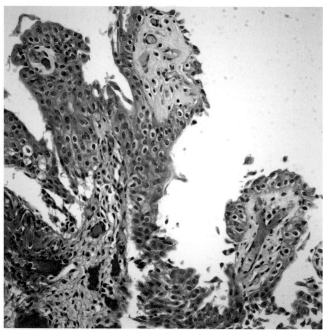

Fig 2. Polypoid urethritis. Broad papillary projections are covered with normal-appearing urothelial cells without atypia.

Definition
- Exophytic or verruciform epithelial proliferation related to human papillomavirus (HPV) infection

Clinical features
Epidemiology
- Incidence is common in sexually active young adults, with a predilection for anogenital areas.
- In males, glans is most frequently affected, followed by foreskin, distal penile urethra (fossa navicularis and meatus), and shaft.
- Low-risk HPV types 6 and 11 are predominant genotypes, other identified types include 16, 18, 30 to 32, 42 to 44, and 51 to 55.

Presentation
- Most are papillary, warty lesions, but can be flat.

Prognosis and treatment
- Benign, rare cases can undergo malignant transformation.
- Risk for anogenital cancers is increased.
- Small lesions are treated with cryotherapy, electro-fulguration, and laser ablation; medium-sized to large lesions require surgical resection.

Pathology
Histology
- Papillomatosis with prominent fibrovascular core and broad pushing base is present.
- There is a variable degree of acanthosis, parakeratosis, and hyperkeratosis.
- Typically displays apparent HPV-related changes (koilocytosis) toward surface—cytoplasmic vacuolization, raisinoid nuclei, and binucleation—but the atypia can vary from prominent to inconspicuous.
- Rarely, SCC arises in a condyloma.

Molecular diagnostics
- Most results are positive for HPV6 or HPV11, or both, by in situ hybridization.

Main differential diagnosis
- Warty carcinoma: higher degree of nuclear atypia, pleomorphism and more mitotic activity; irregular and infiltrative tumor base with stromal invasion; positive for high-risk HPV and p16
- Papillary carcinoma: low-grade verruciform variant of SCC with prominent hyperkeratosis and acanthosis, mild to moderate cytologic atypia, and irregular infiltrative base; often associated squamous hyperplasia and differentiated penile intraepithelial neoplasia; no evidence of HPV-related changes
- Verrucous carcinoma: verruciform growth with prominent acanthosis and hyperkeratosis, in conspicuous fibrovascular cores, minimal cytologic atypia, and a pushing border invasion; often associated squamous hyperplasia and differentiated penile intraepithelial neoplasia; no HPV-related cellular changes
- Warty penile intraepithelial neoplasia (PeIN): undulating or spiky growth, not papillomatosis with well-formed fibrovascular core; epithelium replaced by pleomorphic cells with koilocytic changes and numerous mitosis
- Papillomatosis of glans corona: multiple, pearly gray or white, small papules on the dorsal side of glans corona, also called *pearly penile plaques;* small fibroepithelial papillomas showing hyperkeratosis and fibrovascular stroma; no HPV-related cellular changes

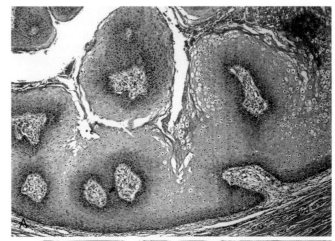

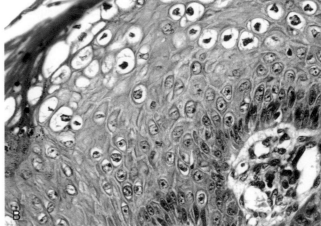

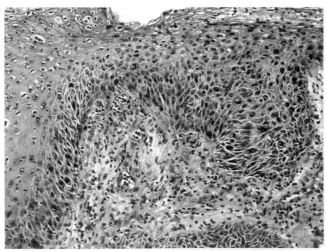

Fig 1. Condyloma with focal marked nuclear atypia and brisk mitotic activity limited to the basal region, which should not be considered as in situ carcinoma (or intraepithelial neoplasia).

Fig 2. **A,** Condyloma shows papillae with acanthosis, parakeratosis, well-formed fibrovascular core and smooth, broad base. **B,** Prominent koilocytic changes are located toward the surface epithelium.

PROSTATIC-TYPE URETHRAL POLYP

Definition
- Uncommon benign polypoid lesion composed of normal prostatic acini and stroma that grows into the prostatic urethra in and around the verumontanum

Clinical features
Epidemiology
- Predominantly affects younger adults (27 to 41 years old), but has been reported in a wide age range

Presentation
- It typically manifests with hematuria, hematospermia, dysuria, and frequency.
- Cystoscopic examination shows a single, polypoid or papillary lesion growing into the prostatic urethra in and around the verumontanum.
- The second most common location is the trigone of the bladder, where the term *ectopic prostatic polyp* is applied.

Prognosis and treatment
- Benign
- Treated by cystoscopic excision and fulguration
- Recurrence uncommon

Pathology
Histology
- Polypoid or papillary growth usually composed of broad-based papillae but occasionally of fingerlike villous projections
- Surface lined by benign urothelial cells and/or benign prostatic epithelial cells
- Submucosal benign prostatic stroma and glands that may be closely packed or cystically dilated at the periphery
- Glands often contain corpora amylacea

Immunohistochemistry
- Positive for prostate-specific markers

Main differential diagnosis
- Prostatic ductal adenocarcinoma: complex glandular structure lined with cytologic atypical cells
- Papillary urothelial neoplasms: papillae lined with urothelial cells; negative for prostate-specific markers
- Villous adenoma: pseudostratified columnar (adenomatous) nuclei with variable cytologic atypia; mucin positivity

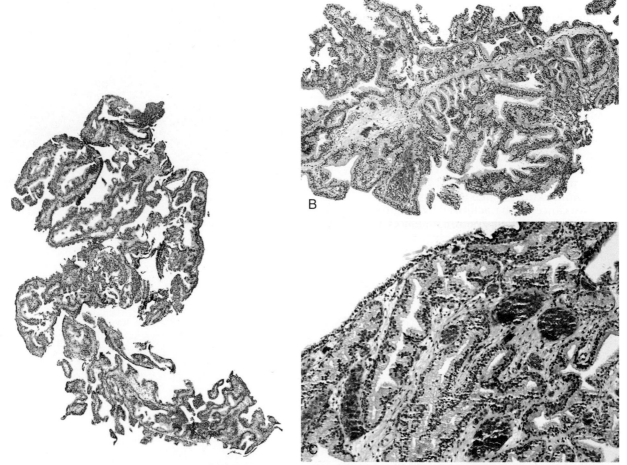

Fig 1. **A,** Low-power view of a prostatic-type urethral polyp growing as polypoid lesion composed of broad-based papillae and submucosal normal prostatic glands. **B,** The papillary projections may be numerous, and rare detached papillae may occasionally be seen *(upper right)*. **C,** The polyp surface is lined by benign prostatic epithelial cells, and the submucosal component is composed of benign prostatic stroma and glands.

URETHRAL UROTHELIAL CARCINOMA ASSOCIATED WITH BLADDER UROTHELIAL CARCINOMA

Definition
- Urothelial carcinoma of the urethra, either by direct extension of the bladder or as a part of multifocal urinary tract tumors

Clinical features
Epidemiology
- Frequent in patients with high-grade multifocal bladder cancer
- Urethral recurrence in 10% of patients after radical cystectomy for urothelial carcinoma, increased in men with bladder cancer involving the prostate and women with bladder cancer involving bladder neck

Presentation
- Hematuria, bloody urethral discharge
- Pain
- Voiding habit change
- Palpable mass

Prognosis and treatment
- Prognosis relatively poor
- Transurethral resection of the tumor or urethrectomy
- Adjuvant chemotherapy and radiotherapy for advanced-stage tumors

Pathology
Histology
- The histologic spectrum is similar to the bladder tumor: noninvasive, invasive, with or without a papillary component, squamous or glandular differentiation, and uncommon morphologic variants.
- Small cell or sarcomatoid differentiation is extremely uncommon.
- Tumor may involve periurethral glands and prostatic ducts, mimicking stromal invasion.
- Invasive cancer is characterized by irregular nests of cells with desmoplasia and inflammatory response.

Main differential diagnosis
- Squamous cell carcinoma: comprises exclusively squamous component without invasive or in situ urothelial carcinoma
- Ductal adenocarcinoma of the prostate: glands or acini lined with columnar cells with prominent nucleoli; often associated with conventional prostate carcinoma; prostate markers positive
- Adenocarcinoma of urethra, including clear cell adenocarcinoma: more common in females; glandular formation; mucin may be seen; glandular metaplasia and urethritis cystica et glandularis often present

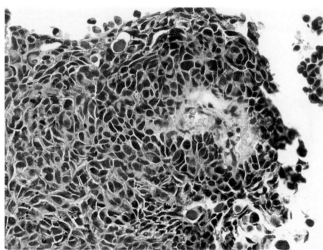

Fig 1. Noninvasive high-grade papillary urothelial carcinoma of penile urethra, in a patient with a history of radical cystectomy for invasive urothelial carcinoma of urinary bladder.

Definition
- Malignant neoplasm arising primarily from the epithelial lining of the urethra

Clinical features
Epidemiology
- Rare
- More common in women than in men
- Age similar to urothelial carcinoma involving other part of the urinary tract (mean age range, 70 to 79 years)

Presentation
- Dysuria, hematuria, and urinary obstruction
- Patients often have a history of infection, diverticulum, stricture, or fistula in the urethra

Prognosis and treatment
- In men, distal tumors are usually treated with partial penectomy and inguinal lymph node dissection, and proximal tumors are treated with cystoprostatectomy, urethrectomy, and inguinal and pelvic lymph node dissection.
- In women, tumors are usually treated with total urethrectomy and inguinal and pelvic lymph node dissection.
- Prognosis correlates with tumor anatomic location and pathologic stage, but not with tumor grade or histologic subtype.
- The distal urethra had a better prognosis (5-year survival, 67%) than the proximal urethra (5-year survival, 21%).

Pathology
Histology
- Urothelial carcinoma is more common in the proximal part, and SCC is more common in the distal part.
- In men, urothelial or SCCs are most common; adenocarcinoma is less common.

- In women, 75% of cases are SCC; urothelial carcinoma and adenocarcinoma are less common.
- Invasion into vascular spaces of the corpus spongiosum or corpora cavernosa is common.

Main differential diagnosis
- Prostatic adenocarcinoma: positive for prostate-specific markers

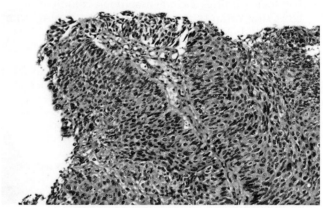

Fig 2. Well-differentiated squamous cell carcinoma in the distal urethra.

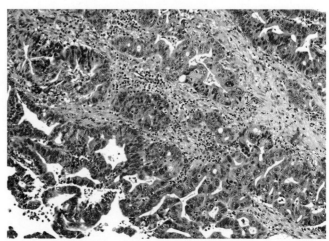

Fig 3. High-grade papillary urothelial carcinoma in the proximal urethra.

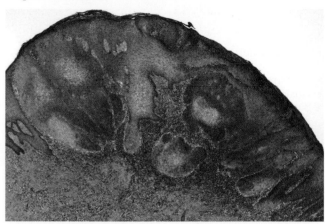

Fig 4. Moderately differentiated adenocarcinoma in the proximal urethra.

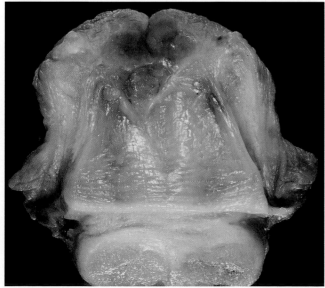

Fig 1. A partial penectomy specimen shows an exophytic tumor in the distal urethra.

Definition
- Adenocarcinoma arising from urothelial lining or surrounding glands of the urethra

Clinical features
Epidemiology
- Represents approximately 10% of all urethral carcinomas
- Female-to-male ratio, 4:1

Presentation
- Urinary frequency
- Dysuria
- Dyspareunia in females
- Obstructive voiding symptoms in males
- Rarely mucosuria

Prognosis and treatment
- Treatment involves surgical resection of the invasive carcinoma followed by chemotherapy in a subset of patients
- May develop distant metastases to soft tissue and lung within 5 years of diagnosis

Pathology
Histology
- Histologic findings include mucinous, colonic-type, signet ring variants, as well as carcinoma arising from Skene glands and clear cell adenocarcinoma.
- Carcinoma may arise in association within a diverticulum, especially in female patients.
- The background urethra may demonstrate intestinal metaplasia with or without high-grade dysplasia or villous adenoma.
- Carcinomas arising in association with Skene glands morphologically resemble prostate cancer and stain for PSA, PSAP, and occasionally produce detectable serum PSA.
- Rarely, Cowper glands give rise to adenoid cystic carcinoma.

Immunopathology
- Similar to bladder adenocarcinoma, including immunoreactivity for cytokeratin 20 and focal reactivity for cytokeratin 7

Main differential diagnosis
- Metastatic adenocarcinoma
- Ductal carcinoma of the prostate: neoplastic papillae lined with relatively uniform columnar cells; positive for prostate-specific markers

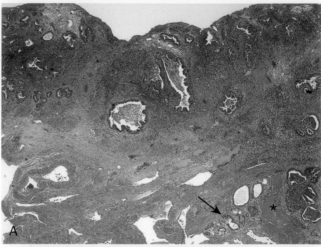

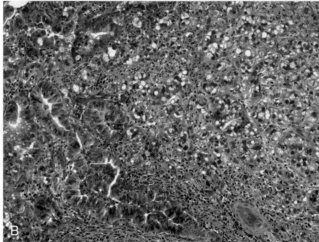

Fig 1. Invasive adenocarcinoma involving the penile urethra. **A,** Carcinoma invades to the level of the corpora spongiosum *(asterisk)* and associated periurethral glands *(arrow).* **B,** High magnification reveals an admixture of colonic-type glands and glands with vacuolated cytoplasm.

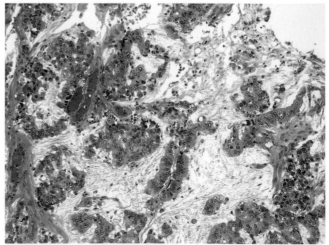

Fig 2. Mucinous adenocarcinoma is characterized by malignant tumor cells floating in pools of extravasated mucin.

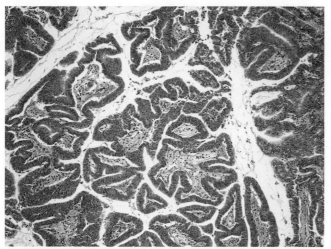

Fig 3. Villous adenomas may occasionally be identified and represent a precursor lesion to invasive adenocarcinoma.

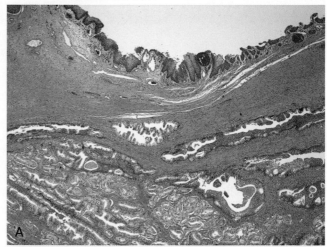

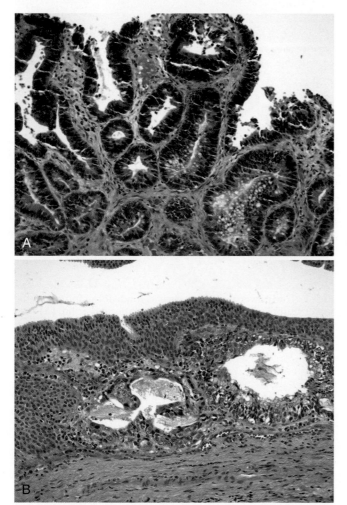

Fig 4. **A,** Glandular change with high-grade dysplasia is another common precursor lesion in this disease. **B,** Occasionally, high-grade dysplasia may be present only in von Brunn nests.

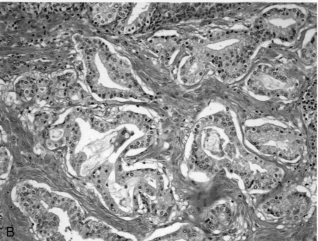

Fig 5. A rare urethral carcinoma arising in a female in Skene glands. **A,** This carcinoma morphologically resembles prostatic adenocarcinoma. **B,** Higher magnification demonstrates classic features of prostatic adenocarcinoma including prominent nucleoli, mucin, and dense pink secretions.

CLEAR CELL ADENOCARCINOMA OF THE URETHRA

Definition
- Unusual variant of urethral adenocarcinoma arising from the urethral mucosa or periurethral glands

Clinical features
Epidemiology
- Exceedingly rare
- Arising through metaplasia of the urethral surface mucosa or from periurethral glands, rather than Müllerian or mesonephric duct remnants

Presentation
- Similar to other tumors of the urethra (hematuria, obstructive voiding symptoms, urinary retention)

Prognosis and treatment
- Prognosis correlates with pathologic stage at presentation.
- Surgical and radiation modalities to abolish the tumor are available.

Pathology
Histology
- Various growth patterns include tubulocystic, tubular, papillary, and diffuse with different patterns often coexisting
- Tumor cells have ample clear cytoplasm or a hobnail appearance, or both.
- Nuclei are large and hyperchromatic, with moderate to marked nuclear atypia.
- Mitotic activity is usually high.

Immunopathology (including immunohistochemistry)
- Positive for CK7 and CA125
- PAX2 positive in some cases
- Positive for prostate-specific antigen and prostate-specific acid phosphatase in female patients in some reports

Main differential diagnosis
- In nephrogenic adenoma, patients usually have a history of urinary tract infection, trauma, or surgery. There is a lack of the nuclear atypical and infiltrative and destructive growth pattern seen in clear cell adenocarcinoma.
- In urothelial carcinoma with clear cell features, focal clear cell changes in an otherwise typical urothelial carcinoma do not warrant a diagnosis of clear cell adenocarcinoma.

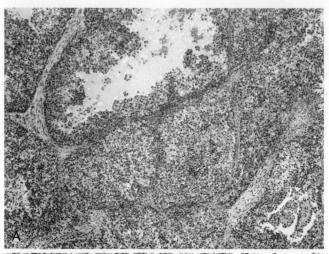

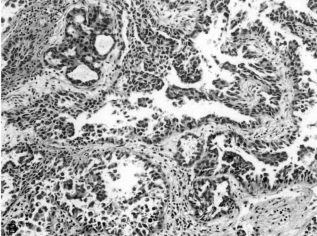

Fig 1. Low-power view of a clear cell adenocarcinoma of the male urethra shows predominantly cystic and solid **(A)** and tubular and papillary patterns of growth **(B).**

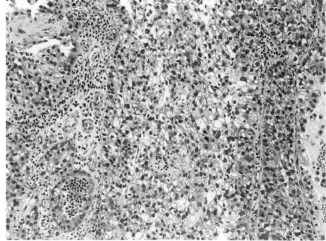

Fig 2. Clear cell adenocarcinoma of the male urethra. Clear cells show ample cytoplasm with distinctive cellular borders, moderate to marked nuclear atypias, and high mitotic rate.

Definition
- Inflammatory condition of the glans penis characterized by a dense plasma cell infiltrate in the upper dermis; also termed *plasma cell balanitis*

Clinical features
Epidemiology
- Typically uncircumcised middle-aged to older men

Presentation
- Chronic, well-circumscribed glistening orange-red lesions on glans penis surrounded by redder pin-point spots ("cayenne pepper spots")

Prognosis and treatment
- Circumcision is often effective.

Pathology
Histology
- Attenuated and spongiotic epidermis with a lichenoid inflammatory infiltrate with plasma cell predominance in the upper dermis
- Ulceration possible
- May be accompanied by dilated capillaries, extravasated red blood cells, and hemosiderin deposition in dermis

Main differential diagnosis
- Squamous cell carcinoma in situ (erythroplasia of Queyrat): plasma cell infiltrate may be present in both conditions; however, epithelial atypia is not a feature of Zoon balanitis.
- Syphilis: lesions of secondary syphilis typically show a more mixed inflammatory infiltrate with granulomas, lack the typical vascular changes of Zoon balanitis, and are often accompanied by psoriasiform epidermal hyperplasia rather than epidermal atrophy.

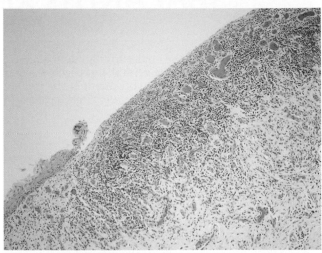

Fig 1. Attenuated epidermis with focal denudation and underlying lichenoid infiltrate in upper dermis in Zoon balanitis.

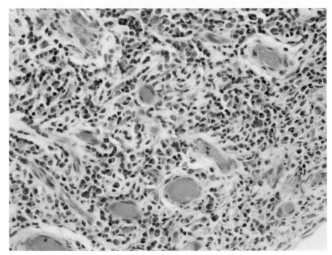

Fig 2. Predominant plasma cellular infiltrate is present in the dermis with dilated capillaries.

LICHEN SCLEROSUS ET ATROPHICUS (BALANITIS XEROTICA OBLITERANS)

Definition
- Atrophic condition of the epidermis and dermal connective tissue involving the genital and perianal skin of both males and females; involvement of the glans penis and prepuce is termed *balanitis xerotica obliterans*

Clinical features
Epidemiology
- Usually found in preputial resections of older men, but can rarely occur in young boys
- Association with autoimmune disorders such as vitiligo and alopecia areata

Presentation
- A well-defined white patch is present on the glans penis or prepuce, which may involve the urethral meatus.
- Chronic lesions may be firm to touch, owing to underlying fibrosis.
- Phimosis can occur as a complication.
- Erosion, ulceration, and bleeding can occur.

Prognosis and treatment
- Treatment is difficult, and various modalities have been attempted: laser therapy, topical steroids, circumcision, and excision.
- There is an association with SCC, in particular those not related to human papilloma virus.

Pathology
Histology
- Orthokeratotic hyperkeratosis and atrophy of the epidermis are the hallmarks of the disease.
- Basal cell vacuolation and clefting of the dermal–epidermal junction can occur.
- Marked edema and collagenization are present in the upper dermis, with a thin band of chronic inflammation beneath.

- Late lesions are characterized by replacement of the dermis by mature collagen, as well as patchy fibrosis alternating with epidermal hyperplasia.

Main differential diagnosis
- Vitiligo usually affects multiple body sites; skin is histologically normal except for the lack of melanocytes.
- Postinflammatory hypopigmentation can be seen as a sequela of an inflammatory dermatosis.
- Scarring can possibly follow a history of trauma or procedure, fibroblastic proliferation and collagen deposition parallel to the epidermis, or vessels perpendicular to the epidermis.

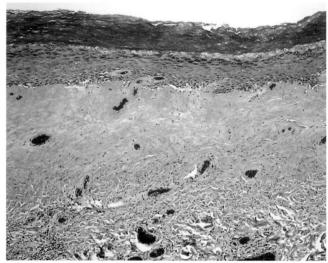

Fig 2. There is vacuolization of the basal layer of the epidermis. The collagen band is paucicellular.

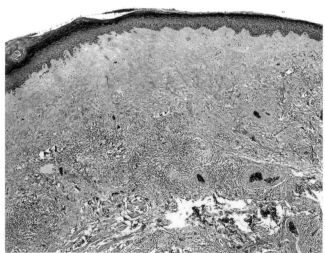

Fig 1. Preputial resection with balanitis xerotica obliterans. The epidermis is atrophic with hyperkeratosis. There is a homogeneous band of collagen in the dermis, just above a layer of chronic inflammatory infiltrates.

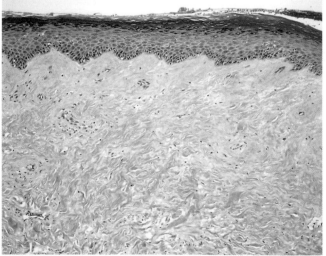

Fig 3. Homogeneous collagen deposition beneath the hyperkeratotic epidermis.

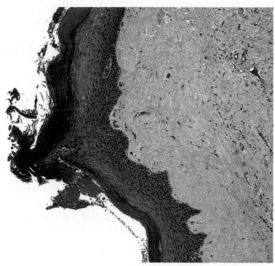

Fig 4. In an advanced case, lichen sclerosis shows epidermal hyperplasia alternating with atrophy. Note the pseudopapillary formation associated with hyperkeratosis.

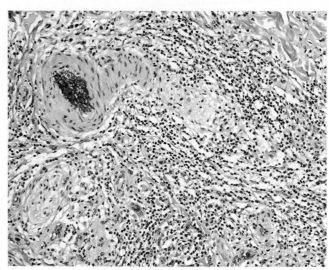

Fig 5. The inflammation is mostly lymphocytic and may be vaguely centered around vessels. In advanced cases, inflammation may be patchy or scant.

PSEUDOEPITHELIOMATOUS KERATOTIC MICACEOUS BALANITIS

Definition
- A rare form of balanitis characterized by hyperkeratotic micaceous growth on the glans penis

Clinical features
Epidemiology
- Rare with only a handful of cases reported
- Patients usually older than 50 years
- Unknown etiology but often associated with a previous adult circumcision, usually for acquired phimosis; or occasionally in uncircumcised men
- No association with HPV infection

Presentation
- Crusty, hyperkeratotic plaques on the glans penis
- Keratotic micaceous scales resembling psoriasis
- Cracking, fissuring, or ulceration possible
- Normal penile shaft, scrotum, and inguinal regions

Prognosis and treatment
- Tends to progress slowly and recur locally
- Considered as an intermediate lesion between benign squamous hyperplasia and SCC
- May be a precursor of verrucous or squamous carcinoma
- Conservative approach for treatment with long-term follow-up when there is no histologic evidence of malignancy
- Surgical excision when there is cytologic atypia
- Excision with wide margin when there is frank malignancy

Pathology
Gross pathology
- Raised micaceous scaling lesions cover the glans penis.

Histology
- Squamous epithelium with acanthosis, papillomatosis, hyperkeratosis, and pseudoepitheliomatous hyperplasia
- Mononuclear inflammatory infiltrates in the stroma
- No cytopathic changes of viral infection

Main differential diagnosis
- Verrucous carcinoma: prominent squamous cell proliferation with papillomatosis, acanthosis and hyperkeratosis; broad-based pushing invasion into the stroma
- Condyloma: prominent papillary growth with hyperkeratosis; HPV-related cellular changes

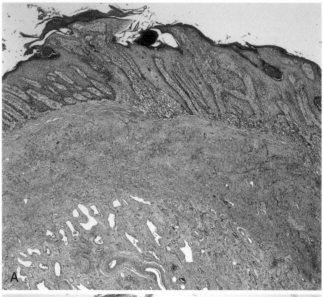

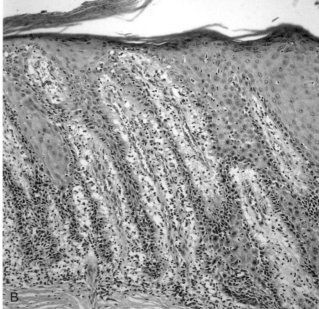

Fig 2. Pseudoepitheliomatous keratotic micaceous balanitis characterized by pseudoepitheliomatous hyperplasia with papillomatosis and hyperkeratosis. **A,** A dense inflammatory infiltrate is present at the interface between the lesion and stroma. **B,** Cytologic atypia and human papilloma virus–related changes are not present.

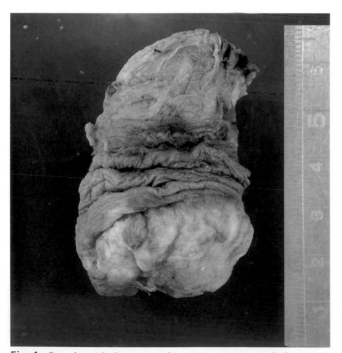

Fig 1. Pseudoepitheliomatous keratotic micaceous balanitis. A raised micaceous scaling lesion covers the glans penis.

Definition
- Localized fibrotic disorder of the penile tunica albuginea

Clinical features
Epidemiology
- Prevalence of approximately 5%; previously estimated at less than 1%
- Etiology unknown; likely multifactorial including chronic minor injury and genetic susceptibility

Presentation
- Penile pain, nodule or induration, penile curvature or shortening during erection, and sexual dysfunction

Prognosis and treatment
- Disease remains stable (40% to 50%) or worsens (40%); spontaneously resolves in only 12% of cases if untreated
- Observation; medical or other physical treatment for mild or early disease; surgery reserved for patients with persistent deformity compromising sexual function

Pathology
Histology
- Fibrous tissue between the corpora cavernosa and tunica albuginea
- Similar to fibromatosis of other sites, but usually more sclerotic and less cellular
- Calcification or ossification in advanced disease
- Perivascular lymphoid infiltrate present in early stage of disease, but rarely seen in surgical specimen

Main differential diagnosis
- Scar formation is more often accompanied by chronic inflammation and foreign body giant cell reaction and a less prominent fibrosis process.

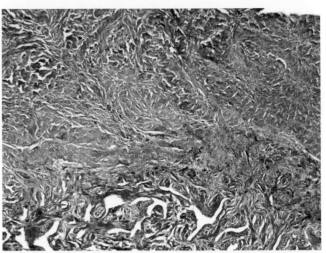

Fig 1. Prominent thickening and fibrosis of tunica albuginea surrounding corpora cavernosa *(bottom)* in an advanced case treated by surgery. The hypocellular fibrosis is composed predominantly of collagen bundles.

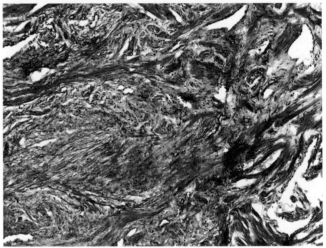

Fig 2. Fibrosis *(center)* extends between vasculatures of corpora cavernosa.

SQUAMOUS HYPERPLASIA OF THE PENIS

Definition
- Benign thickening of squamous epithelium without atypia

Clinical features
Epidemiology
- Most common epithelial change associated with keratinizing penile squamous cell carcinoma
- Usually found adjacent to in situ or invasive SCC (verrucous and low-grade papillary subtypes)

Presentation
- Flat or slightly raised, smooth pearly white plaque
- Equally affecting the glans, coronal sulcus, and foreskin

Prognosis and treatment
- Good outcome
- Excision

Pathology
Histology
- Thickened squamous epithelium with hyperkeratosis, acanthosis, and hypergranulosis
- Normal maturation of squamous epithelium
- Minimal to no parakeratosis
- No cytologic atypia and HPV-related changes
- Several patterns, including flat (most common), papillary, pseudoepitheliomatous, and verrucous

Main differential diagnosis
- Pseudohyperplastic carcinoma: although the neoplastic squamous nests have bland morphologic features, the base of the lesion is irregular and infiltrating.
- Verruciform xanthoma: squamous hyperplasia is present with neutrophilic and histiocytic infiltrate between the long rete ridges.
- Penile intraepithelial neoplasia exhibits cytologic atypia.
- Verruciform carcinomas, including warty, verrucous, and papillary carcinomas, all exhibit varying degree of cytologic atypia.

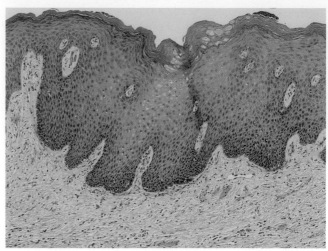

Fig 1. Penile squamous hyperplasia composed of thickened benign squamous epithelium without atypia. Mild hyperkeratosis is also present.

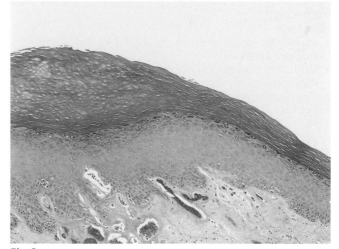

Fig 2. Penile squamous hyperplasia with prominent hyperkeratosis.

PENILE INTRAEPITHELIAL NEOPLASIA, INCLUDING BOWEN DISEASE, ERYTHROPLASIA OF QUEYRAT AND BOWENOID PAPULOSIS

Definition
• Precancerous squamous lesion of the penis

Clinical features
• Low- or intermediate-grade penile intraepithelial neoplasia (PeIN I, II) may be recognized as white patches (leukoplakia)
• Different terms were used for high-grade penile precancerous squamous lesions of different clinicopathologic features
• Bowen disease
  • Occurs on the penile shaft
  • Crusted, sharply demarcated scaly plaque
• Erythroplasia of Queyrat
  • Exclusively in uncircumcised men
  • Occurs on the glans, in the coronal sulcus, or on the inner surface of prepuce
  • Manifested as sharp, demarcated, bright-red, and shiny plaque
• Bowenoid papulosis
  • Usually in young, sexually active adults
  • Usually multiple, small, red papules on penile glans or shaft, foreskin, scrotum, inguinal skin also affected
  • Sometimes diagnosed clinically as a genital wart

Epidemiology
• Most cases are HPV related.
• Some cases are related to lichen sclerosis et atrophicus (non–HPV related).

Prognosis and treatment
• Surgery with adequate margin for high-grade PeIN
• Conservative therapy and follow-up for low-grade PeIN and Bowenoid papulosis; spontaneous regression reported in some cases
• Five percent to 10% of Bowen disease and 10% erythroplasia of Queyrat cases progress to invasive SCC

Pathology
• PeIN is classified based on the thickness of the epithelium occupied by atypical basaloid cells and the degree of cytologic atypia with various loss of polarity.
• The dysplastic squamous cells vary in size and shape with pleomorphic and hyperchromatic nuclei which have lost their polarity. Mitotic figures are usually seen.
• Current World Health Organization classification categorizes PeIN into three grades:
  • Low-grade PeIN (PeIN I): cytologic atypia limited to the lower third of the epithelium
  • Intermediate-grade PeIN (PeIN II): cytologic atypia limited to the lower two thirds of the epithelium
  • High-grade PeIN (PeIN III): cytologic atypia involving more than two thirds or the full thickness of the epithelium, which is equivalent to SCC in situ
• Bowen disease and erythroplasia of Queyrat are equivalent to PeIN III.
• Bowenoid papulosis has a more spotty distribution of atypical cells and greater maturation of keratinocytes than PeIN III.

Main differential diagnosis
• Inflammatory lesions: epithelial cells may have reactive atypia but frank dysplastic changes are absent.

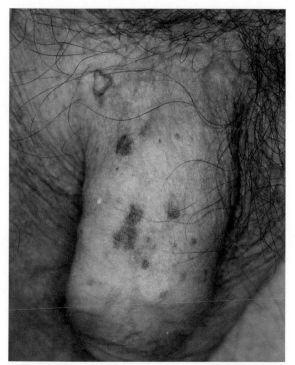

Fig 1. Bowenoid papulosis manifests as multiple, small, red-brown papules on the glans penis. (Courtesy Dr. Yasuhiko Tamada, Nagakute, Japan.)

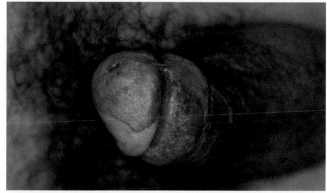

Fig 2. Erythroplasia of Queyrat manifests as a demarcated, bright-red, and shiny plaque on the glans penis. (Courtesy Dr. Takaya Fukumoto, Nara, Japan.)

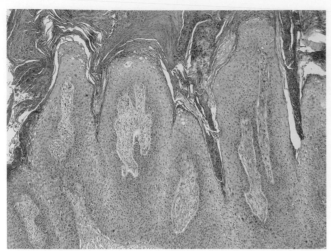

Fig 3. In Bowen disease, the atypical squamous cells involves the full thickness of the epithelium, which has wartlike features.

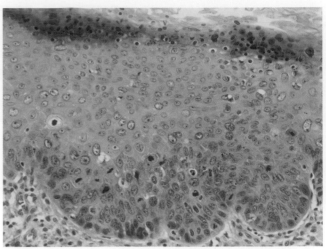

Fig 5. In Bowenoid papulosis, there is full-thickness atypia of the squamous cells with numerous mitosis. Note that maturation is preserved on the surface.

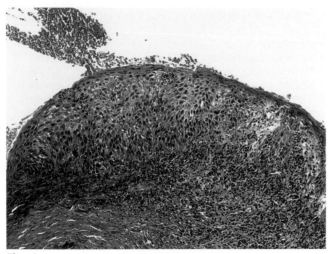

Fig 4. In erythroplasia of Queyrat, atypical squamous cells involves the entire epithelium without polarity. (Courtesy Dr. Akitaka Nonomura, Nara, Japan.)

SQUAMOUS CELL CARCINOMA OF THE PENIS, USUAL TYPE

Definition
- Invasive SCC with a varying degree of keratinization that cannot be classified as other histologic subtypes morphologically; also termed *typical, conventional*, or *SCC, not otherwise specified (NOS)*

Clinical features
Epidemiology
- Low incidence in the United States, but high in developing countries, especially South America
- Accounts for 0.4% to 0.6% of all malignancies in United States and Europe, but represents 20% to 30% of all cancers in men in Asia, Africa, and South America
- Mean age, 60 years
- Rare in circumcised men
- Minority of this subtype of penile cancer associated with HPV (approximately 25%)

Presentation
- Usually as papillary and exophytic lesion
- Flat and ulcerated lesions
- Invasion into corpora and urethra possible; important for management and prognosis
- Ulcerated inguinal metastasis in advanced cases

Prognosis and treatment
- Treatment varies according to the clinical stage and includes radiation and chemotherapy, surgery, or a combination of these modalities.
- The thickness, depth of invasion, degree of squamous differentiation and presence of vascular and perineural invasions are significant prognostic predictors. HPV infection does not seem to correlate with prognosis.

Pathology
Histology
- Tumors are usually well-differentiated or moderately differentiated SCC similar to other sites.
- Squamous cell carcinoma in situ (penile intraepithelial neoplasia) can be seen in the great majority of cases.
- Assessment of depth of invasion, perineural and vascular invasions, involvement of the corpora, glans, and multifocality should be addressed in all reports.

Immunopathology
- This variant is usually negative for HPV by in situ hybridization and p16 by immunostain.

Main differential diagnosis
- Basaloid variant of SCC is an aggressive tumor with strong association with HPV infection. Histologically, the tumor cells have a basaloid appearance with small uniform nuclei and numerous mitosis and apoptosis.
- Pseudoepitheliomatous hyperplasia is a reactive condition characterized by elongated rete ridges and absence of nuclear atypia.

- Urothelial carcinoma should always be included in the differential of penile carcinomas. Centering in the urethra, absence of keratinization, presence of urothelial carcinoma in situ, and tumor in the bladder may aid the differential diagnosis.

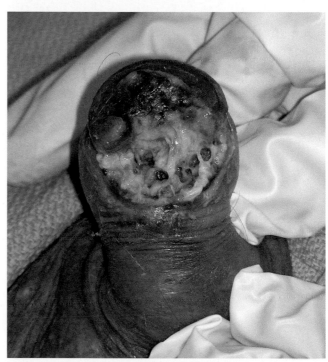

Fig 1. An ulcerated squamous cell carcinoma involves the glans penis.

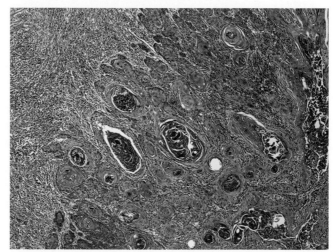

Fig 2. Squamous cell carcinoma, well-differentiated type, shows prominent keratinization and invades the subepithelial connective tissue.

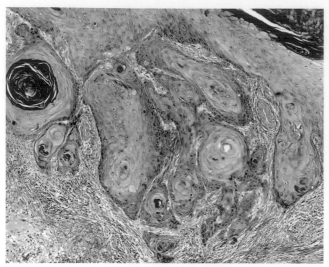

Fig 3. A superficially invasive well-differentiated SCC with extensive keratinization.

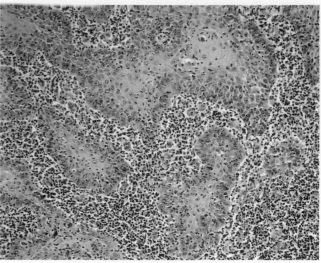

Fig 4. Extensive inflammatory reaction to invasive squamous cell carcinoma with numerous eosinophils.

BASALOID SQUAMOUS CELL CARCINOMA

Definition
- An aggressive variant of SCC with basaloid features

Clinical features
Epidemiology
- Accounts for 5% to 10% of penile SCC
- Most patients are 50 to 59 years old
- Associated with HPV (HPV16 most common)

Presentation
- Ulcerated and infiltrative mass involving the glans
- More than half of patients have inguinal lymph node metastasis

Prognosis and treatment
- Poor prognosis with high cancer-specific mortality rate
- Total penectomy with bilateral inguinal lymph node dissection
- Adjuvant therapy for patients with advanced disease

Pathology
Gross pathology
- Flat, ulcerated, firm, gray-white mass
- Cut surface shows deep infiltration into the underlying soft tissue

Histology
- Monotonous small to medium-sized tumor cells with scanty cytoplasm
- Ovoid nuclei with inconspicuous nucleoli
- Frequent central necrosis (comedonecrosis)
- Occasionally vague peripheral palisading
- Occasional retraction artifact
- Frequent mitoses and apoptotic cells, imparting a "starry sky" appearance
- Focally abrupt keratinization
- Adjacent basaloid carcinoma in situ

Molecular diagnostics
- Most cases positive for high-risk HPV

Main differential diagnosis
- Squamous cell carcinoma, usual type: large, more pleomorphic tumor cells with abundant dense eosinophilic cytoplasm; irregularly distributed keratinization
- Cutaneous basal cell carcinoma: typically involves the skin of the shaft; conspicuous peripheral palisading, lower nuclear grade; lacks comedonecrosis
- Urothelial carcinoma: mass centers around the urethra; invasive and in situ urothelial carcinoma almost always present
- Small cell carcinoma: nuclear molding and streaming; "salt and pepper" chromatin; positive for neuroendocrine markers

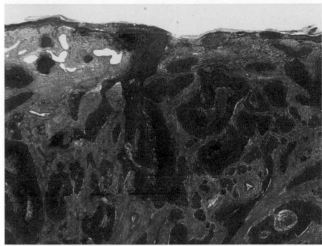

Fig 1. Basaloid carcinoma characterized by deeply infiltrative trabeculae or nests of dark tumor cells.

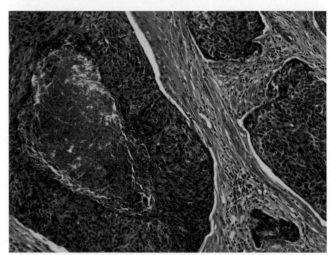

Fig 2. Thick trabeculae with central comedonecrosis and retraction artifact.

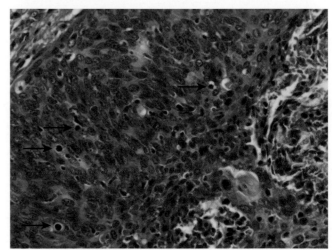

Fig 3. Monotonous tumor cells with eosinophilic cytoplasm and indistinct cell borders. The nuclei are ovoid without prominent nucleoli. Frequently apoptotic bodies are present *(arrows)*.

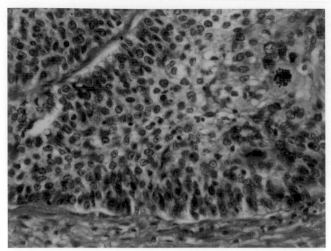

Fig 4. Occasionally the tumor cells have clear cytoplasm. Vague peripheral palisading is seen.

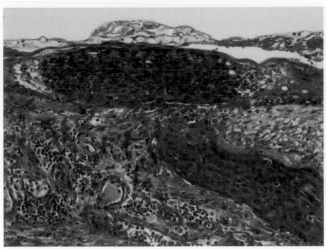

Fig 6. Basaloid carcinoma in situ involves the adjacent epithelium.

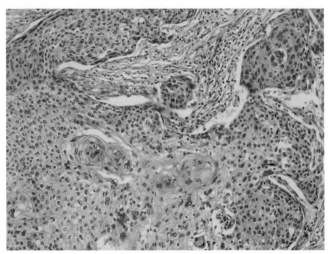

Fig 5. Focal abrupt keratinization.

PENILE WARTY (CONDYLOMATOUS) CARCINOMA

Definition
- A form of squamous carcinoma with verruciform growth pattern; strongly associated with high-risk human papillomavirus infection

Clinical features
Epidemiology
- Six percent of penile carcinomas and 20% to 30% verruciform tumors
- Most commonly involves the glans
- Age distribution similar to conventional squamous carcinoma

Presentation
- Slow-growing lesions; large, firm, and papillary

Prognosis and treatment
- Partial penectomy usually sufficient
- Excellent prognosis for pure tumor; 5-year survival nearly 100%
- Inguinal lymph node metastasis rarely reported; usually associated with deeply invasive lesion

Pathology
Gross pathology
- Exophytic, cauliflower-like, firm, white-gray mass
- May invade subepithelial connective tissue and corpus spongiosum, but cavernosa usually not involved

Histology
- Long, complex, and arborizing papillae with central fibrovascular cores and hyperparakeratosis
- Tumor cells with low- to intermediate-grade cytology and prominent koilocytic atypia
- Base of the tumor usually irregular and the tumor may infiltrate deeply

Molecular diagnostics
- HPV DNA testing demonstrates HPV, almost always high-risk group, in almost all cases.

Main differential diagnosis
- Verrucous carcinoma: papillae straight without obvious fibrovascular cores; tumor base regular, broad, and pushing; minimum cytologic atypia; no HPV-related changes
- Papillary squamous carcinoma: HPV-related changes absent
- Giant condyloma: no invasion, minimum to moderate cytologic atypia; associated with low-risk HPV

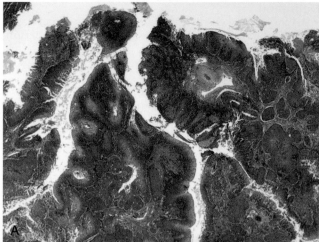
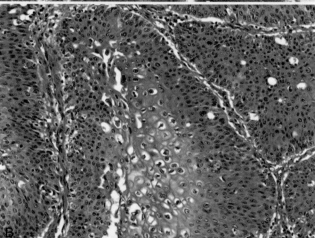
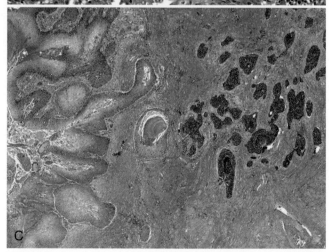

Fig 1. **A,** Low-power view demonstrates complex, undulating papillary structures with thin fibrovascular cores. **B,** The tumor cells have low- to intermediate-grade cytology and prominent koilocytic changes. **C,** The base of the tumor is irregular and invades deeply into the stroma.

SQUAMOUS CELL CARCINOMA, VERRUCOUS

Definition
- A subtype of well-differentiated SCC with broad papillary fronds and pushing base; no apparent association with HPV infection

Clinical features
Epidemiology
- Accounts for 3% to 8% of penile carcinomas
- Mean age, 70 to 80 years
- Precursors not established
- Not associated with HPV infection

Presentation
- Usually involves the glans or foreskin
- Exophytic cauliflower-like gray-white mass
- Slow growing

Prognosis and treatment
- Locally aggressive but biologically indolent
- No metastases reported with pure verrucous carcinoma
- Combined tumors with focal or significant verrucous features (mixed or hybrid verrucous carcinomas) have a metastatic rate of approximately 25%
- Complete local excision with clear margins or partial or total penectomy

Pathology
Histology
- Squamous papillomatous neoplasm is extremely well differentiated with hyperkeratosis and acanthosis.
- Tumors may extend into the underlying stroma with a broad-based pushing border.
- Papillae are straight and lined by well-differentiated neoplastic cells, with surface hyperkeratosis and interpapillary keratin.
- Koilocytosis is not present.
- Occasionally it invades beyond the lamina propria, superficial dartos, or corpus spongiosum.
- Adjacent epithelium may show verrucoid squamous hyperplasia and rarely differentiated penile intraepithelial neoplasia or lichen sclerosus.
- May be associated with urethral low- and high-grade squamous intraepithelial neoplasia, nonkeratinizing hyperplastic, or keratinizing squamous metaplasia.

Main differential diagnosis
- Pseudoepitheliomatous hyperplasia: benign squamous proliferative lesion is typically associated with chronic infections. It may be difficult to differentiate from verrucous carcinoma particularly on a small biopsy specimen. In pseudoepitheliomatous hyperplasia, there is a haphazard proliferation of squamous epithelial nests that lacks the straight papillae with abundant keratin.
- Condyloma acuminatum is a papillomatous lesion that can rarely mimic verrucous carcinoma. The presence of koilocytosis is unlike verrucous carcinoma.
- Low-grade SCC, not otherwise specified: a typical SCC with abundant keratinization that displays destructive invasion.
- Low-grade papillary SCC: a well-differentiated hyperkeratotic tumor with irregular complex papillary structures with or without fibrovascular cores. The base of the tumor is irregular and infiltrative.
- Warty (condylomatous) SCC: a hyperkeratotic papillomatous tumor that displays conspicuous koilocytotic atypia.

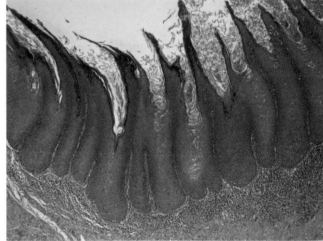

Fig 1. Squamous cell carcinoma, verrucous type with marked hyperkeratosis and papillomatosis. The base of the tumor exhibits broad-front pushing invasion.

Acknowledgment: Brett Delahunt, Wellington School of Medicine and Health Sciences, Wellington, New Zealand

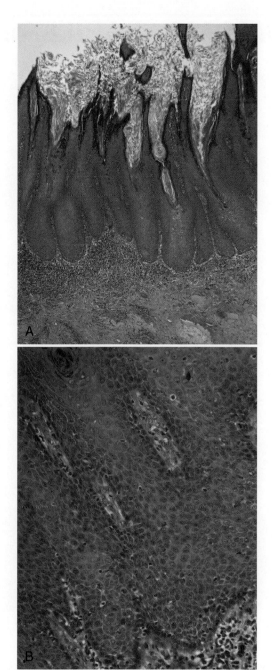

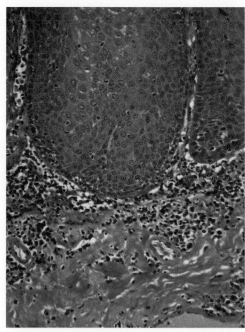

Fig 3. Squamous cell carcinoma, verrucous type with deep, broad-based pushing invasion.

Fig 2. Squamous cell carcinoma, verrucous type. **A,** Papillae are straight and have surface hyperkeratosis and interpapillary keratin. **B,** The tumor cells are well differentiated with minimal nuclear atypia and no koilocytic atypia.

SQUAMOUS CELL CARCINOMA, PAPILLARY

Definition
- A variant of SCC with verruciform growth pattern, not associated with HPV infection

Clinical features
Epidemiology
- Accounts for 5% to 15% of penile SCC
- Affecting patients in fifth and sixth decades of life
- Not associated with HPV

Presentation
- Slow-growing, bulky, cauliflower-like mass involving the glans

Prognosis and treatment
- Less aggressive than usual penile SCC
- Wide local excision or partial penectomy

Pathology
Gross pathology
- Large, cauliflower-like or papillary mass
- Tumor invades into the subepithelial tissue or corpus spongiosum; invasion into cavernosa uncommon

Histology
- Irregular, complex, exophytic papillary growth
- Well-to-moderately differentiated
- Prominent keratinization
- No koilocytic atypia
- Irregular and jagged tumor base with destructive stromal invasion

Main differential diagnosis
- Warty carcinoma: conspicuous HPV-related cellular changes
- Verrucous carcinoma: prominent papillomatosis with broad papillae without fibrovascular cores; minimal cytologic atypia; broadbase pushing invasion
- Giant condyloma: conspicuous HPV-related cellular changes; no frank malignant cytologic features, no invasion

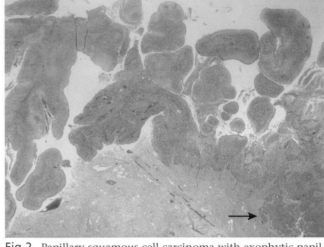

Fig 2. Papillary squamous cell carcinoma with exophytic papillary growth with focal stromal invasion *(arrow)*.

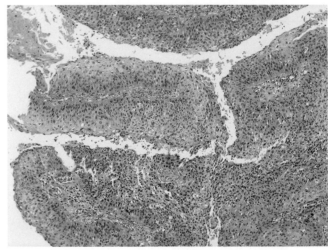

Fig 3. Tumor cells form long papillae with fibrovascular cords.

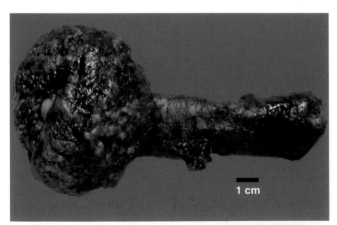

Fig 1. Cauliflower-like tumor involving the glans penis.

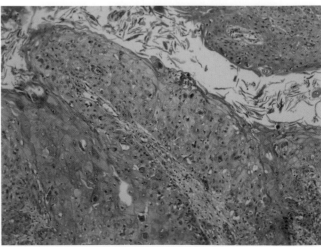

Fig 4. Prominent keratinization with flaky keratin between papillae.

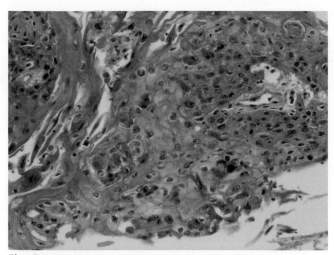

Fig 5. Well-differentiated to moderately differentiated squamous cells with keratin pearls. No HPV-related changes are seen.

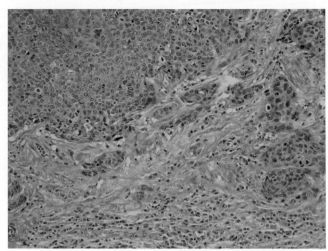

Fig 7. The tumor base shows irregular invasive nests.

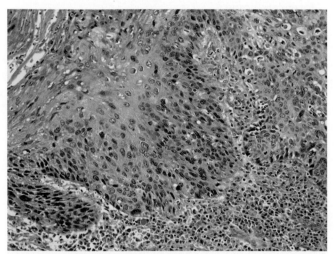

Fig 6. Intense inflammatory reaction at the jagged tumor base.

SQUAMOUS CELL CARCINOMA, PSEUDOHYPERPLASTIC NONVERRUCIFORM

Definition
- A well-differentiated SCC of the penis with an endophytic growth that preferentially involves the foreskin and usually arises in association with lichen sclerosus

Clinical features

Epidemiology
- Rare; only small series and case reports exist
- Affects old patients, between the sixth and eighth decades of life (mean age, 69 years)
- Represents a subgroup of the well-differentiated SCCs not related to HPV infection

Presentation
- Usually arise on the inner side of the foreskin
- Multicentricity common
- Flat or slightly elevated lesion with white and granular surface
- Restricted to the mucosa; involvement of the skin of the foreskin reportedly absent

Prognosis and therapy
- Prognosis is good.
- Resection is curative and can be performed minimally with circumcision or partial penectomy.
- Inguinal lymphadenectomy can be performed for larger lesions, but usually yields only negative nodes.

Pathology

Gross pathology
- Flat or slightly elevated lesion with white and granular surface
- Size ranges from a few millimeters to 3 to 4 cm

Histology
- Nests of highly differentiated squamous cancer cells proliferating downward to involve the lamina propria
- Superficial nests showing keratinization
- Stromal response present but not prominent; inflammation around invasive nests

- Squamous dysplasia and SCC in situ common in the surrounding mucosa
- Lichen sclerosus et atrophicus present in the vast majority of cases

Main differential diagnosis
- Verrucous carcinoma is a well-differentiated SCC, but with pushing borders instead of invasive nests; it also has an exophytic component.
- Pseudoepitheliomatous hyperplasia can mimic nonverruciform tumors especially in biopsy specimens. Careful examination and deeper sections always show invasion in the latter. Cytologic atypia is present, albeit minimal, in pseudohyperplastic nonverruciform carcinoma.

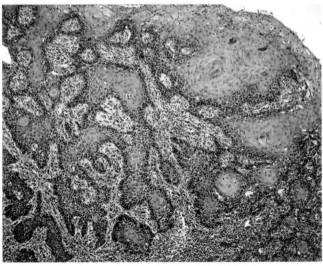

Fig 1. Pseudohyperplastic nonverruciform squamous cell carcinoma of the penis with hyperplastic surface epithelium with subjacent well-differentiated carcinoma. The tumor grows downward in nests with focal keratinization.

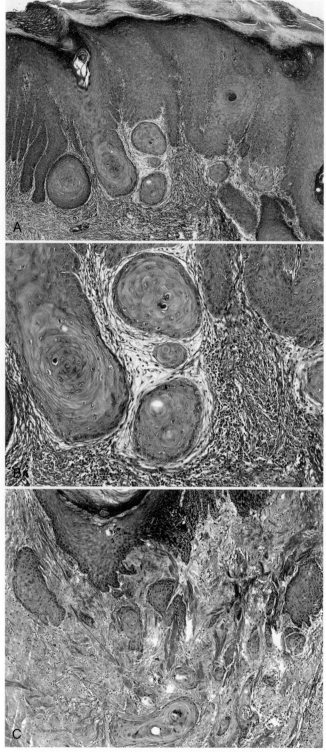

Fig 2. **A,** Pseudohyperplastic nonverruciform squamous cell carcinoma of the penis shows acanthotic and hyperkeratotic surface epithelium. **B,** The invasive component underneath shows only mild atypia. The stroma is slightly desmoplastic. **C,** In the edge of the infiltrating tumors, the overlying epithelium may show only mild hyperplasia. (Courtesy Mathieu Latour, University of Montreal, Montreal, Canada.)

SARCOMATIOD (SPINDLE CELL) SQUAMOUS CELL CARCINOMA OF THE PENIS

Definition
- Squamous cell carcinoma with a malignant spindle cell or sarcomatoid component

Clinical features
- Usually manifests as a white-gray, mixed exophytic and endophytic mass on the glans penis

Epidemiology
- Mean age, 60 years; wide age range of 37 to 80 years

Prognosis and treatment
- Surgery, chemotherapy, radiotherapy
- Clinical course usually aggressive with early lymph node metastasis and distant metastasis (e.g., lung, skin, bone, pleura)

Pathology
Gross pathology
- The tumor usually invades into the corpora spongiosum and cavernosa deeply.

Histology
- The tumor is composed of high-grade SCC and a spindle cell component.
- Spindle cell component shows various histologic features, including myxoid, pseudoangiomatous, malignant fibrous histiocytoma-like, and fibrosarcoma-like.
- Heterologous differentiation into bone, cartilage, and muscle may be found.

Immunohistochemical features
- High-molecular-weight cytokeratin and p63 may be positive in sarcomatoid area.

Main differential diagnosis
- Primary sarcomas of the penis are exceedingly rare. There is no history of penile carcinomas, and no histologic or immunohistochemical evidence of epithelial differentiation.
- In melanoma, epithelioid and spindle cells may be found, but melanin pigment may be present and positive melanocytic markers support the diagnosis.

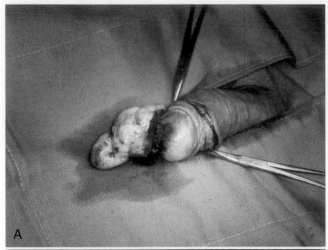
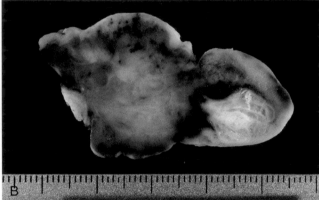

Fig 1. A sarcomatoid squamous cell carcinomas arising from the glans penis **(A)** and deeply invades into the corpora spongiosum and cavernosa **(B).** (Courtesy Dr. Shojiro Morinaga, Tokyo, Japan.)

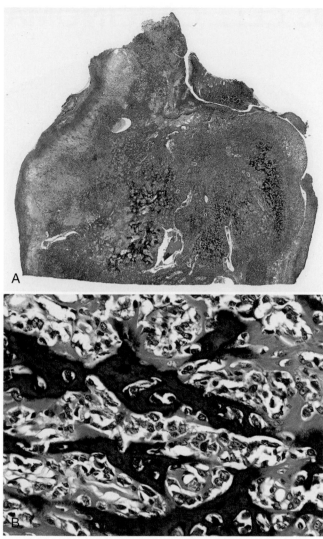

Fig 2. **A,** The exophytic mass contains osteoid component in the center. **B,** Osteosarcoma component is identified at high magnification.

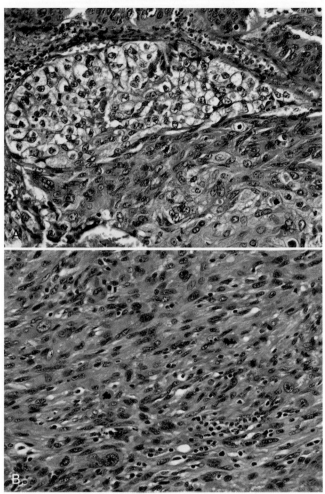

Fig 3. High-grade squamous cell carcinoma component **(A)** and spindle cell component **(B)** in a sarcomatoid squamous cell carcinoma.

Definition
- A form of penile SCC with both squamous and adeno-carcinomatous components, probably arising from the embryologically misplaced glands or metaplastic mucinous glands

Pathology
Histology
- The squamous component predominates over the glandular component
- Squamous component: warty or usual types of squamous carcinoma
- Glandular component: definitive gland formation or mucin producing
- Can invade deeply into muscularis propria and show vascular invasion

Immunohistochemistry
- Glandular component positive for carcinoembryonic antigen (CEA)

Main differential diagnosis
- Acantholytic squamous carcinoma with pseudoglandular formation: no true glandular formation; CEA and mucin negative
- Squamous carcinoma with secondary involvement of periurethral glands: glandular component morphologically benign

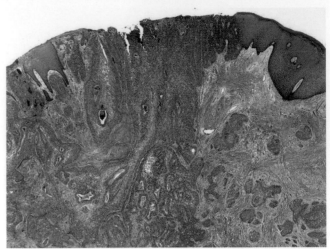

Fig 1. Low-power view of an invasive adenosquamous carcinoma of the penis with glandular differentiation *(center bottom)*.

MIXED CARCINOMAS OF THE PENIS

Definition
• Carcinoma containing more than one histologic subtypes, most commonly hybrid squamous-verrucous carcinoma

Clinical features
Epidemiology
• May be present in up to 25% of penile verrucous carcinoma

Presentation
• A large fungating warty lesion on the penile, commonly on the coronal sulcus

Prognosis and treatment
• Frequently recur but rarely metastasize
• Treated by local resection, partial or total penectomy

Pathology
Histology
• The most common finding is hybrid squamous-verrucous carcinoma, composed of verrucous carcinoma mixed with microfoci of conventional invasive SCC.
• Other combinations are extremely rare, including SCC-adenocarcinoma (or mucoepidermoid carcinoma), adenocarcinoma-basaloid carcinoma (adeno-basaloid carcinoma), warty-basaloid carcinoma, and squamous-neuroendocrine carcinoma.

Main differential diagnosis
• Condyloma acuminatum: shows HPV-related cellular changes; positive for HPV on in situ hybridization test

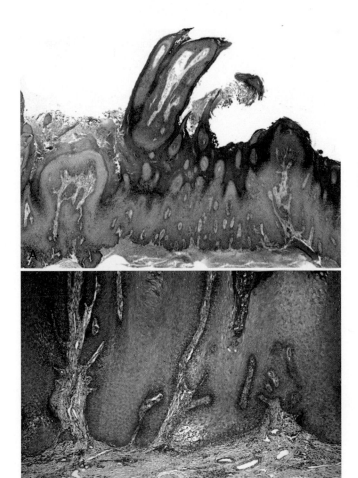

Fig 1. Verrucous carcinoma component in mixed carcinomas shows acanthosis and hyperkeratosis (A) and minimal nuclear atypia and a broad-based pushing growth pattern in the subepithelial tissue (B).

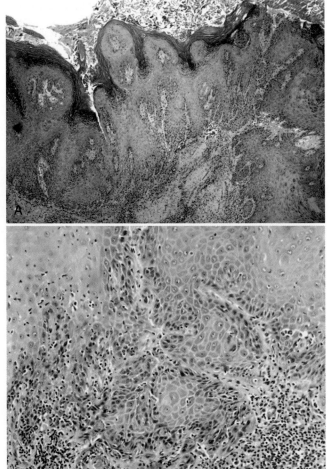

Fig 2. A conventional squamous cell carcinoma component is present at the base of the mixed carcinomas (A) and shows marked nuclear atypia and invades into the subepithelial tissue (B).

Definition
- A rare indolent carcinoma of the penis identical to its cutaneous counterpart

Clinical features
Epidemiology
- Rare; fewer than 50 cases reported even when scrotal tumors included
- Age range, 37 to 87 years (usually greater than 40 years)
- Mostly affects white males
- Etiology includes ultraviolet light, prior trauma, dermatitis, prolonged irritation from truss
- Other risk factors: ionizing radiation, arsenic ingestion, immunosuppression, and inherited syndromes such as nevoid basal cell carcinoma syndrome and xeroderma pigmentosum
- No association with HPV infection

Presentation
- Slowly growing, small, irregular, ulcerated, and hyper-pigmented mass
- Usually localized on the shaft (50% of the cases), rarely on glans (30%), prepuce (14%), and inner surface of foreskin
- Unifocal or multicentric
- Size 1 to 2 cm in diameter

Prognosis and treatment
- Most tumors are superficial lesions with excellent prognosis.
- Metastasis from the primary penile site is extremely rare (scrotal tumors may have higher metastatic potential).
- Wide local surgical excision is the treatment of choice.

Pathology
Gross pathology
- Same as its skin counterpart

Histology
- Same morphology as its skin counterpart
- Bulbous fingerlike projections from the epidermis
- Nests of uniform basaloid cells with peripheral palisading; no intercellular bridges
- Little variation in nuclear size, shape, and intensity of staining; no abnormal mitoses
- Proliferation of young fibroblasts or myxoid stroma adjacent to the tumor; retraction artifact in the stroma around the tumor islands, resulting in cleftlike spaces

Main differential diagnosis
- Basaloid SCC: focal abrupt keratinization; frequent central comedonecrosis

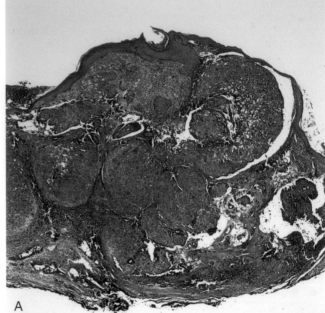

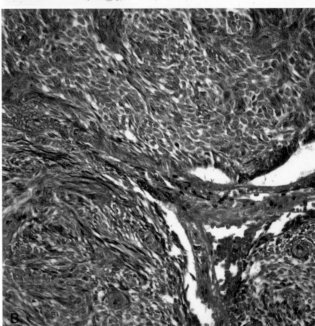

Fig 1. **A,** Basal cell carcinoma in the penile skin composed of nodular proliferation of basaloid cells. The basaloid cells are uniform and show peripheral palisading. The stroma is retracted from the tumor nests. **B,** Mitotic figures are frequent.

EXTRAMAMMARY PAGET DISEASE OF PENIS AND SCROTUM

Definition
- Intraepidermal adenocarcinoma involving the external genitalia

Clinical features
Epidemiology
- Most patients are in sixth to eighth decades of life
- Most cases arise de novo; rarely in association with an underlying malignancy, including colorectal, urogenital, or cutaneous adnexal carcinomas

Presentation
- Red, thick, moist eczema or dermatitis-like plaque with crusting, oozing, or erosion

Prognosis and treatment
- Wide excision with adequate surgical margins
- Good prognosis if completely excised
- Worse prognosis in patients with dermal invasion or Paget disease secondary to underlying carcinoma

Pathology
Histology
- Intraepidermal proliferation of large round atypical cells (Paget cell)
- Paget cells with abundant pale vacuolated cytoplasm, vesicular nuclei with prominent nucleoli
- May extend to the dermal adnexa
- Dermal invasion possible
- Epidermis possibly atrophic, hyperplastic, or ulcerated

Immunohistochemistry
- Intracytoplasmic mucin can be demonstrated by mucicarmine or Alcian blue stain (pH 2.5)
- Positive for CEA, low-molecular-weight cytokeratin, CK7, EMA
- Negative for high-molecular-weight cytokeratin, PSA, S100 protein, HMB45

Main differential diagnosis
- Melanoma: positive for S100 and melanocytic markers, but negative for epithelial markers and CEA
- Pagetoid spreading of urothelial carcinoma: associated with a high-grade urothelial carcinoma in the urethra; positive for high-molecular-weight cytokeratin/p63
- Bowen disease with pagetoid growth pattern: intracytoplasmic mucin not present; CEA negative

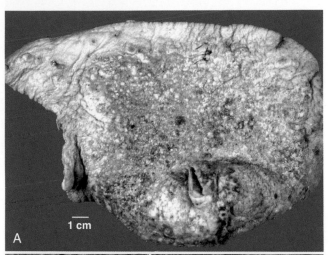
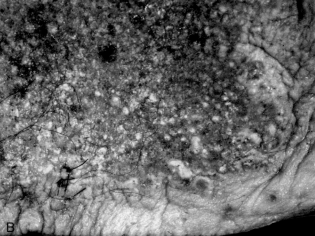

Fig 1. **A,** Paget disease manifests as a dark-colored eczema-like plaque lesion involving the scrotal skin. **B,** A close-up view shows erosion and scaling on the surface.

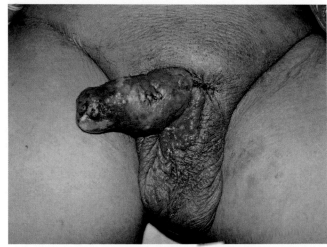

Fig 2. A red, moist, and erosive Paget disease extensively involves the penile shaft and base.

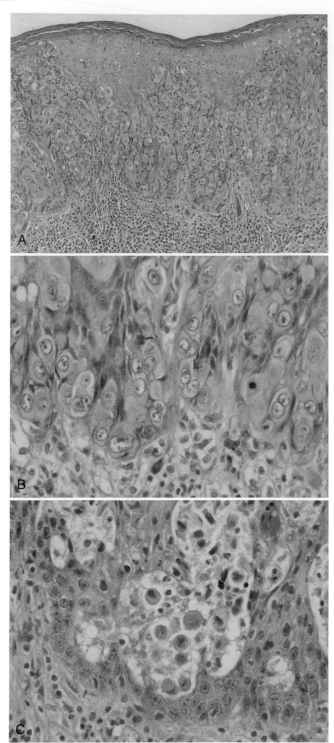

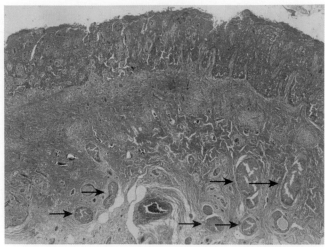

Fig 4. Extensive Paget disease involving whole thickness of epidermis and skin adnexae *(arrows)*.

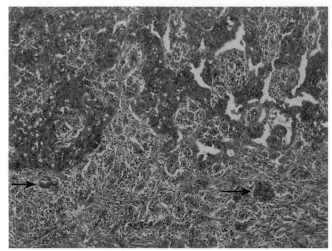

Fig 5. Focal stromal invasion in Paget disease *(arrows)*.

Fig 3. **A,** Aggregates of Paget cells involving the lower half of the epidermis. **B,** High magnification of Paget cells shows abundant pale cytoplasm, large nuclei, and prominent nucleoli. Mitotic figures can be found. **C,** Discrete Paget cells with signet ring or plasmacytoid features.

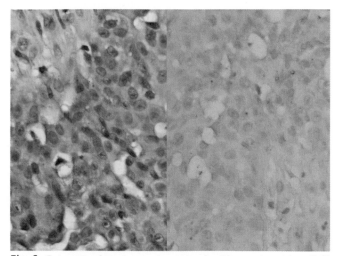

Fig 6. Intracytoplasmic mucin stained with mucicarmine *(left)* and Alcian blue *(right)*.

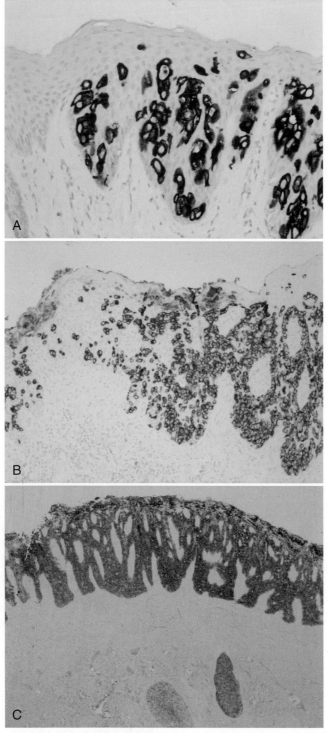

Fig 7. Paget cells are immunoreactive for low-molecular-weight cytokeratin (Cam5.2) **(A),** CK7 **(B),** and carcinoembryonic antigen (CEA) **(C).**

MERKEL CELL CARCINOMA OF THE GENITOURINARY TRACT

Definition
- Aggressive neoplasm of neuroendocrine differentiation, identical to its cutaneous counterpart

Clinical features
Epidemiology
- Primary Merkel cell carcinoma of the genitourinary tract extremely rare, with single case reports in vulva, vagina, penis, and scrotum
- Patient age between third and eighth decades of life

Presentation
- Nodule or rapidly enlarged mass at the affected site
- Hematuria if penile urethra is involved
- Sometimes with regional lymphadenopathy

Prognosis and treatment
- Disease is aggressive with a dire prognosis.
- The patient should be followed closely and managed aggressively.

Pathology
Gross pathology
- Tumor size ranging from 1 to 8 cm
- Well circumscribed but unencapsulated
- Tan and homogenous with focal areas of hemorrhage
- Overlying mucosa may be focally ulcerated

Histology
- Tumor cells are arranged in nests.
- Tumor cells have a scant amount of cytoplasm.
- Nuclei are approximately twofold to threefold the size of a mature lymphocyte with a dispersed chromatin pattern and inconspicuous nucleoli; the nuclei may show molding.
- Mitotic figures and prominent apoptosis are usually identified.
- The tumor may show epidermotropism and prominent angiolymphatic invasion.
- The overlying mucosa or skin may show dysplasia.

Immunohistochemistry
- Positive for keratins such as CK20, AE1, and CAM5.2; perinuclear dot positivity for CK20 and CAM5.2 is characteristic
- Positive for neuroendocrine markers including synaptophysin and chromogranin

Molecular diagnostics
- Merkel cell polyoma virus, a novel polyoma virus, may contribute to the pathogenesis of Merkel cell carcinoma.
- Detection of Merkel cell polyoma viral DNA using PCR-based technology seems to be a specific test for Merkel cell carcinoma.

Main differential diagnosis
- Prostate or urothelial carcinoma with neuroendocrine differentiation: history of prostate or urothelial carcinoma is present. Careful examination reveals prostate or urothelial carcinoma components.
- Metastatic Merkel cell carcinoma from a cutaneous site or metastatic small cell carcinoma from other body sites: history of cutaneous Merkel cell carcinoma should be vigorously sought and the possibility of a metastatic Merkel cell carcinoma should be ruled out in all patients with a diagnosis of Merkel cell carcinoma involving the genitourinary tract.

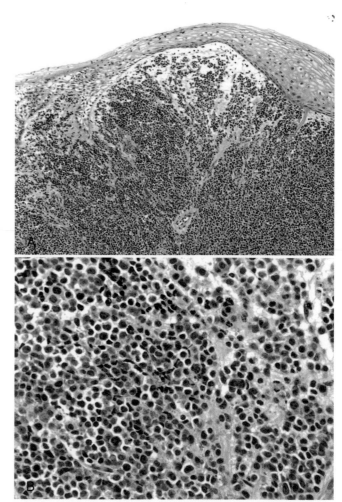

Fig 1. A, Tumor composed of small cells arranged in nests and sheets with overlying squamous epithelium. **B,** The tumor cells show scant cytoplasm, fine chromatin with inconspicuous nucleoli, and molding.

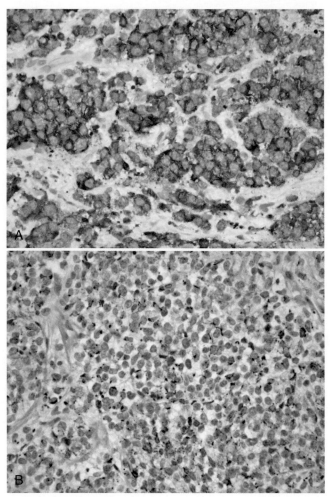

Fig 2. Immunohistochemical profile of Merkel cell carcinoma. The tumor cells are strongly positive for synaptophysin **(A)** and show dotlike cytoplasmic positivity for CAM5.2 **(B).**

Definition
- Granulomatous tissue reaction typically following injection of exogenous lipid-rich substance in male genitalia (penis, scrotum, testis, perineum, or spermatic cord)

Clinical features
Epidemiology
- Typically seen in younger males
- More commonly reported in Japan

Presentation
- Typically a painless, or occasionally painful, mass is present in the genital region.
- Most patients will admit to self-administered injections or topical applications of lipid-rich foreign substance (e.g., silicone, mineral oil, paraffin) in the genital region.
- Presentation can occur following trauma or cold weather in the scrotum.
- Occasionally there is no history of injection trauma (referred to as *primary sclerosing lipogranuloma*).

Prognosis and treatment
- Some cases will spontaneously resolve, whereas others may recur and require surgical resection.

Pathology
Histology
- Cystic-appearing or "Swiss cheese" disruption of subcutaneous adipose tissue
- Widespread, nonnecrotizing granulomatous inflammation, predominantly composed of epithelioid histiocytes and foreign body–type giant cells containing abundant lipid vacuoles
- Extensive fibrosis possibly present depending on the duration of the lesion

Immunopathology
- Histiocytes positive for CD68

Main differential diagnosis
- Infectious granulomatous inflammation: the presence of necrosis in infectious granulomas is helpful. Typically infectious granulomas do not show prominent vacuolization of histiocytes.
- Adenomatoid tumor: low-power appearance may be similar; however, adenomatoid tumors are most often in epididymis while sclerosing lipogranuloma is typically subcutaneous. At higher power, cells lining spaces in sclerosing lipogranuloma appear as foamy histiocytes.

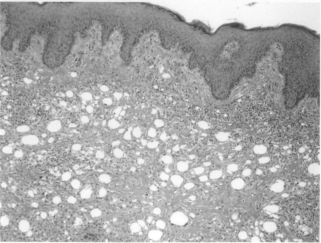

Fig 1. "Swiss cheese" appearance of subcutaneous tissues in sclerosing lipogranuloma.

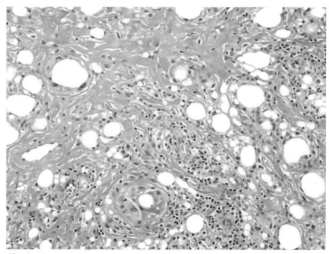

Fig 2. Aggregates of vacuolated histiocytes surround clear spaces where foreign lipid material was once present.

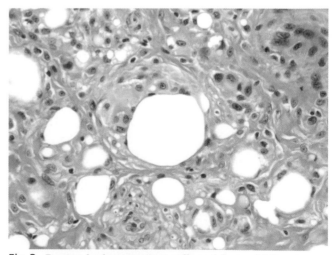

Fig 3. Foreign body–type giant cells and foamy histiocytes are evident at higher power.

Definition
- Calcification of dermal connective tissue of the scrotal skin

Clinical features
Epidemiology
- Usually occurs in young men, with children and older men reportedly also being affected
- Occurs in two settings
  - Calcification of preexisting epidermal or pilar cysts
  - Idiopathic or undetermined etiology (two thirds of cases)

Presentation
- Patients have multiple, firm to hard nodules that vary in size from a few millimeters to 3 cm in the scrotal skin.
- Ulceration may be seen over the nodules with extrusion of "cheesy" material.
- A single nodule may be observed.

Prognosis and treatment
- Treatment may not be required for asymptomatic lesions.
- Surgery is needed for infected, recurrent, or extensive lesions.

Pathology
Histology
- Calcified nodules within the scrotal dermis, seen as hematoxyphilic hardened material
- Foreign body giant cell reaction may be seen

Immunopathology and immunohistochemistry
- Positive reactivity for CEA, suggesting eccrine ducts as an origin for the calcinosis

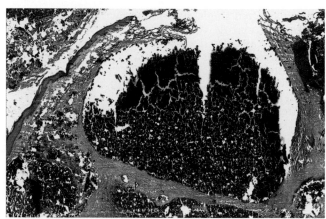

Fig 2. The hematoxyphilic calcified material is surrounded by fibrous stroma.

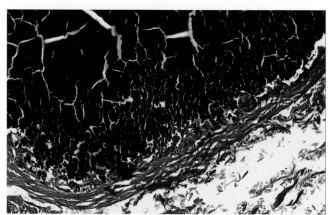

Fig 3. Foreign body multinucleated giant cells and histiocytes form the reaction around the calcified material.

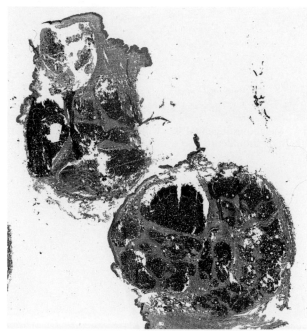

Fig 1. Low-power-magnification of an idiopathic scrotal calcinosis showing a nodular lesion composed of fractured clumps of calcification in the dermis of scrotal skin.

GENITAL MELANOSIS AND LENTIGINOSIS

Definition
- Benign hyperpigmented lesions in the external genitalia area

Clinical features
Epidemiology
- Incidence, 1420 in 10,000 men
- Mean age, 25 years (range, 17 to 66 years)

Presentation
- Genital melanosis
  - Large, often single, flat, dark brown to black pigmented macule
  - May be associated with Laugier-Hunziker syndrome
- Genital lentiginosis
  - Scattered 0.2 to 2 cm, oval to irregular lesions with uniform or variegated dark brown to black pigmentation
  - Areas of depigmentation also present
  - Associations include Cowden's disease and Bannayan-Riley-Ruvalcaba syndrome

Prognosis and treatment
- There is an association with melanoma.
- Treatment is excision.

Pathology
Gross pathology
- Melanosis: irregular darkly pigmented patch
- Lentiginosis: asymmetric, well-demarcated patch of variegated pigmentation with irregular, borders

Histology
- Melanosis: hyperpigmentation of basal epithelium without melanocytic hyperplasia, otherwise normal epithelium
- Lentiginosis: elongated rete ridges with hyperpigmented basal layer, melanocytic hyperplasia, epithelial hyperplasia, and stromal melanophages; no atypia

Main differential diagnosis
- Malignant melanoma and atypical melanocytic hyperplasia: melanocytes exhibit atypical features including pleomorphic large nuclei, prominent nucleoli, and increased mitoses. In contrast, melanocytes in melanosis and lentiginosis do not have cytologic atypia.
- Congenital melanocytic nevus: melanocytic proliferation occurs and often involves reticular dermis, subcutis, skin adnexa, arrector pili muscles, and nerves with single cell permeation of collagen.

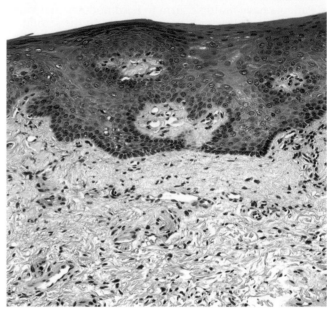

Fig 1. Melanosis of genital skin with hyperpigmentation of basal epithelium, shouldering of rete ridges, and stromal melanophages.

PRIMARY MELANOMA OF THE GENITOURINARY SYSTEM

Definition
- Primary melanoma originating from the genitourinary system

Clinical features
Epidemiology
- Rare
- Most commonly involving urethra, penis, scrotum; rarely reported in prostate, bladder, and ureter
- Mean age, 64 years (range, 50 to 77 years)
- Rare in patients of African ancestry
- Urethral melanoma more common in female patients; no racial difference
- Risk factors: preexisting nevi, exposure to ultraviolet radiation, history of melanoma

Presentation
- Dysuria or hematuria in urethral melanoma
- Papule or nodule that is brown, blue, or red with irregular edges or ulcerated plague on external genitalia

Prognosis and treatment
- Poor prognosis
- Long-term survival in only one third of patients
- Better prognosis for scrotal melanoma

Pathology
Histology
- Similar to melanomas of the skin and other body sites

Immunohistochemistry and special studies
- Positive for S-100, melanocytic markers (e.g., HMB45, Melan-A, tyrosinase, microophthalmia transcriptional factor)
- Masson-Fontana and Prussian blue stains to distinguish melanin pigment from hemosiderin
- Negative for cytokeratins, EMA, and p63
- Ultrastructural studies to document premelanosomes and melanosomes

Molecular diagnostics
- Fifty percent to 60% of advanced-stage cutaneous melanoma harbor *BRAF* mutations; however, it is not known whether the genitourinary melanomas harbor such mutations.

Main differential diagnosis
- Metastatic melanoma should always be ruled out by diligently searching for a history of melanoma of other body sites before a diagnosis of primary genitourinary melanoma is made.
- Bowen disease is characterized by dysplastic and dyskeratotic squamous cells; it is positive for epithelial markers and negative for S-100 and melanocytic markers.
- Extramammary Paget disease is characterized by intraepidermal proliferation of large round atypical cells mimicking melanoma; however, these cells are positive for epithelial markers, CEA, and mucin and negative for S-100 and melanocytic markers.
- Pagetoid spreading of urothelial carcinoma is associated with a high-grade urothelial carcinoma in the urethra; it is positive for high-molecular-weight cytokeratin/p63.

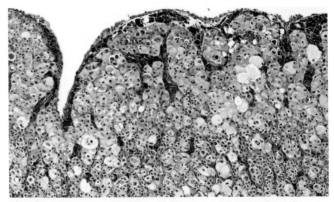

Fig 2. A primary bladder melanoma showing heavily pigmented "balloon cell" melanoma. Note the attenuated overlying urothelium.

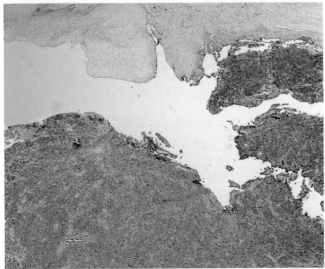

Fig 1. A polypoid urethral melanoma stains positive for S-100 protein.

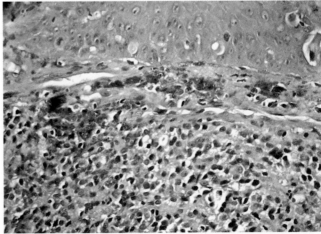

Fig 3. Penile melanoma containing sheets of neoplastic melanocytes. Some neoplastic cells contain melanin pigment. Atypical melanocytes are present in the overlying epidermis.

STAGING FOR PENILE SQUAMOUS CELL CARCINOMA

Definition
- Staging for SCC arising on the shaft and glans penis

Comments
- T1 is subdivided into T1a and T1b based on the presence or absence of lymphovascular invasion or poorly differentiated cancers.
  - Poorly differentiated cancers include poorly differentiated usual SCC, basaloid carcinoma, sarcomatoid carcinoma, and undifferentiated carcinoma.
- Prostatic invasion is considered T4.
- Metastasis to lymph nodes outside of the true pelvis is M1.
- The following stages are from the American Joint Committee on Cancer Staging Manual, seventh edition:
  - Primary tumor (T)
    - TX: primary tumor cannot be assessed
    - T0: no evidence of primary tumor
    - Tis: carcinoma in situ
    - Ta: noninvasive verrucous carcinoma (broad pushing penetration or invasion is permitted; destructive invasion is against this diagnosis)
    - T1a: tumor invades subepithelial connective tissue without lymph vascular invasion and is not poorly differentiated (i.e., grade 3 to 4)
    - T1b: tumor invades subepithelial connective tissue with lymph vascular invasion or is poorly differentiated
    - T2: tumor invades corpus spongiosum or cavernosum
    - T3: tumor invades urethra
    - T4: tumor invades other adjacent structures
  - Regional lymph nodes (N); pathologic stage definition (based on biopsy or surgical excision)
    - pNX: regional lymph nodes cannot be assessed
    - pN0: no regional lymph node metastasis
    - pN1: metastasis in a single inguinal lymph node
    - pN2: metastasis in multiple or bilateral inguinal lymph nodes
    - pN3: extranodal extension of lymph node metastasis or pelvic lymph nodes unilateral or bilateral
  - Distant metastasis (M)
    - M0: no distant metastasis
    - M1: distant metastasis (including lymph node metastasis outside of the true pelvis)

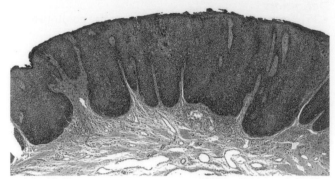

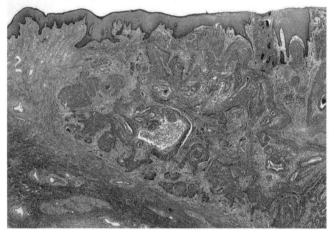

Fig 1. Squamous cell carcinoma in situ of penile shaft, staged as pTis.

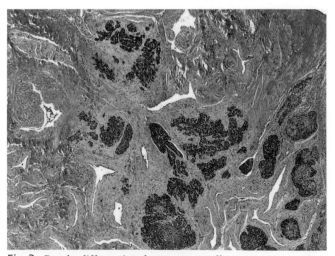

Fig 2. Poorly differentiated squamous cell carcinoma invading the subepithelial connective tissue, staged as pT1b.

Fig 3. Poorly differentiated squamous cell carcinoma invading the erectile tissue of corpora cavernosum, staged as pT2.

STAGING FOR URETHRAL CARCINOMA

Definition
- Staging system for penile carcinomas originated in the distal (penile) urethra

Comments
- Urethral carcinomas are staged using a different TNM system than carcinomas that arise on the penile shaft skin or on the glans penis.
- Most malignant tumors of the urethra are SCCs, followed by urothelial carcinomas and adenocarcinomas. Clear cell adenocarcinomas are rare but more common in female patients.
- In the prostatic urethra, carcinoma of the urethral lining with invasion into subepithelial connective tissue is staged as pT1; invasion arising from the prostatic ducts is designated as at least pT2.
- Tissue sampling and submission
- In transurethral specimens, submit one section per centimeter of tumor diameter (up to 10 cassettes). If the tumor is noninvasive by the initial sampling, then additional submission of tissue (including possibly submitting all tissue) is necessary.
- In urethrectomy specimens, submit one section per centimeter of tumor, including the macroscopically deepest penetration.
- Submit sections to demonstrate the relation between tumor and surrounding anatomic structures.
- 2010 American Joint Committee on Cancer TNM staging for urethral carcinoma
  - Tumor (pT stage)
    - pTX: primary tumor cannot be assessed
    - pTa: noninvasive carcinoma
    - pTis: carcinoma in situ
    - pT1: tumor invades subepithelial connective tissue
    - pT2: tumor invades corpus spongiosum, prostate, periurethral muscle
    - pT3: tumor invades corpus cavernosum, beyond prostatic capsule, anterior vaginal wall, bladder neck
    - pT4: tumor invades other adjacent organs

- Regional lymph node metastasis (pN stage)
  - pNX: regional lymph nodes cannot be assessed
  - pN0: no regional lymph node metastasis
  - pN1: metastasis in a single lymph node 2 cm or less in greatest dimension
  - pN2: metastasis in a single node more than 2 cm in greatest dimension, or in multiple nodes
- Distant metastasis (pM stage)
  - pM0: no distant metastasis
  - pM1: distant metastasis

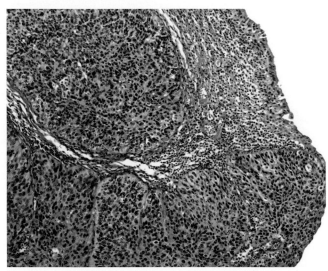

Fig 2. Invasion into the connective tissue beneath the urethral urothelium *(upper right field)* is staged as pT1.

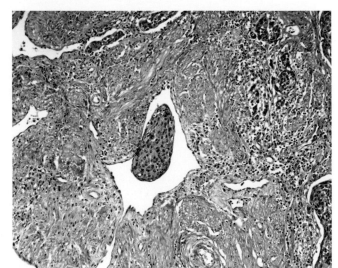

Fig 3. Invasion of the erectile tissue of the corpus spongiosum, either the vascular channels *(center and upper left fields)* or the stroma *(upper right field)* is staged as pT2.

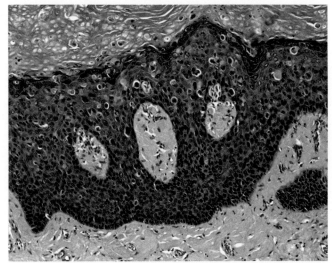

Fig 1. Carcinoma in situ of the penis (penile intraepithelial neoplasia, basaloid type). These lesions are staged as pTis.

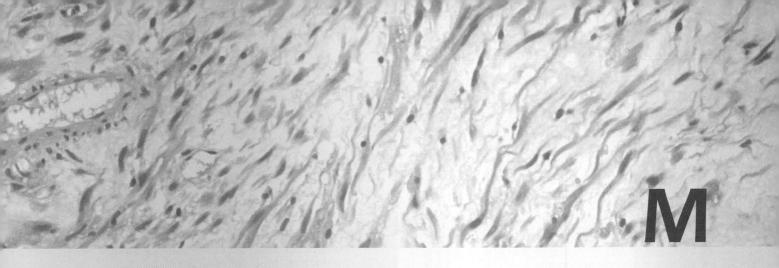

SOFT TISSUE TUMORS AND LYMPHOMAS

INFLAMMATORY MYOFIBROBLASTIC TUMOR OF THE BLADDER

Definition
- Myofibroblastic spindle cell neoplasm of uncertain malignant potential

Clinical features
Epidemiology
- Typically occurs in young adults (9 to 42 years old)
- Slight female preponderance
- History of recent prior instrumentation in a subset of cases

Presentation
- Usually with gross hematuria; also bladder outlet obstruction and dysuria
- Constitutional symptoms such as fever and weight loss reported rarely

Prognosis and treatment
- Rare recurrence has been reported after transurethral resection or partial cystectomy.
- Aggressive therapy (radical cystectomy, radiation, or chemotherapy) is unwarranted given the indolent and often benign clinical course for the majority of cases.
- Routine surveillance and close clinical follow-up are required.

Pathology
Gross pathology
- Typically pedunculated, nodular mass ranging in size from 2 to 5 cm
- May occasionally be sessile and extend into the underlying tissue

Histology
- The proliferation of spindle cells resembling tissue-culture fibroblasts is arranged haphazardly or in fascicles in a loose edematous or vascular myxoid stroma with little to moderate collagen deposition.
- Spindle cells may show focal pleomorphism; atypia is minimal.
- Single, prominent nucleoli may be present.
- Mitotic figures are often conspicuous, but they are not atypical.
- Background usually contains a sparse inflammatory infiltrate consisting of lymphocytes and plasma cells; eosinophils may also be numerous.
- Muscularis propria and perivesical involvement can occur.

Immunopathology (including immunohistochemistry)
- Anaplastic lymphoma kinase (ALK) protein is positive in greater than 80% of cases of inflammatory myofibroblastic tumor of the bladder; ALK rearrangements can be identified in more than half of cases, generally in all cases that are also ALK immunoreactive.
- Cytokeratins show a variable staining pattern.
- Smooth muscle actin is often positive.
- Desmin is typically negative.

Main differential diagnosis
- Carcinosarcoma (sarcomatoid carcinoma): history of urothelial carcinoma or concomitant carcinomatous component; frank cytologic atypia
- Leiomyosarcoma: more uniform in cellularity and exhibits more cytologic atypia; stromal vascularity and inflammation less common

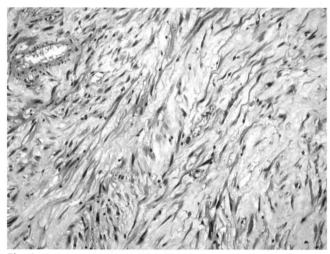

Fig 1. Inflammatory myofibroblastic tumor. The spindle cells are separated by conspicuous myxoid matrix.

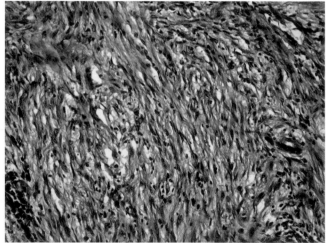

Fig 2. Inflammatory myofibroblastic tumor with spindle cells arranged in hypercellular fascicles focally. Note the lymphocytes and plasma cells in the stroma.

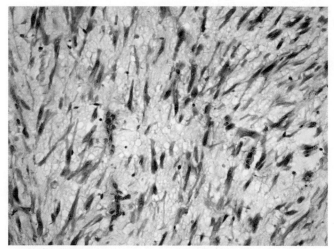

Fig 3. Spindle cells have tissue-culture fibroblast-like appearance with smooth chromatin and single prominent nucleoli.

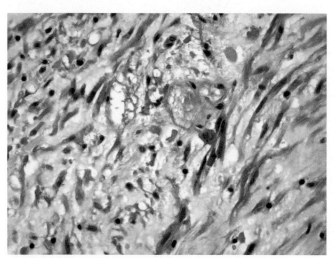

Fig 4. Nuclear atypia is usually minimal. Mitotic figures may be conspicuous, but they are typical.

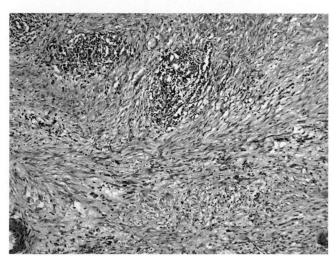

Fig 5. Background stroma contains inflammatory infiltrates consisting of lymphocytes and plasma cells.

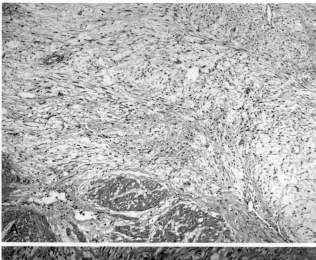

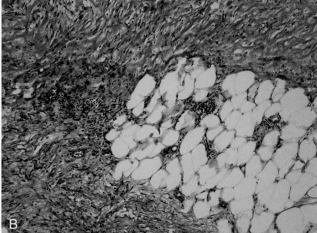

Fig 6. Inflammatory myofibroblastic tumor may extend into muscularis propria **(A)** and perivesical adipose tissue **(B).**

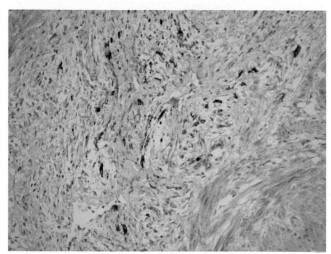

Fig 7. Immunoreactivity for anaplastic lymphoma kinase 1 (ALK1) is useful to confirm the diagnosis of inflammatory myofibroblastic tumor.

Definition
- Benign smooth muscle tumor of the bladder wall

Clinical features
Epidemiology
- Rare, but represents the most common benign mesenchymal tumor of the bladder
- Female predominance
- Most common in middle-aged to older patients
- Rare in children

Presentation
- Obstructive voiding symptoms
- Pelvic pain or ureteral obstruction with hydronephrosis

Prognosis and treatment
- Benign
- May recur if incompletely excised
- Transurethral resection for small tumors, partial cystectomy for larger tumors

Pathology
Gross pathology
- Usually small (less than 2 cm), but may be as large as 25 cm
- Polypoid or pedunculated mass

Histology
- Interlacing bundles of smooth muscle with overlying benign urothelium
- Minimal atypia and few mitosis
- No necrosis

Immunopathology (including immunohistochemistry)
- Positive for smooth muscle actin, desmin, vimentin
- Negative for cytokeratins, S100

Main differential diagnosis
- Leiomyosarcoma: significant cytologic atypia; increased mitosis and atypical mitosis; tumor necrosis; prominent myxoid stromal changes more common
- Inflammatory myofibroblastic tumor: myofibroblastic cells resembling tissue-culture fibroblasts; prominent small vessels in edematous or myxoid stroma; frequently positive for both cytokeratin and smooth muscle actin; negative for desmin

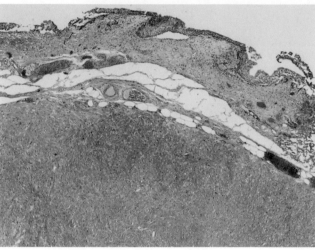

Fig 1. Submucosal leiomyoma of the bladder forms a well-circumscribed nodule in the lamina propria.

LEIOMYOSARCOMA OF THE BLADDER

Definition
- Malignant smooth muscle tumor of the bladder wall

Clinical features
Epidemiology
- Rare, but represents the most common malignant mesenchymal tumor of the bladder in adults
- Male predominance
- Most common in middle-aged to older patients
- Associated with acrolein, a degradation product of cyclophosphamide

Presentation
- Gross hematuria
- Obstructive voiding symptoms
- Ureteral obstruction with hydronephrosis (if close to the ureteral orifice)
- Pelvic mass, abdominal pain

Prognosis and treatment
- Poor
- Recurrence or metastasis resulting in death in half of the patients
- Partial or radical cystectomy

Pathology
Gross pathology
- Usually large tumors (mean size, 7 cm)
- Invasive polypoid mass with surface ulceration
- Fleshy or firm cut surface with myxoid or fibrotic appearance and variable necrosis and hemorrhage

Histology
- Interlacing bundles of malignant smooth muscle cells with overlying benign urothelium
- Increased mitotic activity with frequent atypical mitotic figures
- Marked nuclear pleomorphism
- Variable necrosis and hemorrhage
- Low grade (mild to moderate cytologic atypia, fewer than five mitoses per 10 high-power fields [HPF], minimal necrosis)
- High grade (moderate to marked cytologic atypia, more than five mitoses per 10 HPF, extensive necrosis)
- Variant histology: epithelioid and myxoid

Immunopathology (including immunohistochemistry)
- Positive for smooth muscle actin, desmin, vimentin

Main differential diagnosis
- Sarcomatoid carcinoma (carcinosarcoma): concurrent or history of high-grade urothelial carcinoma; sarcomatous component may be positive for cytokeratin and p63
- Inflammatory myofibroblastic tumor: myofibroblastic cells resembling tissue-culture fibroblasts; prominent small vessels in edematous or myxoid stroma; frequently positive for both cytokeratin and smooth muscle actin; negative for desmin
- Cellular leiomyoma: no cytologic atypia and tumor necrosis

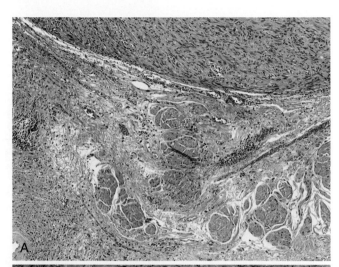

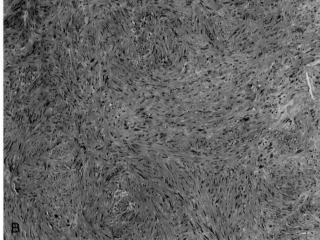

Fig 1. **A,** Leiomyosarcoma of the bladder adjacent to muscularis propria. **B,** Note the marked nuclear pleomorphism and mitotic figures.

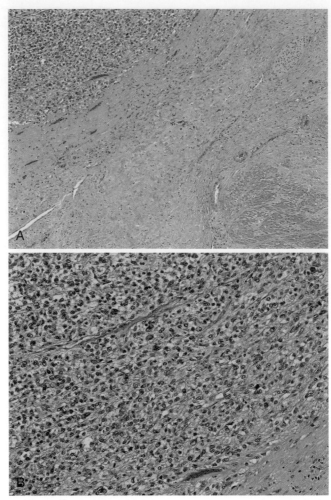

Fig 2. A, Leiomyosarcoma of the bladder with epithelioid features. **B,** Higher magnification shows epithelioid cells with cytoplasmic clearing, pleomorphic nuclei, and mitosis.

SOLITARY FIBROUS TUMOR

Definition
- A benign mesenchymal neoplasm morphologically identical to the namesake tumor occurring at other body sites

Clinical features
Epidemiology
- Rare
- Has been reported in the kidney, bladder, prostate, seminal vesicle, and perirenal pelvic regions

Presentation
- Incidental finding
- Occasionally causes hematuria, pelvic pain, symptoms of urinary obstruction

Prognosis and treatment
- Good prognosis if completely resected; however, recurrence and metastases have been reported in rare cases.
- Transurethral resection or surgical resection is the recommended treatment, depending on the tumor size.

Pathology
Histology
- Bland-looking spindle cells forming irregular interlacing fascicles without an orderly pattern of growth ("patternless pattern")
- Variable amount of intercellular collagen and angulated blood vessels (hemangiopericytoma-like)
- Cellularity varying greatly between different areas of the same tumor
- Presence of marked atypia and high mitotic rate possibly associated with aggressive behavior

Immunopathology (including immunohistochemistry)
- Positive for CD34, vimentin, and BCL2; negative for cytokeratins and S-100

Main differential diagnosis
- Other benign and malignant spindle cell tumors. For any spindle cell neoplasm of the genitourinary tract, solitary fibrous tumor may be considered and immunostains for CD34 may be performed.

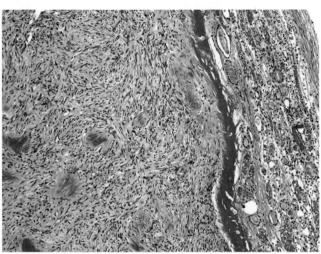

Fig 2. Bland spindle cells forming interlacing fascicles without distinct patterns ("patternless" pattern). Dense intercellular collagen fibers are also present.

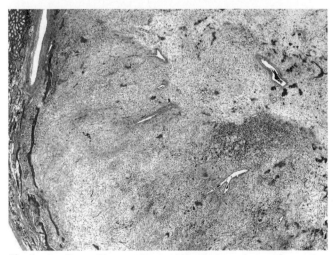

Fig 1. A solitary fibrous tumor of the kidney shows alternating hypocellular and hypercellular areas.

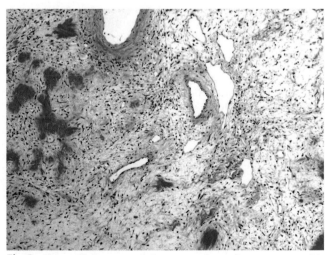

Fig 3. Hypocellular area of the tumor shows loose stroma with many angulated (hemangiopericytoma-like) vessels.

GASTROINTESTINAL STROMAL TUMOR OF THE GENITOURINARY TRACT

Definition
- Gastrointestinal stromal tumors (GIST) secondarily involving, or diagnosed on biopsy specimens of, the genitourinary tract

Clinical features
Epidemiology
- Rare

Presentation
- Most cases represent rectal or perirectal GIST diagnosed on prostate biopsy specimens.
- Rarely, a pelvic GIST compresses on the urinary bladder or extends into the scrotum to form a scrotal mass.
- Hematuria, pelvic pain, and symptoms of urinary obstruction are common.

Prognosis and treatment
- Similar to GIST of other body sites

Pathology
Histology
- Histologic findings are identical to the GISTs of other body sites.
- Most extragastrointestinal GISTs exhibit a spindle cell morphology.
- Several histologic patterns have been described, including spindle (sclerosing, palisading-vacuolated, hypercellular, and sarcomatoid subtypes) and epithelioid (sclerosing, discohesive, hypercellular, and sarcomatoid subtypes).

Immunopathology (including immunohistochemistry)
- Most cases are positive for C-kit (CD117), CD34, and caldesmon.
- Some cases are positive for smooth muscle actin.
- Cases are usually negative for desmin, S-100, and glial fibrillary acidic protein (GFAP).

Main differential diagnosis
- Other benign and malignant spindle cell tumors should be considered. For any spindle cell neoplasm from the genitourinary tract, the possibility of a GIST should be considered and ruled out by performing C-kit immunostaining.

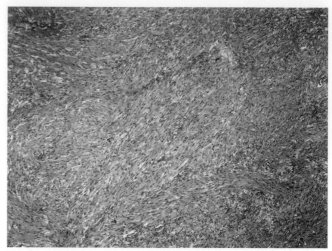

Fig 1. Low-power view of a gastrointestinal stromal tumor of the urinary tract showing interlacing fascicles of spindle cells.

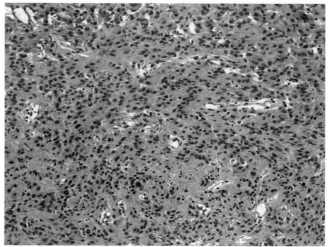

Fig 2. Gastrointestinal stromal tumor of the urinary tract with epithelioid morphology.

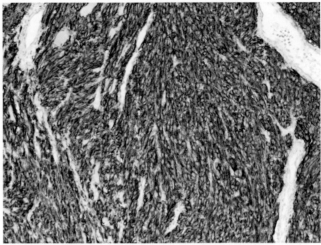

Fig 4. A gastrointestinal stromal tumor of the urinary tract positive for C-kit immunohistochemistry.

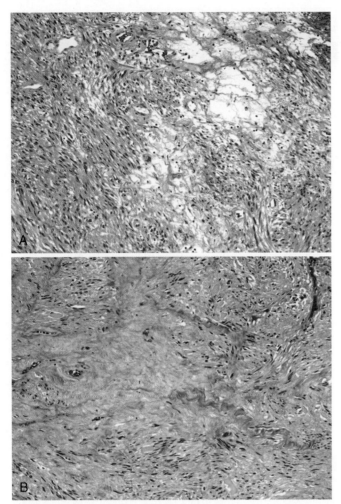

Fig 3. Gastrointestinal stromal tumor of the urinary tract with areas of edema and focal myxoid changes **(A)** and collagenization **(B).**

Definition
- Lymphomas, either primary or secondary, involving the genitourinary organs

Clinical features
Epidemiology
- Incidence is uncommon, accounting for less than 5% of extranodal lymphomas.
- Two thirds are primary, and one third are systemic lymphoma involving the genitourinary organs.
- The kidney is the most common organ reported to be involved; other organs include (in descending order of frequency) testis, prostate, bladder, penis, and ureter.

Presentation
- Variable symptoms according to the site of involvement
- Palpable masses
- Renal insufficiency
- Hematuria
- Abdominopelvic pain
- Voiding difficulty

Prognosis and treatment
- Depending on the lymphoma classification
- Often biopsied or resected by unsuspecting surgeons

Pathology
Gross pathology
- Often indistinct from other epithelial or mesenchymal neoplasms

Histology
- The characteristic histologic feature is interstitial infiltration by lymphoma cells between native structures.
- Diffuse large B cell lymphoma is most common; other subtypes include (in descending order of frequency) Burkitt lymphoma, extranodal marginal zone lymphoma, small lymphocytic lymphoma/chronic lymphocytic leukemia, and follicular lymphoma.

Immunohistochemistry and molecular diagnostics
- Required to classify lymphomas

Main differential diagnosis
- Primary and metastatic neoplasms should be considered. Any atypical histologic features should prompt a consideration of metastatic neoplasm or lymphomas in genitourinary organs. The interstitial pattern of growth is characteristic of but not specific for lymphomas, and the diagnosis of lymphoma should be further supported by characteristic morphologic and immunohistochemical features.

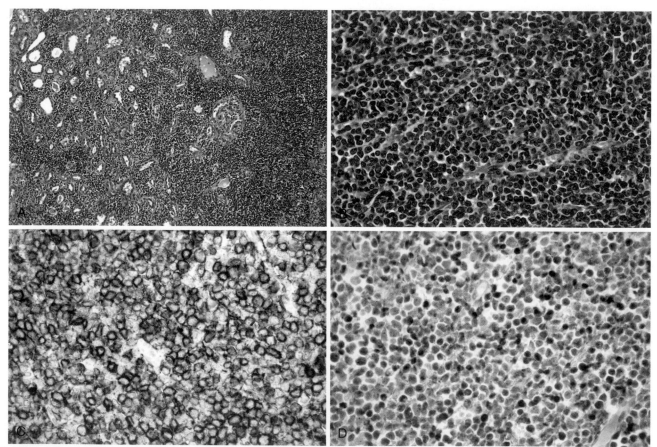

Fig 1. A primary B lymphoblastic leukemia–lymphoma involving the kidney in a 28-year-old woman. Blasts diffusely infiltrate the renal interstitium with sparing of renal tubules and glomeruli **(A).** The blasts are medium to large in size with dispersed chromatin and occasional nucleoli **(B),** and they demonstrate cytoplasmic CD20 staining **(C)** and nuclear TdT staining **(D).**

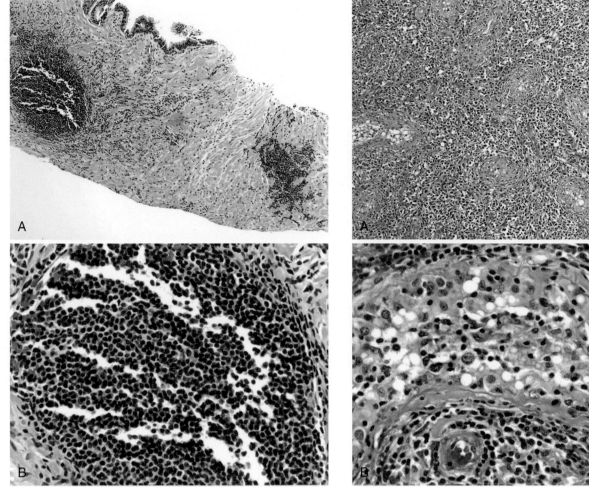

Fig 2. A prostate biopsy specimen secondarily involved by small lymphocytic lymphoma–chronic lymphocytic leukemia. **A,** The biopsy specimen shows patchy lymphocytic infiltrates that spare prostate glands and ducts. **B,** The neoplastic lymphocytes are small and uniform in size and are positive for CD20 and CD5 (not shown).

Fig 3. A diffuse large B cell lymphoma secondarily involving the testis. **A,** At low magnification, the lymphoma cells show characteristic intertubular growth pattern. **B,** Lymphoma cells extend into seminiferous tubules and may mimic intratubular germ cell neoplasia.

Note: Page numbers followed by *f* indicate figures.